STEP-UP to MEDICINE

FOURTH EDITION

EDITORS
Steven S. Agabegi, MD
Elizabeth D. Agabegi, MD

Wolters Kluwer
Philadelphia • Baltimore • New York • London
Buenos Aires • Hong Kong • Sydney • Tokyo

Acquisitions Editor: Tari Broderick
Product Development Editor: Greg Nicholl
Marketing Manager: Joy Fisher-Williams
Design Coordinator: Holly McLaughlin
Compositor: Aptara, Inc.

Fourth Edition

351 West Camden Street
Baltimore, MD 21201

Two Commerce Square
2001 Market Street
Philadelphia, PA 19103

Library of Congress Cataloging-in-Publication Data
Step-up to medicine / editors Steven S. Agabegi, Elizabeth D. Agabegi. — Fourth edition.
p. ; cm.
Includes bibliographical references and index.
ISBN 978-1-4963-0614-2 (alk. paper)
I. Agabegi, Steven S., editor. II. Agabegi, Elizabeth D., editor.
[DNLM: 1. Clinical Medicine—Outlines. 2. Clinical Medicine—Problems and Exercises. WB 18.2]
RC59
616.0076–dc23

2015018774

10 9 8 7 6 5 4 3 2 1

CCS0915

ADVISORY BOARD

REVIEWERS

MOHAMMED ARAFEH
Medical Student
Ross University School of Medicine
Dominica, West Indies

DANA BAIGRIE, DO
Medical Student
Edward Via College of Osteopathic Medicine
Spartanburg, South Carolina

DAVID BALLARD, MD
Medical Student
Louisiana State University Health Sciences Center
Shreveport, Lousiana

JANELLE BLOCKER
Medical Student
University of Sint Eustatius School of Medicine
Sint Maarten, Caribbean

F. BRIAN BOUDI, MD, FACP
Assistant Professor of Medicine
University of Arizona College of Medicine
Phoenix, Arizona

MARIA CANNAROZZI, MD
Associate Professor of Internal Medicine and Pediatrics
University of Central Florida College of Medicine
Orlando, Florida

JIMMY DEMEO
Medical Student
Lake Erie College of Osteopathic Medicine
Erie, Pennsylvania

MATTHEW FITZ, MD
Associate Professor
Clerkship Director, Internal Medicine
Loyola University Stritch School of Medicine
Chicago, Illinois

BRIANNA FOX
Medical Student
Ross University School of Medicine
Dominica, West Indies

ABIGAIL GOODMAN, MD
Resident Physician
Department of Pathology
Midwestern University
Downers Grove, Illinois

KRISTA JOHANSEN, MD
Assistant Professor of Anatomy and Physiology
Edward Via College of Osteopathic Medicine
Blacksburg, Virginia

ASHLEY JONES, MD
Resident Physician
Department of Surgery
Palmetto Health
Columbia, South Carolina

SOOR KOTHARI
Medical Student
St. George's University School of Medicine
Grenada, West Indies

STEVEN MCAFEE, MD
Resident Physician
Department of Anesthesiology
University of Missouri
Columbia, Missouri

LUIS CARLOS MEJIA-RIVERA, MD
Associate Professor of Clinical Pharmacology
San Juan Bautista School of Medicine
Caguas, Puerto Rico

NATE MOORE
Medical Student
Edward via College of Osteopathic Medicine
Blacksburg, Virginia

SHERYL RECINOS, MD
Resident Physician
Department of Family Medicine
Riverside County Regional Medical Center
Moreno Valley, California

KARA RONCIN
Medical Student
Medical University of the Americas
Nevis, West Indies

LESLIE SEIJO
Medical Student
San Juan Bautista School of Medicine
Caguas, Puerto Rico

ARCHANA SHAH
Medical Student
Texas Tech University Health Sciences Center School of Medicine
Lubbock, Texas

VISHAL SHAH
Medical Student
University of Vermont College of Medicine
Burlington, Vermont

MICHAEL SOSTOK, MD
Professor of Medicine
University of Cincinnati College of Medicine
Cincinnati, Ohio

CHRISTINE TRAN
Medical Student
Mayo Clinic College of Medicine
Rochester, Minnesota

BRIAN WU, MD
Medical Student and PhD Candidate
Keck School of Medicine
University of Southern California
Los Angeles, California

PREFACE

We wrote the first edition of *Step-Up to Medicine* during our third year of medical school because we could not find a review book that was concise, yet covered the breadth of pathology encountered during the internal medicine clerkship and the corresponding NBME shelf examinations. Our goal was to create a single "study tool" to spare medical students the hassle and expense of trying to extract pertinent information from multiple sources.

Now in its fourth edition, *Step-Up to Medicine* has been completely revised based on extensive feedback by both faculty and students. In addition, we welcomed an Advisory Board of students and residents to the team that worked collaboratively to enrich the content and ensure that the most tested topics were covered. And, since we know that medical students and interns have no time to waste, we retained and enhanced the high-yield outline format, Quick Hits, and Clinical Pearls. Finally, to pull it all together, we added a new 100-question, clinically-oriented practice exam at the end of the book for self-assessment. Before looking at the answers, take time to answer these questions because these are the questions you will be faced with in clinical practice.

We hope that the new edition of *Step-Up to Medicine* continues to be a valuable tool for students during the clinical years of medical school. However, we recognize the changing nature of science and medicine and encourage you to send comments or suggestions to www.lww.com.

We would like to thank the Advisory Board, and all the reviewers for their efforts in improving the content for this edition. In particular, we would like to give special thanks to Stacey Sebring, with whom we worked for the last eight years, for her tireless efforts and dedication in bringing this and previous editions of Step Up to Medicine to fruition.

Steve and Liz Agabegi

CONTENTS

5 DISEASES OF THE CENTRAL AND PERIPHERAL NERVOUS SYSTEMS

6 CONNECTIVE TISSUE AND JOINT DISEASES

7 DISEASES OF THE RENAL AND GENITOURINARY SYSTEM

8 FLUIDS, ELECTROLYTES, AND ACID–BASE DISORDERS

9 HEMATOLOGIC DISEASES AND NEOPLASMS

10 INFECTIOUS DISEASES

11 DISEASES OF THE SKIN AND HYPERSENSITIVITY DISORDERS

12 AMBULATORY MEDICINE

APPENDIX

DISEASES OF THE CARDIOVASCULAR SYSTEM

1

Ischemic Heart Disease

Stable Angina Pectoris

A. General characteristics

1. Stable angina pectoris is due to fixed atherosclerotic lesions that narrow the major coronary arteries. Coronary ischemia is due to an imbalance between blood supply and oxygen demand, leading to inadequate perfusion. Stable angina occurs when oxygen demand exceeds available blood supply.
2. Major risk factors
   a. Diabetes mellitus (DM)—worst risk factor
   b. Hyperlipidemia—elevated low-density lipoprotein (LDL)
   c. Hypertension (HTN)—most common risk factor
   d. Cigarette smoking
   e. Age (men >45 years; women >55 years)
   f. Family history of premature coronary artery disease (CAD) or myocardial infarction (MI) in first-degree relative: Men <55 years; women <65 years
   g. Low levels of high-density lipoprotein (HDL)
3. Minor risk factors (less clear significance) include obesity, sedentary lifestyle (lack of physical activity), stress, excess alcohol use.
4. Prognostic indicators of CAD
   a. Left ventricular function (ejection fraction [EF])
      - Normal >50%
      - If <50%, associated with increased mortality
   b. Vessel(s) involved (severity/extent of ischemia)
      - Left main coronary artery—poor prognosis because it covers approximately two-thirds of the heart
      - Two- or three-vessel CAD—worse prognosis

B. Clinical features

1. Chest pain or substernal pressure sensation
   a. Lasts less than 10 to 15 minutes (usually 1 to 5 minutes)
   b. Frightening chest discomfort, usually described as heaviness, pressure, squeezing, tightness; rarely described as sharp or stabbing pain
   c. Pain is often gradual in onset
2. Brought on by factors that increase myocardial oxygen demand, such as exertion or emotion
3. Relieved with rest or nitroglycerin
4. Note that ischemic pain does NOT change with breathing nor with body position. Also, patients with ischemic pain do not have chest wall tenderness. If any of these are present, the pain is not likely to be due to ischemia

Quick HIT

CAD can have the following clinical presentations:
- Asymptomatic
- Stable angina pectoris
- USA pectoris
- MI—either NSTEMI or STEMI
- Sudden cardiac death

Quick HIT

In a patient with CAD, goal of LDL is less than 100 mg/dL.

Quick HIT

Typical Anginal Chest Pain
- Substernal
- Worse with exertion
- Better with rest or nitroglycerin

CLINICAL PEARL 1-1

There Are Two Conditions Termed Syndrome X

1. **Metabolic Syndrome X**
   - Any combination of hypercholesterolemia, hypertriglyceridemia, impaired glucose tolerance, diabetes, hyperuricemia, HTN.
   - Key underlying factor is insulin resistance (due to obesity).
2. **Syndrome X**
   - Exertional angina with normal coronary arteriogram: Patients present with chest pain after exertion but have no coronary stenoses at cardiac catheterization.
   - Exercise testing and nuclear imaging show evidence of myocardial ischemia.
   - Prognosis is excellent.

Quick HIT

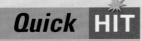

Best initial test for all forms of chest pain is ECG.

Quick HIT

Stress testing is used in the following situations:
- To confirm diagnosis of angina
- To evaluate response of therapy in patients with documented CAD
- To identify patients with CAD who may have a high risk of acute coronary events

Quick HIT

Exercise stress ECG is ideal initial test if able to exercise and normal resting ECG (readily available and relatively inexpensive).

Quick HIT

A stress test is generally considered positive if the patient develops any of the following during exercise: ST segment depression, chest pain, hypotension, or significant arrhythmias.

C. Diagnosis (of CAD)

1. Note that physical examination in most patients with CAD is normal (see Clinical Pearl 1-1)
2. Resting ECG
   a. Usually normal in patients with stable angina
   b. Q waves are consistent with a prior MI
   c. If ST segment or T-wave abnormalities are present during an episode of chest pain, then treat as unstable angina (USA)
3. Stress test—useful for patients with an intermediate pretest probability of CAD based upon age, gender, and symptoms.
   a. Stress ECG
      - Highest sensitivity if patients have normal resting ECG, such that changes can be noted.
      - Test involves recording ECG before, during, and after exercise on a treadmill.
      - 75% sensitive if patients are able to exercise sufficiently to increase heart rate to 85% of maximum predicted value for age. A person's maximum heart rate is calculated by subtracting age from 220 (220—age).
      - Exercise-induced ischemia results in subendocardial ischemia, producing ST segment depression. So the detection of ischemia on an ECG stress test is based on presence of ST segment depression.
      - Other positive findings include onset of heart failure or ventricular arrhythmia during exercise or hypotension.
      - *Patients with a positive stress test result should undergo cardiac catheterization.*
   b. Stress echocardiography
      - Performed before and immediately after exercise. Exercise-induced ischemia is evidenced by wall motion abnormalities (e.g., akinesis or dyskinesis) not present at rest.
      - Favored by many cardiologists over stress ECG. It is more sensitive in detecting ischemia, can assess LV size and function, can diagnose valvular disease, and can be used to identify CAD in the presence of pre-existing ECG abnormalities (see Clinical Pearl 1-2).
      - *Again, patients with a positive test result should undergo cardiac catheterization.*

CLINICAL PEARL 1-2

Types of Stress Tests

Test	Method of Detecting Ischemia
Exercise ECG	ST segment depression
Exercise or dobutamine echocardiogram	Wall motion abnormalities
Exercise or dipyridamole perfusion study (thallium/technetium)	Decreased uptake of the nuclear isotope during exercise

c. Information gained from a stress test can be enhanced by stress myocardial perfusion imaging after IV administration of a radioisotope such as thallium 201 during exercise.
   - Viable myocardial cells extract the radioisotope from the blood. No radioisotope uptake means no blood flow to an area of the myocardium.
   - *It is important to determine whether the ischemia is reversible,* that is, whether areas of hypoperfusion are perfused over time as blood flow eventually equalizes. Areas of *reversible* ischemia may be rescued with percutaneous coronary intervention (PCI) or coronary artery bypass graft (CABG). Irreversible ischemia, however, indicates infarcted tissue that cannot be salvaged.
   - Perfusion imaging increases the sensitivity and specificity of exercise stress tests, but is also more expensive, subjects the patient to radiation, and is often not helpful in the presence of a left bundle branch block.

4. If the patient cannot exercise, perform a *pharmacologic stress test.*
   a. IV adenosine, dipyridamole, or dobutamine can be used. The cardiac stress induced by these agents takes the place of exercise. This can be combined with an ECG, an echocardiogram, or nuclear perfusion imaging.
   b. IV adenosine and dipyridamole cause generalized coronary vasodilation. Since diseased coronary arteries are already maximally dilated at rest to increase blood flow, they receive relatively less blood flow when the entire coronary system is pharmacologically vasodilated.
   c. Dobutamine increases myocardial oxygen demand by increasing heart rate, blood pressure, and cardiac contractility.
5. Holter monitoring (ambulatory ECG) can be useful in detecting silent ischemia (i.e., ECG changes not accompanied by symptoms). The Holter monitor is also used for evaluating arrhythmias, heart rate variability, and to assess pacemaker and implantable cardioverter-defibrillator (ICD) function.
   a. Continuously examines patient's cardiac rhythm over 24 to 72 hours during normal activity
   b. Useful for evaluating unexplained syncope and dizziness as well
6. Cardiac catheterization with coronary angiography (see Clinical Pearl 1-3, Figure 1-1)
   a. Coronary angiography—definitive test for CAD. Often performed with concurrent PCI or for patients being considered for revascularization with CABG.

CLINICAL PEARL 1-3

Cardiac Catheterization

1. Most accurate method of determining a specific cardiac diagnosis.
2. Provides information on hemodynamics, intracardiac pressure measurements, cardiac output, oxygen saturation, etc.
3. Coronary angiography (see below) is almost always performed as well for visualization of coronary arteries.
4. There are many indications for cardiac catheterization (generally performed when revascularization or other surgical intervention is being considered):
   - After a positive stress test.
   - Acute MI with intent of performing angiogram and PCI.
   - In a patient with angina in any of the following situations: When noninvasive tests are nondiagnostic, angina that occurs despite medical therapy, angina that occurs soon after MI, and any angina that is a diagnostic dilemma.
   - If patient is severely symptomatic and urgent diagnosis and management are necessary.
   - For evaluation of valvular disease, and to determine the need for surgical intervention.

Coronary Arteriography (Angiography)

1. Most accurate method of identifying the presence and severity of CAD; the standard test for delineating coronary anatomy.
2. Main purpose is to identify patients with severe coronary disease to determine whether revascularization is needed. Revascularization with PCI involving a balloon and/or a stent can be performed at the same time as the diagnostic procedure.
3. Coronary stenosis >70% may be significant (i.e., it can produce angina).

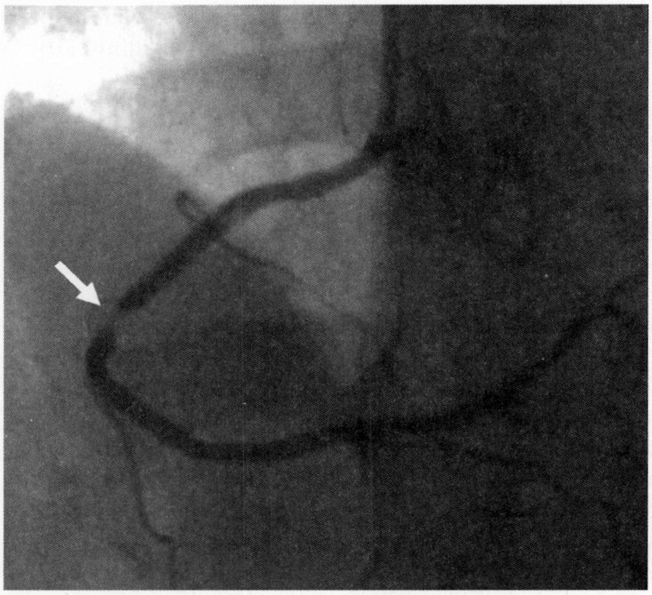

FIGURE 1-1 **Coronary angiogram. Injection of the right coronary artery shows a stenosis in the midportion of the vessel, indicated by the *arrow*.**
(From Lilly LS. *Pathophysiology of Heart Disease*. 5th ed. Philadelphia, PA: Lippincott Williams & Wilkins, 2011:152, Figure 6.8; Courtesy of Dr. William Daley.)

b. Contrast is injected into coronary vessels to visualize any stenotic lesions. This defines the location and extent of coronary disease.
c. Angiography is the most accurate test for detecting CAD.
d. If CAD is severe (e.g., left main or three-vessel disease), refer patient for surgical revascularization (CABG).

D. Treatment

1. Risk factor modification
   a. Smoking cessation cuts coronary heart disease (CHD) risk in half by 1 year after quitting.
   b. HTN—vigorous BP control reduces the risk of CHD, especially in diabetic patients.
   c. Hyperlipidemia—reduction in serum cholesterol with lifestyle modifications and HMG-CoA reductase inhibitors (statins) reduce CHD risk.
   d. DM—type II diabetes is considered to be a cardiovascular heart disease equivalent, and strict glycemic control should be strongly emphasized.
   e. Obesity—weight loss modifies other risk factors (diabetes, HTN, and hyperlipidemia) and provides other health benefits.
   f. Exercise is critical; it minimizes emotional stress, promotes weight loss, and helps reduce other risk factors.
   g. Diet: Reduce intake of saturated fat (<7% total calories) and cholesterol (<200 mg/day).

Quick HIT

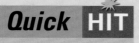

Standard of care for stable angina is aspirin and a β-blocker (only ones that lower mortality), and nitrates for chest pain.

2. Medical therapy
   a. Aspirin
      - Indicated in all patients with CAD
      - **Decreases morbidity—reduces risk of MI**
   b. β-Blockers—block sympathetic stimulation of heart. First-line choices include atenolol and metoprolol.
      - Reduce HR, BP, and contractility, thereby decreasing cardiac work (i.e., β-blockers lower myocardial oxygen consumption)
      - **Have been shown to reduce the frequency of coronary events**
   c. Nitrates—cause generalized vasodilation
      - Relieve angina; reduce preload myocardial oxygen demand
      - May prevent angina when taken before exertion

Quick HIT

Side effects of nitrates:
- Headache
- Orthostatic hypotension
- Tolerance
- Syncope

- Effect on prognosis is unknown; main benefit is symptomatic relief
- Can be administered orally, sublingually, transdermally, intravenously, or in paste form. For chronic angina, oral or transdermal patches are used. For acute coronary syndromes (see below), either sublingual, paste, or IV forms are used

d. Calcium channel blockers
- Cause coronary vasodilation and afterload reduction, in addition to reducing contractility.
- Now considered a **secondary treatment** when β-blockers and/or nitrates are not fully effective. None of the calcium channel blockers have been shown to lower mortality in CAD. In fact, they may increase mortality because they raise heart rates. Do not routinely use these drugs in CAD.

e. If congestive heart failure (CHF) is also present, treatment with ACE inhibitors and/or diuretics may be indicated as well.

3. Revascularization
   a. May be preferred for high-risk patients, although there is some controversy whether revascularization is superior to medical management for a patient with stable angina and stenosis >70%
   b. Two methods—PCI and CABG—see Clinical Pearl 1-4
   c. Revascularization does **not** reduce incidence of MI, but does result in significant improvement in symptoms
4. Management decisions (general guidelines)—risk factor modification and aspirin are indicated in all patients. Manage patients according to overall risk
   a. Mild disease (normal EF, mild angina, single-vessel disease)
      - Nitrates (for symptoms and as prophylaxis) and a β-blocker are appropriate
      - Consider calcium channel blockers if symptoms continue despite nitrates and β-blockers
   b. Moderate disease (normal EF, moderate angina, two-vessel disease)
      - If the above regimen does not control symptoms, consider coronary angiography to assess suitability for revascularization (either PCI or CABG)
   c. Severe disease (decreased EF, severe angina, and three-vessel/left main or left anterior descending disease)
      - Coronary angiography and consider for CABG

Quick HIT

The COURAGE trial showed essentially no difference in all cause mortality and nonfatal MIs between patients with stable angina treated with maximal medical therapy alone versus medical therapy with PCI and bare metal stenting.

Quick HIT

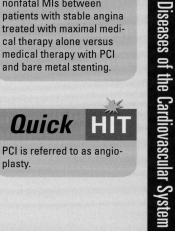

PCI is referred to as angioplasty.

CLINICAL PEARL 1-4

Percutaneous Coronary Intervention

- Consists of both coronary angioplasty with a balloon and stenting.
- Should be considered in patients with one-, two-, or three-vessel disease. Even with three-vessel disease, mortality and freedom from MI have been shown to be equivalent between PTCA with stenting and CABG. The only drawback is the higher frequency of revascularization procedures in patients who received a stent.
- Best if used for proximal lesions.
- Restenosis is a significant problem (up to 40% within first 6 months); however, if there is no evidence of restenosis at 6 months, it usually does not occur. New techniques and technologic improvements such as drug-eluting stents are attempting to reduce this problem.

Coronary Artery Bypass Grafting

- While CABG remains the standard of care at some institutions for patients with high-risk disease, the PRECOMBAT and SYNTAX trails have shown that PTCA with stenting may be as good as CABG even in patients with left main CAD. CABG is still used as the primary method of revascularization in a small number of patients with STEMI. In addition, it may be indicated in patients with cardiogenic shock post-MI, after complications with PCI, in the setting of ventricular arrhythmias, and with mechanical complications after acute MI.
- Main indications for CABG: Three-vessel disease with >70% stenosis in each vessel. Left main coronary disease with >50% stenosis, left ventricular dysfunction.

Quick HIT

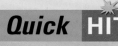

Acute Coronary Syndrome
- The clinical manifestations of atherosclerotic plaque rupture and coronary occlusion
- Term generally refers to USA, NSTEMI, or STEMI

Quick HIT

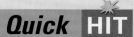

Stress testing only detects flow-limiting high-grade lesions. Thus, can still have MI despite negative stress test because mechanism of MI is acute plaque rupture onto a moderate lesion.

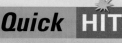

Quick HIT

USA and non-ST segment elevation MI are often considered together because it is very difficult to distinguish the two based on patient presentation. If cardiac enzymes are elevated, then the patient has non-ST segment elevation MI.

Quick HIT

The **ESSENCE** trial showed that in USA and non-ST segment elevation MI, risk of death, MI, or recurrent angina was lower in the enoxaparin group than in the heparin group at 14 days, 30 days, and 1 year. The need for revascularization was also lower in the enoxaparin group.

Quick HIT

Thrombolytic therapy (fibrinolysis) has **not** been proven to be beneficial in **USA.** This is only indicated in STEMI when no access to urgent catheterization for PCI.

Unstable Angina Pectoris

A. General characteristics

1. Pathophysiology
   a. With USA, *oxygen demand is unchanged*. Supply is decreased secondary to **reduced resting coronary flow.** This is in contrast to stable angina, which is due to increased demand.
   b. USA is significant because it indicates stenosis that has enlarged via thrombosis, hemorrhage, or plaque rupture. It may lead to total occlusion of a coronary vessel.
2. The following patients may be said to have USA:
   a. Patients with chronic angina with increasing frequency, duration, or intensity of chest pain
   b. Patients with new-onset angina that is severe and worsening
   c. Patients with angina at rest
3. The distinction between USA and NSTEMI is based entirely on cardiac enzymes. The latter has elevation of troponin or creatine kinase-MB _(CK-MB). Both USA and NSTEMI lack ST segment elevations and pathologic Q waves.

B. Diagnosis (see stable angina)

1. Perform a diagnostic workup to exclude MI in all patients.
2. Patients with USA have a higher risk of adverse events during stress testing. These patients should be stabilized with medical management before stress testing *or* should undergo cardiac catheterization initially.

C. Treatment

1. Hospital admission on a floor with continuous cardiac monitoring. Establish IV access and give supplemental oxygen. Provide pain control with nitrates (below) and morphine.
2. Aggressive medical management is indicated—treat as in MI except for fibrinolysis.
   a. Aspirin
   b. Clopidogrel—shown to reduce the incidence of MI in patients with USA compared with aspirin alone in the CURE trial. This benefit persists whether the patient undergoes revascularization with PCI or not. Patients presenting with USA should generally be treated with aspirin and clopidogrel for 9 to 12 months, in accordance with the CURE trial. This may be altered however, according to the bleeding risk of each patient
   c. β-Blockers—first-line therapy if there are no contraindications
   d. Low–molecular-weight heparin (LMWH) is superior to unfractionated heparin. Goal is to prevent progression or development of a clot
      - Should be continued for at least 2 days
      - Enoxaparin is the drug of choice based on clinical trials (see Quick Hit on ESSENCE trial).
   e. Nitrates are first-line therapy
   f. Oxygen if patient is hypoxic
   g. Glycoprotein IIb/IIIa inhibitors (abciximab, tirofiban) can be helpful adjuncts in USA, especially if patient is undergoing PTCA or stenting
   h. Morphine is controversial—provides good pain relief but may mask worsening symptoms
   i. Replacement of deficient electrolytes, especially K^+ and Mg^{2+}
3. Cardiac catheterization/revascularization
   a. More than 90% of patients improve with the above medical regimen within 1 to 2 days.
   b. The choice of invasive management (early catheterization/revascularization within 48 hours) versus conservative management (catheterization/revascularization only if medical therapy fails) is controversial.
      - No study has shown a significant difference in outcomes between these two approaches.

- If patient responds to medical therapy, perform a stress ECG to assess need for catheterization/revascularization. Many patients with USA that is controlled with medical therapy eventually require revascularization.
- If medical therapy fails to improve symptoms and/or ECG changes indicative of ischemia persist after 48 hours, then proceed directly to catheterization/revascularization. Additional indications for PCI include hemodynamic instability, ventricular arrhythmias, and new mitral regurgitation (MR) or new septal defect.
- The TIMI risk score can be used to guide the decision on conservative versus more aggressive treatment.

4. After the acute treatment
   a. Continue aspirin (or other antiplatelet therapy), β-blockers (atenolol or metoprolol), and nitrates
   b. Reduce risk factors
      - Smoking cessation, weight loss
      - Treat diabetes, HTN
      - Treat hyperlipidemia—patients with any form of CAD (stable angina, USA, NSTEMI, STEMI) should be started on an HMG-CoA reductase inhibitor regardless of LDL level. Clinical trials of statins have shown the efficacy of such therapy for secondary prevention in CAD (see Quick Hit on CARE trial)

Quick HIT

The **CARE** trial: Patients with prior history of MI were randomized to treatment with statins or placebo. The statin group had a reduced risk of death (by 24%), a reduced risk of stroke (by 31%), and a reduction in need for CABG or coronary angioplasty (by 27%).

Variant (Prinzmetal) Angina

- Involves transient coronary vasospasm that usually is accompanied by a fixed atherosclerotic lesion but can also occur in normal coronary arteries.
- Episodes of angina occur at rest and are associated with ventricular dysrhythmias, some of which may be life threatening. The angina classically occurs at night.
- Hallmark is transient ST segment elevation (not depression) on ECG during chest pain, which represents transmural ischemia.
- Coronary angiography is a definitive test—displays coronary vasospasm when the patient is given IV ergonovine or acetylcholine (to provoke vasoconstriction).
- Vasodilators—calcium channel blockers and nitrates have been proven to be helpful. Risk factor modification including smoking cessation and lipid lowering is also indicated where appropriate.

Myocardial Infarction

A. General characteristics

1. MI is due to necrosis of myocardium as a result of an interruption of blood supply (after a thrombotic occlusion of a coronary artery previously narrowed by atherosclerosis).
   a. Most cases are due to acute coronary thrombosis: Atheromatous plaque ruptures into the vessel lumen, and thrombus forms on top of this lesion, which causes occlusion of the vessel.
   b. **MI is associated with a 30% mortality rate; half of the deaths are prehospital.**
   c. Most patients with MI have history of angina, risk factors for CAD, or history of arrhythmias.

B. Clinical features

1. Chest pain
   a. Intense substernal pressure sensation; often described as "crushing" and "an elephant standing on my chest."
   b. Radiation to neck, jaw, arms, or back, commonly to the left side.
   c. Similar to angina pectoris in character and distribution but much more severe and lasts longer. Unlike in angina, pain typically does not respond to nitroglycerin.
   d. Some patients may have epigastric discomfort.
2. **Can be asymptomatic in up to one-third of patients**; painless infarcts or atypical presentations more likely in postoperative patients, the elderly, diabetic patients, and women.

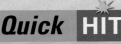

Quick HIT

The combination of substernal chest pain persisting for longer than 30 minutes and diaphoresis strongly suggests acute MI.

Quick HIT

Right ventricular infarct will present with inferior ECG changes, hypotension, elevated jugular venous pressure, hepatomegaly, and **clear lungs.** Preload dependent—do NOT administer nitrates or diuretics as will cause cardiovascular collapse.

Quick HIT

ST segment elevation indicates an infarction 75% of the time. ST segment depression indicates an infarction only 25% of the time.

3. Other symptoms
   a. Dyspnea
   b. Diaphoresis
   c. Weakness, fatigue
   d. Nausea and vomiting
   e. Sense of impending doom
   f. Syncope
4. Sudden cardiac death—usually due to ventricular fibrillation (VFib)

C. Diagnosis

1. ECG (Figure 1-2; see also Table 1-1 and Clinical Pearl 1-5)
   a. Markers for ischemia/infarction include:
      - **Peaked T waves:** Occur very early and may be missed
      - **ST segment elevation** indicates transmural injury and can be diagnostic of an acute infarct
      - **Q waves:** Evidence for necrosis (specific)—Q waves are usually seen late; typically not seen acutely
      - **T-wave** inversion is sensitive but not specific
      - **ST segment depression:** Subendocardial injury

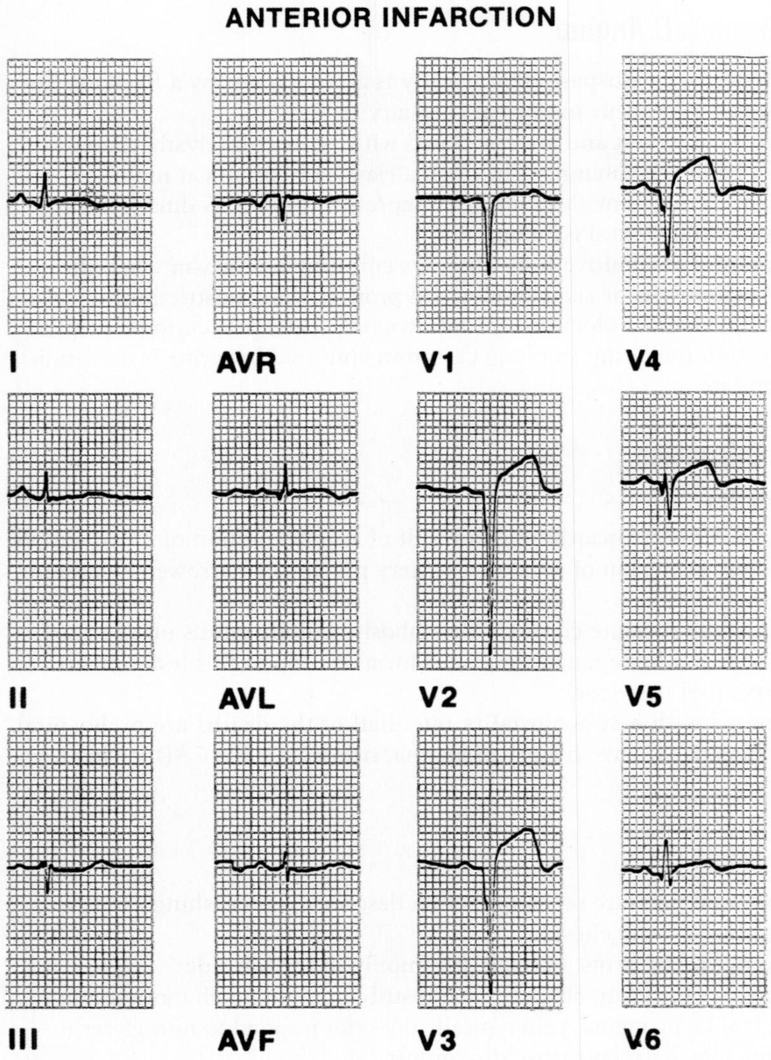

FIGURE 1-2 **ECG showing anterior wall myocardial infarction—all 12 leads.**
(From Davis D. *Quick and Accurate 12-Lead ECG Interpretation*. 3rd ed. Philadelphia, PA: Lippincott Williams & Wilkins, 2000:203.)

TABLE 1-1 **ECG Findings Based on Location of Infarct**

Location of Infarct	ECG Changes
Anterior	ST segment elevation in V1–V4 (acute/active) Q waves in leads V1–V4 (late change)
Posterior	Large R wave in V1 and V2 ST segment depression in V1 and V2 Upright and prominent T waves in V1 and V2
Lateral	Q waves in leads I and aVL (late change)
Inferior	Q waves in leads II, III, aVF (late change)

Note: Augmented ECG leads from aVL indicate the left arm, and from aVF indicate the left foot.

b. Categories of infarcts
   - **ST segment elevation infarct:** Transmural (involves entire thickness of wall); tends to be larger
   - **Non-ST segment elevation infarct:** Subendocardial (involves inner one-third to one-half of the wall); tends to be smaller, and presentation is similar to USA—cardiac enzymes differentiate the two

2. Cardiac enzymes—currently the diagnostic gold standard for myocardial injury (Figure 1-3)
   a. Troponins (Troponin I and T)—most important enzyme test to order
      - Increases within 3 to 5 hours and returns to normal in 5 to 14 days; reaches a peak in 24 to 48 hours.
      - Greater sensitivity and specificity than CK-MB for myocardial injury.
      - Obtain serum levels of either troponin T or troponin I on admission, and again every 8 hours for 24 hours.
      - Troponin I can be falsely elevated in patients with renal failure; thus following trend of levels is important.
   b. CK-MB—less commonly used
      - Increases within 4 to 8 hours and returns to normal in 48 to 72 hours; reaches a peak in 24 hours.
      - When measured within 24 to 36 hours of onset of chest pain, has greater than 95% sensitivity and specificity.
      - Levels of total CK and CK-MB should be measured on admission and every 8 hours thereafter for 24 hours.
      - Most helpful in detecting recurrent infarction given quicker return to baseline than troponin.

Quick HIT

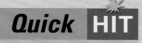

Cardiac enzymes are drawn serially—once on admission and every 8 hours until three samples are obtained. The higher the peak and the longer enzyme levels remain elevated, the more severe the myocardial injury and the worse the prognosis.

Quick HIT

In MI, aspirin, β-blockers, and ACE inhibitors are the only agents shown to reduce mortality.

CLINICAL PEARL 1-5

Cardiac Monitoring for a Patient With an Acute MI

- BP and HR: HTN increases afterload and thus oxygen demand, whereas hypotension reduces coronary and tissue perfusion. Both nitrates and morphine can cause hypotension.
- Rhythm strip with continuous cardiac monitor: Watch for dysrhythmias. Note that PVCs can lower stroke volume and coronary artery filling time. A high frequency of PVCs may predict VFib or VT.
- Auscultate the heart (third and fourth heart sounds, friction rub, and so on) and lungs (crackles may indicate LV failure, pulmonary edema).
- Hemodynamic monitoring (CVP, PCWP, SVR, cardiac index [CI]) with a pulmonary artery catheter is indicated if the patient is hemodynamically unstable. Monitoring is helpful in assessing the need for IV fluids and/or vasopressors.

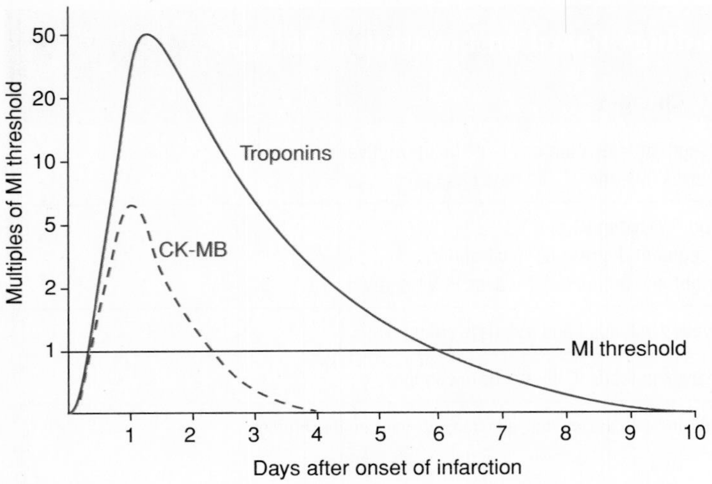

FIGURE 1-3 **Evolution of serum biomarkers in acute MI. Curve M indicates the detection of myoglobin in the serum before other biomarkers. Serum CK (or CK-MB isoenzyme) begins to increase 3 to 8 hours after the onset of the acute infarct and peaks at 24 hours. Cardiac troponins are highly sensitive for myocardial injury and remain detectable in the serum for many days after the acute infarct.**

(From Lilly LS. *Pathophysiology of Heart Disease*. 3rd ed. Philadelphia, PA: Lippincott Williams & Wilkins, 2011:175, Figure 7.9.)

D. Treatment

1. Admit patient to a cardiac monitored floor (CCU) and establish IV access. Give supplemental oxygen and analgesics (nitrates, morphine—see below).
2. Medical therapy
   a. Aspirin
      - Antiplatelet agent reduces coronary reocclusion by inhibiting platelet aggregation on top of the thrombus
      - **Has been shown to reduce mortality and should be part of long-term maintenance therapy**

   b. β-Blockers
      - Block stimulation of HR and contractility to reduce oxygen demand and decrease the incidence of arrhythmias
      - Reduce remodeling of the myocardium post-MI
      - **Have been shown to reduce mortality and should be part of maintenance therapy**

   c. ACE inhibitors
      - Initiate within hours of hospitalization if there are no contraindications
      - **Have been shown to reduce mortality and should be part of long-term maintenance therapy**

   d. Statins
      - **Reduce risk of further coronary events**
      - Stabilize plaques and lower cholesterol
      - The PROVE IT-TIMI 22 trial showed the superiority of starting atorvastatin 80 mg over other statins before discharging a STEMI patient
      - **Should be part of maintenance therapy**

   e. Oxygen
      - May limit ischemic myocardial injury

   f. Nitrates
      - Dilate coronary arteries (increase supply)
      - Venodilation (decrease preload and thus demand)
      - Reduce chest pain, although not as effective as narcotics

   g. Morphine sulfate
      - Analgesia
      - Causes venodilation, which decreases preload and thus oxygen requirements

h. Heparin
   - Initiate in all patients with MI; prevents progression of thrombus; however, has **not** been shown to decrease mortality
   - LMWH, specifically enoxaparin, is preferred over unfractionated heparin, as shown in the ExTRACT TIMI 25 trial as well as a recent meta-analysis. Enoxaparin was shown to decrease the risk of another MI versus unfractionated heparin

3. Revascularization
   a. Benefit highest when performed **early** (within 90 minutes of hospital arrival).
   b. Should be considered in all patients.
   c. Revascularization options include thrombolysis, PCI, or CABG—see Clinical Pearl 1-6.
      - Several studies have shown enhanced survival and lower rates of recurrent MI and intracranial bleeding when PCI performed by skilled personnel is chosen over thrombolysis. For patients with a delayed presentation, fibrinolysis alone may be a better option.
      - Urgent/emergent CABG is typically performed only in the setting of mechanical complications of an acute MI, cardiogenic shock, life-threatening ventricular arrhythmias, or after failure of PCI. It is almost never performed in the acute setting on a stable patient.
   d. Clopidogrel—evidence suggests that benefits of clopidogrel is additive to the effects of aspirin. Clopidogrel therapy should be initiated in all patients who

Quick HIT

The **CAPRICORN** trial showed that the β-blocker carvedilol reduces risk of death in patients with post-MI LV dysfunction.

Quick HIT

The following are indicated in patients with MI:
- Oxygen
- Nitroglycerin
- β-Blocker
- Aspirin
- Morphine
- ACE inhibitor
- IV Heparin

Quick HIT

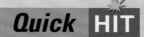

Remember that patients can have a recurrent infarction on same hospital admission. CK-MB is most helpful laboratory test to detect this if patient develops recurrent chest pain.

CLINICAL PEARL 1-6

Methods of Revascularization

Percutaneous Coronary Intervention

- This is the preferred treatment for STEMI as long as it can be performed expeditiously (door to balloon time less than 90 minutes) and by skilled personnel.
- Also preferred in patients with contraindications for thrombolytic therapy; no risk of intracranial hemorrhage.
- PAMI trial showed that PTCA reduces mortality more than t-PA.

Thrombolytic Therapy

- Thrombolytic therapy remains an important treatment modality since PCI is still available only at specialized centers. It is useful for patients who present later, and for those in whom PCI is contraindicated.
- Early treatment is crucial to salvage as much of the myocardium as possible. Administer as soon as possible up to 24 hours after the onset of chest pain. Outcome is best if given within the first 6 hours.
- Indications: **ST segment elevation** in two contiguous ECG leads in patients with pain onset within 6 hours who have been refractory to nitroglycerin.
- Alteplase has been shown to have the best outcomes amongst thrombolytic medications, and is the first choice in many centers, despite its high costs. Alternatives include streptokinase, tenecteplase, reteplase, lanoteplase, and urokinase.
- In ED setting, the main reason to initiate therapy with thrombolytics/angioplasty is whether there is ST segment elevation on ECG.

Absolute Contraindications to Thrombolytic Therapy

- Trauma: Recent head trauma or traumatic CPR
- Previous stroke
- Recent invasive procedure or surgery
- Dissecting aortic aneurysm
- Active bleeding or bleeding diathesis

Coronary Artery Bypass Grafting

- Less often used than the other two in the acute setting.
- Benefits of CABG include low rates of event-free survival and reintervention-free survival.
- It remains the procedure of choice in patients with severe multivessel disease and complex coronary anatomy.

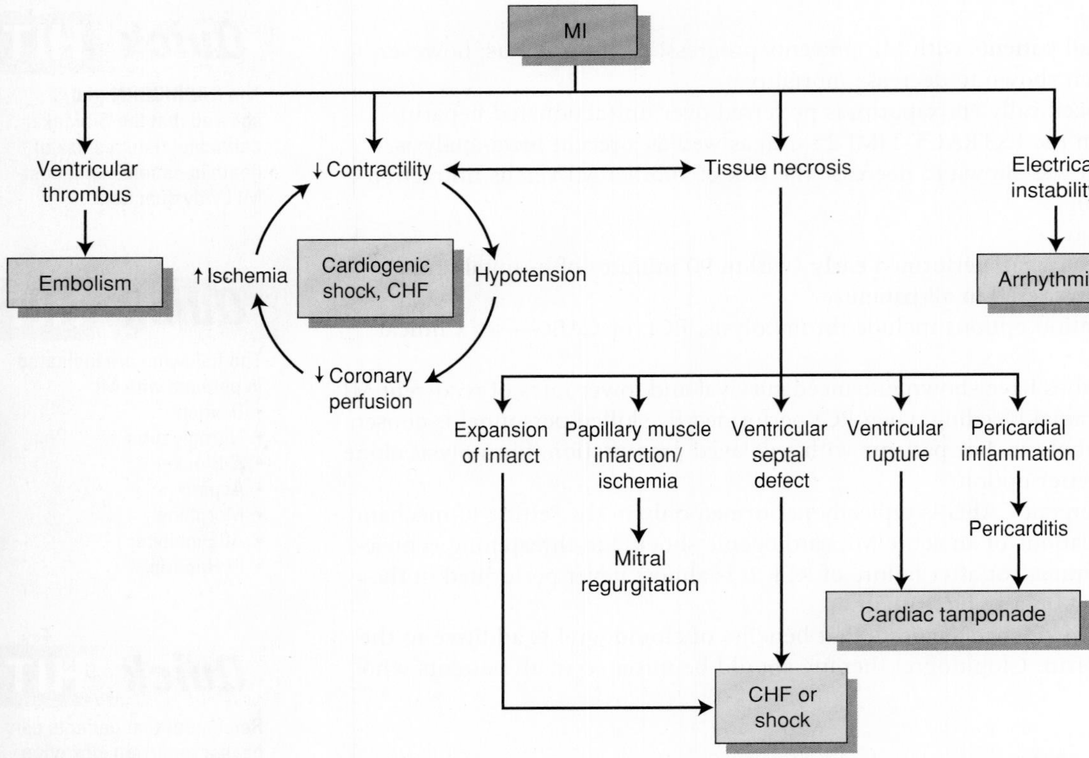

FIGURE **1-4** **Complications of MI.**
(Adapted from Lilly LS. *Pathophysiology of Heart Disease.* 5th ed. Philadelphia, PA: Lippincott Williams & Wilkins, 2011:183, Figure 7.12.)

Quick HIT
Heparin is used for USA and MI (both NSTEMI and STEMI). It is NOT used for stable angina.

Quick HIT
All patients initially treated conservatively for UA/ NSTEMI should have a stress test before leaving the hospital to determine the need for angiography (which in turn determines the need for angioplasty or CABG).

Quick HIT
Patients who suffer an acute MI have a high risk of stroke during the next 5 years. The lower the EF and the older the patient, the higher the risk of stroke.

undergo PCI and receive a stent. Dual antiplatelet treatment with aspirin and clopidogrel should continue for at least 30 days in patients who receive a bare metal stent, and at least 12 months in patients who receive a drug-eluting stent.

4. Rehabilitation
   a. **Cardiac rehabilitation** is a physician-supervised regimen of exercise and risk factor reduction after MI.
   b. **Shown to reduce symptoms and prolong survival.**

E. Complications of acute MI

1. Pump failure (CHF) (Figure 1-4)
   a. Most common cause of in-hospital mortality
   b. If mild, treat medically (ACE inhibitor, diuretic)
   c. If severe, may lead to cardiogenic shock; invasive hemodynamic monitoring may be indicated (see Cardiogenic Shock on page 64)
2. Arrhythmias
   a. Premature ventricular contractions (PVCs)—conservative treatment (observation) indicated; no need for antiarrhythmic agents
   b. Atrial fibrillation (AFib)
   c. Ventricular tachycardia (VT)-sustained VT requires treatment: If patient is hemodynamically unstable, electrical cardioversion is indicated. If patient is hemodynamically stable, start antiarrhythmic therapy (IV amiodarone)—see treatment of VT
   d. VFib—immediate unsynchronized defibrillation and CPR are indicated (see Arrhythmias on page 22)
   e. Accelerated idioventricular rhythm does not affect prognosis; no treatment needed in most cases
   f. Paroxysmal supraventricular tachycardia (PSVT)—for treatment, see Arrhythmias

g. Sinus tachycardia
   - May be caused by pain, anxiety, fever, pericarditis, medications, etc.
   - Worsens ischemia (increases myocardial oxygen consumption)
   - Treat underlying cause (analgesics for pain, aspirin for fever, etc.)

h. Sinus bradycardia
   - A common occurrence in early stages of acute MI, especially right-sided/inferior MI
   - May be a protective mechanism (reduces myocardial oxygen demand)
   - No treatment is required other than observation. If bradycardia is severe or symptomatic (hemodynamic compromise), atropine may be helpful in increasing HR

i. Asystole
   - Very high mortality.
   - Treatment should begin with electrical defibrillation for VFib, which is more common in cardiac arrest and may be difficult to clearly differentiate from asystole.
   - If asystole is clearly the cause of arrest, transcutaneous pacing is the appropriate treatment.

j. AV block
   - Associated with ischemia involving conduction tracts.
   - First-degree and second-degree (type I) blocks do not require therapy.
   - Second-degree (type II) and third-degree blocks: Prognosis is dire in the setting of an **anterior** MI—emergent placement of a temporary pacemaker is indicated (with later placement of a permanent pacemaker). In inferior MI, prognosis is better, and IV atropine may be used initially. If conduction is not restored, a temporary pacemaker is appropriate.

3. Recurrent infarction (extension of existing infarction or reinfarction of a new area)
   a. Both short-term and long-term mortality are increased.
   b. Diagnosis is often difficult.
      - Cardiac enzymes are already elevated from the initial infarction. Troponin levels remain elevated for a week or more, so are not useful here. CK-MB returns to normal faster, and so a reelevation of CK-MB after 36 to 48 hours may be due to recurrent infarction.
      - If there is **repeat ST segment elevation** on ECG within the first 24 hours after infarction, suspect recurrent infarction.
   c. Treatment: Repeat thrombolysis or urgent cardiac catheterization and PCI. Continue standard medical therapy for MI.

4. Mechanical complications
   a. Free wall rupture
      - A catastrophic, usually fatal event that occurs during the first 2 weeks after MI (90% within 2 weeks, most commonly 1 to 4 days after MI)
      - 90% mortality rate
      - Usually leads to hemopericardium and cardiac tamponade
      - Treatment: Hemodynamic stabilization, immediate pericardiocentesis, and surgical repair
   b. Rupture of interventricular septum
      - Greater potential for successful therapy than with a free wall rupture, although this is also a critical event; emergent surgery is indicated
      - Occurs within 10 days after MI
      - Likelihood of survival correlates with size of defect
   c. Papillary muscle rupture
      - **Produces MR** (presents with new murmur)
      - If suspected, obtain an echocardiogram immediately
      - Emergent surgery is needed (mitral valve replacement is usually necessary), as well as afterload reduction with sodium nitroprusside or intra-aortic balloon pump (IABP)
   d. Ventricular pseudoaneurysm
      - Incomplete free wall rupture (myocardial rupture is contained by pericardium)
      - Bedside echocardiogram may show the pseudoaneurysm

Quick HIT

Most common cause of death in first few days after MI is ventricular arrhythmia (either VT or VFib).

Quick HIT

After an MI, all patients should be discharged home with aspirin, β-blocker, statins, and an ACE inhibitor.

- Surgical emergency because ventricular pseudoaneurysms tend to become a free wall rupture

e. Ventricular aneurysm
- Rarely rupture (in contrast to pseudoaneurysms)
- Associated with a high incidence of ventricular tachyarrhythmias
- Medical management may be protective
- Surgery to remove aneurysm may be appropriate in selected patients

5. Acute pericarditis
   a. The incidence has decreased sharply since the introduction of revascularization techniques.
   b. Treatment consists of aspirin (which is already standard in treatment of MI).
   c. NSAIDs and corticosteroids are contraindicated (may hinder myocardial scar formation).
6. *Dressler syndrome* ("postmyocardial infarction syndrome")
   a. Immunologically based syndrome consisting of fever, malaise, pericarditis, leukocytosis, and pleuritis, occurring weeks to months after an MI
   b. Aspirin is the most effective therapy. Ibuprofen is a second option

Chest Pain

A. Differential diagnosis

1. Heart, pericardium, vascular causes
   a. Stable angina, USA, variant angina
   b. MI
   c. Pericarditis
   d. Aortic dissection
2. Pulmonary: Pulmonary embolism (can have pain with pulmonary infarction), pneumothorax, pleuritis (pleural pain), pneumonia, status asthmaticus
3. GI: Gastroesophageal reflux disease (GERD), diffuse esophageal spasm, peptic ulcer disease, esophageal rupture
4. Chest wall: Costochondritis, muscle strain, rib fracture, herpes zoster, thoracic outlet syndrome
5. Psychiatric: Panic attacks, anxiety, somatization
6. Cocaine use can cause angina or MI

Quick HIT

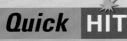

If you suspect a cardiac cause of the pain, sublingual nitroglycerin is appropriate. Also give aspirin if the patient does not have a bleeding disorder.

Quick HIT

Gastrointestinal disorders are the most common cause of noncardiac chest pain that presents in the ED.

B. Approach to treating a patient with chest pain

1. Rule out any life-threatening causes. These include acute MI, USA, aortic dissection, pulmonary embolus, tension pneumothorax, and esophageal rupture
2. Assess vital signs
3. Develop a focused history
   a. Character of the pain (pressure, squeezing, tearing, sharp, stabbing, etc.)
   b. Location of pain
   c. Severity of pain
   d. Duration of pain
   e. Setting in which pain occurred (during exertion, at rest, after meal)
   f. Radiation of pain
   g. Aggravating or alleviating factors (e.g., meal, exertion, rest, respiration)
   h. **Does the patient have a cardiac history?** Ask about results of previous stress tests, echocardiograms, cardiac catheterization, or of any procedures (PCI or CABG)
   i. **If the patient has a history of angina, ask how this episode differs from previous ones (more severe? longer duration?)**
4. Perform a focused physical examination, with attention to cardiopulmonary, abdominal, and musculoskeletal examination
5. Order ancillary tests
   a. Obtain ECG in almost all cases
   b. Cardiac enzymes (CK, CK-MB, troponin) depending on clinical suspicion
   c. Obtain chest radiograph (CXR) in almost all cases
   d. Under appropriate clinical setting, work up the patient for pulmonary embolism (PE) (see pulmonary section)

Quick HIT

If nitroglycerin relieves the pain, a cardiac cause is more likely (although esophageal spasm is still a possibility).

Quick HIT

If pain changes with respiration (pleuritic), changes with body position or if there is tenderness of chest wall, cardiac cause of pain is highly unlikely.

6. Develop a diagnosis
    a. It can be difficult to distinguish between GI causes of chest pain and angina. The decision of whether to initiate a cardiac workup is dependent on a patient's overall risk of CAD and the clinical presentation. If patient is young and without risk factors, treat for GERD and follow up if pain recurs. (Anxiety may be a cause but is difficult to diagnose and usually only considered after ruling out cardiac causes first.) An older patient with risk factors should undergo a cardiac workup.
    b. There is no fail-proof algorithm for approaching chest pain. In general, have a greater index of suspicion for ischemic causes in the elderly, diabetic populations, and those with a history of CAD (see MI section).

Quick HIT

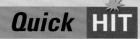

A common presentation is a patient with chronic stable angina who presents with symptoms suggestive of USA. The following are the initial steps:
- Obtain ECG and cardiac enzymes
- Give aspirin
- Begin IV heparin

Congestive Heart Failure

A. General characteristics

1. CHF is a clinical syndrome resulting from the heart's inability to meet the body's circulatory demands under normal physiologic conditions. It is the final common pathway for a wide variety of cardiac diseases (see also Clinical Pearl 1-7).
2. Pathophysiology (Figure 1-5)
    a. Frank–Starling relationship
        - In a normal heart, increasing preload results in greater contractility.
        - When preload is low (at rest), there is little difference in performance between a normal and a failing heart. However, with exertion a failing heart produces relatively less contractility and symptoms occur (Figure 1-6).
3. Systolic dysfunction
    a. Owing to impaired contractility (i.e., the abnormality is decreased EF)
    b. Causes include:
        - Ischemic heart disease or after a recent MI—infarcted cardiac muscle does not pump blood (decreased EF)
        - **HTN resulting in cardiomyopathy**
        - Valvular heart disease
        - Myocarditis (postviral)
        - Less common causes: Alcohol abuse, radiation, hemochromatosis, thyroid disease
4. Diastolic dysfunction
    a. Owing to impaired ventricular filling during diastole (either impaired relaxation or increased stiffness of ventricle or both). Diastolic dysfunction is less common than systolic dysfunction.
    b. Echocardiogram shows impaired relaxation of left ventricle.

Quick HIT

Often, both systolic and diastolic dysfunctions are present simultaneously.

CLINICAL PEARL 1-7

High-output Heart Failure

1. In high-output heart failure, an increase in cardiac output is needed for the requirements of peripheral tissues for oxygen.
2. Causes include:
    - Chronic anemia
    - Pregnancy
    - Hyperthyroidism
    - AV fistulas
    - Wet beriberi (caused by thiamine [vitamin B1] deficiency)
    - Paget disease of bone
    - MR
    - Aortic insufficiency
3. The conditions listed above rarely cause heart failure by themselves. However, if these conditions develop in the presence of underlying heart disease, heart failure can result quickly.

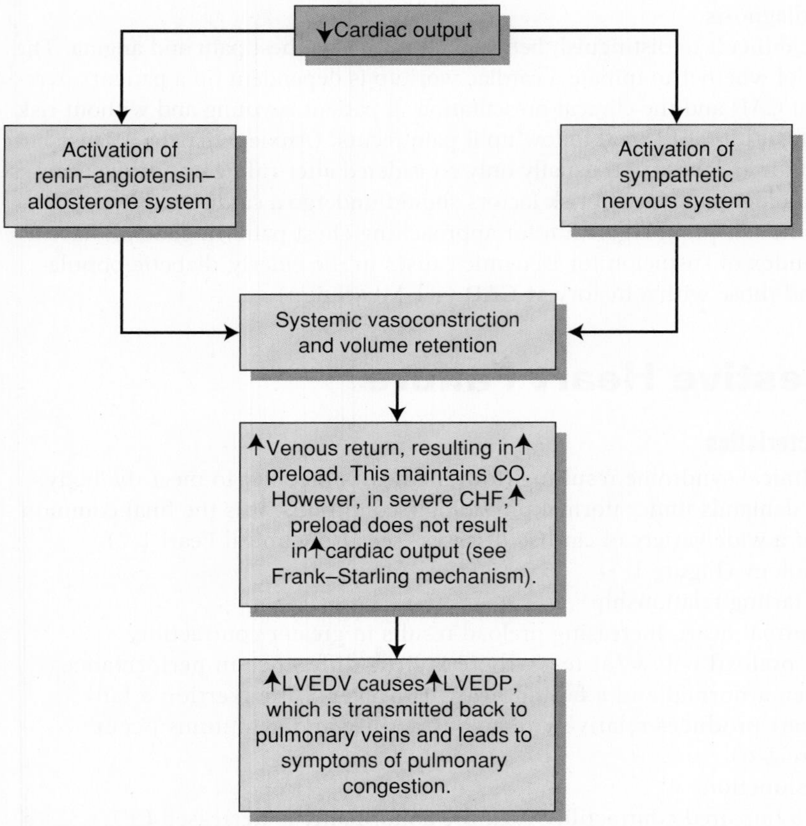

FIGURE 1-5 **Pathophysiology of CHF.**

c. Causes include:
- HTN leading to myocardial hypertrophy—most common cause of diastolic dysfunction
- Valvular diseases such as aortic stenosis (AS), mitral stenosis, and aortic regurgitation
- Restrictive cardiomyopathy (e.g., amyloidosis, sarcoidosis, hemochromatosis)

B. Clinical features

1. Symptoms of left-sided heart failure (see also Clinical Pearl 1-8)
   a. Dyspnea—difficulty breathing secondary to pulmonary congestion/edema
   b. *Orthopnea*—difficulty breathing in the recumbent position; relieved by elevation of the head with pillows

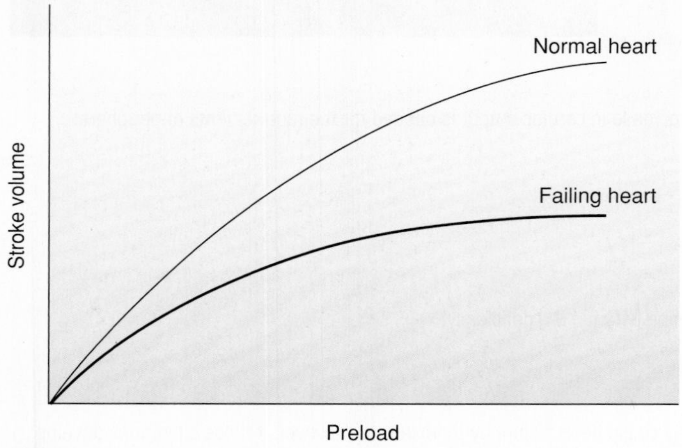

FIGURE 1-6 **Frank–Starling relationship.**

CLINICAL PEARL 1-8

New York Heart Association (NYHA) Classification

- NYHA class I: Symptoms only occur with vigorous activities, such as playing a sport. Patients are nearly asymptomatic.
- NYHA class II: Symptoms occur with prolonged or moderate exertion, such as climbing a flight of stairs or carrying heavy packages. Slight limitation of activities.
- NYHA class III: Symptoms occur with usual activities of daily living, such as walking across the room or getting dressed. Markedly limiting.
- NYHA class IV: Symptoms occur at rest. Incapacitating.

c. *Paroxysmal nocturnal dyspnea* (PND)—awakening after 1 to 2 hours of sleep due to acute shortness of breath (SOB)
d. Nocturnal cough (nonproductive)—worse in recumbent position (same pathophysiology as orthopnea)
e. Confusion and memory impairment occur in advanced CHF as a result of inadequate brain perfusion
f. Diaphoresis and cool extremities at rest—occur in desperately ill patients (NYHA class IV)

2. Signs of left-sided heart failure
   a. Displaced PMI (usually to the left) due to cardiomegaly
   b. Pathologic S_3 (ventricular gallop)
      - Rapid filling phase "into" a noncompliant left ventricular chamber
      - May be normal finding in children; in adults, usually associated with CHF
      - May be difficult to hear, but is among the most specific signs of CHF
      - Heard best at apex with bell of stethoscope
      - The sequence in the cardiac cycle for S_3: S_3 follows S_2 (ken-tuck-**Y**)
   c. S_4 gallop
      - Sound of atrial systole as blood is ejected into a noncompliant, or stiff, left ventricular chamber
      - Heard best at left sternal border with bell of stethoscope
      - The sequence in the cardiac cycle for S_4: S_4 precedes S_1 (**TEN**-nes-see)
   d. Crackles/rales at lung bases
      - Caused by fluid spilling into alveoli; indicates pulmonary edema
      - Rales heard over lung bases suggest at least moderate severity of left ventricular heart failure
   e. Dullness to percussion and decreased tactile fremitus of lower lung fields caused by pleural effusion
   f. Increased intensity of pulmonic component of second heart sound indicates pulmonary HTN (heard over left upper sternal border)
3. Symptoms/signs of right-sided heart failure
   a. Peripheral pitting edema—pedal edema lacks specificity as an isolated finding. In the elderly, it is more likely to be secondary to venous insufficiency
   b. Nocturia—due to increased venous return with elevation of legs
   c. Jugular venous distention (JVD)
   d. Hepatomegaly/hepatojugular reflux
   e. Ascites
   f. Right ventricular heave
4. Given enough time, left-sided heart failure will always lead to right-sided heart failure and vice versa
   a. Patients may present with sign/symptoms of both right- and left-sided HF

Quick HIT

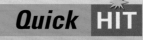

Tests to order for a new patient with CHF:
- Chest x-ray (pulmonary edema, cardiomegaly, rule out COPD)
- ECG
- Cardiac enzymes to rule out MI
- CBC (anemia)
- Echocardiogram (estimate EF, rule out pericardial effusion)

C. Diagnosis

1. Chest x-ray (CXR) (Figures 1-7 and 1-8)
   a. Cardiomegaly

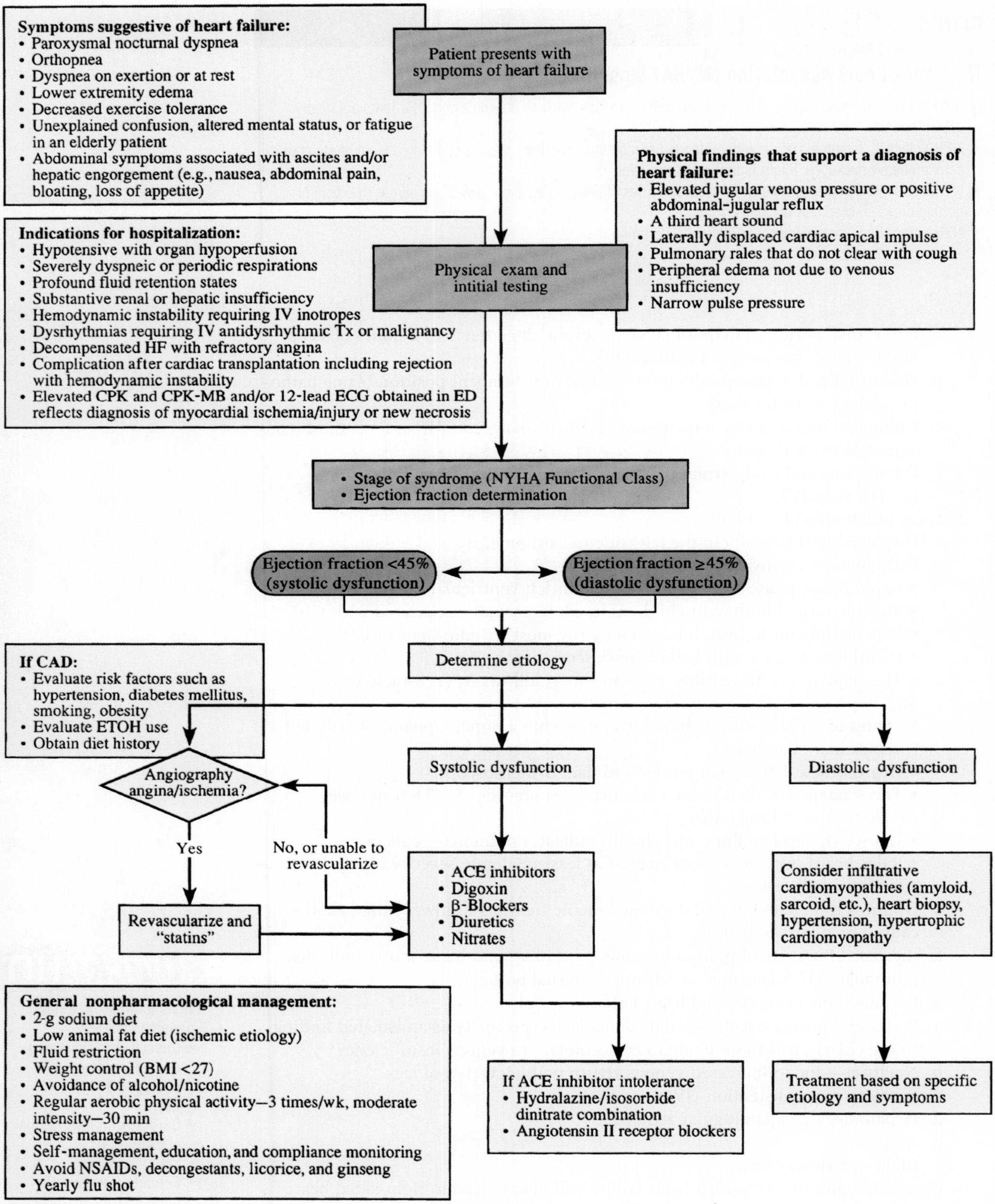
Symptoms suggestive of heart failure:
• Paroxysmal nocturnal dyspnea
• Orthopnea
• Dyspnea on exertion or at rest
• Lower extremity edema
• Decreased exercise tolerance
• Unexplained confusion, altered mental status, or fatigue in an elderly patient
• Abdominal symptoms associated with ascites and/or hepatic engorgement (e.g., nausea, abdominal pain, bloating, loss of appetite)
Patient presents with symptoms of heart failure
Physical findings that support a diagnosis of heart failure:
• Elevated jugular venous pressure or positive abdominal-jugular reflux
• A third heart sound
• Laterally displaced cardiac apical impulse
• Pulmonary rales that do not clear with cough
• Peripheral edema not due to venous insufficiency
• Narrow pulse pressure
Indications for hospitalization:
• Hypotensive with organ hypoperfusion
• Severely dyspneic or periodic respirations
• Profound fluid retention states
• Substantive renal or hepatic insufficiency
• Hemodynamic instability requiring IV inotropes
• Dysrhythmias requiring IV antidysrhythmic Tx or malignancy
• Decompensated HF with refractory angina
• Complication after cardiac transplantation including rejection with hemodynamic instability
• Elevated CPK and CPK-MB and/or 12-lead ECG obtained in ED reflects diagnosis of myocardial ischemia/injury or new necrosis
Physical exam and intitial testing
• Stage of syndrome (NYHA Functional Class)
• Ejection fraction determination
Ejection fraction <45% (systolic dysfunction)
Ejection fraction ≥45% (diastolic dysfunction)
Determine etiology
If CAD:
• Evaluate risk factors such as hypertension, diabetes mellitus, smoking, obesity
• Evaluate ETOH use
• Obtain diet history
Angiography angina/ischemia?
Yes
No, or unable to revascularize
Revascularize and "statins"
Systolic dysfunction
Diastolic dysfunction
• ACE inhibitors
• Digoxin
• β-Blockers
• Diuretics
• Nitrates
Consider infiltrative cardiomyopathies (amyloid, sarcoid, etc.), heart biopsy, hypertension, hypertrophic cardiomyopathy
General nonpharmacological management:
• 2-g sodium diet
• Low animal fat diet (ischemic etiology)
• Fluid restriction
• Weight control (BMI <27)
• Avoidance of alcohol/nicotine
• Regular aerobic physical activity—3 times/wk, moderate intensity—30 min
• Stress management
• Self-management, education, and compliance monitoring
• Avoid NSAIDs, decongestants, licorice, and ginseng
• Yearly flu shot
If ACE inhibitor intolerance
• Hydralazine/isosorbide dinitrate combination
• Angiotensin II receptor blockers
Treatment based on specific etiology and symptoms

FIGURE 1-7 **Diagnosis and management of CHF.**

(Modified from Topol EJ. *Textbook of Cardiovascular Medicine.* 2nd ed. Philadelphia, PA: Lippincott Williams & Wilkins, 2002:1874, Figure 92.4.)

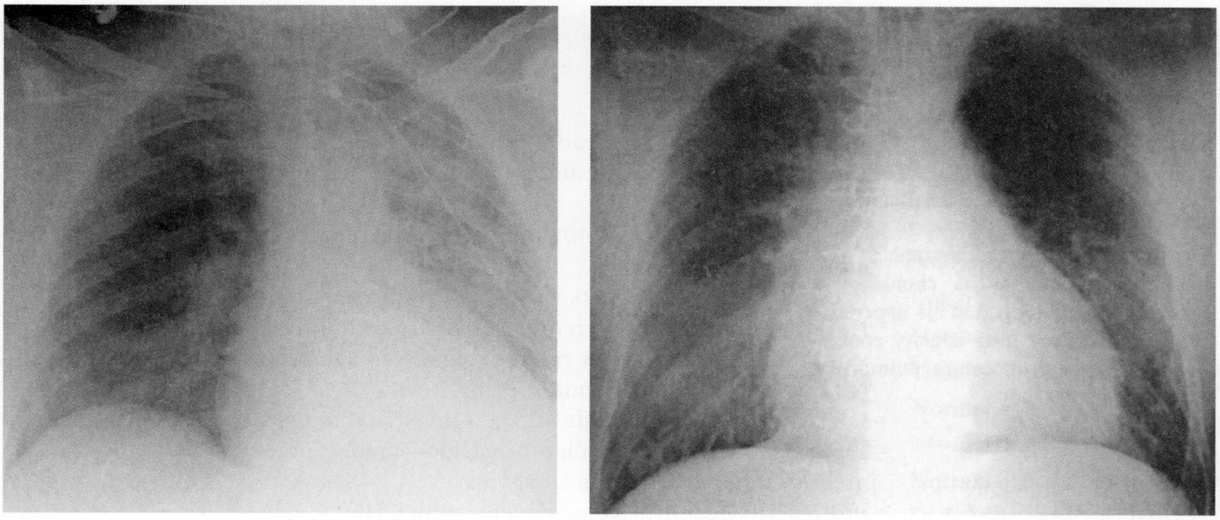

A B

FIGURE 1-8 **A: Chest radiograph showing cardiogenic pulmonary edema. B: Another example of cardiogenic pulmonary edema; note cardiomegaly (patient had CHF).**
(**A** from Mergo PJ. *Imaging of the Chest—A Teaching File.* Philadelphia, PA: Lippincott Williams & Wilkins, 2002:50, Figure 24A.) (**B** from Stern EJ, White CS. *Chest Radiology Companion.* Philadelphia, PA: Lippincott Williams & Wilkins, 1999:38, Figure 5-4.)

b. *Kerley B lines* are short horizontal lines near periphery of the lung near the costophrenic angles, and indicate pulmonary congestion secondary to dilation of pulmonary lymphatic vessels
c. Prominent interstitial markings
d. Pleural effusion

2. Echocardiogram (transthoracic)
   a. Initial test of choice—should be performed whenever CHF is suspected based on history, examination, or CXR.
   b. Useful in determining whether systolic or diastolic dysfunction predominates, and determines whether the cause of CHF is due to a pericardial, myocardial, or valvular process.
   c. Estimates EF (very important): Patients with systolic dysfunction (EF <40%) should be distinguished from patients with preserved left ventricular function (EF >40%).
   d. Shows chamber dilation and/or hypertrophy.
3. ECG is usually nonspecific but can be useful for detecting chamber enlargement and presence of ischemic heart disease or prior MI.
4. Radionuclide ventriculography using technetium-99m ("nuclear ventriculography"). Also called multigated acquisition (MUGA) scan.
5. Cardiac catheterization can provide valuable quantitative information regarding diastolic and systolic dysfunction, and can clarify the cause of CHF if noninvasive test results are equivocal. Consider coronary angiography to exclude CAD as an underlying cause of CHF.
6. Stress testing
   a. Identifies ischemia and/or infarction
   b. Quantitates level of conditioning
   c. Can differentiate cardiac versus pulmonary etiology of dyspnea
   d. Assesses dynamic responses of HR, heart rhythm, and BP

Quick HIT

BNP is released from the ventricles in response to ventricular volume expansion and pressure overload.
- BNP levels >150 pg/mL correlate strongly with the presence of decompensated CHF. (Unit of measurement varies.)
- BNP may be useful in differentiating between dyspnea caused by CHF and COPD.
- N-terminal pro-BNP (NT-proBNP) is a newer assay with similar predictive value as BNP. The normal range for this value depends on the age of the patient, but a NT-proBNP <300 virtually excludes the diagnosis of HF.

D. Treatment

1. Systolic dysfunction
   a. General lifestyle modification:
      - Sodium restriction (less than 4 g/day)
      - Fluid restriction (1.5 to 2.0 L daily)

Quick HIT

HTN is a common cause of CHF and should be treated. Goal is to reduce preload and afterload.

Quick HIT

The **RALES** trial showed that spironolactone reduces morbidity and mortality in patients with class III or IV heart failure. It is contraindicated in renal failure.

Quick HIT

Monitoring a patient with CHF:
- Weight—unexplained weight gain can be an early sign of worsening CHF
- Clinical manifestations (exercise tolerance is key); peripheral edema
- Laboratory values (electrolytes, K, BUN, creatinine levels; serum digoxin, if applicable)

Quick HIT

Standard treatment of CHF includes a loop diuretic, ACE inhibitor, and β-blocker. Depending on severity and patient factors, other medications such as digoxin, hydralazine/nitrate, spironolactone may be added.

Quick HIT

Most common cause of death from CHF is sudden death from ventricular arrhythmias. Ischemia provokes ventricular arrhythmias.

Quick HIT

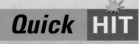

The **COMET** trial compared two β-blockers in the treatment of CHF and showed that carvedilol led to significant improvement in survival compared with metoprolol.

- Weight loss
- Smoking cessation
- Restrict alcohol use
- Exercise program
- All patients should monitor weight daily to detect fluid accumulation
- Annual influenza vaccine and pneumococcal vaccine recommended

b. Diuretics
- Most effective means of providing **symptomatic** relief to patients with moderate to severe CHF
- Recommended for patients with systolic failure and volume overload
- **Have not been shown to reduce mortality or improve prognosis, just for symptom control. Goal is relief of signs and symptoms of volume overload (dyspnea, peripheral edema)**
- Loop diuretics: Furosemide (Lasix)—most potent, usually used
- Thiazide diuretics: Hydrochlorothiazide—modest potency

c. Spironolactone (aldosterone antagonist)
- Prolong survival in selected patients with CHF
- Monitor serum potassium and renal function
- Spironolactone is proven effective only for more advanced stages of CHF (classes III and IV)
- Eplerenone is an alternative to spironolactone (does not cause gynecomastia)

d. ACE inhibitors
- Cause venous and arterial dilation, decreasing preload and afterload.
- Indicated for left ventricular systolic dysfunction (LV EF less than 40%).
- **The combination of a diuretic and an ACE inhibitor should be the initial treatment in most symptomatic patients.**
- **ACE inhibitors reduce mortality** (Cooperative North Scandinavian Enalapril Survival Study [CONSENSUS] and Studies of Left Ventricular Dysfunction [SOLVD] trials), **prolong survival, and alleviate symptoms in mild, moderate, and severe CHF.**
- All patients with systolic dysfunction should be on an ACE inhibitor even if they are asymptomatic.
- Always start at a low dose to prevent hypotension.
- Monitor BP, potassium, BUN, and creatinine.

e. Angiotensin II receptor blockers (ARBs)
- Used in patients unable to take ACE inhibitors due to side effect of cough, but should **not** replace ACE inhibitors if patient tolerates an ACE inhibitor

f. β-Blockers
- **Proven to decrease mortality in patients with post-MI heart failure.**
- Reported to improve symptoms of CHF; may slow progression of heart failure by slowing down tissue remodeling. The decrease in heart rate leads to decreased oxygen consumption. β-Blockers also have antiarrhythmic and anti-ischemic effect.
- Should be given to *stable* patients with mild to moderate CHF (class I, II, and III) unless there is a noncardiac contraindication.
- Not all β-blockers are equal. There is evidence only for metoprolol, bisoprolol, and carvedilol.

g. Digitalis
- Positive inotropic agent.
- Useful in patients with EF <40%, severe CHF, or severe AFib.
- Provides short-term symptomatic relief (used to control dyspnea and will decrease frequency of hospitalizations) but **has *not* been shown to improve mortality.**
- **For patients with EF <40%, who continue to have symptoms despite optimal therapy (with ACE inhibitor, β-blocker, aldosterone antagonist, and a diuretic).**
- Serum digoxin level should be checked periodically.

h. Hydralazine and isosorbide dinitrates
   - Can be used in patients who cannot tolerate ACE inhibitors.
   - The combination of hydralazine and isosorbide dinitrate has been shown to improve mortality in selected patients (African Americans) with CHF. But not as effective as ACE inhibitors and require inconvenient dosing schedules.

i. The following medications are contraindicated in patients with CHF:
   - Metformin—may cause potentially lethal lactic acidosis
   - Thiazolidinediones—causes fluid retention
   - NSAIDs may increase risk of CHF exacerbation
   - Some antiarrhythmic agents that have negative inotropic effects

j. The following devices have been shown to reduce mortality in select patients:
   - An ICD lowers mortality by helping prevent sudden cardiac death (which is the most common cause of death in CHF). It is indicated for patients at least 40 days post-MI, EF <35%, and class II or III symptoms despite optimal medical treatment.
   - Cardiac resynchronization therapy (CRT): This is biventricular pacemaker—indications are similar to ICD except these patients also have prolonged QRS duration >120 msec. Most patients who meet criteria for CRT are also candidates for ICD and receive a combined device.

k. Cardiac transplantation is the last alternative if the above do not control symptoms.

2. Diastolic dysfunction: Few therapeutic options available; patients are treated symptomatically (**NO medications have proven mortality benefit**)
   a. β-Blockers have clear benefit and should be used
   b. Diuretics are used for symptom control (volume overload)
   c. Digoxin and spironolactone should NOT be used.
   d. ACE inhibitors and ARBs—benefit is not clear for diastolic dysfunction
3. General principles in treatment of CHF (see Clinical Pearls 1-9 and 1-10)

Acute Decompensated Heart Failure

A. Acute dyspnea associated with elevated left-sided filling pressures, with or without pulmonary edema.
B. Most commonly due to LV systolic or diastolic dysfunction.

CLINICAL PEARL 1-9

General Principles in the Treatment of CHF

No one simple treatment regimen is suitable for all patients.

The following is a general guideline, but the order of therapy may differ among patients and/or with physician preferences.

Mild CHF (NYHA Classes I to II)

- Mild restriction of sodium intake (no-added-salt diet of 4 g sodium) and physical activity.
- Start a loop diuretic if volume overload or pulmonary congestion is present.
- Use an ACE inhibitor as a first-line agent.

Mild to Moderate CHF (NYHA Classes II to III)

- Start a diuretic (loop diuretic) and an ACE inhibitor.
- Add a **β-blocker** if moderate disease (class II or III) is present and the response to standard treatment is suboptimal.

Moderate to Severe CHF (NYHA Classes III to IV)

- Add digoxin (to loop diuretic and ACE inhibitor).
- Note that digoxin may be added at any time for the relief of symptoms in patients with systolic dysfunction. (It does not improve mortality.)
- In patients with class IV symptoms who are still symptomatic despite the above, adding spironolactone can be helpful.

Quick HIT

Medications that have been shown to lower mortality in systolic heart failure:
- ACE inhibitors and ARBs
- β-Blockers
- Aldosterone antagonists (spironolactone)
- Hydralazine, plus nitrate

Medications that do NOT decrease mortality
- Loop diuretics
- Digoxin

Quick HIT

Signs of digoxin toxicity:
- GI: Nausea/vomiting, anorexia
- Cardiac: Ectopic (ventricular) beats, AV block, AFib
- CNS: Visual disturbances, disorientation

Quick HIT

Calcium channel blockers (CCB) play no role in treatment of CHF and some may actually raise mortality. However, amlodipine and felodipine are safe to use in CHF if CCBs are needed for another indication (e.g., hypertension or angina).

Quick HIT

The overall 5-year mortality for all patients with CHF is about 50%.

CLINICAL PEARL 1-10

- **Ventricular assist device (VAD).** Work on these devices has been occurring for the past five decades, and most of the products on the market now represent research that was done 30 years ago. There is great potential for these devices as more research is conducted and clinicians become more experienced in their advantages and drawbacks.
- VADs may be used to support the left ventricle (LVAD), right ventricle (RVAD, or both ventricles [BiVAD]).
- The pump is implanted in the **abdominal cavity** with cannulation to the heart. The system controller and battery are worn externally.
- These devices may allow for a patient requiring continuous hospitalization to eventually be discharged with relatively straightforward outpatient follow-up. Patients may live with these devices for a year or more.
- Lifelong anticoagulation with heparin or warfarin is essential without exceptions as these devices are very thrombogenic.
- VADs may also be used for hemodynamic support related to the acute treatment of a STEMI or other cardiac pathology (i.e., while recovering from a severe case of myocarditis)

C. Flash pulmonary edema refers to a severe form of heart failure with rapid accumulation of fluid in the lungs.
D. Differential includes pulmonary embolism, asthma, and pneumonia, all of which can cause rapid respiratory distress.
E. Diagnostic tests include ECG, chest x-ray, ABG, B-type natriuretic peptide (BNP), echocardiogram, and possible coronary angiogram if indicated.
F. Hospital admission is indicated.
G. Daily assessment of patient weight is a good method of documenting effective diuresis.
H. **Treatment**
   1. Oxygenation and ventilatory assistance with nonrebreather face mask, NPPV, or even intubation as indicated.
   2. Diuretics to treat volume overload and congestive symptoms—this is the most important intervention. Decreases preload.
   3. Dietary sodium restriction.
   4. Nitrates—IV nitroglycerin (vasodilator) in patients without hypotension. Decreases afterload.
   5. Patients who have pulmonary edema despite use of oxygen, diuretics, and nitrates may benefit from use of inotropic agents (dobutamine). Digoxin takes several weeks to work and is not indicated in an acute setting.
   6. There is limited evidence for use of morphine sulfate.

Arrhythmias

Premature Complexes

A. Premature atrial complexes

1. This early beat arises within the atria, firing on its own.
2. Causes include adrenergic excess, drugs, alcohol, tobacco, electrolyte imbalances, ischemia, and infection.
3. On ECG, look for early P waves that differ in morphology from the normal sinus P wave (because these P waves originate within the atria and not the sinus node).
4. QRS complex is normal because conduction below the atria is normal. There is usually a pause before the next sinus P wave.
5. Premature atrial complexes (PACs) are found in more than 50% of normal adults who undergo Holter monitoring and are of no significance in a normal heart, but may be a precursor of ischemia in a diseased heart.
6. May cause palpitations or give rise to PSVTs.
7. Usually asymptomatic and do not require treatment. Monitor for increased frequency. If symptomatic (e.g., palpitations), β-blockers may be helpful.

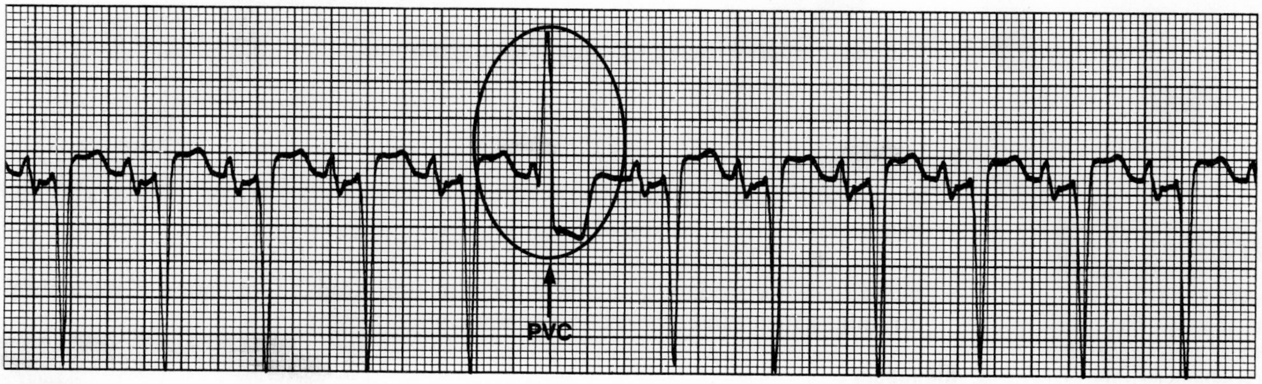

FIGURE **1-9** **Normal sinus rhythm with premature ventricular contraction.**
(From Nettina SM. *The Lippincott Manual of Nursing Practice.* 9th ed. Philadelphia, PA: Lippincott Williams & Wilkins, 2010:433, Figure 13-14.)

B. Premature ventricular complexes

1. This early beat fires on its own from a focus in the ventricle and then spreads to the other ventricle (Figure 1-9).
2. **PVCs can occur in patients with or without structural heart disease.** Causes include hypoxia, electrolyte abnormalities, stimulants, caffeine, medications, and structural heart disease.
3. Since conduction is *not* through normal conduction pathways, but rather through ventricular muscle, it is *slower* than normal, causing a **wide QRS**.
4. Wide, bizarre QRS complexes followed by a compensatory pause are seen; a P wave is not usually seen because it is "buried" within the wide QRS complex.
5. PVCs appear in more than 50% of men who undergo 24-hour Holter monitoring.
6. Most patients are asymptomatic. Some patients may have palpitations and dizziness related to PVCs. If symptomatic, β-blockers may be used.
7. Presence of PVCs in patients with normal hearts is associated with increased mortality.
8. If a patient is found to have frequent PVCs, workup for underlying structural heart disease should be initiated which may require specific treatment.
9. Patients with frequent, repetitive PVCs *and* underlying heart disease are at increased risk for sudden death due to cardiac arrhythmia (especially VFib). Order an electrophysiologic study because patients may benefit from an ICD.

Quick HIT

The Cardiac Arrhythmia Suppression Trial (CAST) I and CAST II studies showed that the use of antiarrhythmic drugs to suppress PVCs after MI increases the risk of death.

Quick HIT

PVCs
- Couplet: Two successive PVCs
- Bigeminy: Sinus beat followed by a PVC
- Trigeminy: Two sinus beats followed by a PVC

Tachyarrhythmias

Atrial Fibrillation

A. General characteristics

1. Multiple foci in the atria fire continuously in a chaotic pattern, causing a totally **irregular, rapid ventricular rate.** Instead of intermittently contracting, the atria quiver continuously.
2. Atrial rate is over 400 bpm, but most impulses are blocked at the AV node so ventricular rate ranges between 75 and 175.
3. Patients with AFib and underlying heart disease are at a markedly increased risk for adverse events, such as thromboembolism and hemodynamic compromise.

B. Causes

1. Heart disease: CAD, MI, HTN, mitral valve disease
2. Pericarditis and pericardial trauma (e.g., surgery)
3. Pulmonary disease, including PE
4. Hyperthyroidism or hypothyroidism
5. Systemic illness (e.g., sepsis, malignancy, DM)

Quick HIT

Patients with AFib **in the presence of underlying heart disease** have an especially high risk of embolization and hemodynamic compromise.

6. Stress (e.g., postoperative)
7. Excessive alcohol intake ("holiday heart syndrome")
8. Sick sinus syndrome
9. Pheochromocytoma

C. Clinical features

1. Fatigue and exertional dyspnea
2. Palpitations, dizziness, angina, or syncope may be seen
3. An **irregularly irregular** pulse
4. Blood stasis (secondary to ineffective contraction) leads to formation of intramural thrombi, which can embolize to the brain.

Quick HIT

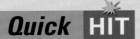

The treatment of AFib and atrial flutter are similar. There are three main goals:
- Control ventricular rate
- Restore normal sinus rhythm
- Assess need for anticoagulation

D. Diagnosis

1. ECG findings: Irregularly irregular rhythm (irregular RR intervals and excessively rapid series of tiny, erratic spikes on ECG with a wavy baseline and no identifiable P waves)

E. Treatment

1. Acute AFib in a hemodynamically *unstable* patient: Immediate electrical cardioversion to sinus rhythm (Figure 1-10; see Clinical Pearl 1-11)
2. Acute AFib in a hemodynamically *stable* patient
   a. Rate control
      - Determine the pulse in a patient with AFib. If it is too rapid, it must be treated. Target rate is 60 to 100 bpm.
      - β-Blockers are preferred. Calcium channel blockers are an alternative.

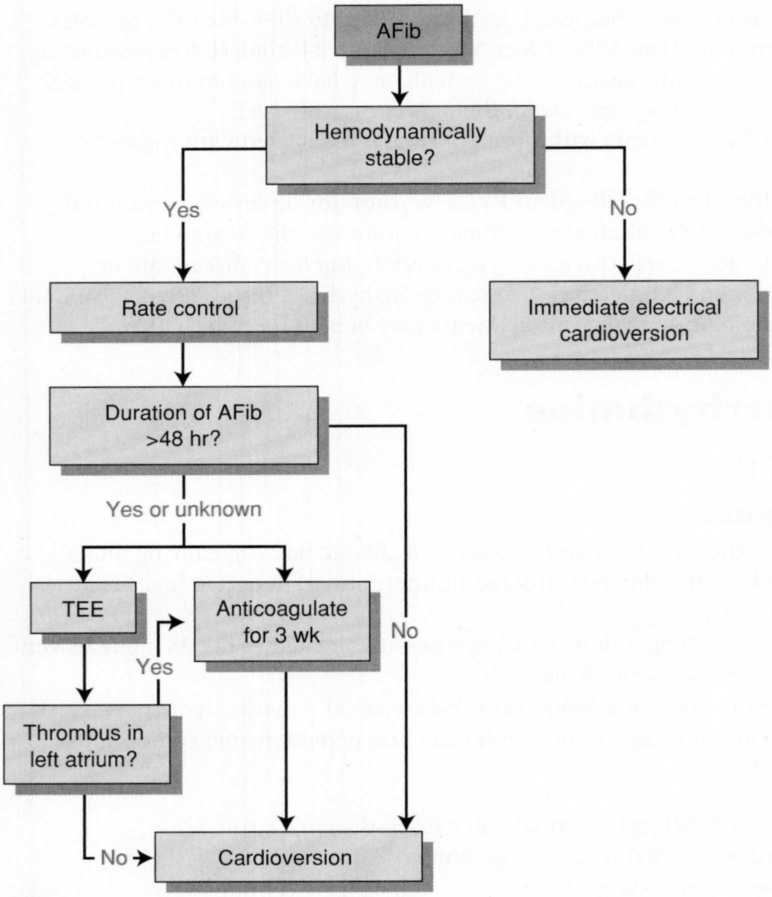

FIGURE 1-10 Acute management of atrial fibrillation.

CLINICAL PEARL 1-11

Cardioversion Versus Defibrillation

Cardioversion

- Delivery of a shock that is **in synchrony** with the QRS complex: Purpose is to terminate certain dysrhythmias such as PSVT or VT; an electric shock during T wave can cause Vfib, so the shock is timed not to hit the T wave.
- Indications: AFib, atrial flutter, VT with a pulse, SVT

Defibrillation

- Delivery of a shock that is **not in synchrony** with the QRS complex: Purpose is to convert a dysrhythmia to normal sinus rhythm.
- Indications: VFib, VT without a pulse.

Automatic Implantable Defibrillator

- Device that is surgically placed: When it detects a lethal dysrhythmia, it delivers an electric shock to defibrillate. It delivers a set number of shocks until the dysrhythmia is terminated.
- Indications: VFib and/or VT that is not controlled by medical therapy.

- If left ventricular systolic dysfunction is present, consider digoxin or amiodarone (useful for rhythm control).

b. Cardioversion to sinus rhythm (after rate control is achieved)
- Candidates for cardioversion include those who are hemodynamically unstable, those with worsening symptoms, and those who are having their first ever case of AFib.
- Electrical cardioversion is preferred over pharmacologic cardioversion. Attempts should be made to control ventricular rate before attempting DC cardioversion.
- Use pharmacologic cardioversion only if electrical cardioversion fails or is not feasible: Parenteral ibutilide, procainamide, flecainide, sotalol, or amiodarone are choices.

c. Anticoagulation to prevent embolic cerebrovascular accident (CVA)
- If AFib present >48 hours (or unknown period of time), risk of embolization during cardioversion is significant (2% to 5%). Anticoagulate patients for 3 weeks before and 4 weeks after cardioversion.
- **An INR of 2 to 3 is the anticoagulation goal range.**
- To avoid waiting 3 weeks for anticoagulation, obtain a transesophageal echocardiogram (TEE) to image the left atrium (LA). If no thrombus is present, start IV heparin and perform cardioversion within 24 hours. Patients still require 4 weeks of anticoagulation after cardioversion.

3. Chronic AFib

a. Rate control with a β-blocker or calcium channel blocker

b. Anticoagulation
- Patients with “lone” AFib (i.e., AFib in the absence of underlying heart disease or other cardiovascular risk factors) **under age 60** do not require anticoagulation because they are at low risk for embolization (aspirin may be appropriate).
- Treat all other patients with chronic anticoagulation (warfarin).

Quick HIT

The **AFFIRM** trial showed that rate control is superior to rhythm control in treatment of AFib.

Quick HIT

Risk of CVA in Patients with AFib
- Patients with “lone AFib”: 1%/yr
- Patients with heart disease: 4%/yr

Atrial Flutter

A. General characteristics

1. Pathophysiology

a. One irritable automaticity focus in the atria fires at about 250 to 350 bpm (typically very close to 300 bpm), giving rise to regular atrial contractions.

b. Atrial rate between around 300 bpm. The long refractory period in the AV node allows only one out of every two or three flutter waves to conduct to the ventricles.

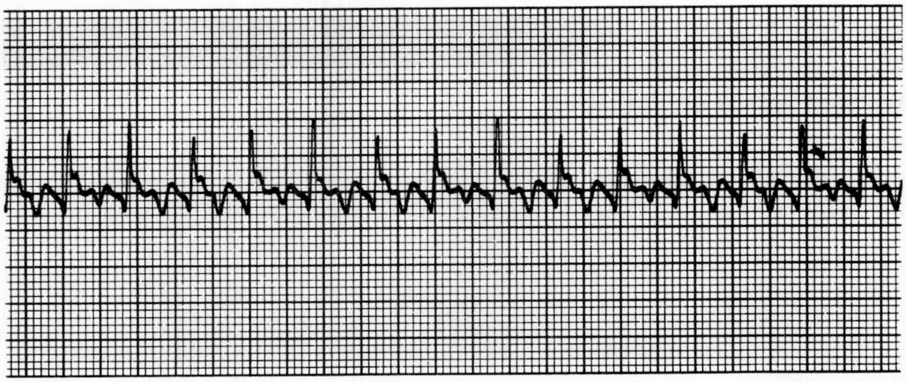

FIGURE 1-11 **Atrial flutter.**
(From Nettina SM. *The Lippincott Manual of Nursing Practice.* 9th ed. Philadelphia, PA: Lippincott Williams & Wilkins, 2010:431, Figure 13-12.)

2. Causes
   a. Heart disease: Heart failure (most common association), rheumatic heart disease, CAD
   b. COPD
   c. Atrial septal defect (ASD)

B. Diagnosis

1. ECG provides a **saw-tooth** baseline, with a QRS complex appearing after every second or third "tooth" (P wave). Saw-tooth flutter waves are best seen in the inferior leads (II, III, aVF). (Figure 1-11)

C. Treatment

1. Similar to treatment for AFib

Multifocal Atrial Tachycardia

- Usually occurs in patients with severe pulmonary disease (e.g., COPD).
- ECG findings: Variable P-wave morphology and variable PR and RR intervals. **At least three different P-wave morphologies are required to make an accurate diagnosis** (Figure 1-12).
- The diagnosis of **wandering atrial pacemaker** is identical except that the heart rate is between 60 and 100 bpm (i.e., not tachycardic).
- Can also be diagnosed by use of vagal maneuvers or adenosine to show AV block without disrupting the atrial tachycardia.
- Treatment directed at the underlying disease, improving oxygenation and ventilation (strong association between MAT and lung disease). If left ventricular function is preserved, acceptable treatments include calcium channel blockers, β-blockers, digoxin, amiodarone, IV flecainide, and IV propafenone. If LV function is not preserved, use digoxin, diltiazem, or amiodarone. Electrical cardioversion is ineffective and should not be used.

Paroxysmal Supraventricular Tachycardia

A. General characteristics

1. Pathophysiology (most often due to reentry) (Figure 1-13)
   a. AV nodal reentrant tachycardia
      - Two pathways (one fast and the other slow) **within the AV node**, so the reentrant circuit is within the AV node
      - Most common cause of supraventricular tachyarrhythmia (SVT)
      - Initiated or terminated by PACs
      - ECG: **Narrow QRS complexes** with no discernible P waves (P waves are buried within the QRS complex). This is because the circuit is short and conduction is rapid, so impulses exit to activate atria and ventricles simultaneously

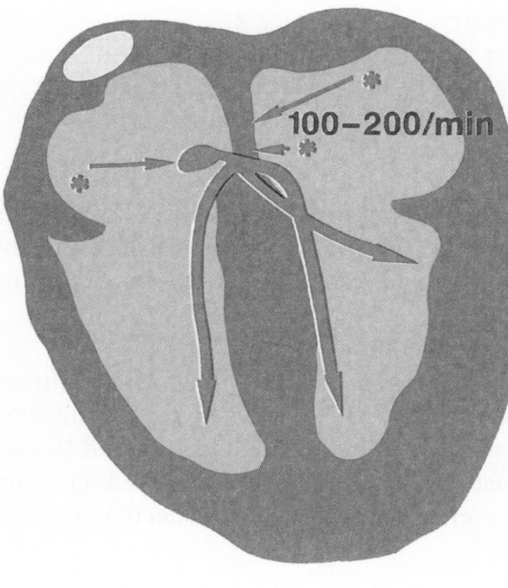

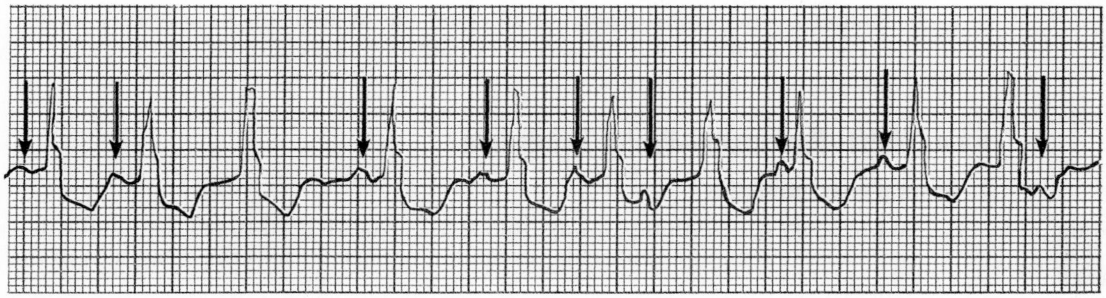

FIGURE 1-12 **ECG of multifocal atrial tachycardia with different P-wave configurations, varying PR intervals, and an irregular rate. Visible ectopic P waves are indicated by *arrows*.**
(From Davis D. *Quick and Accurate 12-Lead ECG Interpretation*. 3rd ed. Philadelphia, PA: Lippincott Williams & Wilkins, 2000:414.)

b. Orthodromic AV reentrant tachycardia
- An accessory pathway between the atria and ventricles that conducts retrogradely
- Called a "concealed bypass tract," and is a common cause of SVTs
- Initiated or terminated by PACs or PVCs
- ECG: **Narrow QRS complexes** with P waves which may or may not be discernible, depending on the rate. This is because the accessory pathway is at some distance from the AV node (reentrant circuit is longer), and there is a difference in the timing of activation of the atria and ventricles

2. Causes
   a. Ischemic heart disease
   b. Digoxin toxicity—paroxysmal atrial tachycardia with 2:1 block is the most common arrhythmia associated with digoxin toxicity

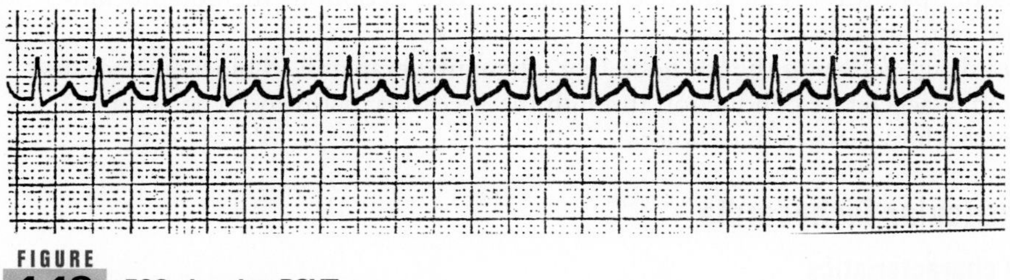

FIGURE 1-13 **ECG showing PSVT.**
(From Harwood-Nuss A, Wolfson AB, Linden CL, et al. *The Clinical Practice of Emergency Medicine*. 5th ed. Philadelphia, PA: Lippincott Williams & Wilkins, 2010:483, Figure 84.1.)

c. AV node reentry
d. Atrial flutter with rapid ventricular response
e. AV reciprocating tachycardia (accessory pathway)
f. Excessive caffeine or alcohol consumption

Quick HIT

In accordance with the electrical conducting system of the heart (SA node, atria, AV node, bundle of His, bundle branches, Purkinje fibers) tachycardias can be quickly separated into two categories based on the width of the QRS complex.
- Narrow QRS complexes suggest that the arrhythmia originates at or above the level of the AV node.
- Wide QRS complexes suggest that the arrhythmia originates outside of the normal conducting system or there is a supraventricular arrhythmia with coexisting abnormality in the His-Purkinje system.

B. Treatment

1. Maneuvers that stimulate the vagus delay AV conduction and thus block the reentry mechanism: The Valsalva maneuver, carotid sinus massage, breath holding, and head immersion in cold water (or placing an ice bag to the face)
2. Acute treatment
   a. Pharmacologic therapy
      - **IV adenosine—agent of choice** due to short duration of action and effectiveness in terminating SVTs; works by decreasing sinoatrial and AV nodal activity.
      - IV verapamil (calcium channel blocker) and IV esmolol (β-blocker) or digoxin are alternatives in patients with preserved left ventricular function.
      - DC cardioversion if drugs are not effective or if unstable; almost always successful.
3. Prevention
   a. Pharmacologic therapy: Verapamil or β-blockers.
   b. Radiofrequency catheter ablation of either the AV node or the accessory tract (depending on which is the accessory pathway) is preferred if episodes are recurrent and symptomatic.

Wolff–Parkinson–White Syndrome

A. General characteristics

1. An accessory conduction pathway from atria to ventricles through the bundle of Kent causes premature ventricular excitation because it lacks the delay seen in the AV node.
2. May lead to a paroxysmal tachycardia, which can be produced by two possible mechanisms:
   a. Orthodromic reciprocating tachycardia
      - The impulse travels through the AV node (anterograde limb) and depolarizes the ventricles. Then it travels back through the accessory pathway (the retrograde limb) and redepolarizes the atria, creating a reentry loop.
      - No delta waves because conduction occurs retrograde over the accessory pathway.
   b. Supraventricular tachycardias (AFib or atrial flutter)
      - Usually, AV node only allows certain impulses to get to ventricles. With an accessory pathway, all or most of the impulses may pass to the ventricles. A fast ventricular rate may occur and cause hemodynamic compromise.

Quick HIT

Side Effects of Adenosine
- Headache
- Flushing
- SOB
- Chest pressure
- Nausea

B. Diagnosis

1. ECG: Narrow complex tachycardia, a short PR interval, and a delta wave (upward deflection seen before the QRS complex)

C. Treatment

1. Radiofrequency catheter ablation of one arm of the reentrant loop (i.e., of the accessory pathway) is an effective treatment. Medical options include procainamide or quinidine.
2. Avoid drugs active on the AV node (e.g., digoxin, verapamil, β-blockers) because they may accelerate conduction through the accessory pathway. Type IA or IC antiarrhythmics are better choices.

Ventricular Tachycardia

A. General characteristics

1. Defined as rapid and repetitive firing of three or more PVCs in a row, at a rate of between 100 and 250 bpm

2. AV dissociation is present, that is, sinus P waves continue with their cycle, unaffected by the tachycardia
3. Originates below the bundle of His
4. Causes
   a. CAD with prior MI is the most common cause
   b. Active ischemia, hypotension
   c. Cardiomyopathies
   d. Congenital defects
   e. Prolonged QT syndrome
   f. Drug toxicity
5. Sustained versus nonsustained VT
   a. Sustained VT (persists in the absence of intervention)
      - **Lasts longer than 30 seconds and is almost always symptomatic**
      - Often associated with marked hemodynamic compromise (i.e., hypotension) and/or development of myocardial ischemia
      - A life-threatening arrhythmia
      - Can progress to VFib if untreated
   b. Nonsustained VT
      - Brief, self-limited runs of VT
      - Usually asymptomatic
      - When CAD and LV dysfunction are present, it is an independent risk factor for sudden death. Therefore, patients with nonsustained VT should be thoroughly evaluated for underlying heart disease and LV dysfunction
6. Prognosis depends on the presence of heart disease and on whether VT is sustained or nonsustained. VT after an MI usually has a poor prognosis, especially if it is sustained. In patients with no underlying heart condition, the prognosis is good

Quick HIT

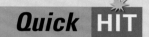

VT or VFib causes 75% of episodes of cardiac arrest.

Quick HIT

Torsades de pointes is a rapid polymorphic VT. It is a dangerous arrhythmia that often can lead to VFib.
- It is associated with many factors that prolong the QT interval (e.g., congenital QT syndromes, tricyclic antidepressants, anticholinergics, electrolyte abnormalities, ischemia).
- IV **magnesium** provides cardiac stabilization.
- Address the underlying cause.

B. Clinical features

1. Palpitations, dyspnea, lightheadedness, angina, impaired consciousness (syncope or near-syncope)
2. May present with sudden cardiac death
3. Signs of cardiogenic shock may be present
4. May be asymptomatic if rate is slow
5. Physical findings include **cannon A waves** in the neck (secondary to AV dissociation, which results in atrial contraction during ventricular contraction) and an S1 that varies in intensity

Quick HIT

In sum, the presence of ventricular irritability (frequent PVCs, VT) is especially worrisome in patients with underlying heart disease and left ventricular dysfunction. These patients are at a high risk for sudden death.

C. Diagnosis

1. ECG: **Wide and bizarre QRS complexes** (Figure 1-14).

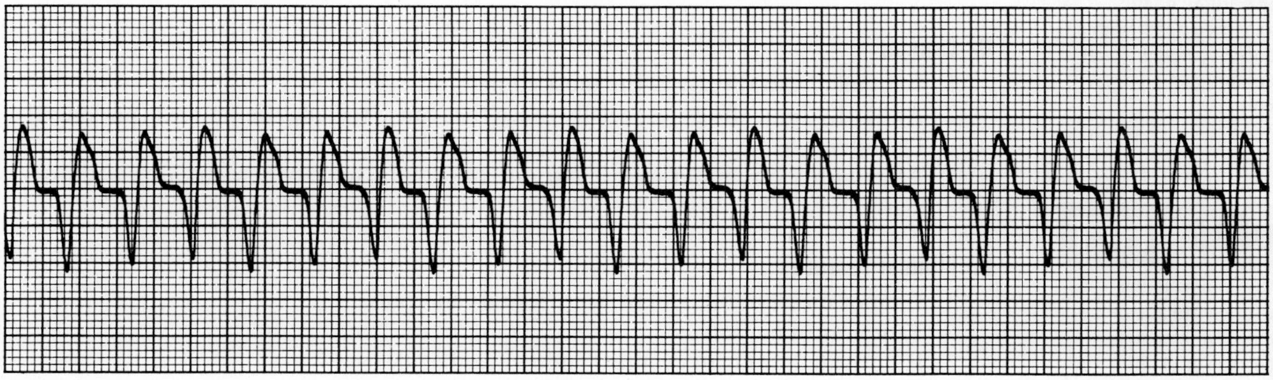

FIGURE **1-14** **Ventricular tachycardia.**
(From Nettina SM. *The Lippincott Manual of Nursing Practice*. 9th ed. Philadelphia, PA: Lippincott Williams & Wilkins, 2010:434, Figure 13-16.)

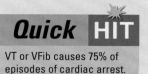

Quick HIT

Always suspect VT in a patient with a wide (>0.12 second) QRS tachycardia.

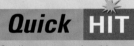

2. QRS complexes may be monomorphic or polymorphic.
   a. In monomorphic VT, all QRS complexes are identical.
   b. In polymorphic VT, the QRS complexes are different.
3. Unlike PSVT, VT does not respond to vagal maneuvers or adenosine.

D. Treatment

1. Identify and treat reversible causes
2. Sustained VT
   a. Hemodynamically stable patients with mild symptoms and systolic BP >90—pharmacologic therapy
      - New advanced cardiac life support (ACLS) guidelines recommend IV amiodarone, IV procainamide, or IV sotalol
   b. Hemodynamically unstable patients or patients with severe symptoms
      - Immediate synchronous DC cardioversion
      - Follow with IV amiodarone to maintain sinus rhythm
   c. Ideally, all patients with sustained VT should undergo placement of an ICD, unless EF is normal (then consider amiodarone)
3. Nonsustained VT
   a. If no underlying heart disease and asymptomatic, do not treat. These patients are *not* at increased risk of sudden death.
   b. If the patient has underlying heart disease, a recent MI, evidence of left ventricular dysfunction, or is symptomatic, order an electrophysiologic study: If it shows inducible, sustained VT, ICD placement is appropriate.
   c. Pharmacologic therapy is second-line treatment. However, amiodarone has the best results of all of the antiarrhythmic agents.

Quick HIT

- It is important to distinguish monomorphic VT from SVT with aberrant conduction.
- Wide complex tachycardia in adults with a history of structural heart disease is much more likely to be due to VT than SVT with aberrancy.

Quick HIT

If a patient with underlying heart disease is found to have nonsustained VT, an implantable defibrillator has been shown to be the most effective treatment.

Ventricular Fibrillation

A. General characteristics

1. Multiple foci in the ventricles fire rapidly, leading to a chaotic quivering of the ventricles and no cardiac output.
2. Most episodes of VFib begin with VT (except in the setting of acute ischemia/infarction).
3. Recurrence
   a. If VFib is not associated with acute MI, recurrence rate is high (up to 30% within the first year). These patients require chronic therapy: Either prophylactic antiarrhythmic therapy (amiodarone) or implantation of an automatic defibrillator.
   b. If VFib develops within 48 hours of an acute MI, long-term prognosis is favorable and the recurrence rate is low (2% at 1 year). Chronic therapy is not required in these patients.
4. Fatal if untreated

Quick HIT

Cardiac arrest and sudden cardiac death are not synonymous:

Cardiac arrest: Sudden loss of cardiac output; potentially reversible if circulation and oxygen delivery are promptly restored.

Sudden cardiac death: Unexpected death within 1 hour of symptom onset secondary to a cardiac cause.

B. Causes

1. Ischemic heart disease is the most common cause
2. Antiarrhythmic drugs, especially those that cause torsades de pointes (prolonged QT intervals)
3. AFib with a very rapid ventricular rate in patients with Wolff–Parkinson–White syndrome

C. Clinical features

1. Cannot measure BP; absent heart sounds and pulse
2. Patient is unconscious
3. If untreated, leads to eventual sudden cardiac death

Quick HIT

Narrow complex tachycardias originate above ventricles. Wide complex tachycardias originate within ventricles and are more ominous because they are more likely to progress to VFib.

D. Diagnosis

1. ECG: No atrial P waves can be identified (Figure 1-15)
2. No QRS complexes can be identified

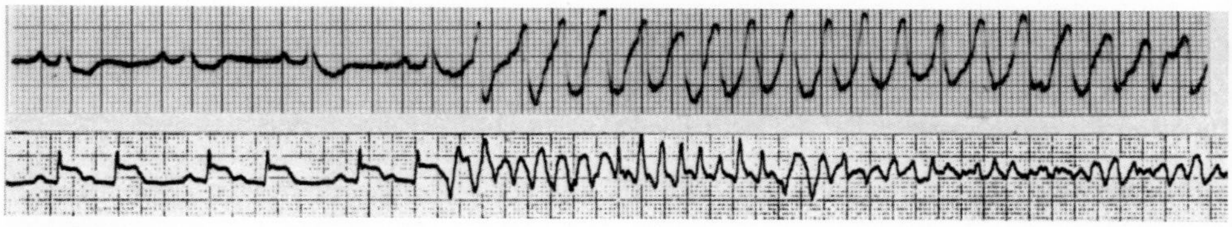

FIGURE 1-15 **Ventricular fibrillation.**
(From Humes DH, DuPont HL, Gardner LB, et al. *Kelley's Textbook of Internal Medicine.* 4th ed. Philadelphia, PA: Lippincott Williams & Wilkins, 2000:499, Figure 76.24.)

3. In sum, no waves can be identified; there is a very irregular rhythm

E. Treatment

1. **This is a medical emergency! Immediate defibrillation and CPR are indicated.**
   a. Initiate unsynchronized DC cardioversion immediately. If the equipment is not ready, start CPR until it is.
   b. Give up to three sequential shocks to establish another rhythm; assess the rhythm between each.
2. If VF persists:
   a. Continue CPR.
   b. Intubation may be indicated.
   c. Epinephrine (1 mg IV bolus initially, and then every 3 to 5 minutes)—this increases myocardial and cerebral blood flow and decreases the defibrillation threshold.
   d. Attempt to defibrillate again 30 to 60 seconds after first epinephrine dose.
3. Other options if the above procedures fail (refractory VFib):
   a. IV amiodarone followed by shock—new ACLS guidelines recommend the use of amiodarone over other antiarrhythmic agents in refractory VFib.
   b. Lidocaine, magnesium, and procainamide are alternative second-line treatments.
4. If cardioversion is successful:
   a. Maintain continuous IV infusion of the effective antiarrhythmic agent. IV amiodarone has been shown to be the most effective.
   b. Implantable defibrillators have become the mainstay of chronic therapy in patients at continued risk for VF. Long-term amiodarone therapy is an alternative.

Quick HIT

- Drugs cannot convert VFib by themselves. Defibrillation is key, along with CPR and epinephrine.
- Defibrillation generally does not work for asystole. Perform CPR and administer epinephrine.

Quick HIT

Pulseless Electrical Activity (PEA)

- Occurs when electrical activity is on the monitor but there are no pulses (even with Doppler), and carries a grim prognosis.
- Treat possible causes (hypoxia, hypovolemia, hypotension, hyperkalemia, tamponade, tension pneumothorax, massive PE, and so on) and medicate according to ACLS guidelines.

Bradyarrhythmias

Sinus Bradycardia

- Sinus rate <60 bpm: Clinically significant when rate is persistently <45 bpm
- Causes include ischemia, increased vagal tone, antiarrhythmic drugs; may be a normal finding in trained athletes
- Can be asymptomatic; patients may complain of fatigue, inability to exercise, angina, or syncope
- Atropine can elevate the sinus rate by blocking vagal stimulation to the sinoatrial node. A cardiac pacemaker may be required if bradycardia persists

Sick Sinus Syndrome

- Sinus node dysfunction characterized by a persistent spontaneous sinus bradycardia. Patients usually elderly.
- Symptoms include dizziness, confusion, syncope, fatigue, and CHF.
- Pacemaker implantation may be required (see Clinical Pearl 1-12).

AV Block

A. First-degree AV block

1. PR interval is prolonged (>0.20 second) (Figure 1-16).
2. A QRS complex follows each P wave.

CLINICAL PEARL 1-12

Cardiac Pacemakers

1. Device that delivers direct electrical stimulation to the heart when the heart's natural pacemaker is unable to do so
2. There are three types:
   - Permanent implantable system for long-term treatment
   - Temporary systems—either transcutaneous (with electrode pads over chest) or transvenous—both use an external pulse generator that patient can secure to waist with straps
3. On ECG, cardiac pacing is noted by presence of a "spike."
4. Indications
   - Sinus node dysfunction is most common indication
   - Symptomatic heart block—Mobitz II second-degree block and complete heart block (even if asymptomatic)
   - Symptomatic bradyarrhythmias
   - Tachyarrhythmias to interrupt rapid rhythm disturbances

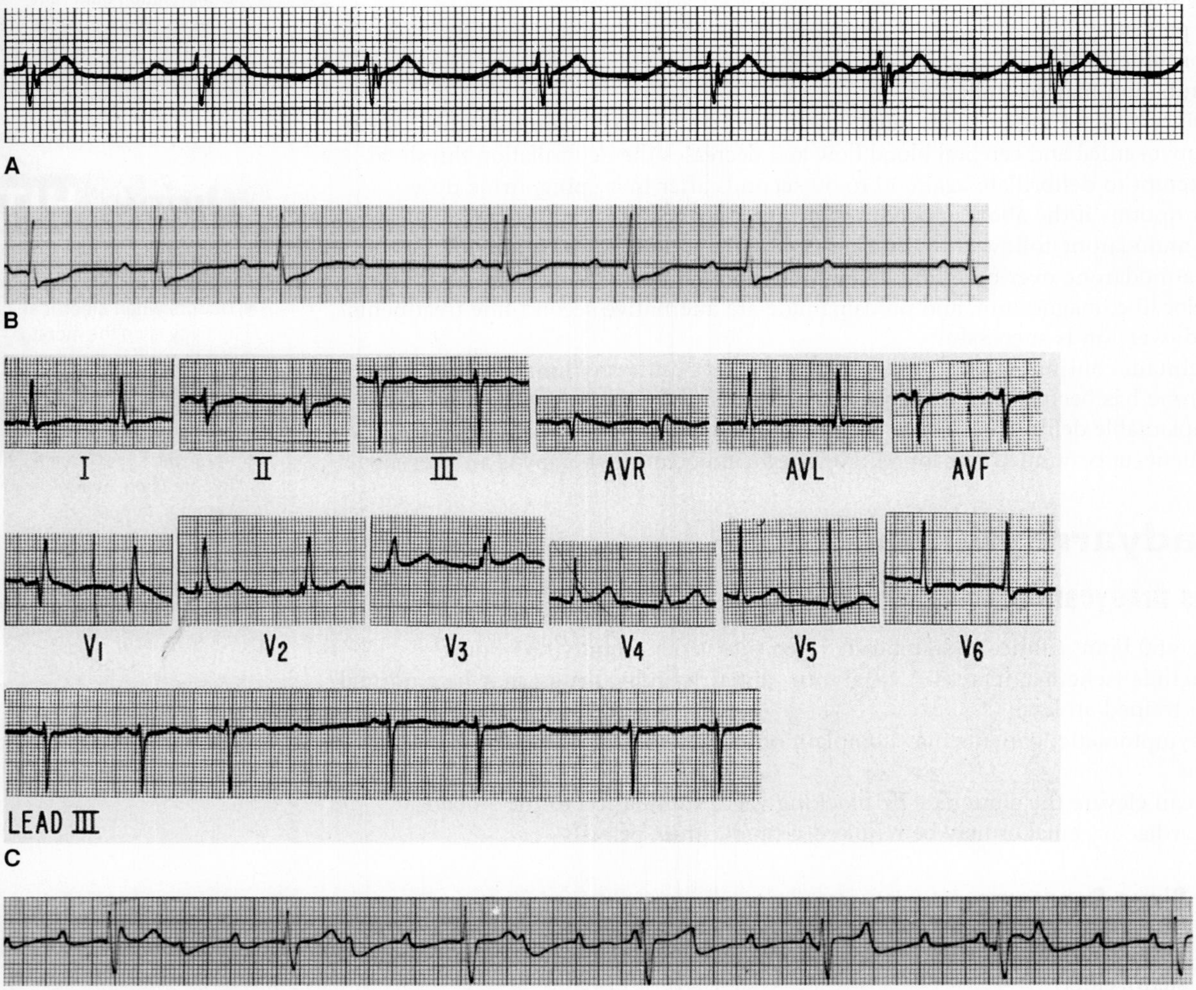

FIGURE 1-16 **A: First-degree AV block. B: Type I second-degree AV block. C: Type II second-degree AV block. D: Type III block.**

(**A** from Nettina SM. *The Lippincott Manual of Nursing Practice.* 9th ed. Philadelphia, PA: Lippincott Williams & Wilkins, 2010:436, Figure 13-18.) (**B** from Humes DH, DuPont HL, Gardner LB, et al. *Kelley's Textbook of Internal Medicine.* 4th ed. Philadelphia, PA: Lippincott Williams & Wilkins, 2000:500, Figure 76.25.) (**C** from Humes DH, DuPont HL, Gardner LB, et al. *Kelley's Textbook of Internal Medicine.* 4th ed. Philadelphia, PA: Lippincott Williams & Wilkins, 2000:501, Figure 76.27.) (**D** from Humes DH, DuPont HL, Gardner LB, et al. *Kelley's Textbook of Internal Medicine.* 4th ed. Philadelphia, PA: Lippincott Williams & Wilkins, 2000:502, Figure 76.30.)

3. Delay is usually in the AV node.
4. Benign condition that does not require treatment.

B. Second-degree AV block (includes Mobitz type I and II)

1. Mobitz type I (Wenckebach)
   a. Characterized by progressive prolongation of PR interval until a P wave fails to conduct
   b. Site of block is usually within the AV node
   c. Benign condition that does not require treatment
2. Mobitz type II
   a. P wave fails to conduct suddenly, without a preceding PR interval prolongation; therefore, the QRS drops suddenly
   b. Often progresses to complete heart block
   c. Site of block is within the His-Purkinje system
   d. **Pacemaker** implantation is necessary

C. Third-degree (complete) AV block

1. Absence of conduction of atrial impulses to the ventricles; no correspondence between P waves and QRS complexes
2. A ventricular pacemaker (escape rhythm) maintains a ventricular rate of 25 to 40 bpm
   a. Characterized by **AV dissociation**
   b. **Pacemaker** implantation is necessary.

> **Quick HIT**
> Second-degree Mobitz type II and third-degree AV blocks require pacemaker implantation.

Diseases of the Heart Muscle

Dilated Cardiomyopathy

A. General characteristics

1. Most common type of cardiomyopathy
2. An insult (e.g., ischemia, infection, alcohol, etc.) causes dysfunction of left ventricular contractility
3. Poor prognosis—many die within 5 years of the onset of symptoms

B. Causes

1. Up to 50% of cases are idiopathic
2. Other causes include:
   a. CAD (with prior MI) is a common cause
   b. Toxic: Alcohol, doxorubicin, Adriamycin
   c. Metabolic: Thiamine or selenium deficiency, hypophosphatemia, uremia
   d. Infectious: Viral, Chagas disease, Lyme disease, HIV
   e. Thyroid disease: Hyperthyroidism or hypothyroidism
   f. Peripartum cardiomyopathy
   g. Collagen vascular disease: SLE, scleroderma
   h. Prolonged, uncontrolled tachycardia
   i. Catecholamine induced: Pheochromocytoma, cocaine
   j. Familial/genetic

C. Clinical features

1. Symptoms and signs of left- and right-sided CHF develop.
2. S_3, S_4, and murmurs of mitral or tricuspid insufficiency may be present.
3. Cardiomegaly is commonly seen.
4. Many patients with DCM will have a coexisting arrhythmia (atrial or ventricular) related to the dilated ventricle.
5. Sudden death.

D. Diagnosis

1. ECG, CXR, and echocardiogram results consistent with CHF.
2. Genetic testing may be warranted if there is a family history of DCM and no other cause can be identified.

E. Treatment

1. Similar to treatment of CHF: Digoxin, diuretics, vasodilators, and cardiac transplantation.
2. Remove the offending agent if possible.
3. Anticoagulation should be considered because patients are at increased risk of embolization.

Hypertrophic Cardiomyopathy

A. General characteristics

1. Most cases are inherited as an **autosomal-dominant** trait. However, spontaneous mutations may account for some cases.
2. Pathophysiology
   a. The main problem is diastolic dysfunction due to a stiff, hypertrophied ventricle with elevated diastolic filling pressures.
   b. These pressures increase further with factors that increase HR and contractility (such as exercise) or decrease left ventricular filling (e.g., the Valsalva maneuver).
   c. Patients may also have a dynamic outflow obstruction due to asymmetric hypertrophy of the interventricular septum.

B. Clinical features

1. Symptoms
   a. Dyspnea on exertion
   b. Chest pain (angina)
   c. Syncope (or dizziness) after exertion or the Valsalva maneuver
   d. Palpitations
   e. Arrhythmias (AFib, ventricular arrhythmias)—due to persistently elevated atrial pressures
   f. Cardiac failure due to increased diastolic stiffness
   g. Sudden death—sometimes seen in a young athlete; may be the first manifestation of disease
   h. Some patients may remain asymptomatic for many years
2. Signs
   a. Sustained PMI
   b. Loud S_4
   c. Systolic ejection murmur
      - Decreases with squatting, lying down, or straight leg raise (due to decreased outflow obstruction)
      - Intensity increases with Valsalva and standing (decreases LV size and thus increases the outflow obstruction)
      - Decreases with sustained handgrip (increased systemic resistance leads to decreased gradient across aortic valve)
      - Best heard at left lower sternal border (LLSB)
   d. Rapidly increasing carotid pulse with two upstrokes (bisferious pulse)

Quick HIT

- Standing, the Valsalva, and leg raise maneuvers diminish the intensity of all murmurs except MVP and hypertrophic cardiomyopathy (HCM). These maneuvers decrease left ventricular volume.
- Squatting increases the intensity of all murmurs except MVP and HCM.
- Sustained handgrip diminishes the intensity of HCM murmur. Sustained handgrip increases systemic resistance.

C. Diagnosis

1. Echocardiogram establishes the diagnosis
2. Clinical diagnosis and family history

D. Treatment

1. Asymptomatic patients generally do not need treatment, but this is controversial. No studies have shown any alteration in the prognosis with therapy, so treatment generally focuses on reducing symptoms.
2. All patients should avoid strenuous exercise, including competitive athletics.
3. Symptomatic patients
   a. β-Blockers should be the initial drug used in symptomatic patients; they reduce symptoms by improving diastolic filling (as HR decreases, duration in diastole increases), and also reduce myocardial contractility and thus oxygen consumption.

b. Calcium channel blockers (verapamil).
   - Can be used if patient is not responding to β-blocker.
   - Reduce symptoms by similar mechanism as β-blockers.

c. Diuretics can be used if fluid retention occurs.

d. If AFib is present, treat accordingly (see Atrial Fibrillation).

e. Surgery
   - Myomectomy has a high success rate for relieving symptoms. It involves the excision of part of the myocardial septum. It is reserved for patients with severe disease.
   - Mitral valve replacement is now rarely performed.

f. Pacemaker implantation has had variable results.

Restrictive Cardiomyopathy

A. General characteristics

1. Infiltration of the myocardium results in impaired diastolic ventricular filling due to decreased ventricular compliance.
2. Systolic dysfunction is variable and usually occurs in advanced disease.
3. Less common than dilated and hypertrophic cardiomyopathies.

B. Causes

1. Amyloidosis
2. Sarcoidosis
3. Hemochromatosis
4. Scleroderma
5. Carcinoid syndrome
6. Chemotherapy or radiation induced
7. Idiopathic

C. Clinical features

1. Elevated filling pressures cause dyspnea and exercise intolerance.
2. Right-sided signs and symptoms are present for the same reason.

D. Diagnosis

1. Echocardiogram
   a. Thickened myocardium and possible systolic ventricular dysfunction
   b. Increased right atrium (RA) and LA size with normal LV and RV size
   c. In amyloidosis, myocardium appears brighter or may have a sparkled appearance
2. ECG: Low voltages or conduction abnormalities, arrhythmias, AFib
3. Endomyocardial biopsy may be diagnostic

E. Treatment

1. Treat underlying disorder
   a. Hemochromatosis: Phlebotomy or deferoxamine
   b. Sarcoidosis: Glucocorticoids
   c. Amyloidosis: No treatment available
   d. Give digoxin if systolic dysfunction is present (except in patients with cardiac amyloidosis, who have increased incidence of digoxin toxicity)
2. Use diuretics and vasodilators (for pulmonary and peripheral edema) cautiously, because a decrease in preload may compromise cardiac output

Myocarditis

- Inflammation of the myocardium, with many possible causes, including viruses (e.g., Coxsackie, parvovirus B19, human herpes virus-6), bacteria (e.g., group A streptococcus in rheumatic fever, Lyme disease, mycoplasma, etc.), SLE, medications (e.g., sulfonamides); can also be idiopathic.
- May be asymptomatic, or may present with fatigue, fever, chest pain, pericarditis, CHF, arrhythmia, or even death

- The classic patient is a young male.
- Look for elevations in cardiac enzyme levels and erythrocyte sedimentation rate.
- Treatment is supportive. Treat underlying causes if possible, and treat any complications.

Pericardial Diseases

Acute Pericarditis

A. General characteristics

1. Inflammation of the pericardial sac—may be an isolated finding or part of an underlying disorder or generalized disease
2. Causes
   a. Idiopathic (probably postviral): Most cases of idiopathic pericarditis are presumed to be postviral, usually preceded by a recent flulike illness or by upper respiratory or GI symptoms
   b. Infectious: Viral (e.g., **Coxsackievirus**, echovirus, adenovirus, EBV, influenza, HIV, hepatitis A or B), bacterial (tuberculosis), fungal, toxoplasmosis
   c. Acute MI (first 24 hours after MI)
   d. Uremia
   e. Collagen vascular diseases (e.g., SLE, scleroderma, rheumatoid arthritis, sarcoidosis)
   f. Neoplasm—especially Hodgkin lymphoma, breast, and lung cancers
   g. Drug-induced lupus syndrome (procainamide, hydralazine)
   h. After MI: (*Dressler syndrome*)—usually weeks to months after MI
   i. After surgery—postpericardiotomy syndrome
   j. Amyloidosis
   k. Radiation
   l. Trauma
3. The majority of patients recover within 1 to 3 weeks. A minority of patients have a prolonged course or recurrent symptoms
4. Complications
   a. Pericardial effusion
   b. Cardiac tamponade—can occur in up to 15% of patients; close observation is important

Quick HIT

Cardinal manifestations of acute pericarditis:
- Chest pain
- Pericardial friction rub
- ECG changes—diffuse ST elevation; PR depression
- Pericardial effusion (with or without tamponade)

B. Clinical features

1. Chest pain (most common finding)
   a. Often severe and **pleuritic** (can differentiate from pain of MI because of association with breathing).
   b. Often localized to the retrosternal and left precordial regions and radiates to the trapezius ridge and neck.
   c. Pain is **positional:** It is aggravated by lying supine, coughing, swallowing, and deep inspiration. **Pain is relieved by sitting up and leaning forward.**
   d. Pain is not always present, depending on the cause (e.g., usually absent in rheumatoid pericarditis).
2. Fever and leukocytosis may be present
3. Patient may give symptoms of preceding viral illness such as a nonproductive cough or diarrhea
4. **Pericardial friction rub**
   a. Not always present, but it is very specific for pericarditis
   b. Caused by friction between visceral and parietal pericardial surfaces
   c. Scratching, high-pitched sound with up to three components. Patients may have any or all of the three components:
      - Atrial systole (presystolic)
      - Ventricular systole (loudest and most frequently heard)
      - Early diastole

d. Heard best during expiration with patient sitting up and with stethoscope placed firmly against the chest
e. Friction rub may come and go over a period of several hours, and can vary greatly in intensity

C. Diagnosis

1. ECG shows four changes in sequence
   a. **Diffuse ST elevation and PR depression**
   b. ST segment returns to normal—typically around 1 week
   c. T wave inverts—does not occur in all patients
   d. T wave returns to normal
2. Echocardiogram if pericarditis with effusion is suspected, but echocardiogram is often normal

D. Treatment

1. Most cases are self-limited and resolve in 2 to 6 weeks.
2. Treat the underlying cause if known.
3. NSAIDs are the mainstay of therapy (for pain and other systemic symptoms). Colchicine is also often used.
4. Glucocorticoids may be tried if pain does not respond to NSAIDs, but should be avoided if at all possible.
5. Relatively uncomplicated cases can be treated as an outpatient. However, patients with more worrisome symptoms such as fever and leukocytosis and patients with worrisome features such as pericardial effusion should be hospitalized.

Constrictive Pericarditis

A. General characteristics

1. **Fibrous scarring of the pericardium** leads to rigidity and thickening of the pericardium, with obliteration of the pericardial cavity.
2. Pathophysiology
   a. A fibrotic, rigid pericardium restricts the diastolic filling of the heart.
   b. Ventricular filling is unimpeded during early diastole because intracardiac volume has not yet reached the limit defined by the stiff pericardium.
   c. When intracardiac volume reaches the limit set by the noncompliant pericardium, ventricular filling is halted abruptly. (In contrast, ventricular filling is impeded **throughout** diastole in cardiac tamponade.)
3. Causes
   a. In most patients, the cause is never identified and is idiopathic or related to a previous viral infection.
   b. Other causes include uremia, radiation therapy, tuberculosis, chronic pericardial effusion, tumor invasion, connective tissue disorders, and prior surgery involving the pericardium.

> **Quick HIT**
> **Diastolic Dysfunction in Constrictive Pericarditis**
> Early diastole: Rapid filling
> Late diastole: Halted filling

B. Clinical features

1. Patients appear very ill
2. Patients with constrictive pericarditis typically present in one of the two ways:
   a. With symptoms characteristic of fluid overload such as edema, ascites, and pleural effusions
   b. With symptoms related to the diminished cardiac output such as dyspnea on exertion, fatigue, decreased exercise tolerance, and cachexia
   c. Patient can present with a combination of both of these findings
3. Signs include:
   a. **JVD**—most prominent physical finding; central venous pressure (CVP) is elevated and displays prominent x and y descents
   b. *Kussmaul sign*—JVD (venous pressure) fails to decrease during inspiration
   c. Pericardial knock—corresponding to the abrupt cessation of ventricular filling
   d. Ascites
   e. Dependent edema

> **Quick HIT**
> If a patient has clinical signs of cirrhosis (ascites, hepatomegaly) and distended neck veins, perform tests to rule out constrictive pericarditis.

Quick HIT

Often, constrictive pericarditis progresses to worsening cardiac output and to hepatic and/or renal failure. Surgical treatment is indicated in most cases.

Quick HIT

Echocardiogram is the imaging study of choice for diagnosis of pericardial effusion and cardiac tamponade (has a high sensitivity).

Quick HIT

Pericardial effusion is important clinically when it develops rapidly because it may lead to cardiac tamponade.

4. May be difficult to distinguish from restrictive cardiomyopathy—may require echo or cardiac catheterization to distinguish these entities

C. Diagnosis

1. ECG
   a. Nonspecific changes such as low QRS voltages, generalized T-wave flattening or inversion, left atrial abnormalities.
   b. **AFib** is more often seen in advanced disease but overall occurs in fewer than half of all patients.
2. Echocardiogram
   a. Increased pericardial thickness is seen in about half of all patients.
   b. A sharp halt in ventricular diastolic filling and atrial enlargement can also be seen.
3. CT scan and MRI may also show pericardial thickening and calcifications, and can aid greatly in the diagnosis.
4. Cardiac catheterization
   a. Elevated and equal diastolic pressures in all chambers.
   b. Ventricular pressure tracing shows a rapid y descent, which has been described as a dip and plateau or a "square root sign."

D. Treatment

1. **Treat the underlying condition**
2. Diuretics may be extremely helpful in treating fluid overload symptoms
3. Surgical pericardiectomy

Pericardial Effusion

A. General characteristics

1. Defined as any cause of acute pericarditis (see above) that can lead to exudation of fluid into the pericardial space
2. Can occur in association with ascites and pleural effusion in salt and water retention states such as CHF, cirrhosis, and nephrotic syndrome
3. Is often asymptomatic and suspected based on the symptoms of the underlying condition
4. May be acute or chronic

B. Clinical features

1. All physical examination signs are extremely nonspecific and often do not aid in the diagnosis but may include
   a. Muffled heart sounds
   b. Soft PMI
   c. Dullness at left lung base (because it may be compressed by pericardial fluid)
   d. Pericardial friction rub may or may not be present

C. Diagnosis

1. Echocardiogram
   a. Imaging procedure of choice: Confirms the presence or absence of a significant effusion
   b. Most sensitive and specific method of determining whether pericardial fluid is present; can show as little as 20 mL of fluid
   c. Should be performed in all patients with acute pericarditis to rule out an effusion
2. CXR
   a. CXR shows enlargement of cardiac silhouette when >250 mL of fluid has accumulated
   b. Cardiac silhouette may have prototypical "water bottle" appearance
   c. An enlarged heart without pulmonary vascular congestion suggests pericardial effusion

3. ECG
   a. Shows low QRS voltages and T-wave flattening but should not be used to diagnose pericardial effusion
   b. Electrical alternans (see definition below under Cardiac Tamponade) suggests a massive pericardial effusion and tamponade
4. CT scan or MRI—very accurate, but often unnecessary given the accuracy of an echocardiogram
5. Pericardial fluid analysis—may clarify the cause of the effusion
   a. Order protein and glucose content, cell count and differential, cytology, specific gravity, hematocrit, Gram stain, acid-fast stains, fungal smear, cultures, LDH content

D. Treatment

1. Depends on patient's hemodynamic stability.
2. Pericardiocentesis is not indicated unless there is evidence of cardiac tamponade. Analysis of pericardial fluid can be useful if the cause of the effusion is unknown.
3. If the effusion is small and clinically insignificant, a repeat echocardiogram in 1 to 2 weeks is appropriate.

Cardiac Tamponade

A. General characteristics

1. Defined as accumulation of pericardial fluid. It is the **rate** of fluid accumulation that is important, not the amount.
   a. Two hundred milliliters of fluid that develops rapidly (i.e., blood secondary to trauma) can cause cardiac tamponade.
   b. Two liters of fluid may accumulate slowly before cardiac tamponade occurs. When fluid accumulates slowly, the pericardium has the opportunity to stretch and adapt to the increased volume (i.e., related to a malignancy).
2. Pathophysiology
   a. Pericardial effusion that mechanically impairs diastolic filling of the heart.
   b. Characterized by the elevation and equalization of intracardiac and intrapericardial pressures.
      - Pressures in the RV, LV, RA, LA, pulmonary artery, and pericardium equalize during diastole.
      - **Ventricular filling is impaired during diastole.**
      - Decreased diastolic filling leads to decreased stroke volume and decreased cardiac output.
3. Causes
   a. Penetrating (less commonly blunt) trauma to the thorax, such as gunshot and stab wounds.
   b. Iatrogenic: Central-line placement, pacemaker insertion, pericardiocentesis, etc.
   c. Pericarditis: Idiopathic, neoplastic, or uremic.
   d. Post-MI with free wall rupture.

B. Clinical features

1. **Elevated jugular venous pressure is the most common finding** (distended neck veins). Venous waveforms: Prominent x descent with absent y descent is seen.
2. Narrowed pulse pressure (due to decreased stroke volume).
3. *Pulsus paradoxus*
   a. Exaggerated decrease in arterial pressure during inspiration (>10 mm Hg drop).
   b. Can be detected by a decrease in the amplitude of the femoral or carotid pulse during inspiration.
      - Pulse gets strong during expiration and weak during inspiration.
4. Distant (muffled) heart sounds.
5. Tachypnea, tachycardia, and hypotension with onset of cardiogenic shock.

Quick HIT

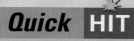

Cardiac Tamponade
Pressures in the RV, LV, RA, LA, pulmonary artery, and pericardium equalize during diastole.

Quick HIT

Beck Triad (Cardiac Tamponade)
- Hypotension
- Muffled heart sounds
- JVD

C. Diagnosis

1. Echocardiogram
   a. Must be performed if suspicion of tamponade exists based on history/examination
   b. Usually diagnostic; the most sensitive and specific noninvasive test
2. CXR
   a. Enlargement of cardiac silhouette when >250 mL has accumulated
   b. Clear lung fields
3. ECG
   a. *Electrical alternans* (alternate beat variation in the direction of the ECG waveforms)—due to pendular swinging of the heart within the pericardial space, causing a motion artifact
   b. Findings are neither 100% sensitive nor specific. ECG should not be used to diagnose tamponade
4. Cardiac catheterization
   a. Shows equalization of pressures in all chambers of the heart
   b. Shows elevated right atrial pressure with loss of the y descent

D. Treatment

1. Nonhemorrhagic tamponade
   a. If patient is hemodynamically stable
      - Monitor closely with echocardiogram, CXR, ECG
      - If patient has known renal failure, dialysis is more helpful than pericardiocentesis
   b. If patient is not hemodynamically stable
      - Pericardiocentesis is indicated
      - If no improvement is noted, fluid challenge may improve symptoms
2. Hemorrhagic tamponade secondary to trauma
   a. If the bleeding is unlikely to stop on its own, emergent surgery is indicated to repair the injury
   b. Pericardiocentesis is only a temporizing measure and is not definitive treatment. Surgery should **not** be delayed to perform pericardiocentesis

Valvular Heart Disease

Mitral Stenosis

A. General characteristics

1. Almost all cases are due to rheumatic heart disease. (Patient may not recall a history of rheumatic fever.)
2. Pathophysiology
   a. Immune-mediated damage to the mitral valve (due to rheumatic fever) caused by cross-reactivity between the streptococcal antigen and the valve tissue leads to scarring and narrowing of the mitral valve orifice.
   b. Mitral stenosis results in elevated left atrial and pulmonary venous pressure leading to pulmonary congestion.
   c. Anything that increases flow across the mitral valve (exercise, tachycardia, and so on) exacerbates the pulmonary venous HTN and associated symptoms.
   d. Long-standing mitral stenosis can result in pulmonary HTN and ultimately can result in right ventricular failure (RVF).
   e. Long-standing mitral stenosis can also lead to AFib due to increased left atrial size pressure and size.
   f. Patients are usually asymptomatic until the mitral valve area is reduced to approximately 1.5 cm^2 (normal valve area is 4 to 5 cm^2).

B. Clinical features

1. Symptoms
   a. Exertional dyspnea, orthopnea, PND
   b. Palpitations, chest pain

c. Hemoptysis—as the elevated LA pressure ruptures anastomoses of small bronchial veins
d. Thromboembolism—often associated with AFib
e. If RVF occurs, ascites and edema may develop

2. Signs
   a. Mitral stenosis murmur.
      - The **opening snap** is followed by a **low-pitched diastolic rumble** and presystolic accentuation. This murmur increases in length as the disease worsens.
      - Heard best with bell of stethoscope in left lateral decubitus position.
   b. S_2 is followed by an opening snap. The distance between S_2 and the opening snap can give an indication as to the severity of the stenosis. The closer the opening snap follows S_2, the worse is the stenosis.
   c. Murmur is followed by a **loud** S_1. A loud S_1 may be the most prominent physical finding.
   d. With long-standing disease, will find signs of RVF (e.g., right ventricular heave, JVD, hepatomegaly, ascites) and/or pulmonary HTN (loud P_2).
   e. All signs and symptoms will increase with exercise and during pregnancy.

C. Diagnosis

1. CXR: Left atrial enlargement (early)
2. Echocardiogram—most important test in confirming diagnosis
   a. Left atrial enlargement
   b. Thick, calcified mitral valve
   c. Narrow, "fish mouth"-shaped orifice
   d. Signs of RVF if advanced disease

D. Treatment

1. Medical
   a. Diuretics—for pulmonary congestion and edema.
   b. β-Blockers—to decrease heart rate and cardiac output.
2. Surgical (for severe disease)
   a. Percutaneous balloon valvuloplasty usually produces excellent results.
   b. Open commissurotomy and mitral valve replacement are other options if valvotomy is contraindicated.
3. Management
   a. No therapy is required in asymptomatic patients.
   b. Diuretics can be used if the patient has mild symptoms.
   c. If symptoms are more severe, surgical treatment is recommended.
   d. If AFib develops at any time, treat accordingly (see discussion on AFib).

Aortic Stenosis

A. General characteristics

1. Pathophysiology
   a. Causes obstruction to LV outflow, which results in left ventricular hypertrophy (LVH).
   b. When the aortic valve area falls below 0.7 cm^2, cardiac output fails to increase with exertion, causing angina (but may be normal at rest).
   c. With long-standing AS, the LV dilates, causing progressive LV dysfunction.
   d. With severe AS, LV dilation pulls the mitral valve annulus apart, causing MR.
2. Causes
   a. Calcification of a congenitally abnormal bicuspid aortic valve.
   b. Calcification of tricuspid aortic valve in elderly.
   c. Rheumatic fever.
3. Course
   a. Patients are often asymptomatic for years (until middle or old age) despite severe obstruction.
   b. Development of angina, syncope, or heart failure is a sign of poor prognosis. Survival is similar to that of the normal population before the development

Diseases of the Cardiovascular System

Quick HIT

Altogether, only one-fourth of patients with **symptomatic** AS survive 3 years in the absence of aortic valve replacement (i.e., the 3-year mortality rate is 75% without surgery).

of these three classic symptoms. Without surgical intervention, the survival is poor:
- Angina (35%)—average survival, 3 years
- Syncope (15%)—average survival, 2 years
- Heart failure (50%)—average survival, 1.5 years

B. Clinical features

1. Symptoms
   a. Angina
   b. Syncope—usually exertional
   c. Heart failure symptoms, such as dyspnea on exertion, orthopnea, or PND
2. Signs
   a. Murmur
      - **Harsh crescendo–decrescendo systolic murmur**
      - Heard in second right intercostal space
      - **Radiates to carotid arteries**

   b. **Soft S2. S2 may also be single since the aortic component may be delayed and merge into P2**
   c. S_4
   d. *Parvus et tardus*—diminished and delayed carotid upstrokes
   e. Sustained PMI
   f. Precordial thrill

C. Diagnosis

1. CXR: Calcific aortic valve, enlarged LV/LA (late)
2. ECG: LVH, LA abnormality
   a. Echocardiogram—diagnostic in most cases. Findings include LVH; thickened, immobile aortic valve; and dilated aortic root
3. Cardiac catheterization
   a. Definitive diagnostic test
   b. Can measure valve gradient and calculate valve area (<0.8 cm^2 indicates severe stenosis); normal aortic valve is 3 to 4 cm^2
   c. Useful in symptomatic patients before surgery

Quick HIT

Management of AS is straightforward:
- If asymptomatic: No treatment
- If symptomatic: Surgery (aortic valve replacement)

D. Treatment

1. Medical therapy has a limited role.
2. Surgical therapy: **Aortic valve replacement is the treatment of choice.** It is indicated in all symptomatic patients.

Aortic Regurgitation

A. General characteristics

1. Pathophysiology
   a. Also called aortic insufficiency, this condition is due to inadequate closure of the aortic valve leaflets. Regurgitant blood flow increases left ventricular end diastolic volume.
   b. LV dilation and hypertrophy occur in response in order to maintain stroke volume and prevent diastolic pressure from increasing excessively.
   c. Over time, these compensatory mechanisms fail, leading to increased left-sided and pulmonary pressures.
   d. The resting left ventricular EF is usually normal until advanced disease.
2. Course
   a. For chronic aortic regurgitation, survival is 75% at 5 years.
      - After the development of angina, death usually occurs within 4 years.
      - After the development of heart failure, death usually occurs within 2 years.

   b. For acute aortic regurgitation, mortality is particularly high without surgical repair.

B. Causes

1. Acute
   a. Infective endocarditis
   b. Trauma
   c. Aortic dissection
   d. Iatrogenic as during a failed replacement surgery
2. Chronic
   a. Primary valvular: Rheumatic fever, bicuspid aortic valve, Marfan syndrome, Ehlers–Danlos syndrome, ankylosing spondylitis, SLE
   b. Aortic root disease: Syphilitic aortitis, osteogenesis imperfecta, aortic dissection, Behçet syndrome, Reiter syndrome, systemic HTN

Quick HIT

Other Physical Findings in Aortic Insufficiency
- De Musset sign: Head bobbing (rhythmical jerking of head)
- Müller sign: Uvula bobs
- Duroziez sign: Pistol-shot sound heard over the femoral arteries

C. Clinical features

1. Symptoms
   a. May be symptomatic for many years
   b. Dyspnea on exertion, PND, orthopnea
   c. Palpitations—worse when lying down
   d. Angina
   e. Cyanosis and shock in acute aortic regurgitation (medical emergency)
2. Physical examination
   a. **Widened pulse pressure**—markedly increased systolic BP, with decreased diastolic BP.
   b. Diastolic decrescendo murmur best heard at left sternal border.
   c. *Corrigan pulse* (water-hammer pulse)—rapidly increasing pulse that collapses suddenly as arterial pressure decreases rapidly in late systole and diastole; can be palpated at wrist or femoral arteries.
   d. *Austin Flint murmur*—low-pitched diastolic rumble due to competing flow anterograde from the LA and retrograde from the aorta. It is similar to the murmur appreciated in mitral stenosis.
   e. Displaced PMI (down and to the left) and S_3 may also be present.
   f. Murmur intensity increases with sustained handgrip. Handgrip increases systemic vascular resistance (SVR), which causes an increased "backflow" through the incompetent aortic valve.

D. Diagnosis

1. CXR: LVH, dilated aorta
2. ECG: LVH
3. Echocardiogram—perform serially in chronic, stable patients to assess need for surgery
   a. Assess LV size and function
   b. Look for dilated aortic root and reversal of blood flow in aorta
   c. In acute aortic regurgitation, look for early closure of mitral valve
4. Cardiac catheterization: To assess severity of aortic regurgitation and degree of LV dysfunction

E. Treatment

1. Conservative if stable and asymptomatic: Salt restriction, diuretics, **vasodilators**, digoxin, afterload reduction (i.e., ACE inhibitors or arterial dilators), and restriction on strenuous activity
2. Definitive treatment is surgery (aortic valve replacement). This should be considered in symptomatic patients, or in those with significant LV dysfunction on echocardiogram.
3. Acute AR (e.g., post-MI): **Medical emergency—perform emergent aortic valve replacement!**

Mitral Regurgitation

A. General characteristics

1. Pathophysiology
   a. Acute
      - Abrupt elevation of left atrial pressure in the setting of normal LA size and compliance, causing backflow into pulmonary circulation with resultant pulmonary edema
      - Cardiac output decreases because of decreased forward flow, so hypotension and shock can occur

   b. Chronic
      - Gradual elevation of left atrial pressure in the setting of dilated LA and LV (with increased left atrial compliance)
      - LV dysfunction occurs due to dilation
      - Pulmonary HTN can result from chronic backflow into pulmonary vasculature
2. Causes
   a. Acute
      - Endocarditis (most often *Staphylococcus aureus*)
      - Papillary muscle rupture (from infarction) or dysfunction (from ischemia)
      - Chordae tendineae rupture

   b. Chronic
      - Mitral valve prolapse (MVP)
      - Rheumatic fever
      - Marfan syndrome
      - Cardiomyopathy
3. Prognosis
   a. Acute form is associated with much higher mortality
   b. Survival is related to extent of LV cavity dilation

B. Clinical features

1. Symptoms
   a. Dyspnea on exertion, PND, orthopnea
   b. Palpitations
   c. Pulmonary edema
2. Signs
   a. **Holosystolic murmur** (starts with S_1 and continues on through S_2) **at the apex**, which radiates to the back or clavicular area, depending on which leaflet is involved
   b. AFib is a common finding
   c. Other findings: Diminished S_1, widening of S_2, S_3 gallop; laterally displaced PMI; loud, palpable P_2

C. Diagnosis

1. CXR: Cardiomegaly, dilated LV, pulmonary edema
2. Echocardiogram: MR; dilated LA and LV; decreased LV function

D. Treatment

1. Medical
   a. Afterload reduction with vasodilators is recommended for symptomatic patients only; they are not recommended in most asymptomatic patients as they may mask progression of the disease
   b. Chronic anticoagulation if patient has AFib
   c. IABP as bridge to surgery for acute MR
2. Surgical
   a. Mitral valve repair or replacement
   b. Must be performed before left ventricular function is too severely compromised

Tricuspid Regurgitation

A. General characteristics

1. Tricuspid regurgitation (TR) results from a failure of the tricuspid valve to close completely during systole, causing regurgitation of blood into the RA. It is estimated that up to 70% of normal adults have mild, physiologic TR as seen on high-resolution echocardiography. A much smaller percentage of people are actually symptomatic.
2. Causes—up to 90% of cases occur in people with anatomically normal valve leaflets and chords.
   a. TR is usually secondary to RV dilation. Any cause of RV dilation can result in enlargement of the tricuspid orifice.
      - Left ventricular failure is the most common cause.
      - Right ventricular infarction.
      - Inferior wall MI.
      - Cor pulmonale, secondary to pulmonary HTN.

   b. Tricuspid endocarditis—seen in **IV drug users.**
   c. May be secondary to rheumatic heart disease; usually accompanied by mitral and aortic valve disease.
   d. Epstein anomaly—congenital malformation of tricuspid valve in which there is downward displacement of the valve into the RV.
   e. Other causes include carcinoid syndrome, SLE, and myxomatous valve degeneration.

B. Clinical features

1. **Usually asymptomatic unless the patient develops symptoms of RHF/pulmonary HTN**
2. Signs and symptoms of RVF (ascites, hepatomegaly, edema, JVD)
3. **Pulsatile liver**
4. Prominent V waves in jugular venous pulse with rapid y descent
5. Inspiratory S_3 along LLSB may be present
6. **Blowing holosystolic murmur**
   a. At LLSB
   b. Intensified with inspiration; reduced during expiration or the Valsalva maneuver
7. Right ventricular pulsation along LLSB
8. AFib is usually present

C. Diagnosis

1. Echocardiogram
   a. Quantifies amount of TR
   b. Identifies prolapse/flail of tricuspid valve leaflets
   c. Measures pulmonary pressures
   d. ECG: RV and RA enlargement

D. Treatment

1. Treat any underlying etiology of symptomatic TR
2. Diuretics for volume overload and venous congestion/edema
3. Treat left-sided heart failure, endocarditis, or pulmonary HTN
4. Severe regurgitation may be surgically corrected if pulmonary HTN is not present
   a. Native valve repair surgery
   b. Valvuloplasty of tricuspid ring
   c. Valve replacement surgery: Rarely performed

Mitral Valve Prolapse

A. General characteristics

1. MVP is defined as the presence of excessive or redundant mitral leaflet tissue due to myxomatous degeneration of mitral valve leaflets and/or chordae tendineae.

Quick HIT

Key Signs of MVP
- Systolic clicks
- Midsystolic rumbling murmur that increases with standing and the Valsalva maneuver and decreases with squatting

The redundant leaflet(s) prolapse toward the LA in systole, which results in the auscultated click and murmur.

2. MVP is common in patients with genetic connective tissue disorders, such as Marfan syndrome, osteogenesis imperfecta, and Ehlers–Danlos syndrome.
3. MVP is the most common cause of MR in developed countries.
4. Arrhythmias and sudden death are very rare.

B. Clinical features

1. Symptoms
   a. Most patients are asymptomatic for their entire lives.
   b. Palpitations and atypical chest pain may occur.
   c. **TIAs** due to emboli from mitral valve have been reported, but are very rare.
2. Signs
   a. **Midsystolic or late systolic click(s).**
   b. **Mid-to-late systolic murmur.**
   c. Some patients have midsystolic click without the murmur; others may have the murmur without the click.
   d. Standing and the Valsalva maneuver **increase** murmur and click because these maneuvers reduce LV chamber size, allowing the click and murmur to occur earlier in systole.
   e. Squatting **decreases** murmur and click because it increases LV chamber size, thus delaying the onset of the click and murmur.

C. Diagnosis

1. Echocardiogram is the most useful.
2. Most patients are asymptomatic, so diagnosis is typically made on the basis of the murmur and echocardiogram alone.

D. Treatment

1. If patient is asymptomatic, reassurance. There is some association between MVP and anxiety, so all patients should be reassured about the benign nature of this condition.
2. For chest pain, β-blockers have been useful, but they are unlikely to be required.
3. Surgery is rarely required. The condition is generally benign.

Rheumatic Heart Disease

A. General characteristics

1. Rheumatic heart disease occurs as a complication of streptococcal pharyngitis (group A streptococcus).
2. Acute rheumatic fever is an immunologically mediated systemic process that may progress to rheumatic heart disease.
3. Rheumatic heart disease describes the chronic valvular abnormalities secondary to acute rheumatic fever.
4. The most common valvular abnormality is mitral stenosis, but patients may have aortic or tricuspid involvement as well.
5. The incidence of rheumatic heart disease has fallen drastically in industrialized countries and with widespread antibiotic usage, but remains a significant cause of morbidity and mortality in developing countries.

B. Diagnosis of acute rheumatic fever (requires two major criteria or one major and two minor criteria)

1. Major criteria
   a. Migratory polyarthritis
   b. Erythema marginatum
   c. Cardiac involvement (e.g., pericarditis, CHF, valve disease)
   d. Chorea
   e. Subcutaneous nodules

2. Minor criteria
   a. Fever
   b. Elevated erythrocyte sedimentation rate
   c. Polyarthralgias
   d. Prior history of rheumatic fever
   e. Prolonged PR interval
   f. Evidence of preceding streptococcal infection

C. Treatment

1. Treat streptococcal pharyngitis with penicillin or erythromycin to prevent rheumatic fever.
2. Acute rheumatic fever is treated with NSAIDs. C-reactive protein is used to monitor treatment.
3. Treat the valvular pathology of rheumatic heart disease.

Infective Endocarditis

A. General characteristics

1. Infective endocarditis is defined as an infection of the endocardial surface of the heart (usually involves the cusps of the valves).
2. Classifications (can be classified as acute or subacute).
   a. Acute endocarditis
      - Most commonly caused by *S. aureus* (virulent)
      - Occurs on a normal heart valve
      - If untreated, fatal in less than 6 weeks
   b. Subacute endocarditis
      - Caused by less virulent organisms, such as *Streptococcus viridans* and *Enterococcus*
      - Occurs on damaged heart valves
      - If untreated, takes much longer than 6 weeks to cause death
3. Organisms
   a. Native valve endocarditis
      - *S. viridans* is the most common organism in native valve endocarditis.
      - Other common organisms include *Staphylococcus* species (*S. aureus* more commonly than *S. epidermidis*) and *Enterococci.*
      - **HACEK** group of organisms: *Haemophilus, Actinobacillus, Cardiobacterium, Eikenella,* and *Kingella.*
   b. Prosthetic valve endocarditis
      - Staphylococci are the most common causes of early-onset endocarditis; symptoms appear within 60 days of surgery (*S. epidermidis* more commonly than *S. aureus*).
      - Streptococci are the most common cause of late-onset endocarditis; symptoms appear 60 days after surgery.
   c. Endocarditis in IV drug users
      - Frequently presents with right-sided endocarditis.
      - *S. aureus* is the most common cause.
      - Other organisms include *Enterococci* and *Streptococci.* Fungi (mostly *Candida*) and gram-negative rods (mostly *Pseudomonas*) are less common causes.
4. Complications
   a. Cardiac failure
   b. Myocardial abscess
   c. Various solid organ damage from showered emboli
   d. Glomerulonephritis

B. Diagnosis

1. Duke clinical criteria (Table 1-2): Two major criteria, one major and three minor criteria, or five minor criteria are required to diagnose infective endocarditis.

Quick HIT

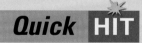

Always suspect endocarditis in a patient with a new heart murmur and unexplained fever or bacteremia.

Quick HIT

TEE is better than transthoracic echocardiography in the diagnosis of endocarditis.

Quick HIT

Infective endocarditis is almost always fatal if left untreated.

TABLE 1-2 Duke Criteria

Major	Minor
• **Sustained bacteremia** by an organism known to cause endocarditis • **Endocardial involvement** documented by either echocardiogram (vegetation, abscess, valve perforation, prosthetic dehiscence) or clearly established **new valvular regurgitation**	• **Predisposing condition** (abnormal valve or abnormal risk of bacteremia) • **Fever** • **Vascular phenomena:** septic arterial or pulmonary emboli, mycotic aneurysms, intracranial hemorrhage, Janeway lesions[a] • **Immune phenomena:** Glomerulonephritis, Osler nodes,[b] Roth spots,[c] rheumatoid factor • **Positive blood cultures** not meeting major criteria • **Positive echocardiogram** not meeting major criteria

From Durack DT, Lukes AS, Bright DK. New criteria for diagnosis of infective endocarditis: utilization of specific echocardiographic findings. Duke Endocarditis Service. *Am J. Med.* 1994;96:200.

Note: Definitive (i.e., highly probable) diagnosis if two major, or one major plus three minor, or five minor criteria are present.

[a]Janeway lesions are painless erythematous lesions on palms and soles.

[b]Osler nodes are painful, raised lesions of fingers, toes, or feet.

[c]Roth spots are oval, retinal hemorrhages with a clear, pale center.

C. Treatment

1. Parenteral antibiotics based on culture results for extended periods (4 to 6 weeks).
2. If cultures are negative but there is high clinical suspicion, treat empirically with a penicillin (or vancomycin) plus an aminoglycoside until the organism can be isolated.

D. Prophylaxis

Scope of patients who qualify for prophylaxis is much narrower than in the past. Must have both a qualifying cardiac indication **AND** procedure to warrant antibiotic prophylaxis.

1. Qualifying cardiac indications
   a. Prosthetic heart valves
   b. History of infective endocarditis
   c. Congenital heart disease
      - Unrepaired cyanotic congenital heart disease
      - Repaired congenital heart disease, with prosthetic material, during first 6 months after procedure
   d. Cardiac transplant with valvulopathy
2. Qualifying procedures
   a. Dental procedures involving manipulation of gingival mucosa or periapical region of teeth (extractions, implants, periodontal surgery, cleaning when bleeding expected)
   b. Procedures involving biopsy or incision of respiratory mucosa
   c. Procedures involving infected skin or musculoskeletal tissue

Quick HIT

Do NOT give antibiotics for endocarditis prophylaxis for:
- Native mitral valve prolapse/stenosis
- Routine GI (colonoscopy/EGD) or GU (cystoscopy) procedures

Nonbacterial Thrombotic Endocarditis (Marantic Endocarditis)

- Associated with debilitating illnesses such as metastatic cancer (found in up to 20% of cancer patients).
- Sterile deposits of fibrin and platelets form along the closure line of cardiac valve leaflets.
- Vegetations can embolize to the brain or periphery.
- Although the use of heparin may be appropriate, no studies have confirmed its efficacy.

Nonbacterial Verrucous Endocarditis (Libman–Sacks Endocarditis)

- Typically involves the aortic valves in individuals with SLE
- Characterized by the formation of small warty vegetations on **both sides** of valve leaflets and may present with regurgitant murmurs

- Rarely gives rise to infective endocarditis, but can be a source of systematic embolization
- Treat underlying SLE and anticoagulate

Congenital Heart Diseases

Atrial Septal Defect

A. General characteristics (types)

1. Ostium secundum (most common—80% of cases)—occurs in central portion of interatrial septum
2. Ostium primum—occurs low in the septum
3. Sinus venosus defects—occurs high in the septum

B. Pathophysiology

1. Oxygenated blood from the LA passes into the RA, increasing right heart output and thus pulmonary blood flow.
2. Leads to increased work of the right side of heart: As shunt size increases, RA and RV dilation occurs with pulmonary-to-systemic flow ratios greater than 1.5:1.0.
3. Pulmonary HTN is a serious sequela, but is rare in ASD.

C. Clinical course

1. Patients are usually asymptomatic until middle age (around 40).
2. Thereafter, symptoms may begin and include exercise intolerance, dyspnea on exertion, and fatigue.
3. If mild, patients can live a normal lifespan.

D. Clinical features

1. Mild systolic ejection murmur at pulmonary area secondary to increased pulmonary blood flow
2. **Fixed split S_2**
3. Diastolic flow "rumble" murmur across tricuspid valve area secondary to increased blood flow
4. In advanced disease, signs of RVF may be seen

E. Diagnosis

1. TEE is diagnostic (better than transthoracic echocardiogram). Contrast echocardiography can improve resolution. A so-called "bubble study" is a type of contrast echo which involves injecting microbubbles and watching them cross the defect via a right-to-left shunt. This is often used to aid in diagnosis of ASDs.
2. CXR: Large pulmonary arteries; increased pulmonary markings (`).
3. ECG: Right bundle branch block and right axis deviation; atrial abnormalities can also be seen (e.g., fibrillation, flutter).

F. Complications

1. Pulmonary HTN—does not occur before 20 years of age, but is a common finding in patients over 40
2. **Eisenmenger disease** is a late complication seen in a minority of patients, in which irreversible pulmonary HTN leads to reversal of shunt, heart failure, and cyanosis
3. Right heart failure
4. Atrial arrhythmias, especially AFib
5. Stroke can result from paradoxical emboli or AFib

G. Treatment

1. Unless they are very large, most defects do not require closure.
2. Surgical repair when pulmonary-to-systemic blood flow ratio is greater than 1.5:1 or 2:1 or if patient is symptomatic.

Quick HIT

Congenital heart disease accounts for only 2% of heart disease in adults.

Ventricular Septal Defect

A. General characteristics

1. Ventricular septal defect is the most common congenital cardiac malformation.
2. Pathophysiology
   a. Blood flows from the LV (high pressure) into the RV (low pressure) through a hole, resulting in increased pulmonary blood flow. As long as the pulmonary vascular resistance (PVR) is lower than the SVR, the shunt is left to right. If the PVR increases above the SVR, the shunt reverses.
   b. Large defects eventually lead to pulmonary HTN, whereas small defects do not change pulmonary vascular hemodynamics.

B. Clinical features

1. Symptoms
   a. A small shunt produces no symptoms. Many of these close spontaneously.
   b. A large shunt without elevated PVR (and thus left-to-right shunt) gives rise to CHF, growth failure, and recurrent lower respiratory infections.
   c. A large shunt with very high PVR (Eisenmenger reaction) gives rise to SOB, dyspnea on exertion, chest pain, syncope, and cyanosis.
2. Signs
   a. Harsh, blowing holosystolic murmur with thrill
      - At fourth left intercostal space
      - Murmur decreases with Valsalva and handgrip
      - The smaller the defect, the louder the holosystolic murmur
   b. Sternal lift (RV enlargement)
   c. As PVR increases, the pulmonary component of S_2 increases in intensity
   d. Aortic regurgitation may be seen in some patients

C. Diagnosis

1. ECG: Biventricular hypertrophy predominates when PVR is high.
2. CXR
   a. Enlargement of the pulmonary artery.
   b. Enlargement of cardiac silhouette: As PVR increases (and left-to-right shunt decreases), heart size decreases, but pulmonary artery size increases.
3. Echocardiogram shows the septal defect.

D. Complications

1. Endocarditis
2. Progressive aortic regurgitation
3. Heart failure
4. Pulmonary HTN and shunt reversal (Eisenmenger)

E. Treatment

1. Endocarditis prophylaxis is important but is NOT currently recommended for patients with uncomplicated VSD and no history of endocarditis.
2. Surgical repair is indicated if the pulmonary flow to systemic flow ratio is greater than 1.5:1 or 2:1, as well as for patients with infective endocarditis.
3. For the asymptomatic patient with a small defect, surgery is not indicated.

Quick HIT

In women, coarctation of the aorta may be associated with Turner syndrome.

Coarctation of the Aorta

A. General characteristics

1. Narrowing/constriction of aorta, usually at origin of left subclavian artery near ligamentum arteriosum, which leads to obstruction between the proximal and distal aorta, and thus to increased left ventricular afterload.

B. Clinical features

1. HTN in upper extremities with hypotension in lower extremities
2. Well-developed upper body with underdeveloped lower half

3. Midsystolic murmur heard best over the back
4. Symptoms include headache, cold extremities, claudication with exercise, and leg fatigue
5. Delayed femoral pulses when compared to radial pulses
6. Prevalence of coarctation of the aorta is increased in patients with Turner syndrome

C. Diagnosis

1. ECG shows LVH
2. CXR
   a. Notching of the ribs
   b. "Figure 3" appearance due to indentation of the aorta at site of coarctation, with dilation before and after the stenosis

D. Complications

1. Severe HTN
2. Rupture of cerebral aneurysms
3. Infective endocarditis
4. Aortic dissection

E. Treatment

1. Standard treatment involves surgical decompression.
2. Percutaneous balloon aortoplasty is also an option in selected cases.

Patent Ductus Arteriosus

A. General characteristics

1. Communication between aorta and pulmonary artery that persists after birth.
2. During fetal life, prostaglandins and low oxygen tension maintain the ductus arteriosus. Blood is shunted away from nonfunctioning lungs; normally closes within days after birth.
3. Becomes a left-to-right shunt in life outside the womb if it remains patent (blood flows from aorta into pulmonary artery).
4. Associated with congenital rubella syndrome, high altitude, and premature births.
5. Pathophysiology
   a. Large left-to-right shunting results in volume overload, pulmonary HTN, and right-sided heart failure.
   b. Cyanosis occurs late.
   c. May eventually see reversal of blood flow.

B. Clinical features

1. May be asymptomatic
2. Signs of heart failure
3. Loud P_2 (sign of pulmonary HTN)
4. LVH: Secondary to left-to-right shunt
5. Right ventricular hypertrophy: Secondary to pulmonary HTN
6. **Continuous "machinery murmur" at left second intercostal space (both systolic and diastolic components)**
7. Wide pulse pressure and bounding peripheral pulses
8. Lower-extremity clubbing: Toes more likely than fingers to be cyanotic (differential cyanosis)

C. Diagnosis

1. CXR
   a. Increased pulmonary vascular markings
   b. Dilated pulmonary artery
   c. Enlarged cardiac silhouette
   d. Sometimes calcifications of ductus arteriosus
2. Echocardiography reveals the patent ductus and/or turbulent blood flow

Quick HIT

The leading causes of death in adults with PDA are heart failure and infective endocarditis.

Quick HIT

Adults with PDA usually have normal pulmonary pressures.

D. Treatment

1. If pulmonary vascular disease is absent: Surgical ligation.
2. If **severe pulmonary HTN or right-to-left shunt** is present, do *not* correct patent ductus arteriosus (PDA). **Surgery is contraindicated.**
3. Indomethacin indicated for closure. Prostaglandin E_1 can be used to keep the PDA open (may be needed in the face of other cardiac abnormalities such as transposition of the great vessels).

Tetralogy of Fallot

A. General characteristics

1. Characterized by a triad of cardiac abnormalities: Ventricular septal defect, right ventricular hypertrophy, pulmonary artery stenosis, and overriding aorta.
2. The exact embryologic variant is unknown, but the four abnormalities likely arise secondary to defects in the development of the infundibular septum.
3. Tetralogy of Fallot (TOF) typically occurs sporadically, but may also be part of a syndrome.

B. Clinical features

1. Cyanosis is the most common symptom.
2. Degree of clinical symptoms depends largely on the degree of right ventricular outflow obstruction.
3. Patients experience Tet spells—they will squat after exertion such as exercise or crying spell in an infant. This maneuver increases SVR, which helps shunt blood from the RV to the lungs instead of the aorta. Oxygen, morphine, and β-blockers may also be needed if the patient continues to be cyanotic.
4. Murmur is typically crescendo–decrescendo in nature and heard best at the left upper sternal border.

C. Diagnosis

1. Echocardiography is the diagnostic modality of choice. This test can clearly define the four abnormalities as well as provide important information about aortic arch anatomy.
2. EKG may show enlarged RA and RV.
3. Chest x-ray classically shows **boot-shaped heart.**
4. Cardiac catheterization may be required in some patients to fully define the anatomy.

D. Treatment

1. Treatment is surgical. Most patients have surgery within the first year of life. Twenty-year survival rates after surgery are above 80%. The most common causes of death are sudden cardiac death and heart failure.
2. Complications after surgery include arrhythmias, pulmonary regurgitation, residual outflow obstruction, and heart failure.

Diseases of the Vasculature

Hypertensive Emergency

A. General characteristics

1. Hypertensive emergency: Systolic BP >220 and/or diastolic BP >120 **in addition to end-organ damage—immediate treatment is indicated** (see Clinical Pearl 1-13).
2. Elevated BP levels alone without end-organ damage—referred to as *hypertensive urgency.* Hypertensive urgencies rarely require emergency therapy and can be managed with attempts to lower BP over a period of 24 hours.
3. Whenever a patient presents with markedly elevated BP, it is critical to assess the following systems for end-organ damage.
   a. Eyes: Papilledema
   b. CNS
      - Altered mental status or intracranial hemorrhage

CLINICAL PEARL 1-13

If a patient presents with severe headache and markedly elevated BP:
- The first step is to lower the BP with an antihypertensive agent.
- The second step is to order a CT scan of the head to rule out intracranial bleeding (subarachnoid hemorrhage is in the differential diagnosis for severe headache).
- If the CT scan is negative, one may proceed to a lumbar puncture.

- Hypertensive encephalopathy may develop (suspect when BP is markedly elevated: 240/140 or higher, along with neurologic findings such as confusion)

c. Kidneys: Renal failure or hematuria
d. Heart: USA, MI, CHF with pulmonary edema, aortic dissection
e. Lungs: Pulmonary edema

4. Hypertensive emergency may lead to posterior reversible encephalopathy syndrome (PRES)—a radiographic condition which is postulated to be caused by autoregulatory failure of cerebral vessels as well as endothelial dysfunction.
   a. Despite the name, the syndrome may not always be reversible and can affect regions other than the posterior region of the brain.
   b. Symptoms include insidious onset of headache, altered level of consciousness, visual changes, and seizures. The classic radiographic finding is posterior cerebral white matter edema.
   c. Most patients are hypertensive, but may be normotensive. Elevated blood pressures overwhelm the autoregulatory mechanisms of the cerebral vessels, leading to arteriolar dilation and extravasation of fluid into the brain.
   d. Diagnose with clinical findings and brain MRI. First treatment step is to lower BP, usually with IV medications. Other treatment steps include correcting electrolyte abnormalities and stopping seizures if they occur.

B. Causes

1. Noncompliance with antihypertensive therapy
2. Cushing syndrome
3. Drugs such as cocaine, LSD, methamphetamines
4. Hyperaldosteronism
5. Eclampsia
6. Vasculitis
7. Alcohol withdrawal
8. Pheochromocytoma
9. Noncompliance with dialysis
10. Renal artery stenosis (atherosclerosis or fibromuscular dysplasia)
11. Polycystic kidney disease

Quick HIT

Lower BP with short acting agents such as hydralazine.

C. Clinical features

1. Severe headache
2. Visual disturbances
3. Altered mentation

D. Treatment

1. Hypertensive emergencies
   a. Reduce mean arterial pressure by 25% in 1 to 2 hours. The goal is not to immediately achieve normal BP, but to get the patient out of danger, then reduce BP gradually.
   b. If severe (diastolic pressure >130) or if hypertensive encephalopathy is present, **IV agents** such as hydralazine, esmolol, nitroprusside, labetalol, or nitroglycerin are appropriate.
   c. In patients who are in less immediate danger, oral agents are appropriate. Options include captopril, clonidine, labetalol, nifedipine, and diazoxide.
2. Hypertensive urgencies: BP should be lowered within 24 hours using **oral agents.**

Quick HIT

Hypertensive emergency—evidence of end-organ damage; use IV medications
Hypertensive urgency—no evidence of end-organ damage; use PO medications

Diseases of the Cardiovascular System

Aortic Dissection

A. General characteristics

1. Predisposing factors
   a. Long-standing systemic HTN (present in 70% of patients)
   b. Cocaine use (may be remote)
   c. Trauma
   d. Connective tissue diseases, such as Marfan and Ehlers–Danlos syndrome
   e. Bicuspid aortic valve
   f. Coarctation of the aorta
   g. Third trimester of pregnancy
2. Daily (Stanford) classification (Figure 1-17)
   a. **Type A (proximal)** involves the ascending aorta (includes retrograde extension from descending aorta).
   b. **Type B (distal)** is limited to the descending aorta (distal to the take-off of the subclavian artery).

Quick HIT

Aortic dissection
- Type A = ascending; treatment is surgical
- Type B = descending; treatment is medical

Quick HIT

The diagnosis of aortic dissection is very difficult to make because the classic clinical findings often are not apparent. The use of thrombolytic therapy in patients with aortic dissection who have been incorrectly diagnosed as having an acute MI can have fatal consequences.

B. Clinical features

1. Severe, tearing/ripping/stabbing pain, typically abrupt in onset, either in the anterior or back of the chest (often the interscapular region)
   a. Anterior chest pain is more common with proximal dissection (type A).
   b. Interscapular back pain is more common with distal dissection (type B).
2. Diaphoresis
3. Most are hypertensive, but some may be hypotensive
4. Pulse or BP asymmetry between limbs
5. Aortic regurgitation (especially proximal dissections)
6. Neurologic manifestations (hemiplegia, hemianesthesia) due to obstruction of carotid artery

C. Diagnosis

1. CXR shows **widened mediastinum** (>8 mm on AP view).
2. TEE has a very high sensitivity and specificity; it is noninvasive and can be performed at the bedside.

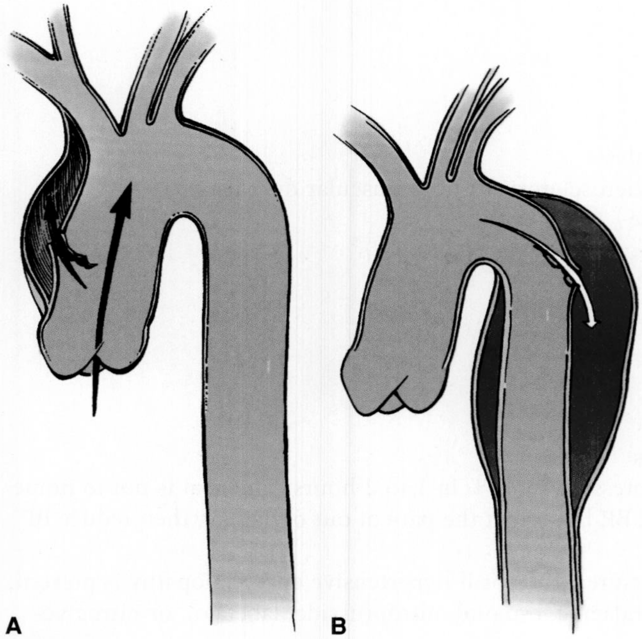

FIGURE 1-17 **Aortic dissection. A: Dissection of ascending aorta. B: Dissection of descending aorta.**
(Modified from Harwood-Nuss A, Wolfson AB, Linden CH, et al. *The Clinical Practice of Emergency Medicine.* 3rd ed. Philadelphia, PA: Lippincott Williams & Wilkins, 2000:212, Figure 51.1.)

3. CT scan and MRI are both highly accurate (MRI more so); MRI takes longer to perform, making it less ideal in the acute setting.
4. Aortic angiography is invasive, but it is the best test for determining the extent of the dissection for surgery.

Quick HIT

TEE and CT scan are the preferred tests in the diagnosis of acute aortic dissection. TEE is very accurate and is ideal in the unstable patient because it can be performed at the bedside.

D. Treatment

1. Initiate medical therapy **immediately**
   a. IV β-blockers to lower heart rate and diminish the force of left ventricular ejection
   b. IV sodium nitroprusside to lower systolic BP below 120 mm Hg
2. For type A dissections—surgical management
   a. Most cases of type A dissections should be treated as surgical emergencies to prevent complications such as MI, aortic regurgitation, or cardiac tamponade
   b. Open surgery is still the standard of care
3. For type B dissections—medical management
   a. Lower blood pressure as quickly as possible. First-line drugs include IV β-blockers such as labetalol, esmolol, or propranolol
   b. Pain control with morphine or dilaudid
   c. Unrelenting symptoms may require surgical treatment—both open and endovascular surgical options exist

Abdominal Aortic Aneurysm

A. General characteristics

1. Abdominal aortic aneurysm (AAA) is an abnormal localized dilation of the aorta. Most AAAs occur between the renal arteries and iliac bifurcation.
2. The incidence increases with age. AAAs are rare before the age of 50. The average age at time of diagnosis is 65 to 70 years.
3. AAAs are much more common in men, though more likely to rupture in women at a given size.

B. Causes

1. Multifactorial—in most cases, there is atherosclerotic weakening of the aortic wall.
2. Other predisposing factors include trauma, HTN, vasculitis, smoking, and positive family history.
3. Syphilis and connective tissue abnormalities (e.g., Marfan disease) are associated with thoracic aneurysms, but they may involve the lower aorta as well.

C. Clinical features

1. Usually asymptomatic and discovered on either abdominal examination or a radiologic study done for another reason
2. Sense of "fullness"
3. Pain may or may not be present—if present, located in the hypogastrium and lower back and usually throbbing in character.
4. Pulsatile mass on abdominal examination
5. Symptoms suggesting expansion and impending rupture include the following:
   a. Sudden onset of severe pain in the back or lower abdomen, radiating to the groin, buttocks, or legs
   b. *Grey Turner sign* (ecchymoses on back and flanks) and *Cullen sign* (ecchymoses around umbilicus)
6. Rupture of an AAA
   a. **The triad of abdominal pain, hypotension, and a palpable pulsatile abdominal mass indicates a ruptured AAA and emergent laparotomy is indicated.** No further diagnostic testing is needed with this constellation of symptoms; however, patients may present with only one or two components of this triad
   b. Cardiovascular collapse
   c. Syncope or near-syncope, secondary to sudden hemorrhage
   d. Nausea and vomiting

D. Diagnosis

1. Ultrasound
   a. Test of choice to evaluate both the location and size of the aneurysm
   b. 100% sensitive in detecting AAAs
2. CT scan
   a. 100% sensitive in detecting AAAs
   b. Takes longer to perform than plain radiographs or ultrasound; should only be used in hemodynamically stable patients
   c. CT is the scan of choice for preoperative planning

E. Treatment

1. Unruptured aneurysms.
   a. Management largely depends on size of aneurysm.
      - **Data from the ADAM and UK-SAT trails have shown that if the aneurysm is >5 cm in diameter or symptomatic, surgical resection with synthetic graft placement is recommended. (The infrarenal aorta is replaced with a fabric tube.) This can often be done endovascularly by accessing the femoral artery.** The diameter of the normal adult infrarenal aorta is about 2 cm.
      - The management of asymptomatic aneurysms <5 cm is controversial. Periodic imaging is recommended to follow up growth. No "safe" size exists, however, and small AAAs **can** rupture.
   b. Other factors to consider are the patient's life expectancy (patient may be more likely to die of other medical illnesses), and the risk of surgery.
2. Ruptured AAAs: Emergency surgical repair is indicated. All of these patients are unstable.
   a. While open repair remains the gold standard, some ruptured AAAs may be repaired endovascularly as well.

Quick HIT

Leriche syndrome: Atheromatous occlusion of distal aorta just above bifurcation causing bilateral claudication, impotence, and absent/diminished femoral pulses.

Peripheral Vascular Disease (Chronic Arterial Insufficiency)

A. General characteristics

1. Peripheral vascular disease (PVD) is an occlusive atherosclerotic disease of the lower extremities (see also Clinical Pearl 1-14)
2. Patients with PVD usually have coexisting CAD (with CHF, history of MI, and so on) and other chronic medical problems (e.g., diabetes, lung disease)
3. Sites of occlusion/stenosis
   a. Superficial femoral artery (in Hunter canal) is the most common site
   b. Popliteal artery
   c. Aortoiliac occlusive disease
4. Risk factors
   a. Smoking is by far the most important risk factor
   b. CAD, hyperlipidemia, HTN
   c. Diabetes—prevalence is markedly increased in these patients
5. Prognosis
   a. If the patient has intermittent claudication, the prognosis is generally good
   b. Patients with rest pain or ischemic ulcers have the worst prognosis (especially in diabetics or smokers)

CLINICAL PEARL 1-14

Evaluation of a Patient with PVD

- Evaluate the cardiovascular system (HTN, carotid bruits, murmurs, AAA).
- Assess arterial pulses.
- Inspect lower extremities for color change, ulcers, muscle atrophy, hair loss, thickened toenails, etc.
- Consider the following tests: ECG, CBC, renal function tests, and coagulation profile (factor V Leiden, antithrombin III, proteins C and S).

B. Clinical features

1. Symptoms (see also Clinical Pearl 1-14)
   a. Intermittent claudication
      - Cramping leg pain that is reliably reproduced by same walking distance (distance is very constant and reproducible)
      - Pain is completely relieved by rest
   b. Rest pain (continuous)
      - Usually felt over the distal metatarsals, where the arteries are the smallest
      - **Often prominent at night**—awakens patient from sleep
      - Hanging the foot over side of bed or standing relieves pain—extra perfusion to ischemic areas due to gravity
      - Rest pain is always worrisome—suggests severe ischemia such that frank gangrene of involved limb may occur in the absence of intervention
2. Signs
   a. Diminished or absent pulses, muscular atrophy, decreased hair growth, thick toenails, and decreased skin temperature
   b. Ischemic ulceration (usually on the toes)
      - Localized skin necrosis
      - Secondary to local trauma that does not heal (due to ischemic limb)
      - Tissue infarction/gangrene in end-stage disease
   c. Pallor of elevation and rubor of dependency (in advanced disease)

Quick HIT

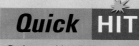

- Femoral or popliteal disease causes calf claudication.
- Aortoiliac occlusive disease causes buttock and hip claudication (in addition to the calves).

C. Diagnosis

1. Ankle-to-brachial index (ABI): Ratio of the systolic BP at the ankle to the systolic BP at the arm
   a. Normal ABI is between 0.9 and 1.3
   b. ABI >1.3 is due to noncompressible vessels and indicates severe disease
   c. Claudication ABI <0.7
   d. Rest pain ABI <0.4
2. Pulse volume recordings
   a. Excellent assessment of segmental limb perfusion
   b. Pulse wave forms represent the volume of blood per heart beat at sequential sites down the leg
   c. A large wave form indicates good collateral blood flow
   d. Noninvasive using pressure cuffs
3. Arteriography (contrast in vessels and radiographs)
   a. Gold standard for diagnosing and locating PVD

Quick HIT

Patients with calcified arteries (especially those with DM) have false ABI readings (vessels are not compressible).

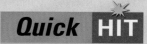

D. Treatment

1. Conservative management for intermittent claudication.
   a. **Stop smoking (the importance of this cannot be overemphasized).** Smoking is linked to progression of atherosclerosis and causes vasoconstriction (further decreasing blood flow).
   b. Graduated exercise program: Walk to point of claudication, rest, and then continue walking for another cycle.
   c. Foot care (especially important in diabetic patients).
   d. Atherosclerotic risk factor reduction (control of hyperlipidemia, HTN, weight, diabetes, and so on).
   e. Avoid extremes of temperature (especially extreme cold).
   f. Aspirin along with ticlopidine/clopidogrel have shown slight improvements in symptom relief. They are often used in these patients for stroke/MI prevention.
   g. Cilostazol is a PDE inhibitor which acts both by suppressing platelet aggregation and by directly dilating arterioles.
2. Surgical treatment
   a. Indications: Rest pain, ischemic ulcerations (tissue necrosis), severe symptoms refractory to conservative treatment that affects quality of life or work.

Quick HIT

Diabetic patients have an amputation rate four times greater than that of nondiabetic patients.

b. Options
- Angioplasty—balloon dilation with or without stenting. Given the minimal risks and good chance of symptomatic relief for patients, this may be performed one or more times before a bypass is done.
- Surgical bypass grafting—has a 5-year patency rate of 70% (immediate success rate is 80% to 90%).

Acute Arterial Occlusion

A. General characteristics

1. Acute occlusion of an artery, usually caused by embolization. The common femoral artery is the most common site of occlusion. Less commonly, in situ thrombosis is the cause.
2. Sources of emboli
   a. Heart (85%)
   - AFib is the most common cause of embolus from the heart
   - Post-MI
   - Endocarditis
   - Myxoma

   b. Aneurysms

   c. Atheromatous plaque

B. Clinical features (remember the six Ps)

1. Pain—acute onset. The patient can tell you precisely when and where it happened. The pain is very severe, and the patient may have to sit down or may fall to the ground (Table 1-3)
2. Pallor
3. Polar (cold)
4. Paralysis
5. Paresthesias
6. Pulselessness (use Doppler to assess pulses)

C. Diagnosis

1. Arteriogram to define site of occlusion
2. ECG to look for MI, AFib
3. Echocardiogram for evaluation of cardiac source of emboli—valves, thrombus, shunts

D. Treatment

1. Main goal: Assess viability of tissues to salvage the limb.
2. Skeletal muscle can tolerate 6 hours of ischemia; perfusion should be reestablished within this time frame.
3. Immediately anticoagulate with IV heparin.
4. Emergent surgical embolectomy is indicated via cutdown and Fogarty balloon. Bypass is reserved for embolectomy failure.
5. Thrombolytics can also be infused intra-arterially. Double blind trials comparing intra-arterial thrombolytics such as recombinant urokinase to surgery showed mixed results.
6. Treat any complications such as compartment syndrome that may occur.

Quick HIT

The Fogarty balloon catheter is used for embolectomy—the catheter is inserted, the balloon is inflated, and the catheter is pulled out—the balloon brings the embolus with it.

TABLE 1-3 Pvd Versus Acute Arterial Occlusion

	Clinical Features	Diagnosis	Treatment
Peripheral vascular disease	Intermittent claudication, rest pain, decreased pulses, ischemic ulcers	Arteriogram	Intermittent claudication—conservative treatment Rest pain—surgery
Acute arterial occlusion	Six Ps—pallor, pain, pulselessness, paresthesias, paralysis, polar (cold)	Arteriogram	Anticoagulation, emergent surgery

Cholesterol Embolization Syndrome

- This syndrome is due to "showers" of cholesterol crystals originating from a proximal source (e.g., atherosclerotic plaque), most commonly the abdominal aorta, iliacs, and femoral arteries.
- It is often triggered by a surgical or radiographic intervention (e.g., arteriogram), or by thrombolytic therapy.
- It presents with small, discrete areas of tissue ischemia, resulting in blue/black toes, renal insufficiency, and/or abdominal pain or bleeding (the latter is due to intestinal hypoperfusion).
- Treatment is supportive. Do **not** anticoagulate. Control BP. Amputation or surgical resection is only needed in extreme cases.

Mycotic Aneurysm

- An aneurysm resulting from damage to the aortic wall secondary to **infection**
- Blood cultures are positive in most cases
- Treatment: IV antibiotics and surgical excision

Luetic Heart

- Luetic heart is a complication of **syphilitic aortitis**, usually affecting men in their fourth to fifth decade of life. Aneurysm of the aortic arch with retrograde extension extends backward to cause aortic regurgitation and stenosis of aortic branches, most commonly the coronary arteries.
- Treatment: IV penicillin and surgical repair.

Deep Venous Thrombosis

A. General characteristics

1. Cause: *Virchow triad* (endothelial injury, venous stasis, hypercoagulability) gives rise to venous thrombosis (see also Table 1-4)
2. Risk factors
   a. Age >60
   b. Malignancy
   c. Prior history of deep venous thrombosis (DVT), PE, or varicose veins
   d. Hereditary hypercoagulable states (factor V Leiden, protein C and S deficiency, antithrombin III deficiency)
   e. Prolonged immobilization or bed rest
   f. Cardiac disease, especially CHF
   g. Obesity
   h. Major surgery, especially surgery of the pelvis (orthopedic procedures)
   i. Major trauma
   j. Pregnancy, oral contraceptives/estrogen use

Quick HIT

If a superficial venous system is patent, the classic findings of DVT (erythema, pain, cords) will not occur because blood drains from these patent veins. This is why only half of all patients with DVT have the classic findings.

TABLE 1-4 Diseases of the Venous System

Disease	Clinical Features	Diagnosis	Treatment
Superficial thrombophlebitis	Local tenderness, erythema along course of a superficial vein	Clinical diagnosis	Analgesics, monitor for spread or cellulitis
Chronic venous insufficiency	Aching of lower extremities, worse at end of day; relieved by elevation of legs and worsened by recumbency; edema, pigmentation, ulcers	Clinical diagnosis	Leg elevation, avoid long periods of standing, elastic stockings; if ulcers develop, Unna boots, wet-to-dry dressings
Deep venous thrombosis	Usually asymptomatic; calf pain may be present	Duplex, d-dimer	Anticoagulation

Quick HIT

Only 50% of patients with the classic DVT findings have a DVT, and only 50% of patients with documented DVT have the classic findings.

B. Clinical features

1. Clinical presentation may be subtle
2. Classic findings (all have very low sensitivity and specificity):
   a. Lower-extremity pain and swelling (worse with dependency/walking, better with elevation/rest)
   b. *Homans sign* (calf pain on ankle dorsiflexion)
   c. Palpable cord
   d. Fever

C. Diagnosis

1. Available studies
   a. Doppler analysis and Duplex ultrasound
      - Initial test for DVT; noninvasive, but highly operator dependent
      - High sensitivity and specificity for detecting proximal thrombi (popliteal and femoral), not so for distal (calf vein) thrombi
   b. Venography
      - Most accurate test for diagnosis of DVT of calf veins
      - Invasive and infrequently used
      - Allows visualization of the deep and superficial venous systems, and allows assessment of patency and valvular competence
   c. Impedance plethysmography
      - A noninvasive alternative to Doppler ultrasound
      - Blood conducts electricity better than soft tissue, so electrical impedance decreases as blood volume increases
      - High sensitivity for proximal DVT, but not for distal DVT (calf veins)
      - Poor specificity because there is a high rate of false positives
      - As accurate as Doppler, but less operator dependent
   d. d-dimer testing
      - Has a very high sensitivity (95%), but low specificity (50%); can be used to rule out DVT when combined with Doppler and clinical suspicion
2. Interpretation of diagnostic tests
   a. Intermediate-to-high pretest probability of DVT
      - If Doppler ultrasound is positive, begin anticoagulation
      - If Doppler ultrasound is nondiagnostic, repeat ultrasound every 2 to 3 days for up to 2 weeks
   b. Low-to-intermediate probability of DVT
      - If Doppler ultrasound is negative, there is no need for anticoagulation; observation is sufficient
      - Repeat ultrasound in 2 days

D. Complications

1. Pulmonary embolus (PE) can originate from the iliofemoral, pelvic, calf, ovarian, axillary, subclavian, and internal jugular veins, as well as the inferior vena cava and cavernous sinuses of the skull—see Chapter 3 for discussion on PE
2. Postthrombotic syndrome (chronic venous insufficiency [CVC])
   a. Occurs in approximately half of all patients with acute DVT
   b. Residual venous obstruction and valvular incompetence lead to ambulatory HTN (see section on chronic venous insufficiency)
3. *Phlegmasia cerulea dolens(painful, blue, swollen leg)*
   a. Occurs in extreme cases of DVT—indicates that major venous obstruction has occurred
   b. Severe leg edema compromises arterial supply to the limb, resulting in impaired sensory and motor function
   c. Venous thrombectomy is indicated

E. Treatment

1. Anticoagulation
   a. Prevents further propagation of the thrombus

b. Heparin bolus followed by a constant infusion and titrated to maintain the PTT at 1.5 to 2 times aPTT
c. Start warfarin once the aPTT is therapeutic and continue for 3 to 6 months. Anticoagulate to INR at 2 to 3
d. Continue heparin until the INR has been therapeutic for 48 hours

2. Thrombolytic therapy (streptokinase, urokinase, tissue plasminogen activator [t-PA])
   a. Speeds up the resolution of clots
   b. Indicated mainly for patients with massive PE who are hemodynamically unstable (hypotension with SBP <90 mm Hg), and with no contraindications for thrombolytics
3. Inferior vena cava filter placement (Greenfield filter)
   a. Indications for treatment of VTE
      - If absolute contraindication to anticoagulation (bleeding)
      - If failure of appropriate anticoagulation
   b. Effective only in preventing PE, not DVT
4. Methods of prophylaxis after surgery
   a. Mechanical
      - Leg elevation, graduated compression stockings, early ambulation
      - Pneumatic compression boots—intermittently inflate and deflate, causing compression of the limb, usually the calves; very effective
      - IVC filter for patients at high risk for DVT/PE who have an absolute contraindication to other forms of prophylaxis; for example, after trauma or spinal/orthopedic surgery and have evidence of bleeding
   b. Pharmacologic
      - Heparin or LMWH: Unfractionated heparin or LMWH postoperatively until patient is ambulatory
      - Combination of pneumatic compression devices and pharmacologic prophylaxis may provide the greatest protection

Quick HIT

Low–Molecular-Weight Heparin
- Has longer half life than unfractionated heparin and can be dosed once daily
- Can be given on outpatient basis
- No need to follow aPTT levels
- Is much more expensive than unfractionated heparin

Chronic Venous Insufficiency (Venous Stasis Disease)

A. General characteristics

1. Also referred to as postphlebitic syndrome
2. CVI may involve the superficial, deep, or both venous systems
3. Anatomy
   a. The lower-extremity venous system consists of three systems: deep, superficial, and perforating systems. Valves exist in all three systems, preventing retrograde blood flow.
   b. The perforating veins connect the superficial and deep systems. Valves allow flow from superficial to deep, but not vice versa.
4. Pathophysiology
   a. History of DVT is the underlying cause in many cases (such a history might not be documented). This has two major effects:
      - It causes destruction of venous valves in the deep venous system. Valvular incompetence results in gravitational pressure of the blood column to be transmitted to ankles.
      - Valves in the perforator veins are also damaged secondary to the chronically elevated deep venous pressure, inhibiting transmission of blood from superficial to deep, as normally occurs.
   b. Leads to **ambulatory venous HTN**, which has two undesirable effects:
      - Interstitial fluid accumulation, resulting in edema.
      - Extravasation of plasma proteins and RBCs into subcutaneous tissues, resulting in brawny induration and pigmentation (a brown-black color) of skin.
   c. Eventually leads to reduced local capillary blood flow and hypoxia of tissues.
      - Even mild trauma may precipitate tissue death and ulcer formation.
      - Venous ulcers usually develop medially from the instep to above the ankle, overlying an incompetent perforator vein.

Quick HIT

Many patients with a history of DVT eventually develop CVI (80%).

B. Clinical features

1. Swelling of the lower leg
   a. When chronic, causes an aching or tightness feeling of the involved leg; often worse at the end of the day
   b. Symptoms are worsened by periods of sitting or inactive standing
   c. Leg elevation provides relief of symptoms (the opposite is true in arterial insufficiency)
2. Chronic changes include:
   a. Skin changes
      - Skin becomes thin, atrophic, shiny, and cyanotic
      - Brawny induration develops with chronicity
   b. Venous ulcers
      - Less painful than ulcers associated with arterial insufficiency
      - Usually located just above the medial malleolus
      - Often rapidly recur

Quick HIT

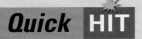

Ulcer formation is directly proportional to the amount of swelling present.

C. Treatment

1. Before the development of ulcers, strict adherence to the following controls stasis sequelae in most patients.
   a. Leg elevation: Periods of leg elevation during the day and throughout the night to a level above the heart.
   b. Avoiding long periods of sitting or standing.
   c. Heavy-weight elastic stockings (knee-length) are worn during waking hours.
2. If ulcers develop, management also entails:
   a. Wet-to-dry saline dressings (three times daily).
   b. Unna venous boot (external compression stocking)—best changed every week to 10 days.
      - Healing occurs in 80% of ulcers. Compliance reduces the rate of recurrence.
      - For ulcers that do not heal with the Unna boot: Apply **split-thickness skin grafts** with or without ligation of adjacent perforator veins.

Quick HIT

When superficial thrombophlebitis occurs in different locations over a short period of time, think of *migratory superficial thrombophlebitis* (secondary to occult malignancy, often of the pancreas–Trousseau syndrome)

Superficial Thrombophlebitis

A. General characteristics

1. Virchow triad is again implicated (but pathophysiology not entirely clear)
2. In upper extremities, usually occurs at the site of an IV infusion
3. In lower extremities, usually associated with **varicose veins** (in the greater saphenous system)—secondary to static blood flow in these veins

Quick HIT

Two conditions that should not be confused with superficial thrombophlebitis are cellulitis and lymphangitis. In these conditions, swelling and erythema are more widespread, and there is no palpable, indurated vein.

B. Clinical features

1. Pain, tenderness, induration, and erythema along the course of the vein
2. A tender cord may be palpated

C. Treatment

1. **No anticoagulation** is required—rarely causes PE. Only if thrombus extends into the deep system
2. Localized thrombophlebitis—a mild analgesic (aspirin or NSAIDs) elevation, and hot compresses; continue activity
3. Suppurative thrombophlebitis—septic phlebitis is usually due to infection of an IV cannula. Redness extends beyond the area of the vein and purulent drainage may be present. Remove the cannula and administer systemic antibiotics.

Cardiac Neoplasms

- Primary tumors of the heart are rare (typically less than 0.1% of the general population).
- Metastases from other primary tumors are more common (75% of cardiac neoplasms). Sites of these primary tumors include the lung, breast, skin, kidney, lymphomas, and Kaposi sarcoma in patients with AIDS.

Atrial Myxoma

- An atrial myxoma is a benign gelatinous growth, usually pedunculated and usually arising from the interatrial septum of the heart in the region of the fossa ovalis. It is the most common primary cardiac neoplasm.
- Although benign, atrial myxomas can embolize, leading to metastatic disease, or can cause relative valvular dysfunction.
- The majority of myxomas are sporadic, but autosomal-dominant transmission has been noted.
- Prototypically present with fatigue, fever, syncope, palpitations, malaise, and a low-pitched diastolic murmur that changes character with changing body positions (**diastolic plop**).
- **Treatment**: Surgical excision.

Shock

Basics of Shock

A. General characteristics

1. Shock is equivalent to **underperfusion of tissues.** It is a medical emergency that needs to be corrected right away, before the condition becomes irreversible.
2. Presents with tachycardia, a decrease in BP, and malfunction of underperfused organ systems, most notably:
   a. Lactic acidosis
   b. Renal (anuria/oliguria)
   c. CNS dysfunction (altered mentation)
3. Shock is characterized by its effect on cardiac output, SVR, and volume status (volume status is assessed via jugular venous pressure or pulmonary capillary wedge pressure [PCWP]). The hemodynamic changes associated with different types of shock are set forth in Table 1-5.

Quick HIT

The following signs and symptoms are common to all forms of shock:
- Hypotension
- Oliguria
- Tachycardia
- Altered mental status

B. Initial approach to a patient in shock

1. A focused history and physical examination to determine possible cause of shock.
   a. Fever and a possible site of infection suggest septic shock.
   b. Trauma, GI bleeding, vomiting, or diarrhea suggests hypovolemic shock.
   c. History of MI, angina, or heart disease suggests cardiogenic shock.
   d. If JVD is present, this suggests cardiogenic shock.
   e. If spinal cord injury or neurologic deficits are present, neurogenic shock likely.
2. Initial steps: Simultaneously stabilize the patient hemodynamically and determine the cause of shock.
   a. Establish two large-bore venous catheters, a central line, and an arterial line.
   b. A fluid bolus (multiple liters of normal saline or lactated Ringer solution) should be given in most cases.
   c. Draw blood: CBC, electrolytes, renal function, PT/PTT.
   d. ECG, CXR.

TABLE 1-5 Hemodynamic Changes in Shock States

Shock	Cardiac Output	SVR	PCWP
Cardiogenic	↓	↑	↑
Hypovolemic	↓	↑	↓
Neurogenic	↓	↓	↓
Septic	↑	↓	↓

Diseases of the Cardiovascular System

e. Continuous pulse oximetry.
f. Vasopressors (dopamine, norepinephrine or phenylephrine) may be given if the patient remains hypotensive despite fluids.
g. If the diagnosis is still in question after the above tests, a pulmonary artery catheter (Swan–Ganz catheter) and/or echocardiogram may help in diagnosis.

C. Treatment

1. **ABCs (airway, breathing, and circulation) should be addressed for all patients in shock.**
2. Specific treatment is described below for each type of shock. With the exception of cardiogenic (and sometimes neurogenic) shock, a generous amount of IV fluid is usually required to resuscitate the patient. The more advanced the stage of shock, the greater the fluid (and blood) requirement.

Cardiogenic Shock

A. General characteristics

1. Occurs when heart is unable to generate a cardiac output sufficient to maintain tissue perfusion
2. Can be defined as a systolic BP <90 with urine output <20 mL/hr and adequate left ventricular filling pressure

B. Causes

1. After acute MI—most common cause
2. Cardiac tamponade (compression of heart)
3. Tension pneumothorax (compression of heart)
4. Arrhythmias
5. Massive PE leading to RVF
6. Myocardial disease (cardiomyopathies, myocarditis)
7. Mechanical abnormalities (valvular defects, ventricular septal defect)

Quick HIT

Note that jugular venous pulse/PCWP is only elevated in cardiogenic shock.

C. Clinical features

1. Typical findings seen in shock (altered sensorium, pale cool skin, hypotension, tachycardia, etc.)
2. Engorged neck veins—Venous pressure is usually elevated
3. Pulmonary congestion

D. Diagnosis

1. ECG—ST segment elevation suggesting acute MI or arrhythmia are the most common findings.
2. Echocardiogram—can diagnose a variety of mechanical complications of MI, identify valve disease, estimate EF, look for pericardial effusion, etc.
3. Hemodynamic monitoring with a Swan–Ganz catheter may be indicated: PCWP, pulmonary artery pressure, cardiac output, cardiac index, SVR—keep cardiac output >4 L/min, cardiac index >2.2, PCWP <18 mm Hg.

E. Treatment

1. ABCs
2. Identify and treat underlying cause
   a. Acute MI
      - Standard treatment with aspirin, heparin (see MI section)
      - Aggressive management, that is, emergent revascularization with PCI (or CABG), has been shown to improve survival
   b. If cardiac tamponade, pericardiocentesis/surgery
   c. Surgical correction of valvular abnormalities
   d. Treatment of arrhythmias
3. Vasopressors or inotropes
   a. Dopamine is often the initial vasopressor used. Norepinephrine is another consideration

CLINICAL PEARL 1-15

Intra-aortic Balloon Pump

- A device that gives "mechanical support" to a failing heart—it works opposite to the normal pumping action of the heart, that is, it serves to "pump" during diastole and "relax" during systole.
- A balloon catheter is positioned in the descending thoracic aorta just distal to subclavian artery. **It facilitates ventricular emptying by deflating just before the onset of systole *(reducing afterload)* and increases coronary perfusion by inflating at the onset of diastole (increasing diastolic pressure).**
- **The net effect is enhanced myocardial oxygenation and increased cardiac output.**
- Indications are angina refractory to medical therapy, mechanical complications of MI, cardiogenic shock, low cardiac output states, and as a bridge to surgery in severe AS.

b. Dobutamine (inotrope) may be used in combination with dopamine to further increase cardiac output

4. Afterload-reducing agents such as nitroglycerin or nitroprusside are typically not used initially because they aggravate hypotension. They may be used later with vasopressors
5. **IV fluids are likely to be harmful if left ventricular pressures are elevated. Patients may in fact need diuretics.**
6. While still controversial, IABPs are often used for hemodynamic support (see Clinical Pearl 1-15). Effects include:
   a. Decreased afterload
   b. Increased cardiac output
   c. Decreased myocardial oxygen demand

Quick HIT

- Compensatory mechanisms begin to fail when more than 20% to 25% of blood volume is lost.
- If CVP is low, hypovolemic shock is most likely present.

Hypovolemic Shock

A. General characteristics

1. Primary pathophysiologic events: Decreased circulatory blood volume leads to decreased preload and cardiac output.
2. The rate of volume loss is very important. The slower the loss, the greater the effectiveness of compensatory mechanisms. Acute loss is associated with higher morbidity and mortality.
3. Patients with significant medical comorbidities (especially cardiac) may be unable to compensate physiologically in the early stages of hypovolemic shock.
4. There are four "classes" of hypovolemic shock, based on the severity of volume loss (Table 1-6).
5. Causes
   a. Hemorrhage
      - Trauma
      - GI bleeding
      - Retroperitoneal

TABLE 1-6 Hemodynamic Changes in Hypovolemic Shock

Class	Blood Volume Lost (%)	Pulse (↑)	Systolic BP (↓)	Pulse Pressure (↓)	Capillary Refill (↓)	Respiratory Rate (↑)	CNS	Urine Output (↓)
I	10–15	Normal	Normal	Normal	Normal	Normal	Normal	Normal
II	20–30	>100	Normal	Decreased	Delayed	Mild tachypnea	Anxious	20–30 mL/hr
III	30–40	>120 weak	Decreased	Decreased	Delayed	Marked tachypnea	Confused	20 mL/hr
IV	>40	>140 nonpalpable	Marked decrease	Marked decrease	Absent	Marked tachypnea	Lethargic, coma	Negligible

b. Nonhemorrhagic
   - Voluminous vomiting
   - Severe diarrhea
   - Severe dehydration for any reason
   - Burns
   - Third-space losses in bowel obstruction

B. Diagnosis: If the diagnosis is unclear from the patient's vital signs and clinical picture, a central venous line or a pulmonary artery catheter can give invaluable information for hemodynamic monitoring: Decreased CVP/PCWP, decreased cardiac output, increased SVR (see Table 1-5).

C. Treatment

1. Airway and breathing—patients in **severe** shock and circulatory collapse generally require intubation and mechanical ventilation.
2. Circulation
   a. If hemorrhage is the cause, apply direct pressure.
   b. IV hydration
      - Patients with class I shock usually do not require fluid resuscitation. Patients with class II shock benefit from fluids, and patients with classes III and IV require fluid resuscitation.
      - Give fluid bolus followed by continuous infusion and reassess.
      - The hemodynamic response to this treatment guides further resuscitative effort.
   c. For nonhemorrhagic shock, blood is not necessary. Crystalloid solution with appropriate electrolyte replacement is adequate.

Quick HIT

Monitoring urine output is the most useful indicator of the effectiveness of treatment. A pulmonary artery catheter and/or central venous line, if available, are very helpful in monitoring as well.

●●● Septic Shock

A. General characteristics

1. Septic shock is defined as hypotension induced by sepsis that persists despite adequate fluid resuscitation. This results in hypoperfusion and can ultimately lead to multiple organ system failure and death.
2. Common causes include (but are not limited to) pneumonia, pyelonephritis, meningitis, abscess formation, cholangitis, cellulitis, and peritonitis.
3. Clinically, there is a progression from systemic inflammatory response syndrome (SIRS), to sepsis, to septic shock, to multiorgan dysfunction syndrome—see Clinical Pearl 1-15.
4. Pathophysiology
   a. **There is a severe decrease in SVR secondary to peripheral vasodilation.** Extremities are often warm due to vasodilation.
   b. Cardiac output is normal or increased (due to maintenance of stroke volume and tachycardia).
   c. EF is decreased secondary to a reduction in contractility.
5. Can be complicated by adult respiratory distress syndrome, ATN, DIC, multiple organ failure, or death.

Quick HIT

Septic shock is associated with severe peripheral vasodilatation (flushing, warm skin).
Hypovolemic shock is associated with peripheral vasoconstriction (cool skin).

B. Clinical features

1. Manifestations related to cause of sepsis (e.g., pneumonia, urinary tract infection, peritonitis)
2. Signs of SIRS (see Clinical Pearl 1-16)
3. Signs of shock (hypotension, oliguria, lactic acidosis)
4. Patient may have a **fever** or may be **hypothermic** (hypothermia is more common in the very young, elderly, debilitated, and immunocompromised)

C. Diagnosis

1. Septic shock is essentially a clinical diagnosis.
2. Confirmed by positive blood cultures, but negative cultures are common.
3. A source of infection can aid in diagnosis, but there may be no confirmed source in some cases.

CLINICAL PEARL 1-16

Systemic Inflammatory Response Syndrome (SIRS)

SIRS

SIRS is **characterized by two or more** of the following:

- Fever (>38°C) or hypothermia (<36°C)
- Hyperventilation (rate >20 bpm) or $PaCO_2$ < 32 mm Hg
- Tachycardia (>90 bpm)
- Increased WBC count (>12,000 cell/hpf, <4,000 cells/hpf, or >10% band forms)

Sepsis

- When have a suspected source of infection and SIRS is present

Septic Shock

- Hypotension induced by sepsis persisting despite adequate fluid resuscitation

Multiple Organ Dysfunction Syndrome (MODS)

- Altered organ function in an acutely ill patient, usually leading to death

D. Treatment

1. Initially, IV antibiotics (broad spectrum) at maximum dosages. Antibiotics for more rare organisms or antifungal medications may be required if there is no clinical response or if suspicion for an atypical organism (i.e., immunocompromised). If cultures are positive, antibiotics can be narrowed based on sensitivity testing.
2. Surgical drainage if necessary.
3. Fluid administration to increase mean BP (may require many liters of fluid).
4. Vasopressors (Norepinephrine, dopamine, phenylephrine) may be used if hypotension persists despite aggressive IV fluid resuscitation.

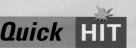

Quick HIT

Septic shock is the most common cause of death in the ICU.

Neurogenic Shock

A. General characteristics

1. Neurogenic shock results from a failure of the sympathetic nervous system to maintain adequate vascular tone (sympathetic denervation)
2. Causes include spinal cord injury, severe head injury, spinal anesthesia, pharmacologic sympathetic blockade
3. Characterized by peripheral vasodilation with decreased SVR

B. Clinical features

1. Warm, well-perfused skin
2. Urine output low or normal
3. Bradycardia and hypotension (but tachycardia can occur)
4. Cardiac output is decreased, SVR low, PCWP low to normal

C. Treatment

1. Judicious use of IV fluids as the mainstay of treatment
2. Vasoconstrictors to restore venous tone, but cautiously
3. Supine or Trendelenburg position
4. Maintain body temperature

2 DISEASES OF THE PULMONARY SYSTEM

Obstructive Lung Diseases

Chronic Obstructive Pulmonary Disease

A. General characteristics

1. There are two classic types of chronic obstructive pulmonary disease (COPD): **chronic bronchitis** and **emphysema** (see Table 2-1 and Clinical Pearl 2-1).
   a. Chronic bronchitis is a clinical diagnosis: chronic cough productive of sputum for at least 3 months per year for at least 2 consecutive years.
   b. Emphysema is a pathologic diagnosis: permanent enlargement of air spaces distal to terminal bronchioles due to destruction of alveolar walls.
   c. **The two often coexist.** Pure emphysema or pure chronic bronchitis is rare.
   d. **COPD is the fourth leading cause of death in the United States.**
2. Risk factors and causes
   a. Tobacco smoke (indicated in almost 90% of COPD cases)
   b. α_1-Antitrypsin deficiency—risk is even worse in combination with smoking
   c. Environmental factors (e.g., second-hand smoke)
   d. Chronic asthma—speculated by some to be an independent risk factor
3. Pathogenesis
   a. Chronic bronchitis
      - Excess mucus production narrows the airways; patients often have a productive cough.
      - Inflammation and scarring in airways, enlargement in mucous glands, and smooth muscle hyperplasia lead to obstruction.
   b. Emphysema
      - Destruction of alveolar walls is due to relative excess in protease (elastase) activity, or relative deficiency of antiprotease (α_1-antitrypsin) activity in the lung. Elastase is released from PMNs and macrophages and digests human lung. This is inhibited by α_1-antitrypsin.
      - Tobacco smoke increases the number of activated PMNs and macrophages, inhibits α_1-antitrypsin, and increases oxidative stress on the lung by free radical production.

> **Quick HIT**
>
> **Pathology**
>
> Centrilobular emphysema:
> - Most common type, seen in smokers (rarely in nonsmokers)
> - Destruction limited to respiratory bronchioles (proximal acini) with little change in distal acini
> - Predilection for upper lung zones
>
> Panlobular emphysema:
> - Seen in patients with α_1-antitrypsin deficiency
> - Destruction involves both proximal and distal acini
> - Predilection for lung bases

> **Quick HIT**
>
> In COPD,
> - The FEV_1/FVC ratio is <0.70.
> - FEV_1 is decreased.
> - TLC is increased.
> - Residual volume is increased.

B. Clinical features

1. Symptoms
   a. Any combination of cough, sputum production, and dyspnea (on exertion or at rest, depending on severity) may be present. Dyspnea is initially during exertion but eventually becomes progressively worse with less exertion and even at rest.
   b. Some patients have very sedentary lifestyles but few complaints. They may avoid exertional dyspnea, which is the most common early symptom of COPD by limiting their activity.

TABLE 2-1 COPD—Emphysema and Chronic Bronchitis

Predominant Emphysema ("Pink Puffers")	Predominant Chronic Bronchitis ("Blue Bloaters")
• Patients tend to be thin due to increased energy expenditure during breathing. • When sitting, patients tend to lean forward. • Patients have a barrel chest (increased AP diameter of chest).	• Patients tend to be overweight and cyanotic (secondary to chronic hypercapnia and hypoxemia). • Chronic cough and sputum production are characteristic. • Signs of cor pulmonale may be present in severe or long-standing disease.
Tachypnea with prolonged expiration through pursed lips is present.	Respiratory rate is normal or slightly increased.
Patient is distressed and uses accessory muscles (especially strap muscles in neck).	Patient is in no apparent distress, and there is no apparent use of accessory muscles.

2. Signs—the following may be present:
   a. **Prolonged expiratory time.**
   b. During auscultation, end-expiratory wheezes on forced expiration, decreased breath sounds, and/or inspiratory crackles
   c. Tachypnea, tachycardia
   d. Cyanosis
   e. Use of accessory respiratory muscles
   f. Hyperresonance on percussion
   g. Signs of cor pulmonale

Quick HIT

FEV_1 is the amount of air that can be forced out of the lungs in 1 second. The lower the FEV_1, the more difficulty one has breathing.

C. Diagnosis

1. Pulmonary function testing (spirometry)—see Table 2-2 and Figure 2-1.
   a. This is the definitive diagnostic test.
   b. Obstruction is evident based on the following:
      - **Decreased FEV_1** and decreased FEV_1/FVC ratio—GOLD staging is based on FEV_1. $FEV_1 \geq 80\%$ of predicted value is mild disease, 50% to 80% is moderate disease, 30% to 50% is severe disease, and <30% is very severe disease.

Quick HIT

To diagnose airway obstruction, one must have a normal or increased TLC with a decreased FEV_1.

Diseases of the Pulmonary System

CLINICAL PEARL 2-1

Key Points in Taking History of COPD Patients

General

- History of cardiopulmonary diseases
- Smoking history (duration, intensity, current smoker)
- Family history—COPD, heart disease, asthma
- Occupation—industrial dusts, fumes
- Overall health
- History of respiratory infections—frequency, severity
- Pulmonary medications

Pulmonary Symptoms

- Dyspnea—quantitate severity
- Cough
- Sputum production—quantity, quality, duration, hemoptysis
- Wheezing

Adapted from Burton GG, Hodgkin JE, Ward JJ, eds. *Respiratory Care—A Guide to Clinical Practice.* 4th ed. Philadelphia, PA: Lippincott Williams & Wilkins, 1997:1026, Table 28-3.

TABLE 2-2 Obstructive Versus Restrictive Lung Disease

Measurement	Obstructive	Restrictive
FEV_1	Low	Normal or slightly low
FEV_1/FVC	Low	Normal or high
Peak expiratory flow rate	Low	Normal
Residual volume	High	Low, normal, or high
Total lung capacity	High	Low
Vital capacity	Low	Low

Quick HIT

One can measure the peak expiratory flow rate using a peak flow meter. If <350 L/min, one should perform pulmonary function testing, because this is a good screening test for obstruction.

Quick HIT

COPD leads to chronic respiratory acidosis with metabolic alkalosis as compensation.

Quick HIT

Clinical monitoring of COPD patients entails the following:
- Serial FEV_1 measurements—this has the highest predictive value
- Pulse oximetry
- Exercise tolerance

- Increased total lung capacity (TLC), residual volume, and functional reserve capacity (FRC) (indicating air trapping) (see Figure 2-2). Although COPD increases TLC, the air in the lung is not useful because it all becomes residual volume and does not participate in gas exchange.
- Decreased vital capacity.

2. Chest radiograph (CXR)
   a. Low sensitivity for diagnosing COPD; only severe, advanced emphysema will show the typical changes, which include:
      - Hyperinflation, flattened diaphragm, enlarged retrosternal space (see Figure 2-3).
      - Diminished vascular markings.
   b. Useful in an acute exacerbation to rule out complications such as pneumonia or pneumothorax.
3. Measure α_1-antitrypsin levels in patients with a personal or family history of premature emphysema (≤50 years old).
4. Arterial blood gas (ABG)—chronic PCO_2 retention, decreased PO_2.

D. Treatment

1. Modalities
   a. **Smoking cessation—the most important intervention.**
      - Disease progression is accelerated by continued smoking and can be greatly slowed by its cessation.
      - At around age 35, FEV_1 decreases approximately 25 to 30 mL/yr. In smokers, the rate of decline is faster (threefold to fourfold). If a smoker quits, the ***rate of decline*** of FEV_1 slows to that of someone of the same age who has never smoked. **However, quitting does *not* result in complete reversal.**

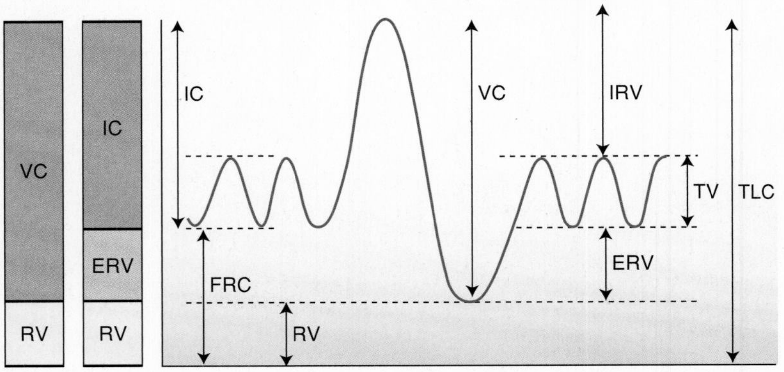

1. TLC (total lung capacity) = volume of air in the lungs after maximum inspiration
2. FRC (functional residual capacity) = volume of air in the lungs after a normal expiration
3. RV (residual volume) = volume of air in the lungs at maximal expiration
4. TV (tidal volume) = volume of air breathed in and out of the lungs during quiet breathing
5. VC (vital capacity) = volume of air expelled from the lungs during a maximum expiration

FIGURE 2-1 **Lung volumes. IC, inspiratory capacity; ERV, expiratory reserve volume.**

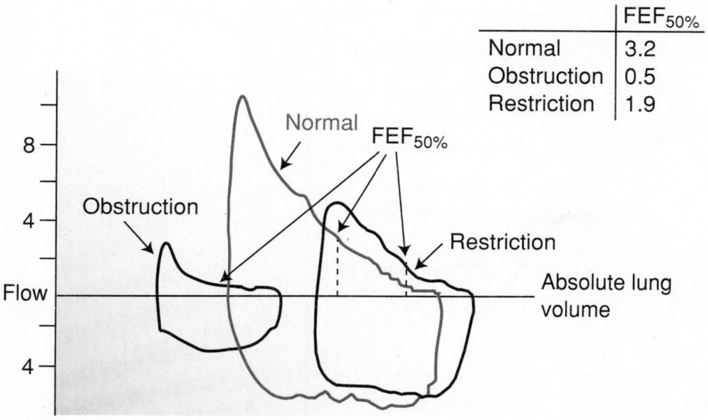

FIGURE 2-2 **Flow volume loops. Examples of flow volume curves in a patient with obstructive disease and a patient with restriction (diffuse interstitial fibrosis), as compared with a healthy person. Volumes on the axis are absolute volumes to better show the relation of flows (e.g., FEF$_{50\%}$) to hyperinflation and restriction.**
(Redrawn from Humes DH, DuPont HL, Gardner LB, et al. *Kelley's Textbook of Internal Medicine.* 4th ed. Philadelphia, PA: Lippincott Williams & Wilkins, 2000:2580, Figure 387.2.)

- **Smoking cessation prolongs the survival rate but does not reduce it to the level of someone who has never smoked** (see Figure 2-4).
- Respiratory symptoms improve within 1 year of quitting.

b. Inhaled anticholinergic drugs (e.g., ipratropium bromide): bronchodilators.
   - Slower onset of action than the β-agonists, but last longer.

c. Inhaled β_2-agonists (e.g., albuterol): bronchodilators.
   - Provide symptomatic relief. Use long-acting agents (e.g., salmeterol) for patients requiring frequent use.

d. Combination of β-agonist albuterol with ipratropium bromide.
   - More efficacious than either agent alone in bronchodilation.
   - Also helps with adherence to therapy (both medications in one inhaler).

e. Inhaled corticosteroids (e.g., budesonide, fluticasone): anti-inflammatory.
   - May minimally slow down the decrease in FEV_1 over time; however, many studies have failed to show any benefit in pulmonary function.

Quick HIT

Smoking cessation and home oxygen therapy are the only interventions shown to lower mortality.

Quick HIT

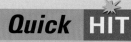

- Treat COPD with bronchodilators (anticholinergics, β_2-agonists, or both).
- Give steroids and antibiotics for acute exacerbations.

Quick HIT

β-Blockers are generally contraindicated in acute COPD or asthma exacerbations.

Diseases of the Pulmonary System

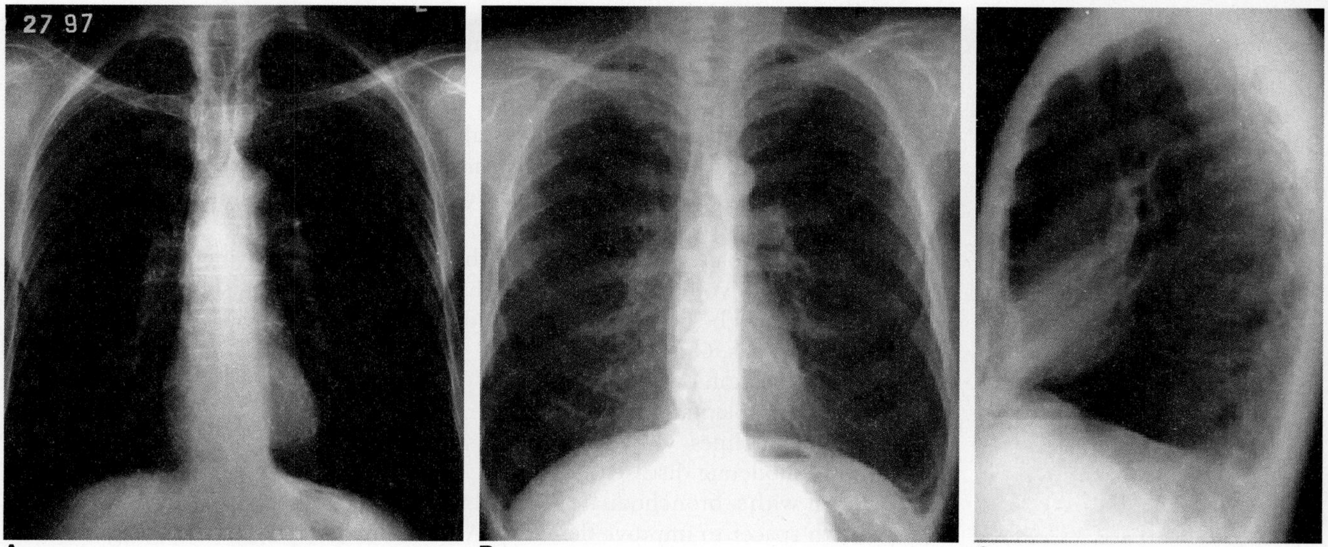

A B C

FIGURE 2-3 **Chest radiographs showing a patient with COPD.**
(**A** from Daffner RH. *Clinical Radiology: The Essentials.* 3rd ed. Philadelphia, PA: Lippincott Williams & Wilkins, 2007:136, Figure 4.87A.) (**B** and **C** from Stern EJ, White CS. *Chest Radiology Companion.* Philadelphia, PA: Lippincott Williams & Wilkins, 1999:189, Figure 13-1A and B.)

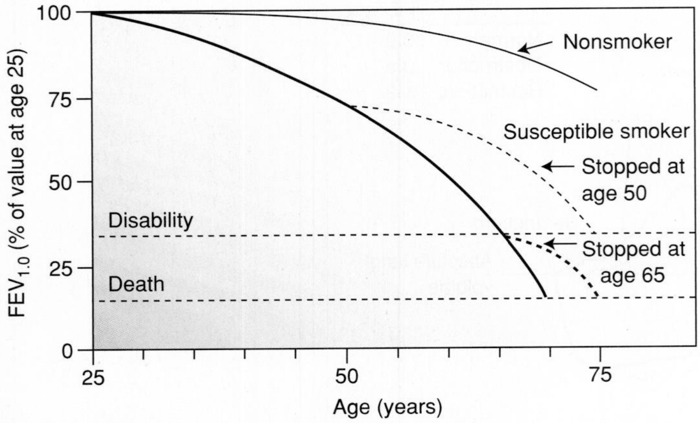

FIGURE 2-4 **Smoking and COPD. Age-related rate of decline in lung function ($FEV_{1.0}$) in a nonsmoker (top) and susceptible smoker (bottom). The *dashed lines* indicate the beneficial effects of smoking cessation with moderate and severe disease. The accelerated decline in lung function approaches the normal rate, significantly delaying the onset of disability and death.** (Redrawn from Fletcher CM, Peto R. The natural history of chronic airflow obstruction. *BMJ* 1977;1:1645.)

- Typically used in combination with a long-acting bronchodilator for patients with significant symptoms or repeated exacerbations.

f. Theophylline (oral)—role is controversial.
- May improve mucociliary clearance and central respiratory drive.
- Narrow therapeutic index, so serum levels must be monitored.
- Only modestly effective and has more side effects than other bronchodilators. Occasionally used for patients with refractory COPD.

g. Oxygen therapy.
- **Shown to improve survival and quality of life in patients with COPD *and* chronic hypoxemia.**
- Some patients need continuous oxygen, whereas others only require it during exertion or sleep. Get an ABG to determine need for oxygen (see Quick Hit).
- Long-standing hypoxemia may lead to pulmonary HTN and ultimately cor pulmonale. Continuous oxygen therapy for ≥18 hr/day has been shown to reduce mortality in patients with these complications by controlling pulmonary HTN.

h. Pulmonary rehabilitation—education, exercise, physiotherapy: A major goal is to improve exercise tolerance. Pulmonary rehabilitation improves functional status and quality of life.

i. Vaccination
- Influenza vaccination annually for all patients.
- Vaccination against *Streptococcus pneumoniae* every 5 to 6 years—should be offered to patients with COPD over 65 years old, or under 65 who have severe disease.

j. Antibiotics are given for acute exacerbations (see below)—increased sputum production in volume or change in character or worsening shortness of breath.

k. Surgery—may be beneficial in selected patients; carefully weigh potential benefits with risks. Options include:
- Lung resection
- Lung transplantation

2. Treatment guidelines

a. Mild to moderate disease.
- Begin with a bronchodilator in a metered-dose inhaler (MDI) formulation (with spacer to improve delivery). Anticholinergic drugs and/or β-agonists are first-line agents.
- Inhaled glucocorticoids may be used as well (see above). Use the lowest dose possible.
- Theophylline may be considered if the above do not adequately control symptoms.

Quick HIT

Systemic glucocorticoids are only used for acute exacerbations and should not be used for long-term treatment, even for patients with severe COPD.

Quick HIT

Criteria for continuous or intermittent long-term oxygen therapy in COPD:
- PaO_2 **55 mm Hg** *OR*
- O_2 **saturation ≤88%** (pulse oximetry) either at rest or during exercise *OR*
- PaO_2 55 to 59 mm Hg plus polycythemia or evidence of cor pulmonale
- Note that the above must be consistent findings despite optimal medical therapy

b. Severe disease
- Medications as above.
- Continuous oxygen therapy (if patient is hypoxemic).
- Pulmonary rehabilitation.
- Triple inhaler therapy (long-acting β-agonist plus a long-acting anticholinergic plus an inhaled glucocorticoid) is an option for severe disease.

3. Acute COPD exacerbation. Definition: Increased dyspnea, sputum production, and/or cough. Acute COPD exacerbation can lead to acute respiratory failure requiring hospitalization, and possibly mechanical ventilation; potentially fatal.
   a. Bronchodilators (β_2-agonist) alone or in combination with anticholinergics are first-line therapy.
   b. Systemic corticosteroids are used for patients requiring hospitalization (IV methylprednisolone is a common choice). Taper with oral prednisone on clinical improvement. Do not use inhaled corticosteroids in acute exacerbations.
   c. Antibiotics (azithromycin, levofloxacin, doxycycline, etc.; no antibiotic superior to another): Studies have shown that patients who receive broad-spectrum antibiotics do slightly better than a placebo group.
   d. Supplemental oxygen is used to keep O_2 saturation 90% to 93%. Start with a nasal cannula; a face mask may need to be used.
      - If SaO_2 is >93%, the patient is at risk of CO_2 retention from worsening V/Q mismatch, loss of hypoxemic respiratory drive, and the Haldane effect.
   e. Noninvasive positive pressure ventilation (NPPV) (bilevel positive airway pressure [BIPAP] or CPAP): Studies have shown a benefit in acute exacerbations. It may decrease the likelihood of respiratory failure requiring invasive mechanical ventilation.
   f. Intubation and mechanical ventilation may be required if the above do not stabilize the patient. Intubate if increasing RR, increasing $PaCO_2$, and worsening acidosis.

E. Complications
1. Acute exacerbations—most common causes are infection, noncompliance with therapy, and cardiac disease
2. Secondary polycythemia (Hct >55% in men or >47% in women)—compensatory response to chronic hypoxemia
3. Pulmonary HTN and cor pulmonale—may occur in patients with severe, longstanding COPD who have chronic hypoxemia

Asthma

A. General characteristics
1. Characteristically defined by the following triad:
   a. Airway inflammation
   b. Airway hyperresponsiveness
   c. Reversible airflow obstruction
2. **Asthma can begin at any age**
3. Extrinsic versus intrinsic asthma
   a. Extrinsic asthma (most cases)
      - Patients are atopic, that is, produce immunoglobulin E (IgE) to environmental antigens. May be associated with eczema and hay fever
      - Patients become asthmatic at a young age
   b. Intrinsic asthma—not related to atopy or environmental triggers
4. Triggers include pollens, house dust, molds, cockroaches, cats, dogs, cold air, viral infections, tobacco smoke, medications (β-blockers, aspirin), and exercise.

B. Clinical features
1. Characterized by intermittent symptoms that include **SOB, wheezing, chest tightness,** and **cough.** Symptoms have variable severity and may not be present simultaneously. Usually occur within 30 minutes of exposure to triggers.
2. Symptoms are typically worse at night.

Quick HIT

- One of the main treatment goals for COPD patients is to reduce the number and severity of exacerbations they experience each year.
- Pulmonary infection (*S. pneumoniae, Haemophilus influenzae, Mycoplasma pneumoniae, Moraxella catarrhalis,* and viruses are the most common organisms) is one of the main precipitants of a COPD exacerbation.

Quick HIT

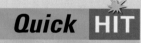

If a patient presents with COPD exacerbation, the following steps are appropriate:
- CXR
- β_2-agonist and anticholinergic inhalers
- Systemic corticosteroids
- Antibiotics
- Supplemental oxygen
- NPPV if needed (see Clinical Pearl 2-9)

Quick HIT

Signs of acute severe asthma attacks:
- Tachypnea, diaphoresis, wheezing, speaking in incomplete sentences, and use of accessory muscles of respiration.
- Paradoxic movement of the abdomen and diaphragm on inspiration is sign of impending respiratory failure.

CLINICAL PEARL 2-2

"All That Wheezes Is Not Asthma"

The most common cause of wheezing is asthma. However, any condition that mimics large-airway bronchospasm can cause wheezing.

- CHF—due to edema of airways and congestion of bronchial mucosa
- COPD—inflamed airways may be narrowed, or bronchospasm may be present
- Cardiomyopathies, pericardial diseases can lead to edema around the bronchi
- Lung cancer—due to obstruction of airways (central tumor or mediastinal invasion)

3. Wheezing (during both inspiration and expiration) is the most common finding on physical examination (see Clinical Pearl 2-2).

Quick HIT

PFTs in asthma:
1. Decreased FEV_1, decreased FVC, decreased FEV_1/FVC ratio
2. Increase in FEV_1 >12% with albuterol
3. Decrease in FEV_1 >20% with methacholine or histamine

Quick HIT

Although asthma can be diagnosed with PFTs and spirometry, in an acute setting (ED) when patient is SOB, peak flow measurement is quickest method of diagnosis.

Quick HIT

During asthma exacerbations, the patient hyperventilates, leading to low $PaCO_2$ levels. If the patient is no longer hyperventilating (CO_2 level is normal or high), this could be a sign that the patient is decompensating (due to fatigue) and that intubation may be required.

Quick HIT

Avoid β-blockers in asthmatics!

C. Diagnosis

1. Pulmonary function tests (PFTs) are required for diagnosis. They show an obstructive pattern: decrease in expiratory flow rates, decreased FEV_1, and decreased FEV_1/FVC ratio (<0.70).
2. Spirometry before and after bronchodilators can confirm diagnosis by proving reversible airway obstruction. If inhalation of a bronchodilator (β_2-agonist) results in an increase in FEV_1 or FVC by at least 12%, airflow obstruction is considered reversible.
3. Peak flow (peak expiratory flow rate)—useful measure of airflow obstruction. Patients should self-monitor their peak flow:
   a. Mild persistent asthma: Periodic monitoring is sufficient. Increase the dose of inhaled steroid if the peak flow decreases.
   b. Moderate persistent asthma: Daily monitoring is required. Increase the dose of inhaled steroid if the peak flow decreases.
   c. Severe persistent asthma: Daily monitoring is required. Initiate prednisone if the peak flow decreases.
4. Bronchoprovocation test.
   a. May be useful when asthma is suspected but PFTs are nondiagnostic.
   b. Measures ease with which airways narrow in response to stimuli.
   c. Measures lung function before and after inhalation of increasing doses of methacholine (muscarinic agonist); hyperresponsive airways develop obstruction at lower doses.
5. Chest x-ray
   a. Normal in mild cases; severe asthma reveals hyperinflation
   b. Only necessary in severe asthma to exclude other conditions (e.g., pneumonia, pneumothorax, pneumomediastinum, foreign body).
6. ABGs
   a. ABGs should be considered if the patient is in significant respiratory distress. **Hypocarbia** is common. Hypoxemia may be present.
   b. If the $PaCO_2$ is normal or increased, respiratory failure may ensue.
      - Remember that patients with an asthma attack have an increased respiratory rate, which should cause the $PaCO_2$ to decrease. Increased $PaCO_2$ is a sign of respiratory muscle fatigue or severe airway obstruction.
      - The patient should be hospitalized and mechanical ventilation considered.

D. Treatment

1. Available modalities (see Table 2-3).
   a. Inhaled β_2-agonists.
      - Short-acting β_2-agonists (e.g., albuterol) are used for acute attacks (rescue). Onset is 2 to 5 minutes, duration is 4 to 6 hours.
      - Long-acting versions (e.g., salmeterol) are especially good with nighttime asthma and exercise-induced asthma.
   b. Inhaled corticosteroids for moderate to severe asthma.
      - Preferred over oral steroids due to fewer systemic side effects. (Oral steroids are reserved for severe, persistent asthma.)

TABLE 2-3 Chronic Treatment of Asthma

Severity	Long-term Control Medications
Mild intermittent (symptoms two or fewer times per week)	None
Mild persistent (symptoms two or more times per week but not every day)	Low dose inhaled corticosteroid
Moderate persistent (daily symptoms; frequent exacerbations)	Daily inhaled corticosteroid (low dose) with long-acting inhaled β-agonist, or daily inhaled corticosteroid (medium dose). Alternatives include adding a leukotriene modifier or theophylline to the daily inhaled corticosteroid (low dose)
Severe persistent (continual symptoms, frequent exacerbations, limited physical activity)	Daily inhaled corticosteroid (medium or high dose) and long-acting inhaled β_2-agonists. Omalizumab (anti-IgE) may be considered additionally. If poor control, systemic corticosteroids should be considered.

Note: All patients should have intermittent short-acting inhaled β_2-agonists as needed plus long-term control medications based on the severity of their asthma.

From The National Asthma Education and Prevention Program, *Expert Panel Report 2*, 1997.

- If used on a regular basis, airway hyperresponsiveness decreases, and the number of asthma exacerbations decreases.

c. Montelukast—leukotriene modifiers—less efficacious than inhaled steroids but useful for prophylaxis of mild exercise-induced asthma and for control of mild to moderate persistent disease. They may allow reductions in steroid and bronchodilator requirements.

d. Cromolyn sodium/nedocromil sodium.
   - Only for prophylaxis (e.g., before exercise); rarely used in adults.

2. Treatment of acute severe asthma exacerbation (hospital admission).

a. Inhaled β_2-agonist (first-line therapy).
   - Via nebulizer or MDI (see Clinical Pearl 2-3).
   - Mainstays of emergency treatment—have an onset of action of minutes.
   - Assess patient response to bronchodilators (clinically and with peak flows).

b. Corticosteroids
   - Traditionally given intravenously initially, but may also be given orally if given in equivalent doses.
   - Taper IV or oral corticosteroids, but only when clinical improvement is seen.
   - Initiate inhaled corticosteroids at the beginning of the tapering schedule.

c. Third-line agent includes IV magnesium—not as effective as β-agonists, magnesium helps with bronchospasm but only used in acute severe exacerbation that has not responded to above medications (albuterol, steroids, oxygen).

CLINICAL PEARL 2-3

MDIs and Nebulizers

- An MDI with a spacer is just as effective as a nebulizer. A spacer is a holding chamber that obviates the need to coordinate inhalation and depression of the canister, and thus makes the use of an MDI easier. Its use leads to a greater bronchodilator effect because more of the drug is deposited in smaller airways and less accumulates in the oropharynx.
- A nebulizer is no more effective than an MDI, but patients may report greater relief of symptoms simply because it provides more medication. It may be preferred by patients with very severe asthma unresponsive to MDIs.

Quick HIT

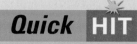

- Side effects of inhaled corticosteroids are due to oropharyngeal deposition and include sore throat, oral candidiasis (thrush), and hoarseness.
- Using a spacer with MDIs and rinsing the mouth after use helps minimize these side effects.

Quick HIT

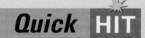

For acute asthma exacerbation, test to order:
1. PEF—decreased
2. ABG—increased A–a gradient
3. Chest x-ray—rule out pneumonia, pneumothorax

Quick HIT

Complications of asthma
1. Status asthmaticus—does not respond to standard medications
2. Acute respiratory failure (due to respiratory muscle fatigue)
3. Pneumothorax, atelectasis, pneumomediastinum

Quick HIT

- Aspirin-sensitive asthma should be considered in patients with asthma and nasal polyps.
- Avoid aspirin or any nonsteroidal anti-inflammatory drugs in these patients because they may cause a severe systemic reaction.

d. Supplemental oxygen (keep oxygen saturation >90%).
e. Antibiotics if severe exacerbation or suspicion of infection.
f. Intubation for patients in respiratory failure or impending respiratory failure.
3. Guidelines for treatment are based on severity.

Bronchiectasis

A. General characteristics

1. There is permanent, abnormal dilation and destruction of bronchial walls with chronic inflammation, airway collapse, and ciliary loss/dysfunction leading to impaired clearance of secretions.
2. Less common today because modern antibiotics are used for respiratory infections.

> **Quick HIT**
> A variety of infections can cause bronchiectasis by destroying and damaging the bronchial walls and interfering with ciliary action.

B. Causes

1. Recurrent infections (airway obstruction, immunodeficiency, allergic bronchopulmonary aspergillosis, mycobacterium)
2. Cystic fibrosis (CF) is most common cause of bronchiectasis (accounts for half of all cases)
3. Primary ciliary dyskinesia (e.g., Kartagener syndrome)
4. Autoimmune disease (rheumatoid arthritis, systemic lupus erythematosus, Crohn disease, etc.)
5. Humoral immunodeficiency (abnormal lung defense), airway obstruction

C. Clinical features

1. Chronic cough with large amounts of mucopurulent, foul-smelling sputum
2. Dyspnea
3. Hemoptysis—due to rupture of blood vessels near bronchial wall surfaces; usually mild and self-limited, but sometimes can be brisk and present as an emergency
4. Recurrent or persistent pneumonia

D. Diagnosis

1. High-resolution CT scan is the diagnostic study of choice.
2. PFTs reveal an obstructive pattern.
3. CXR is abnormal in most cases, but findings are nonspecific.
4. Bronchoscopy applies in certain cases.

E. Treatment

1. Antibiotics for acute exacerbations—superimposed infections are signaled by change in quality/quantity of sputum, fever, chest pain, etc.
2. Bronchial hygiene is very important.
   a. Hydration
   b. Chest physiotherapy (postural drainage, chest percussion) to help remove the mucus
   c. Inhaled bronchodilators

> **Quick HIT**
> The main goal in treating bronchiectasis is to prevent the complications of pneumonia and hemoptysis.

Cystic Fibrosis

- Autosomal recessive condition predominantly affecting Caucasians
- Defect in chloride channel protein causes impaired chloride and water transport, which leads to excessively thick, viscous secretions in the respiratory tract, exocrine pancreas, sweat glands, intestines, and genitourinary tract
- Typically results in obstructive lung disease pattern with chronic pulmonary infections (frequently *Pseudomonas*), pancreatic insufficiency, and other GI complications
- Treatment is pancreatic enzyme replacement, fat-soluble vitamin supplements, chest physical therapy, vaccinations (influenza and pneumococcal), treatment of infections with antibiotics, inhaled recombinant human deoxyribonuclease (rhDNase), which breaks down the DNA in respiratory mucus that clogs the airways
- Traditionally considered a pediatric topic; however, the prognosis has improved significantly, with the median age of death now over 30 years of age

Lung Neoplasms

Lung Cancer

A. General characteristics

1. Pathologic types are divided into two subgroups:
   a. Small cell lung cancer (SCLC)—25% of lung cancers
   b. Nonsmall cell lung cancer (NSCLC)—75% of lung cancers; includes squamous cell carcinoma, adenocarcinoma, large cell carcinoma, and bronchoalveolar cell carcinoma
2. Risk factors
   a. Cigarette smoking—accounts for >85% of cases
      - There is a linear relationship between pack-years of smoking and risk of lung cancer.
      - Adenocarcinoma has the **lowest** association with smoking of all lung cancers.
   b. Second-hand smoke
   c. Asbestos
      - Common in shipbuilding and construction industry, car mechanics, painting
      - Smoking and asbestos in combination synergistically increase the risk of lung cancer
   d. Radon—high levels found in basements
   e. COPD—an independent risk factor after smoking is taken into account
3. **Staging**
   a. NSCLC is staged via the primary TNM system.
   b. SCLC is staged differently (though some recommend TNM saging still be used):
      - Limited—confined to chest plus supraclavicular nodes, but not cervical or axillary nodes
      - Extensive—outside of chest and supraclavicular nodes

Quick HIT

In the diagnosis of lung cancer, it is crucial to differentiate between small cell (25%) and nonsmall cell (75%) types because the treatment approach is completely different (see below). A tissue diagnosis is necessary to make this differentiation.

B. Clinical features

1. Local manifestations (squamous cell carcinoma is most commonly associated with these symptoms)
   a. Airway involvement can lead to cough, hemoptysis, obstruction, wheezing, dyspnea
   b. Recurrent pneumonia (postobstructive pneumonia)
2. Constitutional symptoms
   a. Anorexia, weight loss, weakness
   b. Usually indicative of advanced disease
3. Local invasion
   a. **Superior vena cava (SVC) syndrome**—occurs in 5% of patients
      - Caused by obstruction of SVC by a mediastinal tumor
      - Most commonly occurs with SCLC
      - Findings: facial fullness; facial and arm edema; dilated veins over anterior chest, arms, and face; jugular venous distention (JVD)
   b. Phrenic nerve palsy—occurs in 1% of patients
      - Destruction of phrenic nerve by tumor; phrenic nerve courses through the mediastinum to innervate the diaphragm
      - Results in hemidiaphragmatic paralysis
   c. Recurrent laryngeal nerve palsy (3% of patients)—causes hoarseness
   d. **Horner syndrome**—due to invasion of cervical sympathetic chain by an apical tumor. Symptoms: unilateral facial anhidrosis (no sweating), ptosis, and miosis
   e. **Pancoast tumor**
      - Superior sulcus tumor—an apical tumor involving C8 and T1–T2 nerve roots, causing shoulder pain radiating down the arm
      - Usually squamous cell cancers
      - Symptoms: pain; upper extremity weakness due to brachial plexus invasion; associated with Horner syndrome 60% of the time

Quick HIT

Unfortunately, signs and symptoms are generally nonspecific for lung cancer, and by the time they are present, disease is usually widespread.

Quick HIT

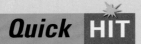

Prognosis of SCLC: For limited disease, 5-year survival is 10% to 13% (median survival ranges from 15 to 20 months). For extensive disease, 5-year survival rate is 1% to 2% (median survival is 8 to 13 months).

Quick HIT

For lung cancer, obtain a CXR, a CT scan, and a tissue biopsy to confirm diagnosis and determine histologic type (SCLC or NSCLC).

Quick HIT

CXR may show pleural effusion, which should be tapped; the fluid should be examined for malignant cells.

Regardless of the findings on CXR or CT scan, pathologic confirmation is required for definitive diagnosis of lung cancer.

Quick HIT

Always perform a biopsy for intrathoracic lymphadenopathy (specificity for metastasis is 60%).

Quick HIT

The prognosis for lung cancer is grim. **Overall 5-year survival for lung cancer patients is 14%;** 85% of patients with SCLC have extensive disease at the time of presentation, and of these almost all die within 2 years.

   f. Malignant pleural effusion—occurs in 10% to 15% of patients
      - Prognosis is very poor—equivalent to distant metastases
4. Metastatic disease—most common sites are brain, bone, adrenal glands, and liver
5. Paraneoplastic syndromes
   a. SIADH: usually seen in small cell carcinoma (10% of SCLC patients)
   b. Ectopic ACTH secretion: small cell carcinoma
   c. PTH-like hormone secretion: most commonly squamous cell carcinoma
   d. Hypertrophic pulmonary osteoarthropathy: adenocarcinoma and squamous cell carcinoma—severe long-bone pain may be present
   e. **Eaton–Lambert syndrome:** most common in SCLC; clinical picture is similar to that of myasthenia gravis, with proximal muscle weakness/fatigability, diminished deep tendon reflexes, paresthesias (more common in lower extremities)
   f. Digital clubbing: loss of normal angle between the fingernail and nail bed due to thickening of subungual soft tissue

C. Diagnosis

1. CXR
   a. Most important radiologic study for diagnosis, but **not** used as a screening test
   b. Demonstrates abnormal findings in nearly all patients with lung cancer
   c. Stability of an abnormality over a 2-year period is almost always associated with a benign lesion
2. CT scan of the chest with IV contrast
   a. Very useful for staging
   b. Can demonstrate extent of local and distant metastasis
   c. Very accurate in revealing lymphadenopathy in mediastinum
3. Cytologic examination of sputum
   a. Diagnoses central tumors (in 80%) but not peripheral lesions
   b. Provides highly variable results; if negative and clinical suspicion is high, further tests are indicated
4. Fiberoptic bronchoscope
   a. Can only be inserted as far as secondary branches of bronchial tree; useful for diagnosing central visualized tumors but not peripheral lesions
   b. The larger and more central the lesion, the higher the diagnostic yield; for visible lesions, bronchoscopy is diagnostic in >90% of cases
5. Whole body positron emission tomography (PET)—provides additional information that primary tumor is malignant, detects lymph node and intrathoracic and distant metastases
6. Transthoracic needle biopsy (under fluoroscopic or CT guidance)
   a. Needle biopsy of suspicious pulmonary masses is highly accurate, and is useful for diagnosing peripheral lesions as well
   b. Needle biopsy is invasive and must be used **only** in selected patients. This is a better biopsy method for peripheral lesions, whereas central, peribronchial lesions should be biopsied using bronchoscopy
7. Mediastinoscopy
   a. Allows direct visualization of the superior mediastinum
   b. Identifies patients with advanced disease who would not benefit from surgical resection

D. Treatment

1. NSCLC
   a. Surgery is the best option.
      - A definitive pathologic diagnosis must be made prior to surgery.
      - Patients with metastatic disease outside the chest are **not** candidates for surgery.
      - Recurrence may occur even after complete resection.
   b. Radiation therapy is an important adjunct to surgery.
   c. Chemotherapy is of uncertain benefit. Some studies show a modest increase in survival. More trials are underway.

2. SCLC
   a. For limited disease, combination of chemotherapy and radiation therapy is used initially.
   b. For extensive disease, chemotherapy is used alone as initial treatment. If patient responds to initial chemotherapy treatment, prophylactic radiation decreases incidence of brain metastases and prolongs survival.
   c. Surgery has a limited role because these tumors are usually nonresectable.

Quick HIT
Most asymptomatic masses are benign.

Solitary Pulmonary Nodule

A. A single, well-circumscribed nodule usually discovered incidentally with no associated mediastinal or hilar lymph node involvement. The main question is whether the lesion is malignant and requires biopsy or resection (see Figure 2-5).

B. Has a wide differential diagnosis (e.g., infectious granuloma, bronchogenic carcinoma, hamartoma, bronchial adenoma), but one must investigate the possibility of malignancy because resection can lead to a cure with early detection

C. Several features favor benign versus malignant nodules:
1. Age—the older the patient, the more likely it is malignant—over 50% chance of malignancy if patient is over 50.
2. Smoking—if history of smoking, more likely to be malignant.
3. Size of nodule—the larger the nodule, the more likely it is malignant. Small is <1 cm, large >2 cm.
4. Borders—Malignant nodules have more irregular borders. Benign lesions have smooth/discrete borders.
5. Calcification—Eccentric asymmetric calcification suggests malignancy. Dense, central calcification suggests benign lesion.
6. Change is size—enlarging nodule suggests malignancy.

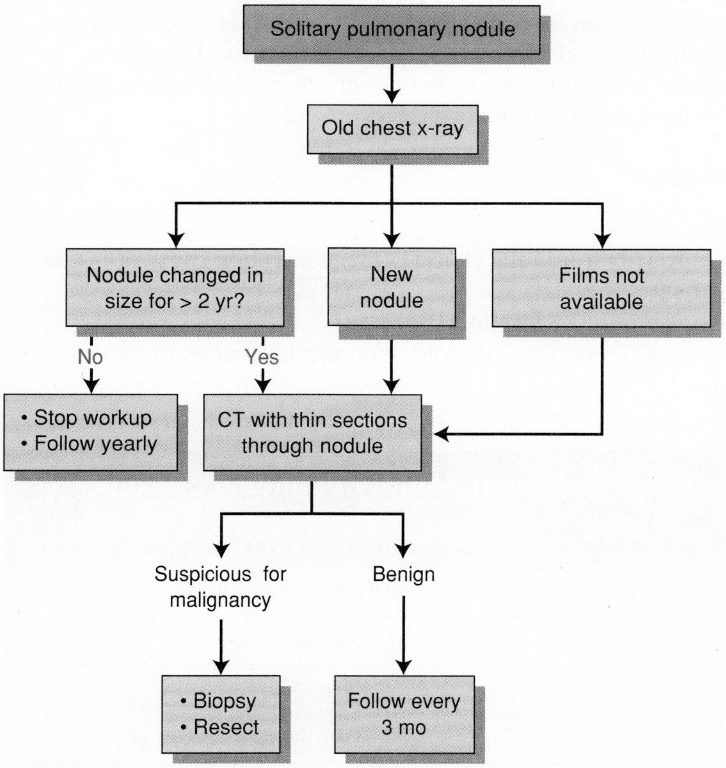

FIGURE 2-5 **Evaluation of a solitary pulmonary nodule.**
(Adapted from Humes DH, DuPont HL, Gardner LB, et al. *Kelley's Textbook of Internal Medicine.* 4th ed. Philadelphia, PA: Lippincott Williams & Wilkins, 2000:2574, Figure 386.6.)

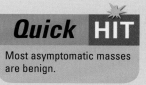

TABLE 2-4 Types of Lung Cancer

Pathologic Type		Incidence	Location	Special Features
NSCLC	Squamous cell carcinoma	30% of all lung cancers	Usually central	Cavitation on CXR
	Adenocarcinoma	35% of all lung cancers—most common type	Often peripheral	• Pleural involvement in 20% of cases • Less closely associated with smoking than other types • Can be associated with pulmonary scars/fibrosis
	Large cell carcinoma	5%–10% of all lung cancers	Usually peripheral	
SCLC		20%–25% of all lung cancers	Central	• Tend to narrow bronchi by extrinsic compression • Widespread metastases are common. 50%–75% of patients have metastases outside the chest at the time of presentation.

D. Considering the above factors, one designates the nodule as low, intermediate, or high probability of being malignant.
1. Low-probability nodules—serial CT scan
2. Intermediate-probability nodule 1 cm or larger—PET scan. If PET positive, biopsy
3. High-probability nodule—biopsy (transbronchial, transthoracic, or video-assisted thoracoscopic surgery) followed by lobectomy if appropriate.

E. Previous CXR is very helpful: Every effort should be made to find a previous CXR for comparison. If the lesion is stable for more than 2 years, it is likely benign. Malignant lesions grow relatively rapidly (growth is usually evident within months) (see Table 2-4). However, growth over a period of days is usually nonmalignant (often infectious/inflammatory) (see Table 2-5).

Mediastinal Masses

A. Causes

1. Metastatic cancer (especially from lung cancer)—most common cause of mediastinal mass in older patients
2. Most common cause according to location:
   a. Anterior mediastinum: "Four T's"—thyroid, teratogenic tumors, thymoma, terrible lymphoma

TABLE 2-5 Benign Versus Malignant Solitary Pulmonary Nodules

Factors That Favor a Benign Diagnosis	Factors That Favor Malignancy
Age <50 yrs	Age >50 yrs
Nonsmoker	Smoker or previous smoker
Size of nodule <2 cm	Size of nodule >3 cm
No growth over 2-yr period	Steady growth over serial radiographs
Nodule circular and regular shaped	Nodule grossly irregular or speculated margin
Central laminated calcification	Stippled or eccentric pattern of calcification

b. Middle mediastinum: lung cancer, lymphoma, aneurysms, cysts, Morgagni hernia
c. Posterior mediastinum: neurogenic tumors, esophageal masses, enteric cysts, aneurysms, Bochdalek hernia

B. Clinical features

1. Usually asymptomatic
   a. When symptoms are present, they are due to compression or invasion of adjacent structures
   b. Cough (compression of trachea or bronchi), sometimes hemoptysis
   c. Chest pain, dyspnea
   d. Postobstructive pneumonia
   e. Dysphagia (compression of esophagus)
   f. SVC syndrome
   g. Compression of nerves
      - Hoarseness (recurrent laryngeal nerve)
      - Horner syndrome (sympathetic ganglia)
      - Diaphragm paralysis (phrenic nerve)

C. Diagnosis

1. Chest CT is test of choice
2. Usually discovered incidentally on a CXR performed for another reason

Quick HIT

If CT scan suggests a benign mass and the patient is asymptomatic, observation is appropriate.

Diseases of the Pleura

Pleural Effusion

A. General characteristics

1. Caused by one of the following mechanisms: increased drainage of fluid into pleural space, increased production of fluid by cells in the pleural space, or decreased drainage of fluid from the pleural space (see Figure 2-6)
2. Transudative effusions—pathophysiology is due to either elevated capillary pressure in visceral or parenteral pleura (e.g., CHF), or decreased plasma oncotic pressure (e.g., hypoalbuminemia)
3. Exudative effusions
   a. Pathophysiology: caused by increased permeability of pleural surfaces or decreased lymphatic flow from pleural surface because of damage to pleural membranes or vasculature (see Clinical Pearl 2-4).

Quick HIT

If the patient has minimal lung compromise, pleural effusions are well tolerated, whereas pleural effusion in the presence of lung disease may lead to respiratory failure.

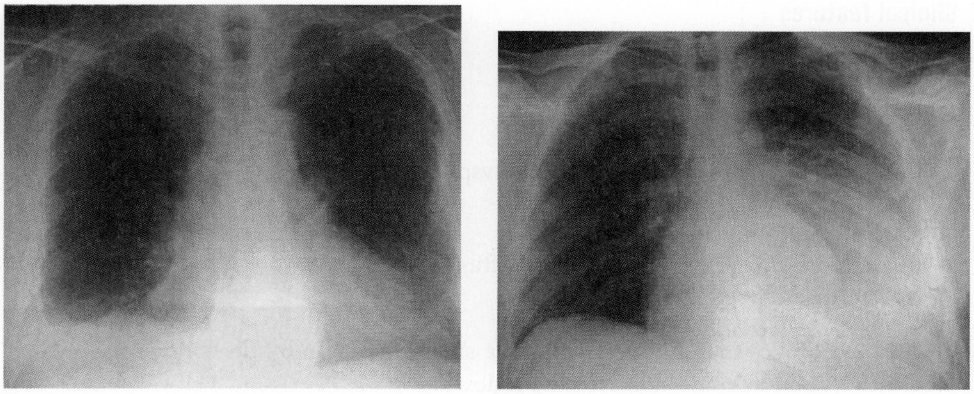

A B

FIGURE 2-6 **A: Upright chest radiograph showing blunting of the right costophrenic angle, typical of a small right pleural effusion (this patient had chronic liver disease). B: Chest radiograph showing left pleural effusion.**

(From Stern EJ, White CS. *Chest Radiology Companion.* Philadelphia, PA: Lippincott, Williams & Wilkins, 1999:375, Figure 22-1A; 376, Figure 22-2A.)

CLINICAL PEARL 2-4

Causes of Transudative and Exudative Pleural Effusions

Transudative

- CHF
- Cirrhosis
- PE
- Nephrotic syndrome
- Peritoneal dialysis
- Hypoalbuminemia
- Atelectasis

Exudative

- Bacterial pneumonia, TB
- Malignancy, metastatic disease
- Viral infection
- PE
- Collagen vascular diseases

Quick HIT

Pleural Fluid Pearls

- Elevated pleural fluid amylase: esophageal rupture, pancreatitis, malignancy
- Milky, opalescent fluid: **chylothorax** (lymph in the pleural space)
- Frankly purulent fluid: **empyema** (pus in the pleural space)
- Bloody effusion: malignancy
- Exudative effusions that are primarily lymphocytic: TB
- pH <7.2: **parapneumonic effusion** or empyema

Quick HIT

If pleural fluid glucose level is <60, consider rheumatoid arthritis. However, glucose in pleural fluid can be low with other causes of pleural effusion: TB, esophageal rupture, malignancy, lupus.

b. If an exudative effusion is suspected, perform the following tests on the pleural fluid: differential cell count, total protein, LDH, glucose, pH, amylase, triglycerides, microbiology, and cytology.

c. Exudative effusions meet at least one of the following of Light's criteria (transudates have none of these):
- Protein (pleural)/protein (serum) >0.5
- LDH (pleural)/LDH (serum) >0.6
- LDH > two-thirds the upper limit of normal serum LDH

B. Causes

1. CHF is most common cause
2. Pneumonia (bacterial)
3. Malignancies: lung (36%), breast (25%), lymphoma (10%)
4. Pulmonary embolism (PE)
5. Viral diseases
6. Cirrhosis with ascites

C. Clinical features

1. Symptoms
   a. Often asymptomatic
   b. Dyspnea on exertion
   c. Peripheral edema
   d. Orthopnea, paroxysmal nocturnal dyspnea
2. Signs
   a. Dullness to percussion
   b. Decreased breath sounds over the effusion
   c. Decreased tactile fremitus

D. Diagnosis: Can confirm presence/evaluate size of effusion by the following:

1. CXR (PA and lateral)—look for the following:
   a. Blunting of costophrenic angle
   b. About 250 mL of pleural fluid must accumulate before an effusion can be detected.
   c. Lateral decubitus films: more reliable than PA and lateral CXRs for detecting small pleural effusions; can also determine whether fluid is free flowing or loculated

2. CT scan—more reliable than CXR for detecting effusions
3. Thoracentesis
   a. Thoracentesis is useful if etiology is not obvious. It provides a diagnosis in 75% of patients, and even when it is not diagnostic it provides important clinical information.
   b. Therapeutic—drainage provides relief for large effusions.
   c. Pneumothorax is a complication seen in 10% to 15% of thoracenteses, but it requires treatment with a chest tube in <5% of cases. Do not perform thoracentesis if effusion is <10-mm thick on lateral internal decubitus CXR.

E. Treatment

1. Transudative effusions
   a. Diuretics and sodium restriction
   b. Therapeutic thoracentesis—only if massive effusion is causing dyspnea
2. Exudative effusions: treat underlying disease
3. Parapneumonic effusions (pleural effusion in presence of pneumonia)
   a. Uncomplicated effusions: antibiotics alone (in most cases)
   b. Complicated effusions or empyema
      - Chest tube drainage
      - Intrapleural injection of thrombolytic agents (streptokinase or urokinase); may accelerate the drainage
      - Surgical lysis of adhesions may be required

Empyema

A. Causes

1. Exudative pleural effusions, if left untreated, can lead to empyema (pus within the pleural space).
2. Most cases occur as a complication of bacterial pneumonia, but other foci of infection can also spread to the pleural space (e.g., mediastinitis, abscess).

B. Clinical features: The clinical features are those of the underlying disease (pneumonia most common).

C. Diagnosis: CXR and CT scan of the chest are the recommended tests.

D. Treatment

1. Treat empyema with aggressive drainage of the pleura (via thoracentesis) and antibiotic therapy.
2. The infection is very difficult to eradicate, and recurrence is common, requiring repeated drainage.
3. If empyema is severe and persistent, rib resection and open drainage may be necessary.

Pneumothorax

A. General characteristics

1. Defined as air in the normally airless pleural space.
2. There are two major categories: spontaneous and traumatic pneumothoraces.
3. Traumatic pneumothoraces are often iatrogenic.
4. Spontaneous pneumothorax occurs without any trauma.
   a. Primary (simple) pneumothorax
      - Occurs without any underlying lung disease—that is, in "healthy" individuals
      - Caused by spontaneous rupture of subpleural blebs (air-filled sacs on the lung) at the apex of lungs—escape of air from the lung into pleural space causes lung to collapse
      - More common in tall, lean young men

Quick HIT

- A parapneumonic effusion is a noninfected pleural effusion secondary to bacterial pneumonia.
- An empyema is a complicated parapneumonic effusion, which means the pleural effusion is infected.

Quick HIT

Spontaneous pneumothorax has a high recurrence rate—50% in **2 years.**

- These patients have sufficient pulmonary reserve, so severe respiratory distress does not occur in most cases.
- Recurrence rate is 50% in 2 years

b. Secondary (complicated) pneumothorax
- Occurs as a complication of underlying lung disease, most commonly COPD; other underlying conditions include asthma, interstitial lung disease (ILD), neoplasms, CF, and tuberculosis (TB)
- Is more life-threatening because of lack of pulmonary reserve in these patients

B. Clinical features

1. Symptoms
   a. Ipsilateral chest pain, usually sudden in onset
   b. Dyspnea
   c. Cough
2. Physical signs
   a. Decreased breath sounds over the affected side
   b. Hyperresonance over the chest
   c. Decreased or absent tactile fremitus on affected side
   d. Mediastinal shift toward side of pneumothorax

C. Diagnosis: CXR confirms the diagnosis—shows the visceral pleural line (see Figure 2-7)

D. Treatment

1. Primary spontaneous pneumothorax
   a. If small and patient is asymptomatic:
      - Observation—should resolve spontaneously in approximately 10 days
      - Small chest tube (with one-way valve) may benefit some patients.
   b. If pneumothorax is larger and/or patient is symptomatic:
      - Administration of supplemental oxygen
      - Needle aspiration or chest tube insertion to allow air to be released and lung to reexpand
2. Secondary spontaneous pneumothorax—chest tube drainage

Tension Pneumothorax

A. General characteristics

1. Accumulation of air within the pleural space such that tissues surrounding the opening into the pleural cavity act as valves, allowing air to enter but not to escape.
2. The accumulation of air under (positive) pressure in the pleural space **collapses the ipsilateral lung** and **shifts the mediastinum away** from the side of the pneumothorax.

B. Causes

1. Mechanical ventilation with associated barotrauma
2. CPR
3. Trauma

Quick HIT

Do not obtain CXR if a tension pneumothorax is suspected. Immediately decompress the pleural space via large-bore needle or chest tube!

C. Clinical features

1. Hypotension—cardiac filling is impaired due to compression of the great veins
2. Distended neck veins
3. Shift of trachea **away** from side of pneumothorax on CXR (see Figure 2-8)
4. Decreased breath sounds on affected side
5. Hyperresonance to percussion on side of pneumothorax

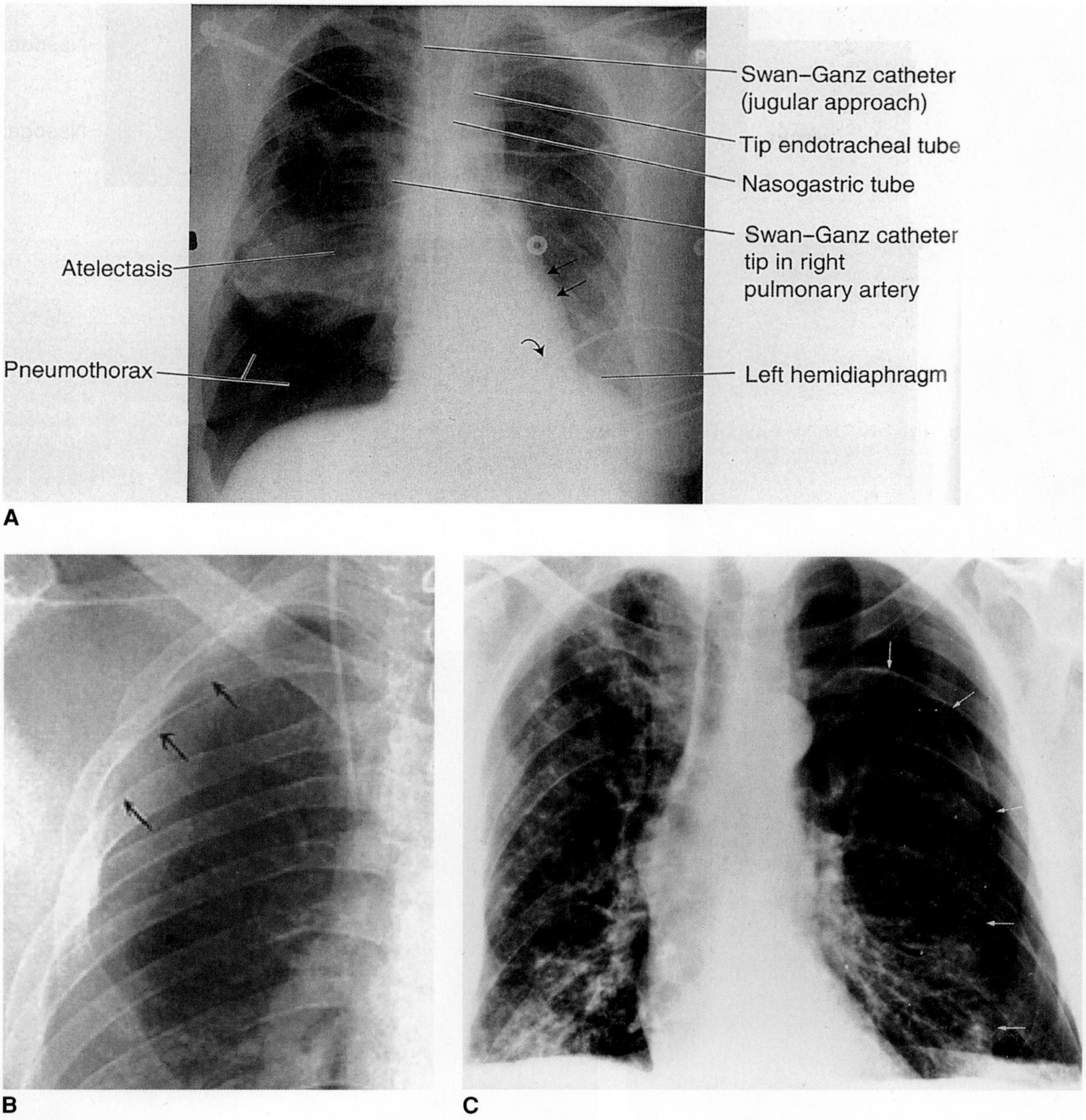

FIGURE 2-7 **A: Right pneumothorax seen in a patient on a ventilator. B: Chest radiograph showing a right pneumothorax that occurred as a complication of placement of a central line. These small pneumothoraces are often difficult to detect. C: Large left pneumothorax.**

(**A** from Erkonen WE, Smith WL. *Radiology 101: The Basics and Fundamentals of Imaging.* Philadelphia, PA: Lippincott Williams & Wilkins, 1998:100, Figure 6-41B.) (**B** from Stern EJ, White CS. *Chest Radiology Companion.* Philadelphia, PA: Lippincott Williams & Wilkins, 1999:381, Figure 22-9.) (**C** from Daffner RH. *Clinical Radiology: The Essentials.* 2nd ed. Philadelphia, PA: Lippincott Williams & Wilkins, 1999:82, Figure 4.11B.)

D. Treatment

1. Must be treated as a **medical emergency**—If the tension in the pleural space is not relieved, the patient is likely to die of hemodynamic compromise (inadequate CO or hypoxemia).
2. Immediately perform chest decompression with a large-bore needle (in the second or third intercostal space in the midclavicular line), followed by chest tube placement.

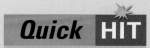

Quick HIT

Not all mesotheliomas are malignant. Benign mesotheliomas have an excellent prognosis (and are unrelated to asbestos exposure).

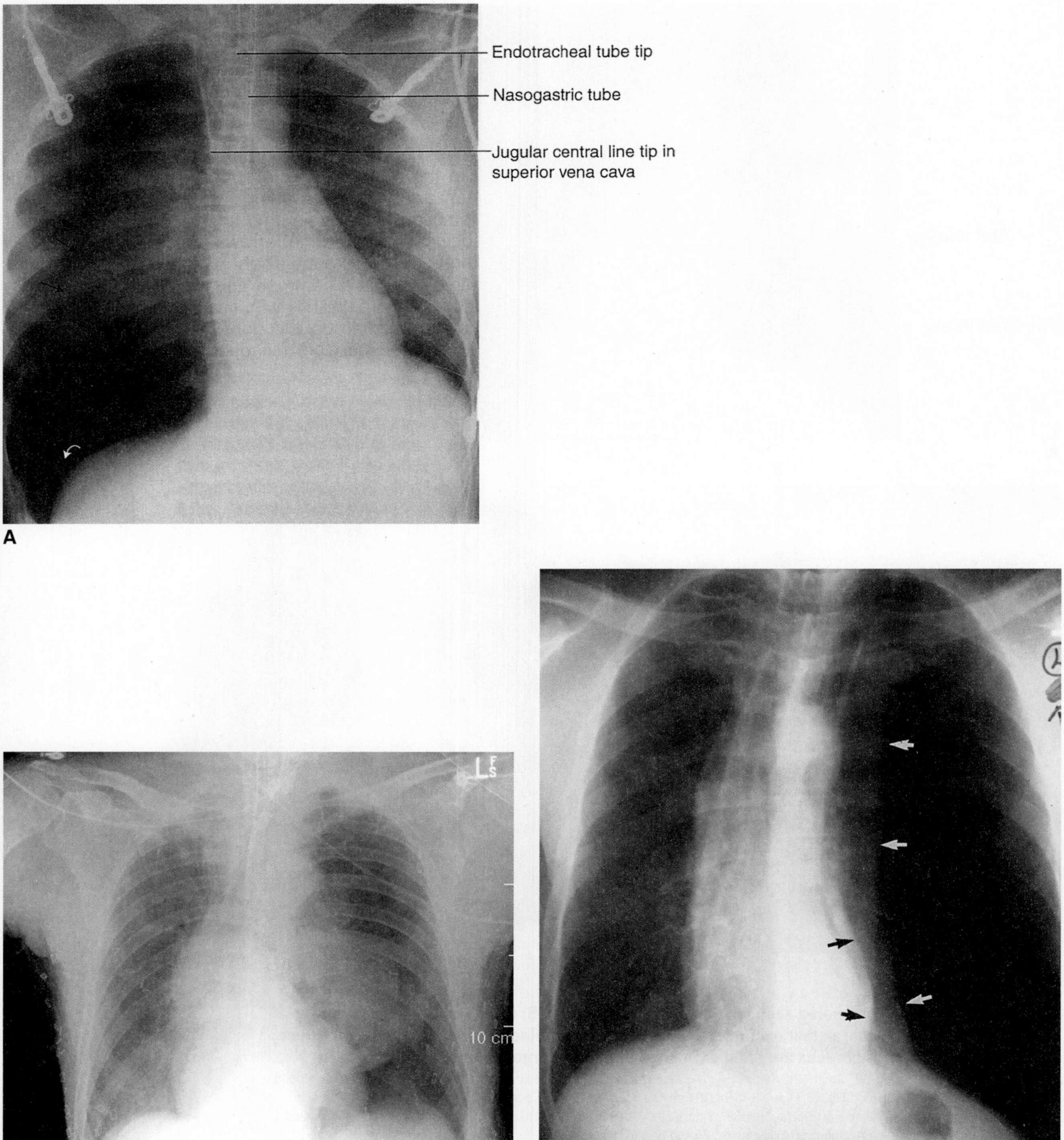

FIGURE 2-8 **A: Example of a right tension pneumothorax. Note that the mediastinum is displaced to the left. B: Tension pneumothorax. C: Tension pneumothorax.**

(**A** from Erkonen WE, Smith WL. *Radiology 101: The Basics and Fundamentals of Imaging.* Philadelphia, PA: Lippincott Williams & Wilkins, 1998:100, Figure 6-41C.) (**B** from Mergo PJ. *Imaging of the Chest—A Teaching File.* Philadelphia, PA: Lippincott Williams & Wilkins, 2002:258, Figure 145.) (**C** from Topol EJ. *Textbook of Cardiovascular Medicine.* 2nd ed. Philadelphia, PA: Lippincott Williams & Wilkins, 2002:1050, Figure 47.2.)

Malignant Mesothelioma

- Most cases are secondary to asbestos exposure.
- Dyspnea, weight loss, and cough are common findings.
- Bloody effusion is common.
- Prognosis is dismal (few months' survival).

Interstitial Lung Disease

Overview

A. General characteristics

1. ILD is defined as an inflammatory process involving the alveolar wall (resulting in widespread fibroelastic proliferation and collagen deposition) that can lead to irreversible fibrosis, distortion of lung architecture, and impaired gas exchange.
2. The prognosis is very variable and depends on the diagnosis.
3. Patients with environmental or occupational lung disease, especially those with asbestosis, are frequently involved in lawsuits against their employers.

B. Classification

1. Classified based on pathologic and clinical characteristics
2. Environmental lung disease
   a. Coal worker's pneumoconiosis
   b. Silicosis
   c. Asbestosis
   d. Berylliosis
3. ILD associated with granulomas
   a. Sarcoidosis—other organs in addition to the lungs are involved.
   b. Histiocytosis X
   c. Wegener granulomatosis
   d. Churg–Strauss syndrome
4. Alveolar filling disease
   a. Goodpasture syndrome
   b. Idiopathic pulmonary hemosiderosis
   c. Alveolar proteinosis
5. Hypersensitivity lung disease
   a. Hypersensitivity pneumonitis
   b. Eosinophilic pneumonitis
6. Drug-induced—amiodarone, nitrofurantoin, bleomycin, phenytoin, illicit drugs
7. Miscellaneous
   a. Idiopathic pulmonary fibrosis
   b. Cryptogenic organizing pneumonia (COP)
   c. ILD associated with connective tissue disorders: rheumatoid arthritis, scleroderma, SLE, mixed connective tissue disease
   d. Radiation pneumonitis

C. Clinical features

1. Symptoms
   a. Dyspnea (at first with exertion; later at rest)
   b. Cough (nonproductive)
   c. Fatigue
   d. Other symptoms may be present secondary to another condition (such as a connective tissue disorder)
2. Signs
   a. Rales at the bases are common
   b. Digital clubbing is common (especially with idiopathic pulmonary fibrosis) (see Figure 2-9 and Clinical Pearl 2-5)
   c. Signs of pulmonary HTN and cyanosis in advanced disease

Quick HIT

If ILD is suspected, ask about the following:
- Medication history, because some drugs are known to be toxic to lungs (chemotherapeutic agents, gold, amiodarone, penicillamine, and nitrofurantoin)
- Previous jobs, because occupational exposure is a cause of ILD (asbestos, silicone, beryllium, coal)

Quick HIT

Over 100 causes of ILD have been identified.
- In general, the clinical findings and imaging study results are nonspecific and do not point to a definitive diagnosis. Often one is confronted with the question of whether to obtain a tissue biopsy.

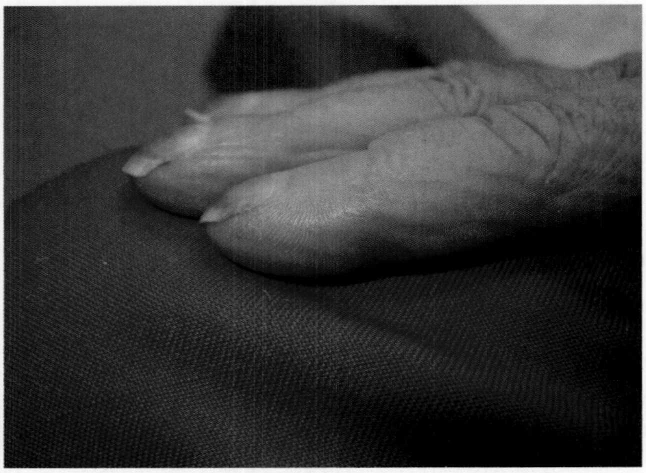

FIGURE
2-9 **Clubbing of the finger.**
(From *Stedman's Medical Dictionary.* 28th ed. Philadelphia, PA: Lippincott Williams & Wilkins, 2005.)

D. Diagnosis

1. CXR (see Figure 2-10)
   a. Findings are usually nonspecific.
   b. Typical diffuse changes are noted (reticular, reticulonodular, ground glass, honeycombing).
2. High-resolution CT scan shows the extent of fibrosis better than other imaging modalities.
3. PFTs
   a. A restrictive pattern is noted: FEV_1/FVC ratio is increased. All lung volumes are low. Both FEV_1 and FVC are low, but the latter more so.
   b. Low diffusing capacity (DL_{CO}).
4. Oxygen desaturation during exercise.
5. Bronchoalveolar lavage (fluid for culture and cytology)—Use is controversial because results are quite variable.
6. Tissue biopsy.
   a. This is often required in patients with ILD, though high-resolution CT can often be used to make the diagnosis without the need for biopsy.
   b. This can be done via fiberoptic bronchoscopy with transbronchial biopsy (a limited amount of tissue can be obtained, which limits its utility), open lung biopsy, or video-assisted thoracoscopic lung biopsy.
7. Urinalysis, if there are signs of glomerular injury (for Goodpasture syndrome and Wegener granulomatosis)

Quick HIT

"Honeycomb lung" refers to a scarred shrunken lung and is an end-stage finding with poor prognosis. Air spaces are dilated, and there are fibrous scars in the interstitium. It can arise from many different types of ILD.

CLINICAL PEARL 2-5

Clubbing of the Fingers

- Increased convexity of the nail—the distal phalanx is enlarged due to an increase in soft tissue.
- If a patient has clubbing, get a CXR because lung disease may be present.
- Chronic hypoxia is the underlying cause in most cases.
- Differential diagnoses vary and include pulmonary diseases (lung cancer, CF, ILD, empyema, sarcoidosis, and mesothelioma), congenital heart disease, bacterial endocarditis, biliary cirrhosis, inflammatory bowel disease, and primary biliary cirrhosis.
- Digital clubbing may be an idiopathic or primary finding, such as in familial clubbing or hypertrophic osteoarthropathy.

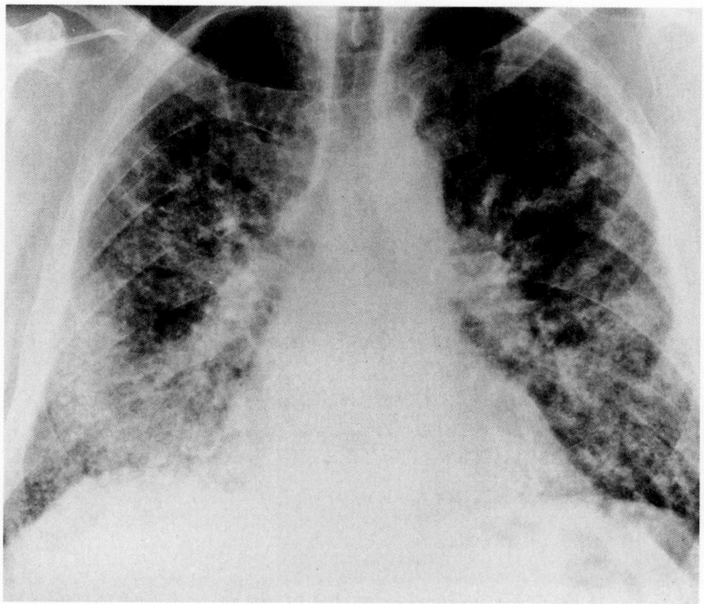

FIGURE
2-10 **Example of interstitial lung disease: Chest radiograph shows extensive pulmonary fibrosis.**
(From Daffner RH. *Clinical Radiology: The Essentials.* 2nd ed. Philadelphia, PA: Lippincott Williams & Wilkins, 1999:152, Figure 4.89A.)

Interstitial Lung Diseases Associated With Granulomas

A. Sarcoidosis

1. **General characteristics**
   a. A chronic systemic granulomatous disease characterized by **noncaseating granulomas**, often involving multiple organ systems. Lungs are almost always involved. Etiology unknown.
   b. Occurs most often in the **African American population**, especially women.
   c. 75% of cases occur when individual is <40 years of age.
   d. Sarcoidosis carries a good prognosis in majority of patients.
2. **Clinical features**
   a. Constitutional symptoms
      - Malaise, fever, anorexia, weight loss
      - Symptoms vary in severity and may be absent in many patients.
   b. Lungs: dry cough, dyspnea (especially with exercise)
   c. Skin (25% of cases)
      - **Erythema nodosum**
      - Plaques, subcutaneous nodules, maculopapular eruptions
   d. Eyes (25% of cases)—may result in significant visual impairment
      - **Anterior uveitis** (75%)
      - Posterior uveitis (25%)
      - Conjunctivitis
   e. Heart (5% of cases)
      - Arrhythmias
      - Conduction disturbances, such as heart block
      - Sudden death
   f. Musculoskeletal system (25% to 50%)
      - Arthralgias and arthritis
      - Bone lesions
   g. Nervous system (5%)
      - Cranial nerve VII involvement (Bell palsy)
      - Optic nerve dysfunction
      - Papilledema
      - Peripheral neuropathy

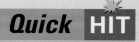

Quick HIT

- Up to two-thirds of patients with sarcoidosis experience resolution/improvement of symptoms over several years.
- Approximately 20% of patients develop chronic disease.
- From 10% to 20% of patients are asymptomatic but have CXR findings.

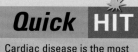

Quick HIT

Cardiac disease is the most common cause of death, although it is not a common finding.

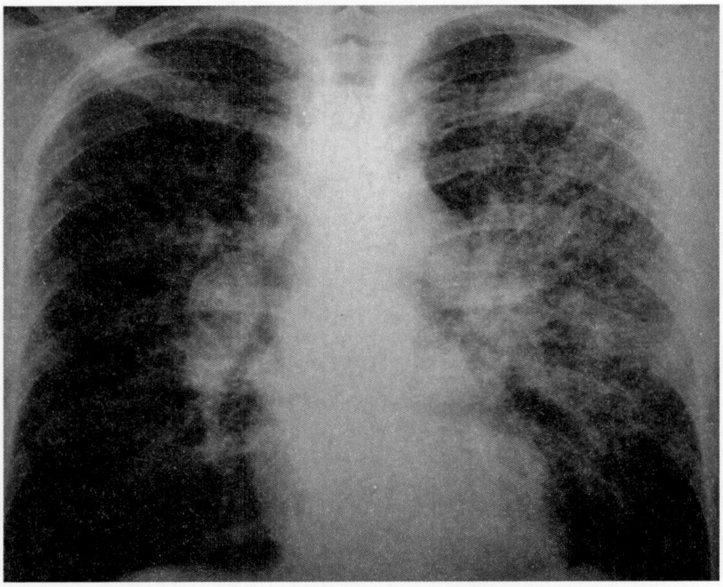

FIGURE 2-11 **Chest radiograph in a patient with sarcoidosis. Note enlargement of mediastinal and hilar lymph nodes, as well as diffuse interstitial disease, especially on the left.**
(From Daffner RH. *Clinical Radiology: The Essentials.* 2nd ed. Philadelphia, PA: Lippincott Williams & Wilkins, 1999:140, Figure 4.75B.)

Quick HIT

Typical presentation of sarcoidosis: young patient with constitutional symptoms, respiratory complaints, erythema nodosum, blurred vision, and bilateral hilar adenopathy.

3. **Diagnosis**
   a. Diagnosis is based on clinical, radiographic, and histologic findings.
   b. CXR—**Bilateral hilar adenopathy** is the hallmark of this disease but is not specific; it is seen in 50% of cases (see Figure 2-11). Four stages have been described based on CXR findings (see below).
   c. Skin anergy—typical finding but not diagnostic
   d. **Angiotensin-converting enzyme (ACE)** is elevated in serum in about 50% to 80% of patients. This test helps support the diagnosis. However, other pulmonary diseases may cause an elevation in this enzyme (lacks sensitivity and specificity).
   e. Hypercalciuria and hypercalcemia are common.
   f. Definitive diagnosis requires transbronchial biopsy:
      - Must see **noncaseating granulomas**
      - By itself is not diagnostic because noncaseating granulomas are found in other diseases
      - Must be used in the context of clinical presentation
   g. PFTs: decreased lung volumes (VC and TLC), decreased DL_{CO} (diffusing capacity for carbon monoxide), decreased FEV_1/FVC ratio
4. **Staging of sarcoidosis (on CXR)**
   a. Stage I: bilateral hilar adenopathy without parenchymal infiltrates (highest rate of remission)
   b. Stage II: hilar adenopathy with parenchymal infiltrates
   c. Stage III: diffuse parenchymal infiltrates without hilar adenopathy (least favorable prognosis)
   d. Stage IV: pulmonary fibrosis with honeycombing and fibrocystic parenchymal changes
5. **Treatment**
   a. Most cases resolve or significantly improve spontaneously in 2 years and do not require treatment.
   b. **Systemic corticosteroids are the treatment of choice.** The indications for treatment are unclear. However, patients who are symptomatic or have active lung disease, pulmonary function deterioration, conduction disturbances, or severe skin or eye involvement should be treated.
   c. Methotrexate used in patients with progressive disease refractory to corticosteroids.

B. Histiocytosis X

1. Chronic interstitial pneumonia caused by abnormal proliferation of histiocytes (related to Langerhans cells of the skin).
2. Most patients (90%) are cigarette smokers.
3. Variants of disease include eosinophilic granuloma (localized to bone or lung), and two systemic forms—Letterer–Siwe disease and Hand–Schüller–Christian syndrome.
4. Common findings include dyspnea and nonproductive cough.
5. Other possible manifestations are spontaneous pneumothorax, lytic bone lesions, and diabetes insipidus.
6. CXR has a honeycomb appearance, and CT scan shows cystic lesions.
7. The prognosis and course are highly variable. Corticosteroids are sometimes effective. Lung transplantation may be necessary.

C. Wegener granulomatosis

1. Rare disease with unknown etiology.
2. Characterized by necrotizing granulomatous vasculitis.
3. Affects vessels of lungs, kidneys, upper airway, and sometimes other organs.
4. Manifestations of the disease include upper and lower respiratory infections, glomerulonephritis, and pulmonary nodules.
5. The gold standard for diagnosis is tissue biopsy, but if the patient tests positive for c-antineutrophilic cytoplasmic antibodies, the likelihood of having this condition is high.
6. Treatment usually includes immunosuppressive agents and glucocorticoids.

Quick HIT

Antineutrophilic cytoplasmic antibodies (ANCA) and associated ILD: c-ANCA: Wegener granulomatosis; **p-ANCA** Churg–Strauss syndrome; may also be positive in Goodpasture syndrome.

D. Churg–Strauss syndrome

1. Granulomatous vasculitis is **seen in patients with asthma.**
2. Typically presents with pulmonary infiltrates, rash, and eosinophilia.
3. Systemic vasculitis may result in skin, muscle, and nerve lesions.
4. Diagnosis.
5. Significant blood eosinophilia is common.
6. Associated with perinuclear antineutrophilic cytoplasmic antibody.
7. Treat with systemic glucocorticoids.

Environmental Lung Disease/Pneumoconiosis

Quick HIT

- Pneumoconiosis is defined as the accumulation of dust in the lungs, and the tissue reaction to its presence.
- Dusts that have been implicated: silica, beryllium, asbestos, coal dust, graphite, carbon black, aluminum, talc.

A. Coal worker's pneumoconiosis

1. Most have simple coal worker's pneumoconiosis, which usually causes no significant respiratory disability.
2. Some patients may develop complicated pneumoconiosis, which is characterized by fibrosis (restrictive lung disease).
3. Causes: inhalation of coal dust, which contains carbon and silica.

B. Asbestosis

1. Characterized by diffuse interstitial fibrosis of the lung caused by inhalation of asbestos fibers; predilection for lower lobes.
2. Develops insidiously many years (>15 to 20 years) after exposure.
3. **Increased risk of bronchogenic carcinoma (smoking is synergistic) and malignant mesothelioma.**
4. Symptoms and physical findings are nonspecific (see above under ILD).
5. Diagnosis made based on clinical findings and history of exposure to asbestos.
6. CXR shows hazy infiltrates with bilateral linear opacities and may show pleural plaques (especially in lower lung regions).
7. No specific treatment is available.

Quick HIT

Classic CXR findings in environmental lung disease:
- Asbestosis: pleural plaques
- Silicosis: "egg shell" calcifications

C. Silicosis

1. **Localized** and **nodular** peribronchial fibrosis (upper lobes more common).
2. Can be acute (massive exposure leading to rapid onset and death), or chronic (symptoms years after exposure—up to 15 years or longer).

3. Associated with an increased risk of TB.
4. **Sources include mining, stone cutting, and glass manufacturing.**
5. Exertional dyspnea is the main symptom; cough with sputum is also seen.
6. There are restrictive pulmonary function abnormalities.
7. Treatment involves removal from exposure to silica.

D. Berylliosis

1. Like silicosis, berylliosis has acute and chronic forms.
2. Acute disease is a diffuse pneumonitis caused by massive exposure to beryllium.
3. Chronic disease is very similar to sarcoidosis: granulomas, skin lesions, and hypercalcemia may be present.
4. The beryllium lymphocyte proliferation test is a useful diagnostic blood test.
5. Give glucocorticoid therapy for both acute and chronic berylliosis.

Quick HIT

Some causes of hypersensitivity pneumonitis:

- Farmer's lung* (moldy hay)
- Bird-breeder's lung (avian droppings)
- Air-conditioner lung*
- Bagassosis* (moldy sugar cane)
- Mushroom worker's lung* (compost)

*Caused by spores of thermophilic actinomycetes.

Interstitial Lung Disease Associated With Hypersensitivity

A. Hypersensitivity pneumonitis (extrinsic allergic alveolitis)

1. Inhalation of an antigenic agent to the alveolar level induces an immune-mediated pneumonitis. Chronic exposure may lead to restrictive lung disease.
2. A variety of organic dusts and chemicals have been implicated.
3. The presence of serum IgG and IgA to the inhaled antigen is a hallmark finding, although many may have these antibodies without developing disease.
4. The acute form has flu-like features (e.g., fever, chills, cough, dyspnea). CXR during the acute phase shows pulmonary infiltrates.
5. The chronic form is more insidious and more difficult to diagnose.
6. Treatment involves removal of the offending agent and sometimes glucocorticoids.

B. Eosinophilic pneumonia

1. Fever and peripheral eosinophilia are features.
2. Eosinophilic pneumonia may be acute or chronic.
3. CXR shows peripheral pulmonary infiltrates.
4. Treatment with glucocorticoids is usually very effective, but relapses may occur.

C. Note that there is significant overlap between this category and the ILD associated with granuloma (e.g., Churg–Strauss syndrome).

Alveolar Filling Disease

A. Goodpasture syndrome

1. Autoimmune disease caused by IgG antibodies directed against glomerular and alveolar basement membranes (type II hypersensitivity reaction).
2. Results in hemorrhagic pneumonitis and glomerulonephritis.
3. Ultimately, renal failure is a complication of proliferative glomerulonephritis.
4. Usually presents with hemoptysis and dyspnea.
5. Diagnosis made by tissue biopsy, serologic evidence of antiglomerular basement membrane antibodies.
6. Prognosis is poor; treat with plasmapheresis, cyclophosphamide, and corticosteroids.

B. Pulmonary alveolar proteinosis

1. Rare condition caused by accumulation of surfactant-like protein and phospholipids in the alveoli.
2. Usually presents with dry cough, dyspnea, hypoxia, and rales.
3. **CXR typically has a ground glass appearance with bilateral alveolar infiltrates that resemble a bat shape.**
4. Lung biopsy is required for definitive diagnosis.
5. Treatment is with lung lavage and granulocyte colony-stimulating factor.
6. Patients are at increased risk of infection, and steroids should not be given.

Miscellaneous Interstitial Lung Disease

A. Idiopathic pulmonary fibrosis

1. General characteristics
   a. Etiology unknown; more common in men and smokers.
   b. Presents with gradual onset of progressive dyspnea, nonproductive cough.
   c. This is a devastating and unrelenting disease. Although the prognosis is variable, the mean survival is only 3 to 7 years after first diagnosis.
2. Diagnosis
   a. CXR: ground glass or a honeycombed appearance; may be normal.
   b. Definitive diagnosis requires open lung biopsy consistent with usual interstitial pneumonia.
   c. Other causes of ILD must be excluded.
3. **Treatment.** No effective treatment is available. The majority of patients (>70%) do not improve with therapy and experience progressive and gradual respiratory failure. The following can benefit some patients:
   a. Supplemental oxygen.
   b. Corticosteroids have been used historically but with little or no benefit and have significant side effects.
   c. Lung transplantation.

B. Cryptogenic organizing pneumonitis (COP)

1. An inflammatory lung disease with similar clinical and radiographic features to infectious pneumonia.
2. Associated with many entities (viral infections, medications, connective tissue disease). Most cases are idiopathic.
3. Features: cough, dyspnea, and flu-like symptoms; bilateral patchy infiltrates on CXR.
4. Antibiotics have not been found to be effective.
5. Spontaneous recovery may occur, but corticosteroids are used most commonly (>60% of patients recover).
6. Relapse may occur after cessation of steroids (requiring resumption of steroids).

C. Radiation pneumonitis

1. Interstitial pulmonary inflammation—occurs in 5% to 15% of patients who undergo thoracic irradiation for lung cancer, breast cancer, lymphoma, or thymoma. Mortality and morbidity are related to the irradiated lung volume, dose, patient status, and concurrent chemotherapy.
2. Acute form occurs 1 to 6 months after irradiation; chronic form develops 1 to 2 years later—characterized by alveolar thickening and pulmonary fibrosis.
3. Features: low-grade fever, cough, chest fullness, dyspnea, pleuritic chest pain, hemoptysis, acute respiratory distress
4. CXR is usually normal.
5. CT scan is the best study: diffuse infiltrates (hallmark), ground glass density, patchy/homogenous consolidation, pleural/pericardial pleural effusions. It is excellent for detecting recurrent cancer in irradiated area.
6. The treatment of choice is corticosteroids. Prophylactic treatment is not useful in humans (useful only in mice).

Quick HIT

- Severe hypoxemia can result in irreversible damage to organs (CNS and cardiovascular systems most affected) and must be corrected rapidly.
- Severe hypercapnia (and respiratory acidosis) can lead to dyspnea and vasodilation of cerebral vessels (with increased intracranial pressure and subsequent papilledema, headache, impaired consciousness, and finally coma).

Respiratory Failure

Acute Respiratory Failure

A. General characteristics

1. Acute respiratory failure results when there is inadequate oxygenation of blood or inadequate ventilation (elimination of CO_2) or both (see Clinical Pearl 2-6 and Clinical Pearl 2-7). The following are general criteria used to define acute respiratory failure:
   a. Hypoxia (PaO_2 <60 mm Hg)
   b. Hypercapnia (partial pressure of CO_2 (PCO_2) >50 mm Hg)

CLINICAL PEARL 2-6

Hypoxemia Pearls

1. To determine the underlying mechanism of hypoxemia, three pieces of information are needed:
   - $PaCO_2$ level
   - A–a gradient
   - Response to supplemental oxygen
2. A–a gradient is normal if hypoventilation or low inspired PO_2 is the only mechanism.
3. If $\dot{V}/\dot{Q}$ mismatch or shunting is present, then both $PaCO_2$ and A–a gradient are elevated; response to supplemental O_2 differentiates between the two mechanisms.

2. The following structures or systems are essential components for maintaining normal respiration. Dysfunction or interruption of any component (causes are listed) can potentially lead to respiratory failure.
   a. CNS (brain and spinal cord) depression or insult—drug overdose, stroke, trauma
   b. Neuromuscular disease—myasthenia gravis, polio, Guillain–Barré syndrome, amyotrophic lateral sclerosis
   c. Upper airway—obstruction due to a number of causes, including stenoses, spasms, or paralysis
   d. Thorax and pleura—mechanical restriction due to kyphoscoliosis, flail chest, hemothorax
   e. Cardiovascular system and blood—CHF, valvular diseases, PE, anemia
   f. Lower airways and alveoli—asthma, COPD, pneumonia, **acute respiratory distress syndrome** (ARDS)
3. Classification—acute respiratory failure can be divided into two major types (overlap often exists)
   a. Hypoxemic respiratory failure.
      - Low PaO_2 with a $PaCO_2$ that is either low or normal—present when O_2 saturation is <90% despite FiO_2 >0.6.
      - Causes include disease processes that involve the lung itself (e.g., ARDS, severe pneumonia, pulmonary edema).
      - $\dot{V}/\dot{Q}$ mismatch and intrapulmonary shunting are the major pathophysiologic mechanisms.
   b. Hypercapnic (hypercarbic) respiratory failure—a failure of alveolar ventilation.
      - Either a decrease in minute ventilation or an increase in physiologic dead space leads to CO_2 retention and eventually results in hypoxemia.
      - May be caused by an underlying lung disease (COPD, asthma, CF, severe bronchitis)
      - May also occur in patients with no underlying lung disease who have impaired ventilation due to neuromuscular diseases, CNS depression, mechanical restriction of lung inflation, or any cause of respiratory fatigue (e.g., prolonged hyperventilation in DKA)
4. Pathophysiology
   a. $\dot{V}/\dot{Q}$ mismatch

CLINICAL PEARL 2-7

Ventilation Versus Oxygenation

- Ventilation is monitored by $PaCO_2$: To ↓ $PaCO_2$, one must either ↑ respiratory rate (RR) or ↑ tidal volume (V_T). Note that minute ventilation = RR × V_T.
- Oxygenation is monitored by O_2 saturation and PaO_2: To ↓ PaO_2 in the ventilated patient, one must either ↓ FiO_2 or ↓ PEEP.

Note that ventilation and oxygenation are unrelated. O_2 saturation may be 100% with a very high $PaCO_2$, and the patient can be in ventilatory failure!

- Caused by a defect in either alveolar ventilation (e.g., pulmonary edema) or perfusion (e.g., PE)
- Typically leads to hypoxia **without hypercapnia** (in fact, $PaCO_2$ levels are often low or normal)
- Most common mechanism of hypoxemia (especially in chronic lung disorders)
- Responsive to supplemental oxygen

b. Shunting
- Little or no ventilation in perfused areas (due to collapsed or fluid-filled alveoli); venous blood is shunted into the arterial circulation without being oxygenated; represents one end of the spectrum in $\dot{V}/\dot{Q}$ mismatch.
- Causes of shunts: atelectasis or fluid buildup in alveoli (pneumonia or pulmonary edema), direct right-to-left intracardiac blood flow in congenital heart diseases.
- **Hypoxia due to a shunt is not responsive to supplemental oxygen.**

c. Hypoventilation—leads to hypercapnia, with secondary hypoxemia.
d. Increased CO_2 production (e.g., sepsis, DKA, hyperthermia) results in hypercapnic respiratory failure.
e. Diffusion impairment (e.g., ILD) causes hypoxemia without hypercapnia.

B. Clinical features

1. Symptoms
   a. Dyspnea—first symptom
   b. Cough may or may not be present, depending on the underlying cause.
2. Signs—the following might be present:
   a. Inability to speak in complete sentences, use of accessory muscles of respiration
   b. Tachypnea, tachycardia
   c. Cyanosis
   d. Impaired mentation (due to fatigue or hypercapnia, or if cause of respiratory failure is CNS depression)

C. Diagnosis

1. ABG analysis—may confirm diagnosis and help severity of condition; should be obtained in most cases of respiratory failure (see Figure 2-12)
   a. Hypoxemia: Mechanisms include $\dot{V}/\dot{Q}$ mismatch, intrapulmonary shunting, or hypoventilation.
   b. Hypercapnia: caused by hypoventilation (secondary to a variety of causes).
   c. Arterial pH: Respiratory acidosis occurs when hypercapnia is present. However, if the respiratory failure is chronic, renal compensation occurs and the acidosis is less severe.

Quick HIT

The alveolar–arterial oxygen difference (A–a gradient) is normal when hypoventilation is the cause of hypoxemia. It is increased in most other causes.

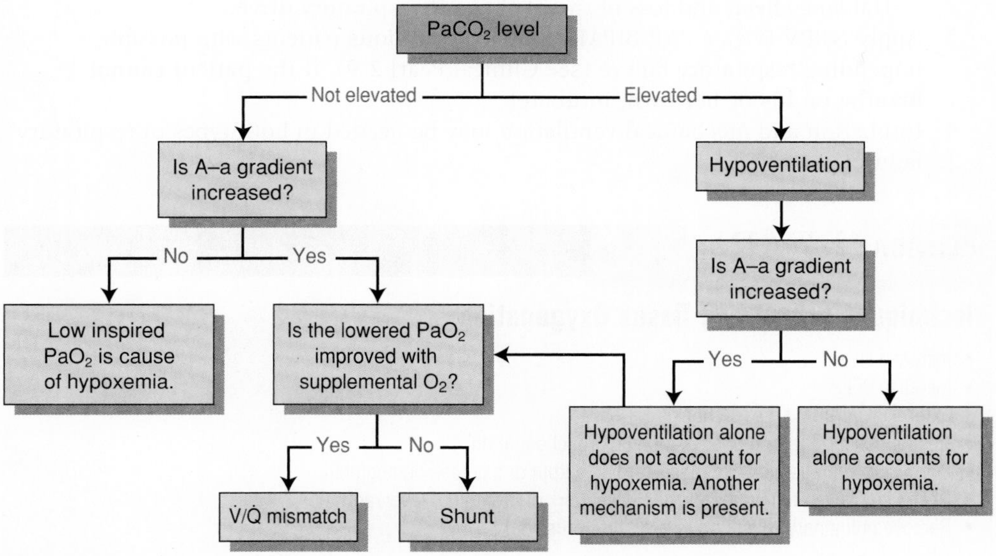

FIGURE 2-12 **Evaluation of a patient with hypoxemia.**

TABLE 2-6 Oxygen Delivery Systems

Oxygen Delivery System[a]		Flow Rate (L/min)	FiO_2 (% Oxygen)	Advantages
Low Flow	Nasal cannula	1–6	Up to 0.40	Easy to use, comfortable
	Simple face mask	5–10	0.40–0.60	Can deliver higher flow rates than nasal cannula
High Flow	Venturi mask	4–10	Up to 0.40, but can determine precise FiO_2 to deliver (24%, 28%, 31%, 35%, 40%)	Preferred in CO_2 retainers because one can more precisely control oxygenation
	Nonrebreathing mask	Up to 15	Variable, up to 0.70–0.90	Can achieve higher FiO_2 at lower flow rates
	High flow nasal cannula	Up to 40	Up to 0.40	Higher flow rates than simple nasal cannula

[a]There are two sources of oxygen in the hospital: wall outlets and oxygen tanks (portable, large green tanks).

2. CXR or CT scan of the chest.
3. CBC and metabolic panel.
4. If cardiogenic pulmonary edema is suspected, consider cardiac enzymes.

D. Treatment

1. Treat underlying disorder (e.g., with bronchodilators, corticosteroids, antibiotics, depending on the cause).
2. Provide supplemental oxygen if patient is hypoxemic (see Table 2-6 and Clinical Pearl 2-8).
   a. Hypoxemic respiratory failure: Use the **lowest concentration of oxygen** that provides sufficient oxygenation to avoid oxygen toxicity, which is due to free radical production.
   b. Hypercapnic respiratory failure: Results from hypoventilation. In COPD patients, excessive administration of oxygen results in V/Q mismatch, the Haldane effect, and loss of the hypoxemic respiratory drive.
3. Apply NPPV (e.g., CPAP, BIPAP) only for **conscious** patients with possible impending respiratory failure (see Clinical Pearl 2-9). **If the patient cannot breathe on his or her own, intubate!**
4. Intubation and mechanical ventilation may be needed in both types of respiratory failure.

Quick HIT

Do not ignore hypoxia in a patient with hypercarbic respiratory failure!

CLINICAL PEARL 2-8

Techniques to Improve Tissue Oxygenation

- Increase FiO_2
- Increase PEEP
- Extend inspiratory time fraction
- Decubitus, upright, or prone positioning bronchodilation
- Improve oxygen delivery: increase cardiac output or increase hemoglobin
- Decrease oxygen requirements: decrease work of breathing, fever, agitation
- Remove pulmonary vasodilators (e.g., nitroprusside)

Adapted from Baum GL, Crapo JD, Celli BR, et al., eds. *Textbook of Pulmonary Diseases.* Vol. II. 7th ed. Philadelphia, PA: Lippincott Williams & Wilkins, 2003 (*was* p. 926, Table 2 in 6th ed.).

CLINICAL PEARL 2-9

Noninvasive Positive Pressure Ventilation

- NPPV is delivered as either BIPAP or CPAP. BIPAP can be set at separate inspiratory and expiratory pressures (the inspiratory is higher than the expiratory).
- Both can be given via nasal mask or full-face mask.
- NPPV is indicated in patients in impending respiratory failure in an attempt to avoid intubation and mechanical ventilation.
- Success rates are highest in patients with hypercapnic respiratory failure (especially COPD patients).
- Note that NPPV should not be used for life support ventilation, only to temporarily support the patient's own spontaneous breathing.
- To use NPPV, the patient must be neurologically intact, awake and cooperative, and able to protect the airway. If no improvement is seen, BIPAP should be discontinued and conventional endotracheal intubation and mechanical ventilation initiated.

Acute Respiratory Distress Syndrome

A. General characteristics

1. ARDS is a diffuse **inflammatory process** (not necessarily infectious) involving both lungs—neutrophil activation (due to a variety of causes) in the systemic or pulmonary circulations is the primary mechanism (see Clinical Pearl 2-10).
2. ARDS is not a primary disease, but rather a disorder that arises due to other conditions that cause a widespread inflammatory process.
3. New 2012 Berlin definition:
   a. Acute onset (<1 week).
   b. Bilateral infiltrates on chest imaging.
   c. Pulmonary edema not explained by fluid overload or CHF (e.g., no clinical evidence of CHF or pulmonary capillary wedge pressure (PCWP) <18 mm Hg).
   d. Abnormal PaO_2/FiO_2 ratio.
      - 200 to 300: mild ARDS
      - 100 to 200: moderate ARDS
      - 100: severe ARDS
4. Pathophysiology
   a. Massive intrapulmonary shunting of blood is a key pathophysiologic event in ARDS—severe hypoxemia with **no significant improvement on 100% oxygen (requires high PEEP to prop open airways).** Shunting is secondary to widespread atelectasis, collapse of alveoli, and surfactant dysfunction.
      - Interstitial edema and alveolar collapse are due to an increase in lung fluid, which leads to stiff lungs, an increase in alveolar–arterial oxygen difference (A–a gradient), and ineffective gas exchange.
      - Note that the **effects** of the increase in pulmonary fluid are identical to those seen in cardiogenic pulmonary edema, but the **cause** is different: An increase in alveolar capillary permeability causes ARDS, whereas congestive hydrostatic forces cause cardiogenic pulmonary edema.

Quick HIT

Patients with sepsis or septic shock have the highest risk of developing ARDS.

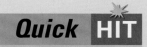

Quick HIT

ARDS can progress rapidly over several hours. Initially, the dyspnea may be exertional, but it can rapidly advance in severity.

CLINICAL PEARL 2-10

Remember the Following When Examining a Patient With ARDS

- Physical findings are usually nonspecific.
- Because the patient is usually intubated and on a ventilator, decreased unilateral breath sounds may be due to the ET being in the right main bronchus or possibly a pneumothorax.
- Look for potential sources of sepsis and check for any signs of infection: acute abdomen, IV lines, wounds, decubiti, etc.
- Keep in mind that cardiogenic pulmonary edema has to be distinguished from ARDS—look for signs of volume overload, CHF, JVD, edema, and hepatomegaly.

b. Decreased pulmonary compliance—leads to increased work of breathing.
c. Increased dead space—secondary to obstruction and destruction of pulmonary capillary bed.
d. Low vital capacity, low FRC.

B. Causes

1. Sepsis is most common risk factor—can be secondary to a variety of infections (e.g., pneumonia, urosepsis, wound infections)
2. Aspiration of gastric contents
3. Severe trauma, fractures (e.g., femur, pelvis), acute pancreatitis, multiple or massive transfusions, near-drowning
4. Drug overdose, toxic inhalations
5. Intracranial HTN
6. Cardiopulmonary bypass

Quick HIT

2012 Berlin criteria for diagnosing ARDS:
- Hypoxemia that is refractory to oxygen therapy: ratio of PaO_2/FiO_2 200 to 300 is mild, 100 to 200 is moderate, and <100 is severe
- Bilateral diffuse pulmonary infiltrates on CXR
- No evidence of CHF clinically or PCWP ≤18 mm Hg

C. Clinical features

1. Dyspnea, tachypnea, and tachycardia due to increased work of breathing.
2. Progressive hypoxemia—not responsive to supplemental oxygen.
3. Patients are difficult to ventilate because of high peak airway pressures due to stiff, noncompliant lungs.

D. Diagnosis

1. CXR—**shows diffuse bilateral pulmonary infiltrates** (see Figure 2-13)
   a. There is a variable correlation between findings on CXR and severity of hypoxemia or clinical response. Diuresis improves and volume overload worsens the infiltrates—regardless of CXR findings, the underlying ARDS may or may not be improved.
   b. CXR improvement follows clinical improvement after 1 to 2 weeks or more.
2. ABG
   a. Hypoxemia (PaO_2 <60)
   b. Initially, respiratory alkalosis ($PaCO_2$ <40) is present, which gives way to respiratory acidosis as the work of breathing increases and $PaCO_2$ increases.
   c. If the patient is septic, metabolic acidosis may be present, with or without respiratory compensation.
3. Pulmonary artery catheter—enables a determination of PCWP. PCWP reflects left heart filling pressures and is an indirect marker of intravascular volume status.
   a. PCWP is the most useful parameter in differentiating ARDS from cardiogenic pulmonary edema.
   b. If PCWP is low (<18 mm Hg), ARDS is more likely, whereas if PCWP is high (>18 mm Hg), cardiogenic pulmonary edema is more likely.
   c. **However, routine placement of pulmonary artery catheters has not been shown to be beneficial in ARDS or sepsis.**
4. Bronchoscopy with bronchoalveolar lavage
   a. This may be considered if patient is acutely ill and infection is suspected.
   b. Fluid collected can be cultured and analyzed for cell differential, cytology, Gram stain, and silver stain.

E. Treatment

1. Oxygenation—try to keep O_2 saturation >90%.
2. Mechanical ventilation is based on the ARDSNet studies. The most important principles include using a high PEEP with low tidal volumes.
3. Fluid management
   a. Volume overload should be avoided. A low-normal intravascular volume is preferred; the goal should be a CVP 4 to 6 cm H_2O. Vasopressors may be needed to maintain BP.
   b. On the other hand, patients with sepsis have high fluid requirements, so determining the appropriate fluid management may be difficult.
4. Treat the underlying cause, for example, infection.

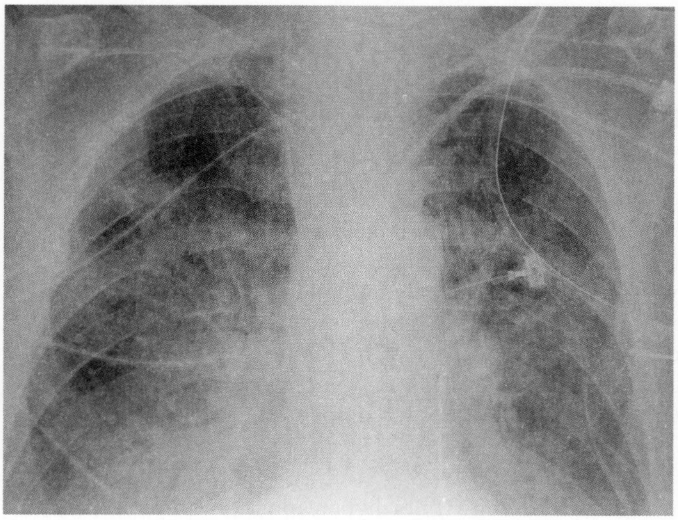

A

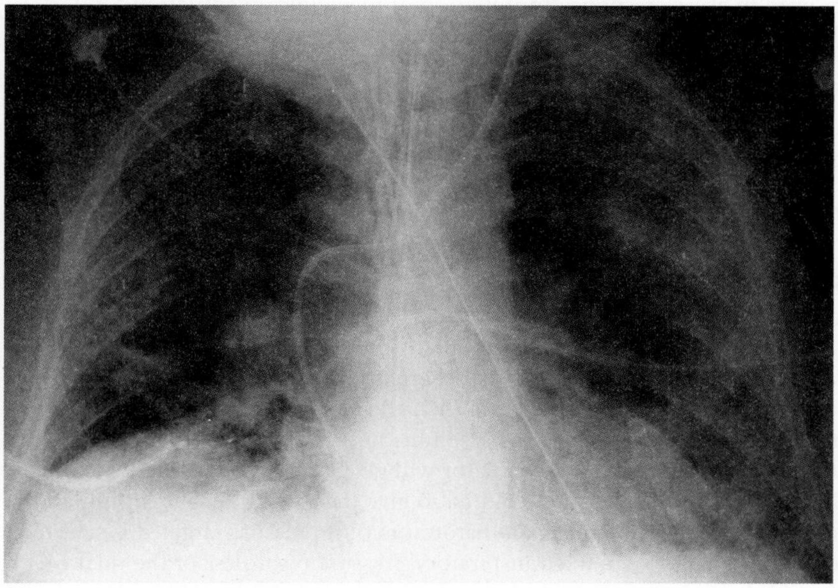

B

FIGURE 2-13 **A: Chest radiograph showing typical findings in ARDS. B: Another example of ARDS. Also note presence of an ET and Swan–Ganz central venous catheter.**
(**A** from Miller WT, Miller WT Jr. *Field Guide to the Chest X-Ray.* Philadelphia, PA: Lippincott Williams & Wilkins, 1999:4, Figure 1.2B.) (**B** from Daffner RH. *Clinical Radiology: The Essentials.* 2nd ed. Philadelphia, PA: Lippincott Williams & Wilkins, 1999:175, Figure 4.117A.)

5. Do not forget to address the patient's nutritional needs. Tube feedings are preferred over parenteral nutrition (see Appendix).

F. Complications

1. Permanent lung injury—resulting in lung scarring or honeycomb lung
2. Complications associated with mechanical ventilation
   a. Barotrauma secondary to high-pressure mechanical ventilation, possibly causing a pneumothorax or pneumomediastinum
   b. Nosocomial pneumonia
3. Line-associated infections: central lines and pulmonary artery catheters (line infection sepsis), urinary catheters (UTI), and nasal tubes (sinus infection)
4. Renal failure—may be due to nephrotoxic medication, sepsis with hypotension, or underlying disease
5. Ileus, stress ulcers

6. Multiple organ failure
7. Critical illness myopathy

Mechanical Ventilation

A. General characteristics

1. In treating respiratory failure, mechanical ventilation has two major goals: to maintain alveolar ventilation and to correct hypoxemia
2. The decision to initiate mechanical ventilation should be a clinical one. Generally, patients with the following require mechanical ventilation:
   a. Significant respiratory distress (e.g., high RR) or respiratory arrest
   b. Impaired or reduced level of consciousness with inability to protect the airway (look for absent gag or cough reflex)
   c. Metabolic acidosis (if the patient is unable to compensate with adequate hyperventilation)
   d. Respiratory muscle fatigue
   e. Significant hypoxemia (PaO_2 <70 mm Hg) or hypercapnia ($PaCO_2$ >50 mm Hg); respiratory acidosis (pH <7.2) with hypercapnia
3. ABGs are used to assess response to initiation of mechanical ventilation. Acceptable ranges of gas values include a PaO_2 of 50 to 60 with $PaCO_2$ of 40 to 50, and pH between 7.35 and 7.50.
4. General principles
   a. Initial settings should rest the respiratory muscles.
   b. The goal is to reduce the likelihood of barotraumas (high static airway pressures, overinflation) and atelectasis (low static airway pressures, underinflation).
   c. A volume-cycled ventilator is most commonly used.

Quick HIT

In general, err on the side of caution when deciding whether to initiate mechanical ventilation. Intubation does not mean the patient will have to remain on the ventilator indefinitely!

B. Ventilator settings

1. Assist control (AC) ventilation
   a. This is the initial mode used in most patients with respiratory failure.
   b. Guarantees a "backup" minute ventilation that has been preset, but the patient can still initiate breaths at a faster rate than the backup rate.
   c. AC and other ventilator modes can be volume targeted or pressure targeted. If volume targeted is selected, the ventilator will give a preset tidal volume for each breath regardless of the pressure required to give that breath (ensures ventilation but could lead to high pressures and barotrauma); if pressure targeted is selected, the ventilator will deliver a fixed inspiratory pressure regardless of the tidal volume (avoids barotraumas but adequate ventilation may not be achieved).
   d. All breaths are supported by the ventilator (in contrast to intermittent mandatory ventilation).
2. Synchronous intermittent mandatory ventilation (SIMV)
   a. Patients can breathe on their own above the mandatory rate **without** help from the ventilator (i.e., the tidal volume of these extra breaths is **not** determined by the ventilator, as it is in the assisted controlled mode).
   b. If no spontaneous breath is initiated by the patient, the predetermined mandatory breath is delivered by the ventilator.
   c. May increase respiratory fatigue and prolonged mechanical ventilation.
3. Continuous positive airway pressure (CPAP)
   a. Positive pressure (0 to 20 cm H_2O) is delivered continuously (during expiration and inspiration) by the ventilator, but no volume breaths are delivered (patient breathes on his or her own).
4. Pressure support ventilation (PSV)
   a. Inspiratory pressure is set to support each patient-triggered breath, with a constant PEEP. This is mostly used during weaning trials (Clinical Pearl 2-11).
5. Noninvasive mechanical ventilation
   a. CPAP: Positive pressure (0 to 20 cm H_2O) is delivered continuously (during expiration and inspiration) by the ventilator, but no volume breaths are delivered (patient breathes on his or her own).

Quick HIT

- Always confirm correct ET placement by listening for bilateral breath sounds **and** checking a postintubation CXR.
- On CXR, the tip of the ET tube should be approximately 2 to 5 cm above the carina.

Diseases of the Pulmonary System

CLINICAL PEARL 2-11

Parameters to Consider in Extubation or Weaning From the Ventilator: The More Criteria That Are Met, the More Likely That Extubation will be Tolerated

- Whether patient has an adequate respiratory drive and is hemodynamically stable
- Intact cough (when suctioning secretions)
- PaO_2/FiO_2 >200, $PaCO_2$ <45
- O_2 saturation of >90%, PEEP of ≤5 cm H_2O, FiO_2 <40%, RR <35 breaths/min, minute ventilation ≤12 L/min, vital capacity >10 mL/kg
- Rapid shallow breathing index (RSBI, RR divided by tidal volume) <105
- Negative inspiratory pressure <–20 cm H_2O or more negative

b. BiPAP: Similar to PSV but done with a face or nasal mask rather than intubation. Delivers a set inspiratory pressure with a constant PEEP.

C. Key parameters

1. Settings that affect $PaCO_2$: Minute ventilation (RR × V_T)
   a. This should be adjusted to achieve the patient's baseline $PaCO_2$.
   b. An initial tidal volume (V_T) of 4 to 8 mL/kg is appropriate in most cases (lower tidal volumes are recommended in patients with ARDS and COPD).
   c. A rate of 10 to 12 breaths/min is appropriate.
2. Settings that affect PaO_2: FiO_2 and PEEP
   a. FiO_2: The initial FiO_2 should be 100%. Quickly titrate down and use the lowest possible FiO_2 to maintain a PaO_2 of 50 to 60 or higher (or saturation >90%) to avoid oxygen toxicity (theoretical, FiO_2 < 60% is usually safe).
   b. PEEP is positive pressure maintained at the end of a passive exhalation—keeps alveoli open—5 cm H_2O is an appropriate initial setting. High levels of PEEP increase the risk of barotrauma (injury to airway = pneumothorax) and decrease cardiac output (decreased venous return from increased intrathoracic pressure).

D. Complications

1. Anxiety, agitation, discomfort
   a. Both sedation and analgesia are important; paralytics should be used during intubation and can be used after intubation if the patient continues to be agitated and fight the ventilator.
2. Difficulty with tracheal secretions—suction on a regular basis.
3. Ventilator-associated pneumonia (risk is ~1% per day).
4. Barotrauma—caused by high airway pressures.
5. **Tracheomalacia** (softening of the tracheal cartilage)—due to the prolonged presence of an endotracheal tube (ET).
6. Laryngeal damage during intubation.
7. Gastrointestinal effects (stress ulcers and cholestasis)—increased risk in mechanically ventilated patients. All patients should be on a PPI or H_2 blocker.

Quick HIT

The presence of an ET tube does not prevent aspiration from occurring.

Quick HIT

When a patient is ventilator-dependent for 2 or more weeks, a tracheostomy is usually performed to prevent tracheomalacia.

Diseases of the Pulmonary Vasculature

Pulmonary Hypertension

A. General characteristics

1. Defined as a mean pulmonary arterial pressure greater than 25 mm Hg at rest
2. There are multiple pathophysiologic processes that can cause pulmonary hypertension (Clinical Pearl 2-12):
   a. Passive due to resistance in the pulmonary venous system (e.g., left heart failure, mitral stenosis, atrial myxoma)

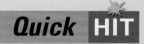

CLINICAL PEARL 2-12

How to Determine the Cause of Pulmonary HTN

- Perform a series of tests (CXR, PFTs, ABGs, serology, echocardiogram, cardiac catheterization). These tests will give you enough information to recognize heart disease or lung disease as the cause of pulmonary HTN.
- If the cause is not revealed (neither heart nor lung), then obtain a V/Q scan: this indicates either PE or primary pulmonary hypertension (pulmonary arterial hypertension, PAH). Note that PAH is a diagnosis of exclusion.

   b. Hyperkinetic (left-to-right cardiac shunts such as ASD or PDA)
   c. Obstruction (e.g., PE, pulmonary artery stenosis)
   d. Pulmonary vascular obliteration (e.g., collagen vascular diseases)
   e. Pulmonary vasoconstriction (e.g., chronic hypoxemia, COPD, OSA)
3. Classification of pulmonary hypertension is based on the revised WHO classification system:
   a. Group 1: Pulmonary arterial hypertension (PAH)
      - Idiopathic, familial, veno-occlusive disease, and PAH with associated conditions (connective tissue disorders, congenital shunting, HIV)
      - An abnormal increase in pulmonary arteriolar resistance leads to thickening of pulmonary arteriolar walls. This worsens the pulmonary HTN, which in turn causes further wall thickening, thus leading to a vicious cycle.
      - The cause is unknown; it usually affects young or middle-aged women.
      - The prognosis is poor. Mean survival is 2 to 3 years from the time of diagnosis.
   b. Group 2: Left heart disease
      - Secondary to any cause of left heart failure, including mitral stenosis and mitral regurgitation
   c. Group 3: Lung disease and/or chronic hypoxemia
      - Causes include ILD, COPD, OSA, and any other cause of chronic hypoxemia
   d. Group 4: Chronic thromboembolic disease
      - Recurrent PE (many patients do not have symptoms of PE), including non-thrombotic etiologies (e.g., tumor emboli)
   e. Group 5: Miscellaneous
      - Pulmonary vascular compression (e.g., tumors or lymphadenopathy), sarcoidosis, histiocytosis X, etc.

B. Clinical features

1. Symptoms
   a. Dyspnea on exertion
   b. Fatigue
   c. Chest pain—exertional
   d. Syncope—exertional (with severe disease)
2. Signs
   a. Loud pulmonic component of the second heart sound (P_2) and subtle lift of sternum (sign of RV dilatation)—**These may be the only findings, and yet the patient may still have a devastating disease!**
   b. When right ventricular failure occurs, the corresponding signs and symptoms appear (JVD, hepatomegaly, ascites, peripheral edema).

C. Diagnosis

1. ECG: Often suggests right ventricular hypertrophy—specifically, right axis deviation and right atrial abnormality are frequently present
2. CXR: Enlarged pulmonary arteries with or without clear lung fields based on the cause of pulmonary hypertension
3. Echocardiogram
   a. Dilated pulmonary artery
   b. Dilatation/hypertrophy of RA and RV
   c. Abnormal movement of IV septum (due to increased right ventricular volume)
4. Right heart catheterization: reveals increased pulmonary artery pressure

D. Treatment

1. One specific treatment plan cannot be recommended due to the variety of causes of pulmonary HTN. If the pulmonary hypertension is secondary to another disease process (e.g., recurrent PE), then the underlying disease should be treated and optimized.
2. Vasoactive agents are typically used in PAH (Group 1), since the trials have been done in this group.
   a. Right heart catheterization with a trial of vasodilators should precede the use of these agents.
   b. Vasoactive agents may lower pulmonary vascular resistance in some patients. Available options include inhaled phosphodiesterase inhibitors (e.g., sildenafil), oral CCBs, prostacyclins (e.g., epoprostenol), and endothelin receptor antagonists (e.g., bosentan).
3. Many patients require home oxygen, diuretics, and occasionally inotropes (e.g., digoxin).
4. Lung transplantation in qualified patients.

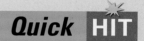

Quick HIT

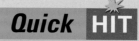

Cor pulmonale is best thought of as the right-sided counterpart to left ventricular heart disease due to systemic HTN.

Quick HIT

Death due to cor pulmonale: Many COPD patients die of right ventricular failure secondary to chronic pulmonary HTN. Many deaths due to PE result from acute pulmonary HTN and right ventricular failure.

Cor Pulmonale

A. General characteristics

1. Cor pulmonale is defined as right ventricular hypertrophy with eventual RV failure resulting from pulmonary HTN, **secondary to pulmonary disease.**
2. The definition does not encompass any of the causes of pulmonary HTN due to left-sided heart disease (such as mitral stenosis or left-to-right shunts).

B. Causes

1. It is most commonly secondary to COPD.
2. Other causes include recurrent PE, ILD, asthma, CF, sleep apnea, and pneumoconioses.

C. Clinical features

1. Decrease in exercise tolerance
2. Cyanosis and digital clubbing
3. Signs of right ventricular failure: hepatomegaly, edema, JVD
4. Parasternal lift

D. Diagnosis

1. CXR: enlargement of the RA, RV, and pulmonary arteries
2. ECG: right axis deviation, P pulmonale (peaked P waves), right ventricular hypertrophy
3. Echocardiogram: right ventricular dilatation, but normal LV size and function; useful in excluding LV dysfunction

E. Treatment

1. Treat the underlying pulmonary disorder.
2. Use diuretic therapy cautiously because patients may be preload-dependent.
3. Apply continuous long-term oxygen therapy if the patient is hypoxic.
4. Administer digoxin only if there is coexistent LV failure.
5. A variety of vasodilators have been studied; no definite improvement has been shown with their use.

Quick HIT

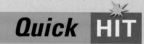

Other sources of emboli to the lungs:
- Fat embolism (long-bone fractures)
- Amniotic fluid embolism (during or after delivery)
- Air embolism (trauma to thorax, indwelling venous/arterial lines)
- Septic embolism (IV drug use)
- Schistosomiasis

Quick HIT

If a patient with long-bone fracture develops dyspnea, mental status change, and petechiae, think **fat embolism**. Respiratory failure and death can ensue rapidly.

Pulmonary Embolism

A. General characteristics

1. A PE occurs when a thrombus in another region of the body embolizes to the pulmonary vascular tree via the RV and pulmonary artery. Blood flow distal to the embolus is obstructed.
2. Consider PE and deep venous thrombosis (DVT) as a continuum of one clinical entity (venous thromboembolism)—diagnosing either PE or DVT is an indication for treatment.

Quick HIT

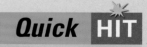

Complications in patients with PE who survive the initial event include:
- Recurrent PE
- Pulmonary HTN (up to two-thirds of patients)

CLINICAL PEARL 2-13

Risk Factors for DVT/PE

- Age >60 years
- Malignancy
- Prior history of DVT, PE
- Hereditary hypercoagulable states (factor V Leiden, protein C and S deficiency, antithrombin III deficiency)
- Prolonged immobilization or bed rest, long-distance travel
- Cardiac disease, especially CHF
- Obesity
- Nephrotic syndrome
- Major surgery, especially pelvic surgery (orthopedic procedures)
- Major trauma
- Pregnancy, estrogen use (oral contraceptives)

Quick HIT

Two important studies to know:
1. The Prospective Investigation of Pulmonary Embolism Diagnosis (PIOPED) is a landmark study (*JAMA.* 1990;263:2753). Guides treatment if V/Q̇ is performed.
2. The Christopher Study (*JAMA.* 2006;295:72–179). Guides treatment if spiral CT is performed.

3. Sources of emboli
   a. Lower extremity DVT—PE is the major complication of DVT.
      - Most pulmonary emboli arise from thromboses in the deep veins of lower extremities above the knee (iliofemoral DVT).
      - Pulmonary emboli can also arise from the deep veins of the pelvis.
      - Although calf vein thrombi have a low incidence of embolizing to the lungs, in many patients these thrombi progress into the proximal veins, increasing the incidence of PE.
   b. Upper extremity DVT is a rare source of emboli (it may be seen in IV drug abusers).
4. Risk factors are those for DVT (see Clinical Pearl 2-13).
5. Pathophysiology
   a. Emboli block a portion of pulmonary vasculature, leading to increased pulmonary vascular resistance, pulmonary artery pressure, and right ventricular pressure. If it is severe (large blockage), acute cor pulmonale may result.
   b. Blood flow decreases in some areas of the lung. Dead space is created in areas of the lung in which there is ventilation but no perfusion. The resulting hypoxemia and hypercarbia drive respiratory effort, which leads to tachypnea.
   c. If the size of the dead space is large (large PE), clinical signs are more overt (SOB, tachypnea).
6. Course and prognosis
   a. Most often, PE is clinically silent. **Recurrences are common**, which can lead to development of chronic pulmonary HTN and chronic cor pulmonale.
   b. When PE is undiagnosed, mortality approaches 30%. A significant number of cases are undiagnosed (as many as 50%).
   c. When PE is diagnosed, mortality is 10% in the first 60 minutes. **Of those who survive the initial event, approximately 30% of patients will die of a recurrent PE if left untreated. Most deaths are due to recurrent PE within the first few hours of the initial PE. Treatment with anticoagulants decreases the mortality to 2% to 8%.**

B. Clinical features

1. Symptoms (frequency per the PIOPED study)
   a. Dyspnea (73%)
   b. Pleuritic chest pain (66%)
   c. Cough (37%)
   d. Hemoptysis (13%)
   e. Note that only one-third of patients with PE will have signs and symptoms of a DVT
   f. Syncope seen in large PE
2. Signs (frequency per the PIOPED study)
   a. Tachypnea (70%)

CLINICAL PEARL 2-14

Workup of PE

It is often difficult to definitively diagnose or rule out PE. The following tests provide an adequate basis for treating PE with anticoagulation:

- Intraluminal filling defects in central, segmental, or lobular pulmonary arteries on CTA
- DVT diagnosed with ultrasound and clinical suspicion
- Positive pulmonary angiogram (definitely proves PE)

The following can essentially rule out PE:

- Low-probability V̇/Q̇ scan (*or* normal helical scan) and low clinical suspicion
- Negative pulmonary angiogram (definite)
- Negative D-dimer assay plus low clinical suspicion

Adapted from PIOPED data. *JAMA.* 1990;263:2753.

b. Rales (51%)
c. Tachycardia (30%)
d. S_4 (24%)
e. Increased P_2 (23%)
f. Shock with rapid circulatory collapse in massive PE
g. Other signs: low-grade fever, decreased breath sounds, dullness on percussion

Quick HIT

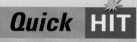

Signs and symptoms are not a reliable indicator of the presence of PE. This often leads to confusion and delay in diagnosis and treatment. If, however, **a patient has symptoms of PE and a DVT is found,** one can make the diagnosis of PE without further testing.

C. Diagnosis

1. ABG levels are not diagnostic for PE (see Clinical Pearl 2-14).
   a. PaO_2 and $PaCO_2$ are low (the latter due to hyperventilation) and pH is high; thus, there is typically a respiratory alkalosis.
   b. The A–a gradient is usually elevated. A normal A–a gradient makes PE less likely, but cannot be relied on to exclude the diagnosis.
2. CXR—usually normal.
   a. Atelectasis or pleural effusion may be present.
   b. The main usefulness is in excluding alternative diagnoses.
   c. Classic radiographic signs such as *Hampton hump* or *Westermark sign* are rarely present.
3. Venous duplex ultrasound of the lower extremities.
   a. If there is a positive result, treat with IV anticoagulation (heparin); treatment of DVT is the same as for PE. Keep in mind that with this approach, a false positive ultrasound will result in anticoagulation of some patients who do not have DVT or PE. Also, a negative result is not helpful, as patient may still have a PE despite no DVT on ultrasound.
   b. This test is very helpful when positive, but of **little value when negative** (negative results occur in 50% of patients with proven PE).
4. V̇/Q̇ (Ventilation–perfusion lung) scan
   a. Traditionally, this was the most common test used when PE is suspected, but has been replaced by CT angiography (CTA) as the initial study of choice in many medical centers.
   b. Plays an important role in diagnosis when there is a contraindication to CTA.
      - May be useful when the chest x-ray is clear and when there is no underlying cardiopulmonary disease.
   c. Interpretation of results: can be either normal, low-probability, intermediate-probability, or high-probability (treatment guidelines based on PIOPED study).
      - A normal V̇/Q̇ scan virtually rules out PE—no further testing is needed—but a scan is almost never "normal" in anyone.
      - A high-probability V̇/Q̇ scan has a very high sensitivity for PE; treat with heparin.
      - **If there is low or intermediate probability, clinical suspicion determines the next step.** If clinical suspicion is high, pulmonary angiography is indicated. Alternatively, perform a lower extremity duplex ultrasound to avoid

Quick HIT

If CTA is negative for PE, and clinical probability of PE is high, there is a 5% incidence of PE. So negative results should be interpreted with caution if patient has a high clinical probability of PE.

pulmonary angiography. If the duplex is positive, treatment for DVT is the same as for PE. If the duplex is negative/uncertain, then pulmonary angiography is indicated to exclude PE.

5. CTA
   a. Has been found to have good sensitivity (>90%) and specificity.
   b. Can visualize very small clots (as small as 2 mm); may miss clots in small subsegmental vessels (far periphery).
   c. The test of choice in most medical centers.
   d. In combination with clinical suspicion, guides treatment (see Figure 2-14).
   e. CTA cannot be performed in patients with significant renal insufficiency because of the IV contrast that is required.
6. Pulmonary angiography is the gold standard.
   a. **Definitively diagnoses or excludes PE, but is invasive. Contrast injected into pulmonary artery branch after percutaneous catheterization of femoral vein.**
   b. **Consider when noninvasive testing is equivocal and risk of anticoagulation is high, or if the patient is hemodynamically unstable and embolectomy may be required. Angiography is rarely performed because it carries a 0.5% mortality.**
7. D-dimer assay
   a. D-dimer is a specific fibrin degradation product; levels can be elevated in patients with PE and DVT.
   b. D-dimer assay is a fairly sensitive test (90% to 98%). **If results are normal and clinical suspicion is low,** PE is very unlikely.

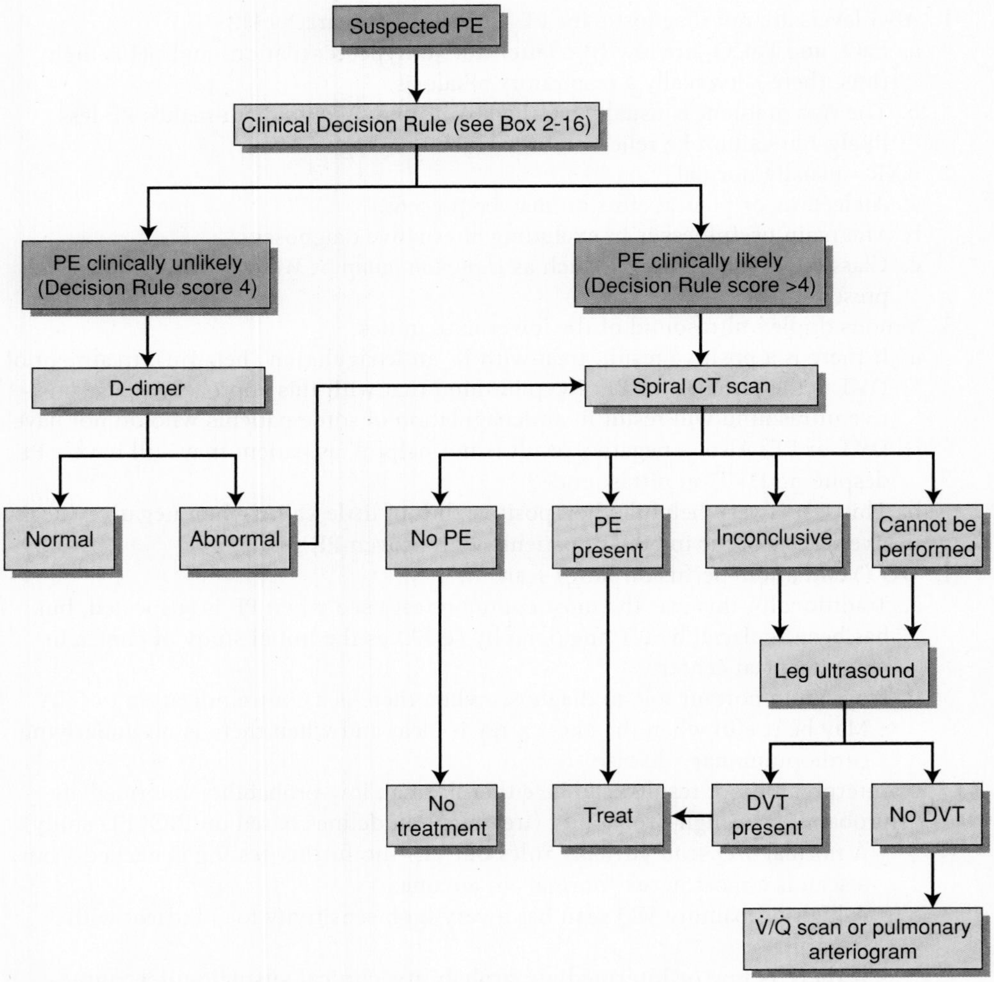

FIGURE 2-14 **Workup in a patient with suspected pulmonary embolism.**

CLINICAL PEARL 2-15

Dichotomized Clinical Decision Rule for Suspected Acute Pulmonary Embolism (Modified Wells Criteria)

Factor	Points
Symptoms and signs of DVT	3.0
Alternative diagnosis less likely than PE	3.0
Heart rate >100 beats/min	1.5
Immobilization (>3 days) or surgery in previous 4 weeks	1.5
Previous DVT or PE	1.5
Hemoptysis	1.0
Malignancy (current therapy, or in previous 6 months, or palliative)	1.0

Score ≤4 indicates that PE is unlikely, score >4 indicates that PE is likely

Adapted from Van Belle A, Büller HR, Huisman MV, et al. Effectiveness of managing suspected pulmonary embolism using an algorithm combining clinical probability, D-dimer testing, and computed tomography. *JAMA.* 2006;295:172–179; Wells PS, Anderson DR, Rodger M, et al. Derivation of a simple clinical model to categorize patients probability of pulmonary embolism: increasing the models utility with the SimpliRED D-dimer. *Thromb Haemost.* 2000;83:416–420.

c. Specificity is low—D-dimer results may also be elevated in MI, CHF, pneumonia, and the postoperative state. Any cause of clot or increased bleeding can elevate the D-dimer level.

8. Overall, the workup of suspected PE is based on pretest probability. The Wells criteria (Clinical Pearl 2-15) is a scoring system that takes this into account and helps guide the workup.
   a. IF PE is unlikely based on the scoring system, then the pretest probability for PE is low and D-dimers can be ordered to exclude PE. If PE is likely, CTA should be performed given its high sensitivity and specificity.

Quick HIT

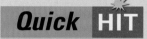

If pretest probability of PE is low, D-dimer test is a good noninvasive test to rule out PE. So if D-dimer is negative, you can rule out a clot. But if it is positive, this does not help you.

D. Treatment

1. Supplemental oxygen to correct hypoxemia. Severe hypoxemia or respiratory failure requires intubation and mechanical ventilation.
2. Acute anticoagulation therapy with either unfractionated or low-molecular-weight heparin to prevent another PE. Anticoagulation prevents further clot formation, but does not lyse existing emboli or diminish thrombus size.
   a. Start immediately on a basis of clinical suspicion. **Do not wait for studies to confirm PE if clinical suspicion is high.**
   b. Give one bolus, followed by a continuous infusion for 5 to 10 days. The goal is an aPTT of 1.5 to 2.5 times control.
      - Heparin acts by promoting the action of antithrombin III.
      - Contraindications to heparin include active bleeding, uncontrolled HTN, recent stroke, and heparin-induced thrombocytopenia (HIT).
      - Low-molecular-weight heparin has better bioavailability and lower complication rates than unfractionated heparin. It has been shown to be at least as effective or more effective than unfractionated heparin.
3. Oral anticoagulation with warfarin or one of the novel oral anticoagulants (e.g., rivaroxaban) for long-term treatment.
   a. Can start with heparin on day 1
   b. Therapeutic INR is 2 to 3.
   c. Continue for 3 to 6 months or more, depending on risk factors. Some patients at significant risk for recurrent PE (e.g., malignancy, hypercoagulable state) may be considered for lifelong anticoagulation.
4. Thrombolytic therapy—for example, streptokinase, tissue plasminogen activator (tPA).
   a. Speeds up the lysis of clots.
   b. There is no evidence that thrombolysis improves mortality rates in patients with PE. Therefore, its use is not well defined at this point.

Quick HIT

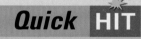

Start therapeutic heparin as initial treatment. Also start warfarin at same time. Goal is therapeutic INR of 2 to 3.

Quick HIT

Why PE and DVT are problematic for physicians:
- Clinical findings are sometimes subtle in both.
- Noninvasive imaging tests do not always detect either condition.
- Anticoagulation carries significant risk.

Quick HIT

INR is a way of reporting the PT in a standardized fashion.
- Warfarin increases INR values.
- "Therapeutic" INR is usually between 2 and 3. Notable exceptions are certain prosthetic mechanical heart valves, prophylaxis of recurrent MI, and treatment of antiphospholipid antibody syndrome, for which 2.5 to 3.5 is recommended.

Quick HIT

If anticoagulation is contraindicated in a patient with PE, a vena cava filter is indicated.

Quick HIT

Aspiration pneumonia develops in 40% of patients who aspirate, usually 2 to 4 days after aspiration. Organisms are often mixed (aerobic–anaerobic).

c. Situations in which thrombolysis should be considered:
   - Patients with massive PE who are hemodynamically unstable (persistent hypotension).
   - Patients with evidence of right heart failure (thrombolysis can reverse this).

d. Catheter-directed thrombolysis has lower systemic side effects and should be considered in patients at high risk for systemic fibrinolysis or surgery.

5. Inferior vena cava interruption (IVC filter placement).
   a. Use has become more common but reduction in mortality has not been conclusively demonstrated.
   b. Patients who have IVC filter placed are at higher risk of recurrent DVT (but lower risk of recurrent PE).
   c. Complications of IVC filter placement (rare): filter migration or misplacement, filter erosion and perforation of IVC wall, and IVC obstruction due to filter thrombosis.
   d. Indications include:
      - Contraindication to anticoagulation in a patient with documented DVT or PE.
      - A complication of current anticoagulation.
      - Failure of adequate anticoagulation as reflected by recurrent DVT or PE.
      - A patient with low pulmonary reserve who is at high risk for death from PE.
6. Surgical thrombectomy
   a. Consider in patients with hemodynamic compromise, a large, proximal thrombus, and who are poor candidates for fibrinolytics.

Miscellaneous Topics

Pulmonary Aspiration

A. General characteristics

1. Pulmonary aspiration syndromes can be due to different types of aspirates.
   a. Acidic gastric contents, which are especially damaging to the lungs.
   b. Aspiration of oropharyngeal flora, which can lead to infection.
   c. Foreign body/fluids (e.g., chemicals).
2. **The right lung is most often involved due to anatomy** (right main bronchus follows a more straight path down), **particularly the lower segments of the right upper lobe and the upper segments of the right lower lobe.**
3. Predisposing factors
   a. Reduced level of consciousness (e.g., seizures, stroke, sedating drugs)
   b. Alcoholism
   c. Extubation (impaired pharyngeal or laryngeal function)
   d. Excessive vomiting, ileus
   e. Tube feeding, tracheostomy tubes
   f. Anesthesia/surgery
   g. Neuromuscular diseases
   h. Esophageal disorders (e.g., achalasia, GERD, cancer)

B. Clinical features

1. Presentation is variable. Some patients develop acute onset of respiratory distress. However, most often, the patient appears well, but later develops respiratory dysfunction (cough, shortness of breath, fever, tachypnea, hypoxemia, or frothy sputum).
2. It may be initially silent, with development of acute respiratory failure with no obvious cause.
3. Fever may or may not be present.
4. May lead to obstruction of the airways with localized wheezing.

C. Diagnosis

1. Findings on CXR are variable and resemble infiltrates that mimic bacterial pneumonia. Atelectasis and local areas of collapse may also be present.

2. Differentiating between aspiration pneumonitis and aspiration pneumonia can be difficult. Aspiration pneumonitis will show infiltrates acutely on CXR, whereas aspiration pneumonia takes a few days to develop. However, many physicians treat empirically with antibiotics since it is often difficult to predict which patients will also develop pneumonia when aspiration pneumonitis is present (controversial).

D. Treatment

1. If aspiration was witnessed: ABCs (airway, breathing, and circulation), supplemental oxygen, and supportive measures.
2. If aspiration pneumonia is suspected, give antibiotics that have anaerobic activity (e.g., clindamycin).
3. If obstruction is present, early bronchoscopy is indicated.
4. Prevention is critical in patients at high risk for aspiration: Keep the head of the bed elevated, and place a nasogastric tube to decompress the stomach.

Quick HIT

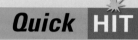

Aspiration can lead to lung abscess if untreated. Poor oral hygiene predisposes to such infections. Foul-smelling sputum often indicates anaerobic infection.

Dyspnea

A. General characteristics

1. Distinguish acute from chronic dyspnea.
2. Patients with chronic dyspnea usually have either heart or lung disease or both. It may be difficult to distinguish between the two.
3. The most common causes of acute dyspnea include CHF exacerbation, pneumonia, bronchospasm, PE, and anxiety.
4. Assess the patient's baseline level of activity, whether the dyspnea is new in onset, and its association with exertion.
5. If the patient has a history of smoking, cough, sputum, repeated infections, or occupational exposure, lung disease is likely to be the reason for chronic dyspnea.

Quick HIT

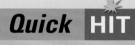

Depending on patient presentation, any of the following tests may be helpful in distinguishing between lung and heart disease:

- CXR
- Sputum Gram stain and culture (if patient has sputum)
- PFTs
- ABGs
- ECG, echocardiogram

B. Causes

1. Cardiovascular causes
   a. CHF
   b. Ischemic heart disease, acute myocardial infarction
   c. Pericarditis, cardiac tamponade
   d. Arrhythmias
   e. Valvular disease
   f. Congenital heart disease
2. Pulmonary causes
   a. Obstructive lung diseases—COPD, asthma, bronchiectasis
   b. PE
   c. ARDS
   d. Pneumonia, TB, bronchitis
   e. Pleural effusion, pulmonary edema
   f. Pneumothorax
   g. Upper airway obstruction, foreign body aspiration
   h. ILD
   i. Chest wall abnormalities (kyphoscoliosis), rib fracture
3. Psychiatric disease—generalized anxiety disorder, panic attacks, hyperventilation
4. Systemic causes—severe chronic anemia, sepsis, DKA, GERD, medication (narcotic overdose)
5. Chest wall abnormalities—kyphoscoliosis, rib fracture, ankylosing spondylitis
6. Neuromuscular diseases that weaken respiratory muscles—myasthenia gravis, muscular dystrophy

Quick HIT

Patients with chronic COPD can also experience paroxysmal nocturnal dyspnea. Their excessive airway secretions accumulate at night causing airway obstruction, resulting in dyspnea that awakens the patient and forces him or her to clear the airway. Therefore, paroxysmal nocturnal dyspnea is not specific to heart disease.

C. Diagnosis

1. Thorough history and physical examination, vital signs.
2. Pulse oximetry—normal is 96% to 100% on room air. Be aware that the baseline oxygen saturation of many COPD patients is chronically low.
3. ABG—may be indicated if oxygen saturation is low on pulse oximetry, if hypercarbia is suspected, or to evaluate for acid–base abnormalities.

Quick HIT

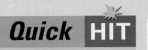

A chronic CO_2 retainer (common in COPD patients) usually has normal pH and increased HCO_3 levels. If CO_2 retention is acute, pH will be decreased and HCO_3 will be closer to normal levels.

4. CXR—can reveal pneumothorax, pleural effusion, pulmonary vascular congestion secondary to CHF, infiltrates due to pneumonia, ILD, and so on.
5. CBC—evaluate for anemia, infection.
6. ECG—may show ventricular hypertrophy or evidence of ischemic heart disease.
7. Echocardiogram—for further evaluation of CHF, valvular heart disease.
8. PFTs—perform if all of the above are normal or if obstructive lung disease is suspected. See Table 2-7.
9. V/Q scan or spiral CT scan—perform if PE is suspected.
10. Bronchoscopy—indicated if foreign body aspiration is suspected.

D. Treatment

1. Treat the underlying cause.
2. Use intubation and mechanical ventilation in the following situations:
   a. If impending respiratory failure is suspected
   b. If patient is unable to protect airway (e.g., decreased mental status, stroke, drug overdose)
   c. Severe hypoxia despite supplemental oxygen (PO_2 <50 to 60)
   d. Severe hypercarbia (PCO_2 > 50)
3. Exercise and conditioning may improve perception of dyspnea.

Quick HIT

Massive Hemoptysis

- Defined as more than 600 mL of blood in 24 hours.
- The most common causes are bronchiectasis and bleeding diathesis.
- Airway protection is key. Intubate if necessary.
- Bronchoscopy can help identify the bleeding source.
- Use bronchial artery embolization or balloon tamponade of the airway if indicated.

Hemoptysis

A. General characteristics

1. Defined as expectoration of blood, hemoptysis varies widely in severity and medical significance. The amount of blood does not necessarily correspond with the gravity of the underlying cause.
2. Differential diagnosis
   a. Most common causes include:
      - Bronchitis (50% of cases)
      - Lung cancer (bronchogenic carcinoma)
      - TB
      - Bronchiectasis
      - Pneumonia
      - Many times the etiology remains idiopathic after thorough evaluation (up to 30% of cases)
   b. Other causes include:
      - Goodpasture syndrome
      - PE with pulmonary infarction
      - Aspergilloma within cavities
      - Mitral stenosis (elevated pulmonary venous pressure)
      - Hemophilia

Quick HIT

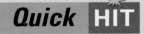

Evaluation of hemoptysis:
- CXR
- Fiberoptic bronchoscopy
- CT scan of chest

B. Diagnosis

1. Verify that hemoptysis has truly occurred. For example, superficial mouth lacerations or hematemesis may be confused with hemoptysis.
2. History and physical
   a. Fever, night sweats, and weight loss suggest TB.
   b. Fevers and chills or a history of HIV suggests either pneumonia or TB.
   c. Look for risk factors for PE.
   d. In the presence of acute renal failure or hematuria, Goodpasture syndrome should be considered.
3. Diagnostic studies
   a. CXR
      - May be a clear indicator of a pathogenic process or even diagnostic—for example, if fungus ball, irregular mass, granuloma, or opacity consistent with pulmonary infarction is present.
      - A normal CXR does not exclude a serious condition, especially PE and even lung cancer.

TABLE 2-7 **Important Pulmonary Studies**

Test	Explanation of Test	Use	Comments
Pulse oximetry	• Measures percentage of oxygenated hemoglobin • Follows a sigmoid curve in relationship to partial pressure of oxygen (PaO_2) in the arterial blood • Oxygen saturation of ≤88% is the established criterion for receiving home oxygen	• Useful in most categories of patients in whom pulmonary disease is suspected • Also helpful in assessing a patient with dyspnea, whether acute or chronic	• Useful as a screening test because it is very sensitive for detecting gas exchange abnormalities • Not very specific • Sensitivity is increased during exercise
Arterial blood gas (ABG)	Measures the partial pressures of oxygen and carbon dioxide as well as the pH of the arterial blood • Normal pH: 7.35–7.45 • Normal PaO_2: decreases with age (90 is normal in a 20-yr-old person) • Normal $PaCO_2$: 35–45 mm Hg	For every 10 mm Hg increase or decrease in $PaCO_2$, there should be a corresponding increase or decrease in pH by 0.08. In general, if the change in pH is in the same direction as change in $PaCO_2$, then the primary disorder is metabolic. When there is an inverse relationship, the primary disorder is respiratory.	• ABG is not necessary in all patients with pulmonary dysfunction. Ask yourself whether the results of the ABG are going to influence what you do for the patient before performing it. • ABG is painful, and radial artery spasm can result in ischemia of the hand in patients with radial-dominant circulation.
Spirometry	• From maximum inspiration, the patient exhales as rapidly and forcibly as possible to maximum expiration. • Spirometer plots the change in lung volume against time (see lung volumes below).	• Helps to distinguish obstructive from restrictive lung disease • Useful in assessing degree of functional impairment as well as monitoring effectiveness of treatment (e.g., during asthma exacerbation) • May detect respiratory impairment in asymptomatic patients (e.g., smokers)	• Volumes are measured as percentages of predicted values based on age, height, and sex. • Incorrect measurement or technique may lead to false positives.
DL_{CO}	• The patient breathes in a small, specific amount of CO, and the amount transferred from alveolar air to pulmonary capillary blood is measured. • CO is a diffusion limited gas, so other variables are eliminated. • Essentially measures the surface area of the alveolar-capillary membrane	• Can often distinguish between asthma, emphysema, and COPD • Useful in monitoring various conditions, such as sarcoidosis and emphysema	1. Causes for low DL_{CO} include: • Emphysema • Sarcoidosis • Interstitial fibrosis • Pulmonary vascular disease • Also lower with anemia due to reduced binding of CO to hemoglobin 2. Causes for high DL_{CO}: • Asthma (increased pulmonary capillary blood volume) • Obesity • Intracardiac left-to-right shunt • Exercise • Pulmonary hemorrhage (alveolar RBCs bind with CO)
Ventilation–perfusion ($\dot{V}/\dot{Q}$) scan	• Compares the degree of ventilation to perfusion of the lungs; an exact match would correspond to a $\dot{V}/\dot{Q}$ ratio of 1 • A high $\dot{V}/\dot{Q}$ ratio occurs when there is inadequate perfusion of an adequately ventilated lung. Thus, dead space is increased. • The normal ratio of ventilation to perfusion is 0.8, so there is normally some degree of $\dot{V}/\dot{Q}$ mismatch, with some degree of shunting	Diagnosis of PE	It is very rare to have a "normal" or "negative" $\dot{V}/\dot{Q}$ scan. When $\dot{V}/\dot{Q}$ scans are ordered for evaluation of suspected PE, the result is usually "low," "indeterminate," or "high probability"
Methacholine challenge	Assesses degree of airway hyperreactivity	Patients in whom asthma or COPD is suspected	Sensitive in detecting airway hyperresponsiveness in mild asthma

b. Fiberoptic bronchoscopy
   - Should be performed even if CXR is normal if there is a significant clinical suspicion for lung carcinoma.
   - Look for a small tumor that may not be evident on a radiograph.
   - May localize the site of bleeding.

4. CT of chest—performed as a complement to bronchoscopy or as a substitute if there are contraindications to bronchoscopy.

C. Treatment

1. Treat the underlying cause.
2. Suppress the cough if it is aggravating the hemoptysis.
3. Correct bleeding diathesis (although anticoagulation is the treatment for PE).

DISEASES OF THE GASTROINTESTINAL SYSTEM

3

Diseases of the Colon

Colorectal Cancer

A. General characteristics

1. Third most common cancer in the United States (in men and women)
2. **Virtually, all colorectal tumors arise from adenomas. Majority are endoluminal adenocarcinomas arising from the mucosa. Rarely, carcinoid tumors, lymphomas, and Kaposi sarcoma may be present but majority are adenocarcinomas**
3. Screening—refer to Chapter 12, Ambulatory Medicine
   a. Fecal occult blood testing (FOBT) has poor sensitivity and specificity. Positive predictive value is only about 20%, but all patients with positive FOBT need a colonoscopy regardless
   b. Digital rectal examination: Only about 10% of tumors are palpable by rectal examination
   c. Colonoscopy
      - **Most sensitive and specific test**; the diagnostic study of choice for patients with a positive FOBT
      - Diagnostic and therapeutic (e.g., biopsy, polypectomy)
   d. Flexible sigmoidoscopy
      - Can be used to reach the area where approximately 50% to 70% of polyps and cancers occur (with a 60-cm scope)
      - Can be diagnostic in about two-thirds of all colorectal cancers (CRCs)
   e. Barium enema
      - Evaluates entire colon; complementary to flexible sigmoidoscopy
      - Disadvantage is that any abnormal finding needs to be evaluated by colonoscopy
   f. Carcinoembryonic antigen (CEA)—not useful for screening; useful for establishing baseline, monitoring treatment efficacy, and recurrence surveillance. CEA does have prognostic significance: Patients with preoperative CEA >5 ng/mL have a worse prognosis
4. Clinical staging done with CT scan of chest, abdomen, and pelvis and by physical examination (ascites, hepatomegaly, lymphadenopathy)
5. Pattern of spread
   a. Direct extension—circumferentially and then through the bowel wall to later invade other abdominoperineal organs
   b. Hematogenous
      - Portal circulation to liver—**liver is most common site of distant spread**
      - Lumbar/vertebral veins to lungs
   c. Lymphatic—regionally
   d. Transperitoneal and intraluminal

Quick HIT

Note that some CRCs may bleed intermittently or not at all.

Quick HIT

Colon cancer screening begins at age 50. If one family member has colon cancer, begin at age 40, or 10 years before age of onset of family member.

Quick HIT

About 20% of patients have distant metastatic disease at presentation.

B. Risk factors

1. Age—everyone over the age of 50 years is at increased risk
2. Adenomatous polyps
   a. These are premalignant lesions, but most do not develop into cancer.
   b. Villous adenomas have higher malignant potential than tubular adenomas.
   c. The larger the size, and the greater the number of polyps, the higher the risk of cancer.
3. Personal history of prior CRC or adenomatous polyps
4. Inflammatory bowel disease (IBD)
   a. Both ulcerative colitis (UC) and Crohn disease pose an increased risk for CRC, but UC poses a greater risk than Crohn disease.
   b. Incidence of CRC is 5 % to 10% at 20 years and 12% to 20% at 30 years with UC. Begin surveillance colonoscopy for CRC 8 years following the diagnosis of IBD.
5. Family history
   a. Multiple first-degree relatives with CRC.
   b. Any first-degree relative diagnosed with CRC or adenoma under age 60.
6. Dietary factors—high-fat, low-fiber diets associated with a higher risk of CRC
7. Major polyposis syndromes
   a. **Familial adenomatous polyposis (FAP)**
      - Autosomal dominant disease caused by hereditary mutations in the APC tumor suppressor gene.
      - Characterized by hundreds of adenomatous polyps in the colon. The colon is always involved, and the duodenum is involved in 90% of cases. Polyps may also form in the stomach, jejunum, and ileum.
      - The risk of CRC is 100% by the third or fourth decade of life (in 100% of FAP cases).
      - Prophylactic colectomy is usually recommended.

   b. **Gardner syndrome**
      - Variant of FAP, autosomal dominant.
      - Polyps plus osteomas, dental abnormalities, benign soft tissue tumors, desmoid tumors, sebaceous cysts.
      - Risk of CRC is 100% by approximately age 40.

   c. **Turcot syndrome**
      - Can be inherited as autosomal dominant or recessive.
      - Polyps plus cerebellar medulloblastoma or glioblastoma multiforme.

   d. **Peutz–Jeghers**
      - Autosomal dominant.
      - Single or multiple hamartomas that may be scattered through entire GI tract: in small bowel (78%), colon (60%), stomach (30%).
      - **Pigmented spots around lips, oral mucosa, face, genitalia, and palmar surfaces.**
      - Unlike adenomas, hamartomas have very low malignant potential.
      - Slightly increased incidence in various carcinomas (e.g., stomach, ovary, breast, cervix, testicle, lung).
      - Intussusception or GI bleeding may occur.

   e. **Familial juvenile polyposis coli**
      - Rare; presents in childhood; only small risk of CRC.
      - More than 10 and up to hundreds of juvenile colon polyps.

   f. **Hereditary nonpolyposis CRC**—without adenomatous polyposis
      - **Lynch syndrome I** (site-specific CRC)—early-onset CRC; absence of antecedent multiple polyposis.
      - **Lynch syndrome II** (cancer family syndrome)—all features of Lynch I plus increased number and early occurrence of other cancers (e.g., female genital tract, skin, stomach, pancreas, brain, breast, biliary tract)

C. Clinical features

1. The presence of symptoms is typically a manifestation of relatively advanced disease. Most symptoms have melena or hematochezia, abdominal pain, change in bowel habits, or unexplained iron deficiency anemia

2. Signs and symptoms potentially common to all locations
   a. **Abdominal pain** is most common presenting symptom. Can be caused by partial obstruction or peritoneal dissemination. Remember that **CRC is the most common cause of large bowel obstruction in adults.** Colonic perforation can lead to peritonitis and is the most life-threatening complication
   b. Weight loss
   c. Blood in stool
   d. May be asymptomatic
3. Signs and symptoms based on specific location of tumor
   a. Right-sided tumors
      - Obstruction is unusual because of the **larger luminal diameter** (the cecum has the largest luminal diameter of any part of the colon), allowing for large tumor growth to go undetected.
      - Common findings: occult blood in stool, iron deficiency anemia, and **melena.**
      - **Change in bowel habits is uncommon.**
      - Triad of anemia, weakness, RLQ mass (occasionally) is present.
   b. Left-sided tumors
      - Smaller luminal diameter—signs of obstruction more common
      - Change in bowel habits more common—alternating constipation/diarrhea; narrowing of stools ("pencil stools")
      - Hematochezia more common
4. Rectal cancer (20% to 30% of all CRCs)
   a. Hematochezia—most common symptom
   b. Tenesmus
   c. Rectal mass; feeling of incomplete evacuation of stool (due to mass)

Quick HIT

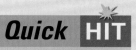

The sensitivity of individual symptoms for diagnosing CRC is poor.

Quick HIT

Right side: Melena is more common. Left side: Hematochezia is more common.

Quick HIT

Rectal cancer has a higher recurrence rate and a lower 5-year survival rate than colon cancer.

D. Treatment

1. Surgery is only curative treatment of CRC. Surgical resection of tumor-containing bowel as well as resection of regional lymphatics
2. CEA level should be obtained before surgery (see below)
3. Utility of adjuvant therapy (chemotherapy or radiation therapy) depends on stage of tumor and is beyond scope of this book
4. Follow-up is important, and varies among physicians
   a. Stool guaiac test
   b. Annual CT scan of abdomen/pelvis and CXR for up to 5 years
   c. Colonoscopy at 1 year and then every 3 years
   d. CEA levels are checked periodically (every 3 to 6 months)
      - A subsequent increase in CEA is a sensitive marker of recurrence
      - Often, second-look operations are based on high CEA levels postresection
      - Very high elevations of CEA suggest liver involvement
5. About 90% of recurrences occur within 3 years after surgery

Quick HIT

Radiation therapy is **not** indicated in the treatment of colon cancer, although it is used in treating rectal cancer.

Colonic Polyps

A. Nonneoplastic polyps—benign lesions with no malignant potential

1. Hyperplastic (metaplastic) polyps are the most common (90%) nonneoplastic polyps; generally remain small and asymptomatic.
2. No specific therapy required, but they can be difficult to distinguish from neoplastic polyps and so are commonly removed.
3. Juvenile polyps (typically in children younger than 10 years) are highly vascular and common, so they should be removed.
4. Inflammatory polyps (pseudopolyps) are associated with UC.

Quick HIT

Polyps may be isolated or may occur as part of inherited polyposis syndromes, which have a very high malignant potential.

B. Adenomatous polyps—benign lesions, but have significant malignant potential; precursors of adenocarcinoma

1. Can be one of three types of adenoma
   a. Tubular (most common; up to 60% to 80% of cases)—smallest risk of malignancy
   b. Tubulovillous—intermediate risk of malignancy
   c. Villous—greatest risk of malignancy

2. Can determine malignant potential by the following:
   a. Size—the larger the polyp, the greater the malignant potential
   b. Histologic type
   c. Atypia of cells
   d. Shape—sessile (flat, more likely to be malignant) versus pedunculated (on a stalk)

C. Treatment: complete removal of polyp

Diverticulosis

A. General characteristics

1. Caused by **increased intraluminal pressure**—inner layer of colon bulges through focal area of weakness in colon wall (usually an area of blood vessel penetration).
2. Risk factors
   a. **Low-fiber diets:** Constipation causes intraluminal pressures to increase.
   b. Positive family history.
3. Prevalence increases with age.
4. **The most common location is the sigmoid colon.** However, diverticula may occur anywhere in the colon.

B. Clinical features

1. Usually asymptomatic and discovered incidentally on barium enema or colonoscopy done for another reason.
2. Vague left lower quadrant (LLQ) discomfort, bloating, constipation/diarrhea may be present.
3. Only 10% to 20% become symptomatic (i.e., develop complications—see below).

C. Diagnosis

1. **Barium enema is the test of choice.**
2. Abdominal x-rays are usually normal and are not diagnostic for diverticulosis.

D. Treatment

1. High-fiber foods (such as bran) to increase stool bulk
2. Psyllium (if the patient cannot tolerate bran)

E. Complications

1. Painless rectal bleeding (up to 40% of patients)
   a. Bleeding is usually clinically insignificant and stops spontaneously. No further treatment is necessary in these patients.
   b. Bleeding can be severe in about 5% of patients. In many cases, the bleeding stops spontaneously. Colonoscopy may be performed to locate site of bleeding (mesenteric angiography in certain cases). If bleeding is persistent and/or recurrent, surgery may be needed (segmental colectomy).
2. **Diverticulitis** (15% to 25% of patients)
   a. Occurs when feces become impacted in the diverticulum, leading to erosion and microperforation.
   b. Can be complicated (see also Clinical Pearl 3-1) or uncomplicated. Uncomplicated diverticulitis accounts for most cases and refers to diverticulitis without the complications listed in Clinical Pearl 3-1.

CLINICAL PEARL 3-1

Complications of Diverticulitis

- Abscess formation (can be drained either percutaneously under CT guidance or surgically)
- Colovesical fistula—accounts for 50% of fistulas secondary to diverticulitis; 50% close spontaneously
- Obstruction—due to chronic inflammation and thickening of bowel wall
- Free colonic perforation—uncommon but catastrophic (leads to peritonitis)

Quick HIT

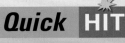

- Most polyps are found in the rectosigmoid region.
- Most patients are asymptomatic.
- In symptomatic patients, rectal bleeding is the most common symptom.

Quick HIT

Diverticulosis (pouches in the colon wall) should be distinguished from diverticulitis, which refers to inflammation or infection of the diverticula and is a complication of diverticulosis.

Quick HIT

- Complications of **diverticulosis** include painless rectal bleeding and diverticulitis.
- Complications of **diverticulitis** include bowel obstruction, abscess, and fistulas.

Quick HIT

- Diverticulitis recurs in about 30% of patients treated medically, usually within the first 5 years.
- Lower GI bleeding is very rare in diverticulitis, but common in diverticulosis.

c. Clinical features: fever, LLQ pain, leukocytosis.
  - Other possible features: alteration in bowel habits (constipation or diarrhea), vomiting, and sometimes a painful mass on rectal examination if inflammation is near the rectum.

d. Diagnostic tests
  - **CT scan (abdomen and pelvis) with oral and IV contrast is the test of choice**; it may reveal a swollen, edematous bowel wall or an abscess.
  - Abdominal radiographs help in excluding other potential causes of LLQ pain, and can rule out ileus or obstruction (indicated by air–fluid levels, distention), and perforation (indicated by free air).
  - **Barium enema and colonoscopy are contraindicated in acute diverticulitis due to the risk of perforation.**

e. Treatment
  - Uncomplicated diverticulitis is managed with IV antibiotics, bowel rest (NPO), IV fluids. Mild episodes can be treated on outpatient basis if patient is reliable and has few or no comorbid conditions. If symptoms persist after 3 to 4 days, surgery may be necessary. Antibiotics continued for 7 to 10 days. After successful treatment, about one-third have recurrence. Surgery recommended for recurrent episodes (resection of involved segment).
  - Complicated diverticulitis—surgery indicated.

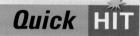

> **Quick HIT**
> - Diverticulosis—barium enema is test of choice
> - Diverticulitis—CT scan is test of choice (barium enema and colonoscopy contraindicated)

> **Quick HIT**
> As many as 25% of patients with bleeding arteriovenous malformations have aortic stenosis. However, no cause-and-effect relationship has been proven.

Angiodysplasia of the Colon (Arteriovenous Malformations, Vascular Ectasia)

- Tortuous, dilated veins in submucosa of the colon (usually proximal) wall.
- A common cause of lower GI **bleeding** in patients over age 60.
- Bleeding is usually low grade, but 15% of patients may have massive hemorrhage if veins rupture.
- Diagnosed by colonoscopy (preferred over angiography).
- In about 90% of patients, **bleeding stops spontaneously**.
- It can frequently be treated by colonoscopic coagulation of the lesion. If bleeding persists, a right hemicolectomy should be considered.

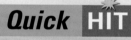

> **Quick HIT**
> - Acute mesenteric ischemia is much more common than chronic mesenteric ischemia.
> - Patients with acute mesenteric ischemia often have pre-existing heart disease (e.g., congestive heart failure, CAD).

Acute Mesenteric Ischemia

A. Introduction

1. Results from a compromised blood supply, usually to the superior mesenteric vessels.
2. There are four types (three are due to arterial disease, one due to venous disease):
   a. **Arterial embolism** (50% of cases): Almost all emboli are of a cardiac origin (e.g., atrial fibrillation, MI, valvular disease).
   b. **Arterial thrombosis** (25% of cases).
      - Most of these patients have atherosclerotic disease (e.g., coronary artery disease [CAD], PVD, stroke) at other sites.
      - Acute occlusion occurs over pre-existing atherosclerotic disease. The acute event may be due to a decrease in cardiac output (e.g., resulting from MI, CHF) or plaque rupture.
      - Collateral circulation has usually developed.
   c. **Nonocclusive mesenteric ischemia** (20% of cases).
      - Splanchnic vasoconstriction secondary to low cardiac output.
      - Typically seen in critically ill elderly patients.
   d. **Venous thrombosis** (<10% of cases).
      - Many predisposing factors—for example, infection, hypercoagulable states, oral contraceptives, portal HTN, malignancy, pancreatitis.
3. The overall mortality rate for all types is about 60% to 70%. If bowel infarction has occurred, the mortality rate can exceed 90%.

> **Quick HIT**
> **Differences in Presentation of Types of Acute Mesenteric Ischemia**
> - Embolic—symptoms are more sudden and painful than other causes
> - Arterial thrombosis—symptoms are more gradual and less severe than embolic causes
> - Nonocclusive ischemia—typically occurs in critically ill patients
> - Venous thrombosis—symptoms may be present for several days or even weeks, with gradual worsening

Quick HIT

- Signs of intestinal infarction include hypotension, tachypnea, lactic acidosis, fever, and altered mental status (eventually leading to shock).
- Check the lactate level if acute mesenteric ischemia is suspected.

B. Clinical features

1. Classic presentation is acute onset of **severe abdominal pain disproportionate to physical findings.** Pain is due to ischemia and possibly infarction of intestines, analogous to MI in CAD.
   a. The abdominal examination may appear benign even when there is severe ischemia. This can lead to a delay in diagnosis.
   b. The acuteness and the severity of pain vary depending on the type of acute mesenteric ischemia (see Quick Hit).
2. Anorexia, vomiting.
3. GI bleeding (mild).
4. Peritonitis, sepsis, and shock may be present in advanced disease.

C. Diagnosis

1. **Mesenteric angiography** is the definitive diagnostic test.
2. Obtain a plain film of the abdomen to exclude other causes of abdominal pain.
3. "Thumbprinting" on barium enema due to thickened edematous mucosal folds.

D. Treatment

1. Supportive measures: IV fluids and broad-spectrum antibiotics
2. Direct intra-arterial infusion of papaverine (vasodilator) into the superior mesenteric system during arteriography is the therapy of choice for all arterial causes of acute mesenteric ischemia. This relieves the occlusion and vasospasm.
3. Direct intra-arterial infusion of thrombolytics or embolectomy may be indicated in some patients with embolic acute mesenteric ischemia.
4. Heparin anticoagulation is the treatment of choice for venous thrombosis.
5. Surgery (resection of nonviable bowel) may be needed in all types of acute mesenteric ischemia if signs of peritonitis develop.

Quick HIT

Avoid vasopressors in mesenteric ischemia because they worsen the ischemia.

Chronic Mesenteric Ischemia

- Caused by **atherosclerotic occlusive disease** of main mesenteric vessels (celiac artery, superior and inferior mesenteric arteries).
- Abdominal angina—dull pain, typically **postprandial** (when there is increased demand for splanchnic blood flow); analogous to anginal pain of CAD.
- Significant **weight loss** may occur due to abdominal angina.
- Mesenteric arteriography confirms the diagnosis.
- Surgical revascularization is definitive treatment and leads to pain relief in 90% of cases.

Quick HIT

Patients with Ogilvie syndrome are usually ill and commonly have a history of recent surgery or medical illness.

Ogilvie Syndrome

- An unusual problem in which signs, symptoms, and radiographic evidence of large bowel obstruction are present, but **there is no mechanical obstruction.**
- Common causes include recent surgery or trauma, serious medical illnesses (e.g., sepsis, malignancy), and medications (e.g., narcotics, psychotropic drugs, anticholinergics).
- The diagnosis cannot be confirmed until mechanical obstruction of the colon is excluded.
- Treatment consists of stopping any offending agent (e.g., narcotics) and supportive measures (IV fluids, electrolyte repletion).
- Decompression with gentle enemas or nasogastric suction may be helpful. Colonoscopic decompression is usually successful if the above measures fail.
- Surgical decompression with cecostomy or colostomy is a last resort.

Quick HIT

Whenever there is colonic distention and when the colon diameter exceeds 10 cm, bowel is at risk of impending rupture leading to peritonitis and even death; **decompress immediately.**

Pseudomembranous Colitis

A. General characteristics

1. This is also referred to as **antibiotic-associated colitis** because many patients do not have grossly visible pseudomembranes.
2. Antibiotic treatment kills organisms that normally inhibit growth of *Clostridium difficile*, leading to overgrowth of *C. difficile* and toxin production.

3. Almost all antibiotics have been associated, but the most frequently implicated antibiotics are clindamycin, ampicillin, and cephalosporins.
4. Symptoms usually begin during first week of antibiotic therapy. However, up to 6 weeks may elapse after stopping antibiotics before clinical findings become apparent.
5. Disease severity varies widely.

Quick HIT

Complications of severe pseudomembranous colitis (may require surgery):
- Toxic megacolon
- Colonic perforation
- Anasarca, electrolyte disturbances

B. Clinical features

1. Profuse watery diarrhea (usually no blood or mucus)
2. Crampy abdominal pain
3. **Toxic megacolon** (in severe cases) with risk of perforation

C. Diagnosis

1. Demonstration of *C. difficile* toxins in stool is diagnostic, but results take at least 24 hours (95% sensitivity).
2. Flexible sigmoidoscopy is the most rapid test and is diagnostic, but because of discomfort/expense, it is infrequently used (usually reserved for special situations).
3. Abdominal radiograph (to rule out toxic megacolon and perforation).
4. Leukocytosis (very common).

D. Treatment

1. Discontinue the offending antibiotic, if possible.
2. Metronidazole is drug of choice (cannot be used in infants or pregnant patients)
3. Oral vancomycin used if patient is resistant to metronidazole or cannot tolerate it.
4. Regardless of choice of antibiotic, recurrence may occur within 2 to 8 weeks after stopping the antibiotic. This occurs in 15% to 35% of successfully treated patients.
5. Cholestyramine may be used as an adjuvant treatment to improve diarrhea.

Colonic Volvulus

A. General characteristics

1. Defined as twisting of a loop of intestine about its mesenteric attachment site.
2. May result in obstruction or vascular compromise (with potential for necrosis and/or perforation if untreated).
3. The **most common site is the sigmoid colon** (75% of all cases).
4. Cecal volvulus accounts for 25% of all cases.
5. Risk factors
   a. Chronic illness, age, institutionalization, and CNS disease increase risk of sigmoid volvulus.
   b. Cecal volvulus is due to congenital lack of fixation of the right colon and tends to occur in younger patients.
   c. Chronic constipation, laxative abuse, antimotility drugs.
   d. Prior abdominal surgery.

B. Clinical features

1. Acute onset of colicky abdominal pain
2. Obstipation, abdominal distention
3. Anorexia, nausea, vomiting

C. Diagnosis

1. Plain abdominal films.
   a. Sigmoid volvulus—*Omega loop sign* (or bent inner-tube shape) indicates a dilated sigmoid colon.
   b. Cecal volvulus (distention of cecum and small bowel)—*Coffee bean sign* indicates a large air–fluid level in RLQ.
2. Sigmoidoscopy—preferred diagnostic and therapeutic test for **sigmoid volvulus** (not for cecal volvulus); leads to successful treatment (untwisting and decompression) in many cases.
3. Barium enema—reveals the narrowing of the colon at the point where it is twisted (*"bird's beak"*).

Quick HIT

Do not perform a barium enema if strangulation is suspected!

D. Treatment

1. Sigmoid volvulus: Nonoperative reduction (decompression via sigmoidoscopy) is successful in >70% of cases. The recurrence rate is high, so elective sigmoid colon resection is recommended.
2. Cecal volvulus: Emergent surgery is indicated.

Diseases of the Liver

Cirrhosis

A. General characteristics

1. Cirrhosis is a chronic liver disease characterized by fibrosis, disruption of the liver architecture, and widespread nodules in the liver. The fibrous tissue replaces damaged or dead hepatocytes.
2. Cirrhosis is generally irreversible when advanced. In early stages, specific treatment of the cause of cirrhosis may improve or reverse the condition. The point at which the disease becomes irreversible is not clear.
3. The distortion of liver anatomy causes two major events.
   a. Decreased blood flow through the liver with subsequent hypertension in portal circulation **(portal hypertension)**—this has widespread manifestations, including ascites, peripheral edema, splenomegaly, and varicosity of veins "back stream" in the circulation (e.g., gastric/esophageal varices, hemorrhoids).
   b. Hepatocellular failure that leads to impairment of biochemical functions, such as decreased albumin synthesis and decreased clotting factor synthesis.
4. Assessment of hepatic functional reserve.
   a. **Child–Pugh Score** (see Table 3-1) estimates hepatic reserve in liver failure. It is used to measure disease severity and is a predictor of morbidity and mortality.
   b. Child's class C indicates most severe disease, and Child's class A indicates milder disease.

Quick HIT

Cirrhosis
- The most common causes of cirrhosis are alcoholic liver disease and chronic viral infection (especially hepatitis C).
- **Liver biopsy** is the gold standard for diagnosis of cirrhosis.

B. Causes

1. **Alcoholic liver disease—most common cause**
   a. Refers to a range of conditions from fatty liver (reversible, due to acute ingestion) to cirrhosis (irreversible)
   b. Fifteen percent to 20% of heavy drinkers develop alcoholic cirrhosis
2. **Chronic hepatitis B and C infections—next most common causes**
3. Drugs (e.g., acetaminophen toxicity, methotrexate)
4. Autoimmune hepatitis
5. Primary biliary cirrhosis (PBC), secondary biliary cirrhosis

TABLE 3-1 **Child–Pugh Classification to Assess Severity of Liver Disease**

	POINTS		
	1	**2**	**3**
Ascites	None	Mild–Moderate	Severe
Bilirubin(mg/dL)	<2.0	2.0–3.0	>3.0
Encephalopathy	None	Mild–Moderate	Severe
INR ratio	<1.7	1.7–2.3	>2.3
Albumin	>3.5	2.8–3.5	<2.8

Class A—5 to 6 points total (least severe liver disease), 85% 2-year survival
Class B—7 to 9 points total (moderate severe liver disease), 57% 2-year survival
Class C—10 to 15 points total (severe liver disease), 35% 2-year survival

6. Inherited metabolic diseases (e.g., hemochromatosis, Wilson disease)
7. Hepatic congestion secondary to right-sided heart failure, constrictive pericarditis
8. α_1-Antitrypsin (AAT) deficiency
9. Hepatic venoocclusive disease—can occur after bone marrow transplantation
10. Nonalcoholic steatohepatitis (NASH)

C. Clinical features

1. Some patients have no overt clinical findings, especially early in the disease.
2. Patients may have signs or symptoms suggestive of one or more of the complications of cirrhosis (see Complications section).

D. Complications

1. Portal HTN
   a. Clinical features are listed above. **Bleeding** (hematemesis, melena, hematochezia) secondary to esophagogastric varices is the most life-threatening complication of portal HTN (see below).
   b. Diagnose based on above features. Paracentesis can help in diagnosis.
   c. Treat the specific complication. **Use transjugular intrahepatic portal-systemic shunt (TIPS)** to lower portal pressure.
2. Varices
   a. Esophageal/gastric
      - Variceal hemorrhage has a high mortality rate. Patients with cirrhosis should be evaluated to document presence of varices and risk of hemorrhage. **If varices present, prophylactic measures indicated (such as nonselective β-blocker).**
      - Clinical features include massive hematemesis, melena, and exacerbation of hepatic encephalopathy.
      - Esophageal varices account for 90% of varices, and gastric varices for 10%.
      - Initial treatment is hemodynamic stabilization (give fluids to maintain BP). See Clinical Pearl 3-2 for methods aimed at stopping bleeding.
      - IV antibiotics are given prophylactically.
      - IV octreotide is initiated and continued for 3 to 5 days
      - Perform **emergent upper GI endoscopy** (once patient is stabilized) for diagnosis and to treat the hemorrhage either with variceal ligation or sclerotherapy.
      - Give nonselective β-blockers (propranolol, timolol, nadolol) as long-term therapy to prevent rebleeding.

Quick HIT

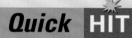

Classic signs of chronic liver disease:
- Ascites
- Varices
- Gynecomastia, testicular atrophy
- Palmar erythema, spider angiomas on skin
- Hemorrhoids
- Caput medusa

Quick HIT

Once a patient develops complications of cirrhosis, they have "decompensated" disease, with high morbidity and mortality.

Quick HIT

Treatment of bleeding esophageal varices involves pharmacologic treatment with IV octreotide in addition to endoscopic treatment (sclerotherapy or variceal ligation).

CLINICAL PEARL 3-2

Treatment of Bleeding Esophageal Varices

- **Variceal ligation/banding**
  - Initial endoscopic treatment of choice.
  - Effective control of active bleeding.
  - Lower rate of rebleeding than sclerotherapy.
- **Endoscopic sclerotherapy**
  - Sclerosing substance is injected into varices during endoscopy.
  - This controls acute bleeding in 80% to 90% of cases.
  - Up to 50% of patients may have rebleeding.
- **IV vasopressin**
  - This is an alternative to octreotide, but is rarely used due to the risk of complications.
  - Vasoconstriction of mesenteric vessels reduces portal pressure.
- **IV octreotide infusion**
  - Has replaced vasopressin as first-line therapy; causes splanchnic vasoconstriction and reduces portal pressure.
  - Fewer side effects than vasopressin.
- **Other options** include esophageal balloon tamponade (Sengstaken–Blakemore tube is a temporary measure), repeat sclerotherapy, TIPS, surgical shunts, and liver transplantation.

CLINICAL PEARL 3-3

Differential Diagnosis of Ascites

- Cirrhosis, portal HTN
- CHF
- Chronic renal disease
- Massive fluid overload
- Tuberculous peritonitis
- Malignancy
- Hypoalbuminemia
- Peripheral vasodilation secondary to endotoxin-induced release of nitrous oxide, which leads to increased renin secretion (and thus secondary hyperaldosteronism)
- Impaired liver inactivation of aldosterone

Quick HIT

Ascites can be managed by salt restriction and diuretics in most cases.

Quick HIT

Complications of Liver Failure (note the mnemonic AC, 9H)
- Ascites
- Coagulopathy
- Hypoalbuminemia
- Portal hypertension
- Hyperammonemia
- Hepatic encephalopathy
- Hepatorenal syndrome
- Hypoglycemia
- Hyperbilirubinemia/jaundice
- Hyperestrinism
- HCC

b. Rectal hemorrhoids
c. *Caput medusae* (distention of abdominal wall veins)

3. Ascites (see also Clinical Pearl 3-3)
   a. Accumulation of fluid in the peritoneal cavity due to **portal HTN** (increased hydrostatic pressure) and **hypoalbuminemia** (reduced oncotic pressure). Ascites is the most common complication of cirrhosis. Patients without portal hypertension do not develop ascites.
   b. Clinical features: abdominal distention, shifting dullness, and fluid wave.
   c. Abdominal ultrasound can detect as little as 30 mL of fluid.
   d. Diagnostic **paracentesis** determines whether ascites is due to portal HTN or another process.
      - Indications include new-onset ascites, worsening ascites, and suspected spontaneous bacterial peritonitis (SBP) (see below).
      - Examine cell count, ascites albumin, Gram stain, and culture to rule out infection (e.g., SBP).
      - Measure the **serum ascites albumin gradient.** If it is >1.1 g/dL, portal HTN is very likely. If <1.1 g/dL, portal HTN is unlikely, and other causes must be considered.
   e. Treatment
      - Bed rest, a low-sodium diet, and diuretics (furosemide and spironolactone)
      - Perform therapeutic paracentesis if tense ascites, shortness of breath, or early satiety is present.
      - Peritoneovenous shunt or TIPS to reduce portal HTN
4. Hepatic encephalopathy
   a. Toxic metabolites (there are many, but **ammonia** is believed to be most important) that are normally detoxified or removed by the liver accumulate and reach the brain.
   b. Occurs in 50% of all cases of cirrhosis, with varying severity.
   c. Precipitants include alkalosis, hypokalemia (e.g., due to diuretics), sedating drugs (narcotics, sleeping medications), GI bleeding, systemic infection, and hypovolemia.
   d. Clinical features
      - Decreased mental function, confusion, poor concentration, even stupor or coma.
      - *Asterixis* ("flapping tremor")—Have the patient extend the arms and dorsiflex the hands. (However, this is not a specific sign.)
      - Rigidity, hyperreflexia.
      - *Fetor hepaticus*—musty odor of breath.
   e. Treatment
      - Lactulose prevents absorption of ammonia. Metabolism of lactulose by bacteria in colon favors formation of NH^{4+}, which is poorly absorbed from GI tract, thereby promoting excretion of ammonia.

- Rifaximin (antibiotic): kills bowel flora, so decreases ammonia production by intestinal bacteria. Historically, neomycin was used but rifaximin has less side effects with same efficacy.
- Diet—limit protein to 30 to 40 g/day.

5. **Hepatorenal syndrome**—indicates end-stage liver disease
   a. Progressive renal failure in advanced liver disease, secondary to renal hypoperfusion resulting from vasoconstriction of renal vessels.
   b. Often precipitated by infection or diuretics.
   c. This is a functional renal failure—kidneys are normal in terms of morphology, and no specific causes of renal dysfunction are evident. This condition does not respond to volume expansion.
   d. Clinical features: azotemia, oliguria, hyponatremia, hypotension, low urine sodium (<10 mEq/L).
   e. Treatment: Liver transplantation is the only cure. In general, the prognosis is very poor, and the condition is usually fatal without liver transplantation.
6. SBP—infected ascitic fluid; occurs in up to 20% of patients hospitalized for ascites.
   a. Usually occurs in patients with ascites caused by end-stage liver disease; associated with high mortality rate (20% to 30%).
   b. Has a high recurrence rate (up to 70% in first year).
   c. Etiologic agents.
      - *Escherichia coli* (most common)
      - *Klebsiella*
      - *Streptococcus pneumoniae*
   d. Clinical features: abdominal pain, fever, vomiting, rebound tenderness. SBP may lead to sepsis.
   e. **Diagnosis is established by paracentesis and examination of ascitic fluid for WBCs (especially PMNs)**, Gram stain with culture, and sensitivities.
      - WBC >500, PMN >250.
      - Positive ascites culture; culture-negative SBP is common as well.
   f. Treatment
      - Broad-spectrum antibiotic therapy: Give specific antibiotic once organism is identified.
      - Clinical improvement should be seen in 24 to 48 hours. Repeat paracentesis in 2 to 3 days to document a decrease in ascitic fluid PMN (<250).
7. Hyperestrinism occurs due to reduced hepatic catabolism of estrogens
   a. *Spider angiomas*—dilated cutaneous arterioles with central red spot and reddish extensions that radiate outward like a spider's web
   b. Palmar erythema
   c. Gynecomastia
   d. Testicular atrophy
8. Coagulopathy occurs secondary to decreased synthesis of clotting factors.
   a. Prolonged prothrombin time (PT); PTT may be prolonged with severe disease.
   b. Vitamin K ineffective because it cannot be used by diseased liver.
   c. Treat coagulopathy with fresh frozen plasma.
9. Hepatocellular carcinoma (HCC)—present in 10% to 25% of patients with cirrhosis

E. Treatment

1. Treat underlying cause—for example, abstinence from alcohol, interferons for hepatitis B and C.
2. Avoid agents that may cause injury to liver, such as acetaminophen, alcohol.
3. Once cirrhosis develops, aim treatment at managing any complications that arise, as described above. The most serious complications are variceal bleeding, ascites, and hepatic encephalopathy.
4. Liver transplantation is the only hope for a cure. Abstinence from alcohol for more than 6 months is required before a patient is eligible for transplantation. Decision to proceed to liver transplantation depends on quality of life, severity of disease, and absence of contraindications.

Quick HIT

Monitoring Patients with Cirrhosis
- Order periodic laboratory values every 3 to 4 months (CBC, renal function tests, electrolytes, LFTs, and coagulation tests).
- Perform an endoscopy to determine the presence of esophageal varices.
- If HCC is suspected, perform a CT-guided biopsy for diagnosis.

Quick HIT

SBP: Look for fever and/or change in mental status in a patient with known ascites.

Quick HIT

If SBP is not treated early, mortality is high. Therefore, index of suspicion should be high and diagnostic paracentesis be done early.

Quick HIT

Signs of Acute Liver Failure (any of the following may be present):
- Coagulopathy
- Jaundice
- Hypoglycemia (liver stores glycogen)
- Hepatic encephalopathy
- Infection
- Elevated LFT values
- Any complication associated with cirrhosis

●●● Wilson Disease

A. General characteristics

1. An autosomal recessive disease of **copper metabolism.**
2. Mutations in the ATP7B gene lead to impairment of copper excretion into bile, and incorporation of copper into ceruloplasmin, a copper-binding protein that is necessary for copper excretion.
3. Therefore, copper accumulates in liver cells. As hepatocytes die, copper leaks into plasma and accumulates in various organs, including kidney, cornea, and brain.
4. The disease is most often apparent during childhood/adolescence (after age 5), and the majority of cases present between ages 5 and 35.

B. Clinical features

1. Clinical features are due to copper deposition in various organs.
2. Liver disease (most common initial manifestation): Manifestations vary and may include acute hepatitis, cirrhosis, and fulminant hepatic failure.
3. *Kayser–Fleischer rings* (yellowish rings in cornea) are caused by copper deposition in cornea; they do not interfere with vision (Figure 3-1).
4. CNS findings are due to copper deposition in the CNS.
   a. Extrapyramidal signs—parkinsonian symptoms (resting tremor, rigidity, bradykinesia), chorea, drooling, incoordination due to copper deposition in basal ganglia.
   b. Psychiatric disturbances—depression, neuroses, personality changes, psychosis.
5. Renal involvement—aminoaciduria, nephrocalcinosis.

C. Diagnosis

1. Diagnosis is made by determining the following (patients may have many or only a few of these findings):
   a. Hepatic disease—elevated aminotransferases; impaired synthesis of coagulation factors and albumin.
   b. Decreased serum ceruloplasmin levels (seen in 90% of patients), although ranges within normal do not exclude the diagnosis.
   c. Liver biopsy—significantly elevated copper concentration.
2. If diagnosed, first-degree relatives must be screened as well.

D. Treatment

1. Chelating agents—for example, d-penicillamine, which removes and detoxifies the excess copper deposits
2. Zinc
   a. Prevents uptake of dietary copper
   b. Given alone (presymptomatic or pregnant patients) or in conjunction with chelating agents (to symptomatic patients)

Quick HIT

Secondary hemochromatosis (or iron overload) can occur with multiple transfusions or in chronic hemolytic anemias.

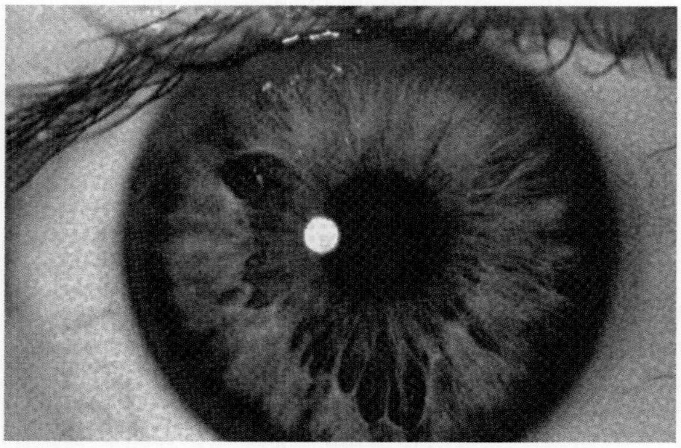

FIGURE 3-1 **Kayser–Fleischer ring.**

(From Humes DH, DuPont HL, Gardner LB, et al. *Kelley's Textbook of Internal Medicine.* 4th ed. Philadelphia, PA: Lippincott Williams & Wilkins, Figure 105.4).

Diseases of the Gastrointestinal System

3. Liver transplantation (if unresponsive to therapy or fulminant liver failure)
4. Monitor patient's copper levels, urinary copper excretion, ceruloplasmin, and liver function; physical examination for signs of liver or neurologic disease; psychological health

Hemochromatosis

A. General characteristics

1. An autosomal recessive disease of iron absorption.
2. Excessive iron absorption in the intestine leads to increased accumulation of iron (as ferritin and hemosiderin) in various organs. Over many years, fibrosis in involved organs occurs secondary to hydroxyl free radicals that are generated by the excess iron.
3. Affected organs
   a. Liver (primary organ)
   b. Pancreas
   c. Heart
   d. Joints
   e. Skin
   f. Thyroid, gonads, hypothalamus
4. This is an inherited disease, so screen the patient's siblings. Early diagnosis and treatment before development of complications (primarily cirrhosis, but also heart disease and diabetes) improves survival.

B. Clinical features

1. Most patients are asymptomatic initially.
2. Findings may include signs of liver disease, fatigue, arthritis, impotence/amenorrhea, abdominal pain, and cardiac arrhythmias.

C. Complications

1. Cirrhosis
   a. Cirrhosis increases the risk of HCC by 200-fold.
   b. The presence of liver disease is a primary factor in determining the prognosis.
2. Cardiomyopathy—CHF, arrhythmias
3. Diabetes mellitus—due to iron deposition in the pancreas
4. Arthritis—most common sites are the second and third metacarpophalangeal joints, hips, and knees
5. Hypogonadism—impotence, amenorrhea, loss of libido
6. Hypothyroidism
7. Hyperpigmentation of skin (resembles suntan, "bronzelike")

D. Diagnosis

1. Markedly elevated serum iron and serum ferritin
2. Elevated iron saturation (transferrin saturation)
3. Decreased total iron-binding capacity (TIBC)
4. **Liver biopsy (determines hepatic iron concentration) required for diagnosis**
5. Genetic testing for chromosomal abnormalities

E. Treatment

1. **Perform repeated phlebotomies**—this is the treatment of choice and improves survival dramatically if initiated early in the course of the disease.
2. Treat any complications (e.g., CHF, diabetes, hypothyroidism, arthritis).
3. Consider liver transplantation in advanced cases.

> **Quick HIT**
>
> Hemochromatosis: Early in the disease course, mild elevation of ALT and AST levels may be the only abnormalities that are noted because the patient is usually asymptomatic. Obtain iron studies. If the iron level is elevated, order a liver biopsy to confirm the diagnosis.

Hepatocellular Adenoma

- Benign liver tumor, most often seen in young women (15 to 40 years of age). Oral contraceptive use, female sex, and anabolic steroid use are the main risk factors.
- Patient may be asymptomatic; hepatocellular adenoma may be discovered incidentally on abdominal imaging studies. RUQ pain or fullness may be present.

- Malignant potential is very low (<1%). However, the adenoma may rupture, leading to hemoperitoneum and hemorrhage.
- Diagnosis made by CT scan, ultrasound, or hepatic arteriography (most accurate but invasive)
- Treatment: Discontinue oral contraceptives; surgically resect tumors >5 cm that do not regress after stopping oral contraceptives (otherwise there is a risk of rupture).

Cavernous Hemangiomas

- Vascular tumors are usually small and asymptomatic. They are the **most common type of benign liver tumor.**
- As the size of the tumor increases (e.g., due to pregnancy or use of oral contraceptives), the symptoms increase and include RUQ pain or mass.
- Complications (uncommon unless tumor is very large) include rupture with hemorrhage, obstructive jaundice, coagulopathy, CHF secondary to a large AV shunt, and gastric outlet obstruction.
- Diagnose with ultrasound or CT scan with IV contrast. Biopsy contraindicated because of risk of rupture and hemorrhage.
- Most cases do not require treatment. Consider resection if the patient is symptomatic or if there is a high risk of rupture (as with large tumors).

Focal Nodular Hyperplasia

- This benign liver tumor without malignant potential occurs in women of reproductive age. There is **no association** with oral contraceptives.
- It is usually asymptomatic. Hepatomegaly may be present. Treatment not necessary in most cases.

Hepatocellular Carcinoma (Malignant Hepatoma)

A. General characteristics

1. HCC accounts for more than 80% of primary liver cancers and, although rare in the United States, accounts for most deaths due to cancers worldwide. High-risk areas include Africa and Asia
2. There are two pathologic types
   a. Nonfibrolamellar (most common)
      - Usually associated with hepatitis B or C and cirrhosis
      - Usually unresectable with very short survival time (months)
   b. Fibrolamellar
      - Usually **not** associated with hepatitis B or C or cirrhosis
      - More often resectable; relatively longer survival time
      - Seen most commonly in adolescents and young adults

> **Quick HIT**
> The most common malignant liver tumors are HCCs and cholangiocarcinomas. The most common benign liver tumor is the hemangioma.

B. Risk factors

1. **Cirrhosis**, especially in association with alcohol or hepatitis B or C; HCC develops in 10% of cirrhotic patients
2. Chemical carcinogens: e.g., aflatoxin, vinyl chloride, Thorotrast
3. AAT deficiency
4. Hemochromatosis, Wilson disease
5. Schistosomiasis
6. Hepatic adenoma (10% risk of malignant transformation)
7. Cigarette smoking
8. Glycogen storage disease (type 1)

> **Quick HIT**
> **Prognosis of HCC**
> - If unresectable: less than 1 year
> - If resectable: 25% of patients are alive at 5 years

C. Clinical features

1. Abdominal pain (painful hepatomegaly)
2. Weight loss, anorexia, fatigue
3. Signs and symptoms of chronic liver disease—portal HTN, ascites, jaundice, splenomegaly

4. Paraneoplastic syndromes—erythrocytosis, thrombocytosis, hypercalcemia, carcinoid syndrome, hypertrophic pulmonary osteodystrophy, hypoglycemia, high cholesterol

D. Diagnosis

1. Liver biopsy—required for definitive diagnosis
2. Laboratory tests—hepatitis B and C serology, liver function tests (LFTs), coagulation tests
3. Imaging studies—ultrasound, CT scan (chest, abdomen, pelvis); MRI or MRA if surgery is an option (they provide more detail about the anatomy of the tumor)
4. Tumor marker elevation (AFP) is useful as a screening tool. AFP level may be elevated in 40% to 70% of patients with HCC, and is also helpful in monitoring response to therapy

Quick HIT

HCC is likely in a patient with cirrhosis who has a palpable liver mass and elevated AFP level.

E. Treatment

1. Liver resection (in the 10% of patients who have resectable tumors)
2. Liver transplantation if diagnosis is made early
3. If unresectable, consider transcatheter arterial chemoembolization (TACE), radiofrequency ablation, or selective internal radiation therapy

Nonalcoholic Steatohepatitis

- Histology of the liver is identical to that in patients with alcoholic liver disease, but these patients do not have a history of alcohol use!
- Associated with obesity, hyperlipidemia, diabetes mellitus (some patients have none of these).
- Usually asymptomatic and a benign course (but cirrhosis develops in 10% to 15%).
- Typically discovered on routine laboratory tests (mild elevation in alanine aminotransferase [ALT] and aspartate aminotransferase [AST]).
- Treatment is not clearly established.

Hemobilia

- Refers to blood draining into the duodenum via the common bile duct (CBD). The source of bleeding can be anywhere along the biliary tract, the liver, or the ampullary region.
- Causes—trauma (most common), papillary thyroid carcinoma, surgery (e.g., cholecystectomy, CBD exploration), tumors, infection.
- Clinical features include GI bleeding (melena, hematemesis), jaundice, and RUQ pain.
- Arteriogram is diagnostic. Upper GI endoscopy shows blood coming out of ampulla of Vater.
- Treatment—resuscitation (may require transfusion). If bleeding is severe, surgery is necessary (options include ligation of hepatic arteries or arteriogram with embolization of vessel).

Liver Cysts

Polycystic Liver Cysts

- Autosomal dominant, usually associated with polycystic kidney disease. Polycystic kidney disease often results in renal failure and is the main determinant of prognosis, whereas liver cysts **rarely** lead to hepatic fibrosis and liver failure.
- Usually asymptomatic; some patients have abdominal pain and upper abdominal mass.
- Treatment unnecessary in most cases.

Hydatid Liver Cysts

- Caused by infection from the tapeworm *Echinococcus granulosus* or, less commonly, *Echinococcus multilocularis*. Cysts most commonly occur in the right lobe of the liver.
- Small cysts are asymptomatic; larger cysts may cause RUQ pain and rupture into the peritoneal cavity, causing fatal anaphylactic shock.
- Treatment is surgical resection (caution to avoid spilling contents of the cyst into the peritoneal cavity). Mebendazole is given after surgery.

Quick HIT

The most common location for liver abscess (both pyogenic and amebic) is the right lobe.

Liver Abscess

Pyogenic Liver Abscess

- Most common cause is biliary tract obstruction—obstruction of bile flow allows bacterial proliferation. Other causes include GI infection (e.g., diverticulitis, appendicitis), with spread via portal venous system, and penetrating liver trauma (e.g., gunshot wound, surgery).
- Causative organisms include *E. coli, Klebsiella, Proteus, Enterococcus,* and anaerobes.
- Clinical features include fever, malaise, anorexia, weight loss, nausea, vomiting, RUQ pain, and jaundice. Patients appear quite ill.
- Diagnosed by ultrasound or CT scan; elevated LFTs.
- Fatal if untreated. Treatment (IV antibiotics and percutaneous drainage of abscess) reduces mortality to about 5% to 20%. Surgical drainage is sometimes necessary.

Amebic Liver Abscess

- Most common in men (9:1), particularly homosexual men. Transmitted through fecal–oral contact.
- Caused by intestinal amebiasis *(Entamoeba histolytica)*—the amoebae reach the liver via the hepatic portal vein.
- Clinical features—fever, RUQ pain, nausea/vomiting, hepatomegaly, diarrhea.
- Serologic testing (immunoglobulin G enzyme immunoassay) establishes diagnosis. LFTs are often elevated. The *E. histolytica* stool antigen test (detects protozoa in stool) is not sensitive. Imaging studies (ultrasound, CT) identify the abscess, but it is difficult to distinguish from a pyogenic abscess.
- IV metronidazole is effective treatment in most cases. Therapeutic aspiration of the abscess (image-guided percutaneous aspiration) may be necessary if the abscess is large (high risk of rupture), or if there is no response to medical therapy.

Quick HIT

Pyogenic and amebic abscesses are potentially life-threatening if not detected early.

Budd–Chiari Syndrome

A. General characteristics

1. Liver disease caused by occlusion of hepatic venous outflow, which leads to hepatic congestion and subsequent microvascular ischemia
2. The course is variable, but most cases are indolent, with gradual development of portal HTN and progressive deterioration of liver function.
3. Rarely, disease is severe and leads to acute liver failure, which may be fatal without immediate therapy.

B. Causes—hypercoagulable states, myeloproliferative disorders (e.g., polycythemia vera), pregnancy, chronic inflammatory diseases, infection, various cancers, trauma. Condition is idiopathic in up to 40% of cases.

C. Clinical features (resemble those of cirrhosis)—hepatomegaly, ascites, abdominal pain (RUQ), jaundice, variceal bleeding

D. Diagnosis—hepatic venography; serum ascites albumin gradient >1.1 g/dL

E. Treatment

1. Medical therapy is usually unsatisfactory (e.g., anticoagulation, thrombolytics, diuretics)
2. Surgery is eventually necessary in most cases (balloon angioplasty with stent placement in inferior vena cava, portacaval shunts)
3. Liver transplantation if cirrhosis is present

Quick HIT

Three Major Causes of Jaundice

- Hemolysis
- Liver disease
- Biliary obstruction

Jaundice

A. General characteristics

1. Yellow coloration of skin, mucous membranes, and sclerae due to overproduction or underclearance of bilirubin (see also Clinical Pearl 3-4)

CLINICAL PEARL 3-4

Bilirubin Metabolism

- Eighty percent of bilirubin is derived from hemoglobin (RBC breakdown). The rest comes from myoglobin breakdown and liver enzymes.
- Hemoglobin is converted to bilirubin in the spleen. This unconjugated bilirubin circulates in plasma, bound to albumin. This bilirubin–albumin complex is not water soluble; therefore, it is not excreted in urine. In the liver, it dissociates from albumin, and the bilirubin is conjugated and excreted into the intestine, where bacteria act on it to produce urobilinogen and urobilin.
- Therefore, unconjugated hyperbilirubinemia results when there is a defect before hepatic uptake. Conjugated hyperbilirubinemia results when there is a defect after hepatic uptake.

2. Clinical jaundice usually becomes evident when total bilirubin is >2 mg/dL
3. Conjugated versus unconjugated bilirubin
   a. Conjugated (direct)
      - Loosely bound to albumin and therefore water soluble
      - When present in excess, it is excreted in urine. **Therefore, dark urine is only seen with conjugated bilirubin!**
      - Nontoxic
   b. Unconjugated (indirect)
      - Tightly bound to albumin and therefore not water soluble
      - Cannot be excreted in urine even if blood levels are high
      - Toxic—unbound form can cross blood–brain barrier and cause neurologic deficits

Quick HIT

Dark urine and pale stools signal a diagnosis of conjugated hyperbilirubinemia.

B. Causes

1. **Conjugated hyperbilirubinemia—urine positive for bilirubin** (see also Clinical Pearl 3-5)
   a. Decreased intrahepatic excretion of bilirubin
      - Hepatocellular disease (viral or alcoholic hepatitis, cirrhosis)
      - Inherited disorders (**Dubin–Johnson syndrome, Rotor syndrome**)
      - Drug-induced (oral contraceptives)
      - PBC
      - Primary sclerosing cholangitis (PSC)
   b. Extrahepatic biliary obstruction
      - Gallstones
      - Carcinoma of head of pancreas
      - Cholangiocarcinoma
      - Periampullary tumors
      - Extrahepatic biliary atresia
2. **Unconjugated hyperbilirubinemia—urine negative for bilirubin**
   a. Excess production of bilirubin—hemolytic anemias

CLINICAL PEARL 3-5

Cholestasis

- This refers to blockage of bile flow (whether intrahepatic or extrahepatic) with a resultant increase in conjugated bilirubin levels.
- Clinical findings
  - Jaundice, gray stools, dark urine
  - Pruritus (bile salt deposition in skin)
  - Elevated serum alkaline phosphatase
  - Elevated serum cholesterol (impaired excretion)
  - Skin xanthomas (local accumulation of cholesterol)
  - Malabsorption of fats and fat-soluble vitamins

b. Reduced hepatic uptake of bilirubin or impaired conjugation
   - **Gilbert syndrome**
     - Occurs in up to 7% of the population—autosomal dominant condition in which there is decreased activity of hepatic uridine diphosphate glucuronyl transferase activity
     - Common cause of isolated elevation of unconjugated bilirubin
     - Exacerbated by fasting (crash diets), fever, alcohol, and infection
     - Asymptomatic in most cases, but occasionally mild jaundice may be present
     - Liver biopsy results are normal, and usually no treatment is necessary
   - Drugs (e.g., sulfonamides, penicillin, rifampin, radiocontrast agents)
   - **Crigler–Najjar syndrome**
     - Type 1—Complete absence of UDP glucuronosyltransferase in hepatic tissue. Severe unconjugated bilirubinemia, often resulting in brain damage at birth.
     - Type 2—Reduced UDP glucuronosyltransferase activity, but can detected in hepatic tissue. Not as severe as type 1.
   - Physiologic jaundice of the newborn (immaturity of conjugating system)
   - Diffuse liver disease (hepatitis, cirrhosis)

Quick HIT

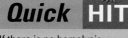

If there is no hemolysis, isolated hyperbilirubinemia (unconjugated) may indicate Gilbert syndrome, which is usually asymptomatic.

C. Diagnosis

1. Serum levels of total conjugated and unconjugated bilirubin (Figure 3-2)
2. If unconjugated hyperbilirubinemia, CBC, reticulocyte count, haptoglobin, LDH, peripheral smear may aid in diagnosis of hemolysis as the cause of jaundice
3. If conjugated hyperbilirubinemia, LFTs may point to the cause
4. Ultrasound (or CT scan) to assess biliary tract for obstruction or anatomic changes
5. Additional tests (e.g., endoscopic retrograde cholangiopancreatography [ERCP], percutaneous transhepatic cholangiography [PTC])—depending on the findings of the above tests
6. Liver biopsy may be indicated in some cases to determine cause of hepatocellular injury

Quick HIT

- ALT is primarily found in the liver.
- AST is found in many tissues (e.g., skeletal muscle, heart, kidney, brain).

D. Treatment: Treat the underlying cause

Liver Function Tests

A. Aminotransferases (ALT and AST)

1. ALT is more sensitive and specific than AST for liver damage.
2. ALT and AST usually have a similar increase. The exception is in alcoholic hepatitis, in which the AST–ALT ratio may be >2:1.
3. If ALT and AST levels are mildly elevated (low hundreds), think of chronic viral hepatitis or acute alcoholic hepatitis.
4. If ALT and AST levels are moderately elevated (high hundreds to thousands), think of acute viral hepatitis.
5. If ALT and AST levels are **severely elevated** (>10,000), extensive hepatic necrosis has occurred. Typical cases are:
   a. Ischemia, shock liver (prolonged hypotension or circulatory collapse)
   b. Acetaminophen toxicity
   c. Severe viral hepatitis
6. Note that liver transaminases are often normal or even low in patients with cirrhosis (without any active cell necrosis) or metastatic liver disease, because the number of healthy functioning hepatocytes is markedly reduced.
7. The following can cause an elevation in ALT or AST levels in asymptomatic patients (note the mnemonic):
   a. **A**utoimmune hepatitis
   b. Hepatitis **B**
   c. Hepatitis **C**
   d. **D**rugs or toxins
   e. **E**thanol

Quick HIT

- In alcoholic hepatitis, the AST level is almost never >500, and the ALT level is almost never >300.
- The higher the AST–ALT ratio, the greater the likelihood that alcohol is contributing to the abnormal LFTs.

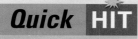

Quick HIT

LFT Pearls

- Cholestatic LFTs: markedly elevated alkaline phosphatase and GGT; ALT and AST slightly elevated
- Hepatocellular necrosis or inflammation: normal or slightly elevated alkaline phosphatase; markedly elevated ALT and AST

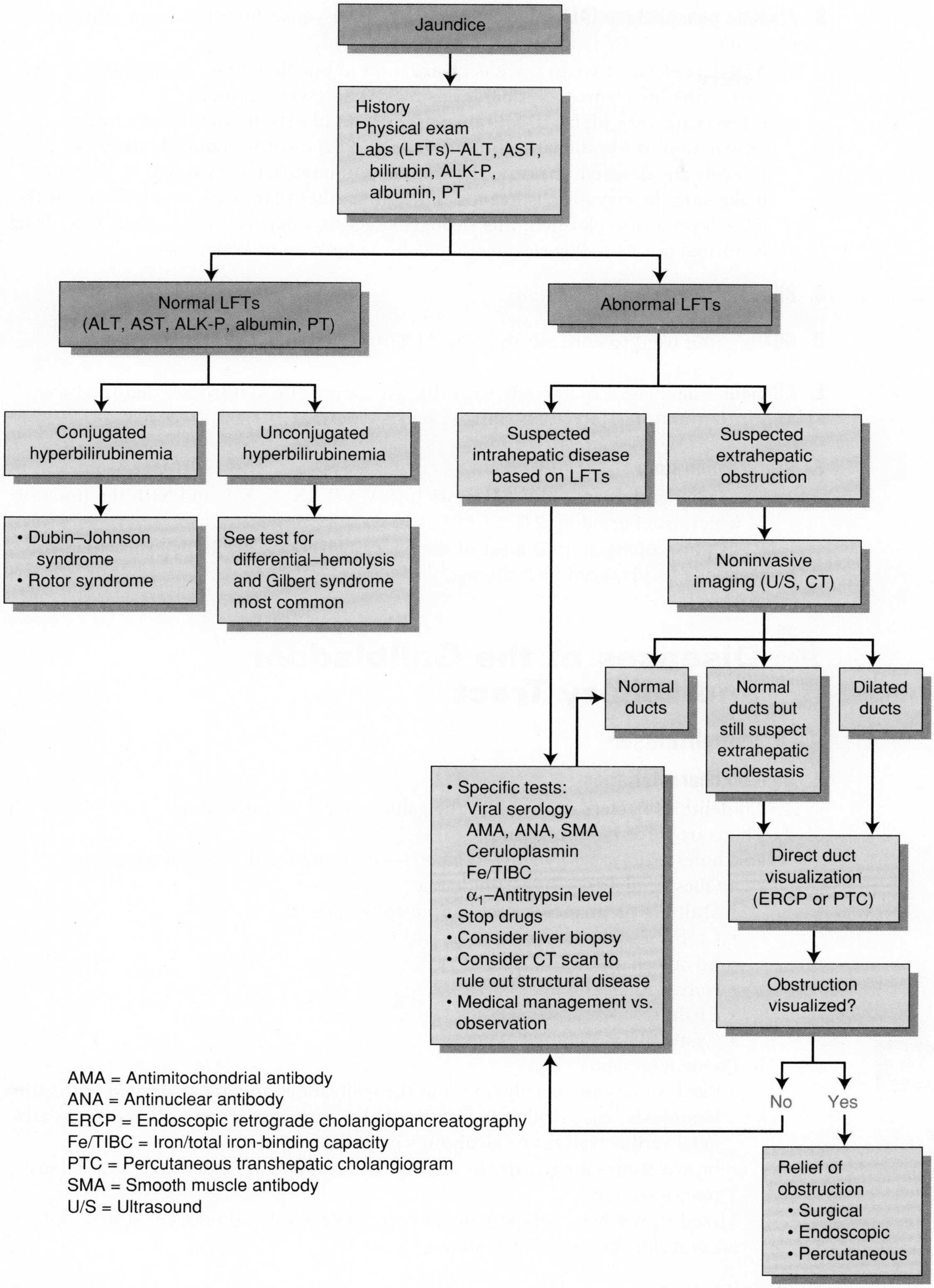

FIGURE 3-2 **Evaluation of jaundice.**

f. **F**atty liver (triglyceridemia)
g. **G**rowths (tumors)
h. **H**emodynamic disorders (e.g., CHF)
i. **I**ron (hemochromatosis), copper (Wilson disease), or AAT deficiency

B. Alkaline phosphatase (ALK-P): Not specific to liver—also found in bone, gut, and placenta

1. ALK-P is elevated when there is obstruction to bile flow (e.g., cholestasis) in any part of the biliary tree. Normal levels make cholestasis unlikely.
2. If levels are **very high** (10-fold increase), think of extrahepatic biliary tract obstruction or intrahepatic cholestasis (e.g., PBC or drug-induced cirrhosis).
3. If levels are **elevated**, measure the gamma-glutamyl-transferase (GGT) level to make sure the elevation is hepatic in origin (rather than bone or intestinal). If the GGT level is also elevated, this strongly suggests a hepatic origin. If the GGT level is normal but ALK-P is elevated, consider pregnancy or bone disease.

C. Bilirubin (see Jaundice section)

D. GGT is often used to confirm that the ALK-P elevation is of hepatic origin

E. Albumin—decreased in chronic liver disease, nephrotic syndrome, malnutrition, and inflammatory states (e.g., burns, sepsis, trauma)

F. Prothrombin time

1. The liver synthesizes clotting factors I, II, V, VII, IX, X, XII, and XIII, the function of which is reflected by PT.
2. PT is not prolonged until most of the liver's synthetic capacity is lost, which corresponds to advanced liver disease.

Diseases of the Gallbladder and Biliary Tract

Cholelithiasis

A. General characteristics

1. Cholelithiasis refers to stones in the gallbladder (i.e., gallstones).
2. There are three types of stones.
   a. Cholesterol stones (yellow to green)—associated with the following:
      - Obesity, diabetes, hyperlipidemia
      - Multiple pregnancies, oral contraceptive use
      - Crohn disease, ileal resection
      - Advanced age
      - Native American ancestry
      - Cirrhosis
      - Cystic fibrosis

   b. Pigment stones
      - Black stones are usually found in the gallbladder and are associated with either **hemolysis** (e.g., sickle cell disease, thalassemia, hereditary spherocytosis, artificial cardiac valves) or **alcoholic cirrhosis.**
      - Brown stones are usually found in bile ducts and are associated with biliary tract infection.

   c. Mixed stones have components of both cholesterol and pigment stones and account for the majority of stones.

Quick HIT

Cholestasis refers to obstruction of bile flow from any cause. If LFTs reveal cholestasis, obtain an abdominal or RUQ ultrasound.

B. Clinical features

1. Most cases are asymptomatic. Majority of patients found to have incidental gallstones will remain asymptomatic.
2. Biliary colic is the cardinal symptom of gallstones and is due to temporary obstruction of cystic duct by a gallstone. Pain occurs as the gallbladder contracts against this obstruction.
   a. Pain is typically located in the RUQ or epigastrium and may be mild, moderate, or severe.

Quick HIT

One-third of patients with biliary colic develop acute cholecystitis within 2 years.

b. Patients classically report pain after eating and at night.
c. *Boas sign*—referred right subscapular pain of biliary colic.

C. Complications

1. Cholecystitis (chronic or acute) with prolonged obstruction of cystic duct
2. Choledocholithiasis with its associated complications—see below
3. Gallstone ileus
4. Malignancy

D. Diagnosis

1. RUQ ultrasound has high sensitivity and specificity (>95%) for stones >2 mm.
2. CT scan and MRI are alternatives.

E. Treatment

1. No treatment if the patient is asymptomatic.
2. Elective cholecystectomy for patients with recurrent bouts of biliary colic.

Acute Cholecystitis

A. General characteristics

1. Obstruction of the cystic duct (**not** infection) induces acute inflammation of the gallbladder wall.
2. Chronic cholecystitis may develop with recurrent bouts of acute cholecystitis.
3. Ten percent of patients with gallstones develop acute cholecystitis.

B. Clinical features

1. Symptoms
   a. Pain is always present and is located in RUQ or epigastrium; it may radiate to the right shoulder or scapula.
   b. Nausea and vomiting, anorexia
2. Signs
   a. RUQ tenderness, rebound tenderness in RUQ
   b. *Murphy sign* is pathognomonic—inspiratory arrest during deep palpation of the RUQ; not present in many cases
   c. Hypoactive bowel sounds
   d. Low-grade fever, leukocytosis

C. Diagnosis

1. RUQ ultrasound is the test of choice.
   a. High sensitivity and specificity.
   b. Findings include thickened gallbladder wall, pericholecystic fluid, distended gallbladder, and presence of stone(s).
2. CT scan is as accurate as ultrasound but is more sensitive in identifying complications of acute cholecystitis (e.g., perforation, abscess, pancreatitis).
3. Radionuclide scan (hepatoiminodiacetic acid [HIDA]).
   a. Used when ultrasound is inconclusive. Its sensitivity and specificity parallel that of ultrasound. If HIDA scan is normal, acute cholecystitis can be ruled out.
   b. A positive HIDA scan means the gallbladder is not visualized.
   c. If gallbladder is not visualized 4 hours after injection, diagnosis of acute cholecystitis is confirmed.

D. Treatment

1. Patient should be admitted. Conservative measures include hydration with IV fluids, bowel rest (NPO), IV antibiotics, analgesics, correction of electrolyte abnormalities.
2. Surgery—Cholecystectomy is indicated in most patients with symptomatic gallstones. Early cholecystectomy is preferred (first 24 to 48 hours). Recurrence rate with nonsurgical treatment is as high as 70%. Timing of surgery depends

Quick HIT

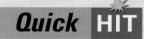

Pain in acute cholecystitis is secondary to gallbladder wall inflammation, whereas the pain of biliary colic is secondary to the contraction of the gallbladder against the obstructed cystic duct. Also, the pain of acute cholecystitis persists for several days, whereas the pain of biliary colic lasts only a few hours.

Quick HIT

Signs of Biliary Tract Obstruction

- Elevated alkaline phosphatase, increased GGT
- Elevated conjugated bilirubin
- Jaundice
- Pruritus
- Clay-colored stools
- Dark urine

Quick HIT

Acute cholecystitis is a syndrome of RUQ pain, fever, and leukocytosis associated with gallbladder inflammation.

Quick HIT

Complications of Cholecystitis

- Gangrenous cholecystitis
- Perforation of gallbladder
- Emphysematous cholecystitis
- Cholecystoenteric fistula with gallstone ileus
- Empyema of gallbladder

on severity of symptoms and patient's risk assessment for surgery, but in most patients, early cholecystectomy is preferred.

> **Quick HIT**
> Gallstone ileus
> - Gallstone enters bowel lumen via cholecystoenteric fistula—gets "stuck" in terminal ileum and causes obstruction
> - Accounts for 1% to 2% of bowel obstructions

Acalculous Cholecystitis

- Acute cholecystitis without stones obstructing the cystic duct (up to 10% of patients with acute cholecystitis).
- Usually idiopathic and seen in patients with severe underlying illness; possibly associated with dehydration, ischemia, burns, severe trauma, and a postoperative state.
- Signs and symptoms are the same as for acute cholecystitis.
- Diagnosis may be difficult because patients with this condition are often severely ill and have other medical problems, so clinical features are less apparent.
- Emergent cholecystectomy is the treatment of choice. For patients who are too ill for surgery, perform percutaneous drainage of the gallbladder with cholecystostomy.

> **Quick HIT**
> Complications of acute cholecystitis include gangrene and gallbladder perforation, which can be life-threatening.

Choledocholithiasis

A. General characteristics

1. Refers to gallstones in the CBD (see Table 3-2)
2. Primary versus secondary stones
   a. Primary stones originate in the CBD (usually pigmented stones).
   b. Secondary stones originate in the gallbladder and then pass into the CBD (usually cholesterol or mixed stones). These account for 95% of all cases.

> **Quick HIT**
> **Complications of CBD Stones**
> - Cholangitis
> - Obstructive jaundice
> - Acute pancreatitis
> - Biliary colic
> - Biliary cirrhosis

B. Clinical features

1. Patients may be asymptomatic for years.
2. Symptoms, when present, include RUQ or epigastric pain and jaundice.

C. Diagnosis

1. Laboratory tests—Total and direct bilirubin levels are elevated, as well as ALK-P.
2. RUQ ultrasound is usually the initial study, but is not a sensitive study for choledocholithiasis. It detects CBD in only 50% of cases, so it cannot be used to rule out this diagnosis.
3. ERCP is the gold standard (sensitivity and specificity of 95%) and should follow ultrasound. ERCP is diagnostic and therapeutic (see below).
4. PTC is an alternative to ERCP.

> **Quick HIT**
> Patients with CBD stones may be asymptomatic for years. However, unlike patients with cholelithiasis, in which biliary colic may lead to acute cholecystitis, the **onset of symptoms** in **choledocholithiasis** can signal the development of **life-threatening** complications such as cholangitis and acute pancreatitis.

D. Treatment

1. ERCP with sphincterotomy and stone extraction with stent placement (successful in 90% of patients)
2. Laparoscopic choledocholithotomy (in select cases)

TABLE 3-2 Cholelithiasis Versus Choledocholithiasis

	Cholelithiasis	Choledocholithiasis
Abnormality	Stone in gallbladder	Stone in CBD
Clinical features	Asymptomatic; biliary colic	Asymptomatic, RUQ/epigastric pain, jaundice
Complications	Cholecystitis, choledocholithiasis, gallstone ileus, malignancy	Cholangitis, obstructive jaundice, acute pancreatitis, biliary cirrhosis
Diagnosis	RUQ ultrasound is highly sensitive	ERCP is test of choice; RUQ ultrasound is not sensitive
Treatment	No treatment in most cases; elective cholecystectomy if biliary colic is severe or recurrent	Removal of stone via ERCP and sphincterotomy

> **Quick HIT**
> Do the following in patients with cholangitis:
> - Blood cultures
> - IV fluids
> - IV antibiotics after blood cultures obtained
> - Decompress CBD when patient stable

Cholangitis

A. General characteristics

1. Infection of biliary tract secondary to obstruction, which leads to biliary stasis and bacterial overgrowth.
   a. Choledocholithiasis accounts for 60% of cases.
   b. Other causes include pancreatic and biliary neoplasm, postoperative strictures, invasive procedures such as ERCP or PTC, and choledochal cysts.
2. Cholangitis is potentially life-threatening and requires emergency treatment.

B. Clinical features

1. *Charcot triad:* RUQ pain, jaundice, and fever—this classic triad is present in only 50% to 70% of cases.
2. *Reynolds pentad:* Charcot triad plus septic shock and altered mental status (CNS depression—e.g., coma, disorientation).
3. Patient is acutely ill, and abdominal symptoms may be lacking or may go unrecognized.

Quick HIT

Reynolds pentad is a highly toxic state that requires emergency treatment. **It can be rapidly fatal.**

C. Diagnosis

1. RUQ ultrasound is the initial study.
2. Laboratory findings—hyperbilirubinemia, leukocytosis, mild elevation in serum transaminases.
3. Cholangiography (PTC or ERCP).
   a. This is the definitive test, but it should not be performed during the acute phase of illness. Once cholangitis resolves, proceed with PTC or ERCP to identify the underlying problem and plan treatment.
   b. Perform PTC when the duct system is dilated (per ultrasound) and ERCP when the duct system is normal.

Quick HIT

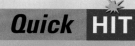

RUQ ultrasound is very accurate in detecting gallstones and biliary tract dilatation, but not very accurate in detecting CBD stones.

D. Treatment

1. IV antibiotics and IV fluids
   a. Close monitoring of hemodynamics, BP, and urine output is important.
   b. Most patients respond rapidly. Once the patient has been afebrile for 48 hours, cholangiography (PTC or ERCP) can be performed for evaluation of the underlying condition.
2. Decompress CBD via PTC (catheter drainage); ERCP (sphincterotomy), or laparotomy (T-tube insertion) once the patient is stabilized, or emergently if the condition does not respond to antibiotics.

Quick HIT

Hepatic abscess is the most serious and dreaded complication of acute cholangitis—**it has a high mortality rate.**

Carcinoma of the Gallbladder

- Most are adenocarcinomas and typically occur in the elderly.
- Associated with gallstones in most cases; other risk factors include cholecystoenteric fistula and porcelain gallbladder (Figure 3-3).
- Clinical features are nonspecific and suggest extrahepatic bile duct obstruction: jaundice, biliary colic, weight loss, anorexia, and RUQ mass. Palpable gallbladder is a sign of advanced disease.
- Difficult to remove with surgery: cholecystectomy versus radical cholecystectomy (with wedge resection of liver and lymph node dissection) depending on depth of invasion.
- Prognosis is dismal—more than 90% of patients die of advanced disease within 1 year of diagnosis. Disease often goes undetected until it is advanced.

Quick HIT

Porcelain Gallbladder
- Definition: intramural calcification of the gallbladder wall
- Prophylactic cholecystectomy is recommended because approximately 50% of patients with porcelain gallbladder will eventually develop cancer of the gallbladder.

Primary Sclerosing Cholangitis

A. General characteristics

1. A chronic idiopathic progressive disease of intrahepatic and/or extrahepatic bile ducts characterized by thickening of bile duct walls and narrowing of their lumens; leads to cirrhosis, portal hypertension, and liver failure (Table 3-3).

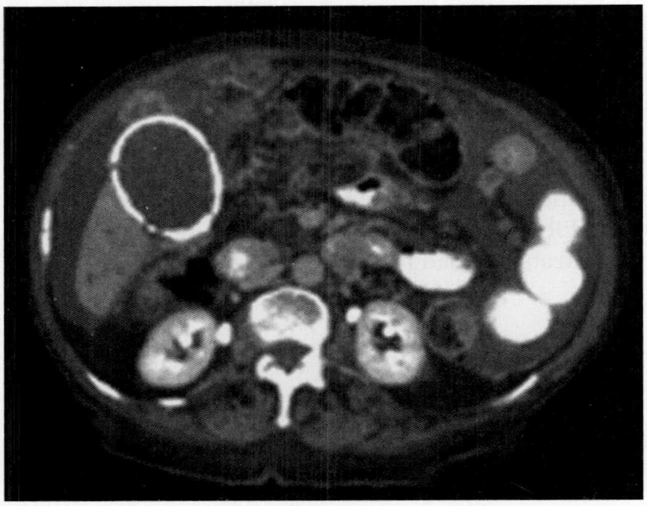

FIGURE 3-3 **Porcelain gallbladder. Note the thin layer of mineralization surrounding the gallbladder wall.**
(Courtesy of Dr Frank Gaillard, Radiopaedia.org.)

Quick HIT

Complications of PSC
- Cholangiocarcinoma (in up to 20% to 30% of patients)
- Recurrent bouts of cholangitis (in about 15% of patients)
- Can progress to secondary biliary cirrhosis, portal HTN, and liver failure

2. There is a strong association with UC (less so with Crohn disease). UC is present in 50% to 70% of patients with PSC; often the UC may dominate the clinical picture. (Note: The course of PSC is unaffected by a colectomy done for UC.)

B. Clinical features
1. Signs and symptoms begin insidiously.
2. Chronic cholestasis findings, including jaundice and pruritus; all patients eventually present with chronic obstructive jaundice
3. Other symptoms: fatigue, malaise, weight loss

C. Diagnosis
1. ERCP and PTC are diagnostic studies of choice—see multiple areas of bead-like stricturing and bead-like dilatations of intrahepatic and extrahepatic ducts.
2. Laboratory tests show cholestatic LFTs.

D. Treatment
1. There is no curative treatment other than liver transplantation.

TABLE 3-3 Primary Biliary Cirrhosis Versus Primary Sclerosing Cholangitis

	Primary Biliary Cirrhosis	Primary Sclerosing Cholangitis
Pathology	Intrahepatic bile duct destruction	Intra- and extrahepatic bile duct thickening and lumenal narrowing
Demographics	Female > Male 9:1	Male > Female
Association with Inflammatory Bowel Disease	None	Strong association with ulcerative colitis (UC) and also Crohn Disease
Diagnosis	+ antimitochondrial antibodies (AMAs) in 90%–95% of patients. Liver biopsy to confirm diagnosis	ERCP will show bead-like dilations in intra- and extrahepatic bile ducts
Treatment	Ursodeoxycholic acid slows progression, liver transplantation	Liver transplantation

2. When a dominant stricture causes cholestasis, ERCP with stent placement for biliary drainage and bile duct dilatation may relieve symptoms.
3. Use cholestyramine for symptomatic relief (to decrease pruritus).

Primary Biliary Cirrhosis

A. General characteristics

1. PBC is a chronic and progressive cholestatic liver disease characterized by **destruction of intrahepatic bile ducts** with portal inflammation and scarring (Table 3-3).
2. It is a slowly progressive disease with a variable course. It may progress to cirrhosis and end-stage liver failure.
3. It is an **autoimmune disease** that is often associated with other autoimmune disorders.
4. It is most common in **middle-aged women.**

B. Clinical features

1. Fatigue
2. Pruritus (early in course of disease)
3. Jaundice (late in course of disease)
4. RUQ discomfort
5. Xanthomata and xanthelasmata
6. Osteoporosis
7. Portal HTN (with resultant sequelae)

C. Diagnosis

1. Laboratory findings
   a. Cholestatic LFTs (elevated ALK-P)
   b. **Positive antimitochondrial antibodies (AMAs) found in 90% to 95% of patients.** This is the hallmark of the disease (specificity of 98%). If serum is positive for AMAs, perform a liver biopsy to confirm diagnosis
   c. Elevated cholesterol, HDL
   d. Elevated immunoglobulin M
2. Liver biopsy (percutaneous or laparoscopic) to confirm the diagnosis
3. Abdominal ultrasound or CT scan to rule out biliary obstruction

D. Treatment

1. Treatment is symptomatic for pruritus (cholestyramine) and osteoporosis (calcium, bisphosphonates, vitamin D).
2. Ursodeoxycholic acid (a hydrophilic bile acid) has been shown to slow progression of the disease.
3. Liver transplantation is the only curative treatment available.

> **Quick HIT**
>
> **Etiology of Secondary Biliary Cirrhosis.** This disease occurs in response to chronic biliary obstruction from the following:
> - Long-standing mechanical obstruction
> - Sclerosing cholangitis
> - Cystic fibrosis
> - Biliary atresia

Cholangiocarcinoma

A. General characteristics

1. Tumor of intrahepatic or extrahepatic bile ducts: most are adenocarcinomas.
2. Mean age of diagnosis is in the seventh decade.
3. Located in three regions: proximal third of the CBD (most common, also called Klatskin tumor), distal extrahepatic (best chance of resectability), intrahepatic (least common).
4. Prognosis is dismal—survival is less than 1 year after diagnosis.
5. Risk factors
   a. PSC is the major risk factor in the United States.
   b. Other risk factors include UC, choledochal cysts, and *Clonorchis sinensis* infestation (in Hong Kong).

B. Clinical features

1. Obstructive jaundice and associated symptoms: dark urine, clay-colored stools, and pruritus
2. Weight loss

> **Quick HIT**
>
> **Klatskin Tumors**
> - Tumors in proximal third of CBD—involve the junction of right and left hepatic ducts
> - Very poor prognosis because they are unresectable

C. Diagnosis

1. Cholangiography (PTC or ERCP) for diagnosis and assessment of resectability.
2. If the patient has an unresectable tumor (more likely the case with proximal than distal bile duct tumors), stent placement is an option during either PTC or ERCP and may relieve biliary obstruction.

D. Treatment

1. Most patients do not have resectable tumors at diagnosis.
2. The survival rate is low despite aggressive chemotherapy, stenting, or biliary drainage.

Choledochal Cysts

- Cystic dilatations of biliary tree involving either the extrahepatic or intrahepatic ducts, or both; more common in women (4:1)
- Clinical features: epigastric pain, jaundice, fever, and RUQ mass
- Complications: cholangiocarcinoma (most feared complication—risk is about 20% over 20 years), hepatic abscess, recurrent cholangitis/pancreatitis, rupture, biliary obstruction, cirrhosis, and portal HTN
- Ultrasound is the best noninvasive test, and ERCP is definitive for diagnosis
- Treatment is surgery: complete resection of the cyst with a biliary-enteric anastomosis to restore continuity of biliary system with bowels

Bile Duct Stricture

- Most common cause is iatrogenic injury (e.g., prior biliary surgery such as cholecystectomy, liver transplantation); other causes include recurring choledocholithiasis, chronic pancreatitis, and PSC.
- Clinical features are those of obstructive jaundice.
- Complications can be life-threatening: secondary biliary cirrhosis, liver abscess, and ascending cholangitis.
- Treatment involves endoscopic stenting (preferred) or surgical bypass if obstruction is complete or if endoscopic therapy fails.

Biliary Dyskinesia

- Motor dysfunction of the sphincter of Oddi, which leads to recurrent episodes of biliary colic without any evidence of gallstones on diagnostic studies such as ultrasound, CT scan, and ERCP
- Diagnosis is made by HIDA scan. Once the gallbladder is filled with labeled radionuclide, give cholecystokinin (CCK) intravenously, then determine the ejection fraction of the gallbladder. If the ejection fraction is low, dyskinesia is likely.
- Treatment options include laparoscopic cholecystectomy and endoscopic sphincterotomy.

Quick HIT

CCK is the hormone that relaxes the sphincter of Oddi and contracts the gallbladder.

Diseases of the Appendix

Acute Appendicitis

A. General characteristics

1. Pathogenesis
   a. The lumen of the appendix is obstructed by hyperplasia of lymphoid tissue (60% of cases), a fecalith (35% of cases), a foreign body, or other rare causes (parasite or carcinoid tumor [5% of cases]).
   b. Obstruction leads to stasis (of fluid and mucus), which promotes bacterial growth, leading to inflammation.
   c. Distention of the appendix can compromise blood supply. The resulting ischemia can lead to infarction or necrosis if untreated. Necrosis can result in appendiceal perforation, and ultimately peritonitis.

Quick HIT

Perforation of Appendix
- Complicates 20% of cases
- Risk factors: delay in treatment (>24 hours) and extremes of age
- Signs of appendiceal rupture (high fever, tachycardia, marked leukocytosis, peritoneal signs, toxic appearance)

2. Peak incidence is in the teens to mid-20s. Prognosis is far worse in infants and elderly patients (higher rate of perforation).

B. Clinical features

1. Symptoms
   a. Abdominal pain—Classically starts in the epigastrium, moves toward umbilicus, and then to the RLQ. With distention of the appendix, the parietal peritoneum may become irritated, leading to sharp pain.
   b. Anorexia always present. Appendicitis is unlikely if patient is hungry.
   c. Nausea and vomiting (typically follow pain).
2. Signs
   a. Tenderness in RLQ (maximal tenderness at *McBurney point:* two-thirds of the distance from the umbilicus to the right anterior superior iliac spine).
   b. Rebound tenderness, guarding, diminished bowel sounds.
   c. Low-grade fever (may spike if perforation occurs).
   d. *Rovsing sign:* Deep palpation in LLQ causes referred pain in RLQ.
   e. *Psoas sign:* RLQ pain when right thigh is extended as patient lies on left side.
   f. *Obturator sign:* Pain in RLQ when flexed right thigh is internally rotated when patient is supine.

C. Diagnosis

1. Acute appendicitis is a clinical diagnosis.
2. Laboratory findings (mild leukocytosis) are only supportive.
3. Imaging studies may be helpful if diagnosis uncertain or in atypical presentations.
   a. CT scan (sensitivity 98% to 100%)—lowers the false-positive rate significantly.
   b. Ultrasound (sensitivity of 90%).

D. Treatment is an appendectomy (usually laparoscopic). Up to 20% of patients who are diagnosed with acute appendicitis are found to have a normal appendix during surgery. Because the illness is potentially life-threatening, this is an acceptable risk even during pregnancy.

Carcinoid Tumors and Carcinoid Syndrome

- Carcinoid tumors originate from **neuroendocrine cells** and secrete **serotonin.**
- The most common site for these tumors is the appendix, but they can be found in a variety of locations (e.g., small bowel, rectum, bronchus, kidney, pancreas).

Diseases of the Pancreas

Acute Pancreatitis

A. General characteristics

1. There is inflammation of the pancreas resulting from prematurely activated pancreatic digestive enzymes that invoke pancreatic tissue autodigestion.
2. Most patients with acute pancreatitis have mild to moderate disease but up to 25% have severe disease. There are two forms of acute pancreatitis, mild and severe:
   a. Mild acute pancreatitis is most common and responds well to supportive treatment.
   b. Severe acute pancreatitis (necrotizing pancreatitis) has significant morbidity and mortality.

B. Causes

1. Alcohol abuse (40%)
2. Gallstones (40%)—the gallstone passes into the bile duct and blocks the ampulla of Vater
3. Post-ERCP—pancreatitis occurs in up to 10% of patients undergoing ERCP
4. Viral infections (e.g., mumps, Coxsackievirus B)

Quick HIT

Acute appendicitis is a clinical diagnosis. Laboratory findings (mild leukocytosis) are only supportive. Radiographs or other imaging studies are unnecessary unless the diagnosis is uncertain or the presentation is atypical.

Quick HIT

Carcinoid syndrome develops in 10% of patients with carcinoid tumors.

- Excess serotonin secretion can lead to **carcinoid syndrome,** which is manifested by cutaneous flushing, diarrhea, sweating, wheezing, abdominal pain, and heart valve dysfunction.
- Risk factors of metastasis increase with the size of the tumor. Metastases are rare with appendiceal tumors. Ileal tumors have the greatest likelihood of malignancy.
- Surgical resection is the treatment of choice.

Quick HIT

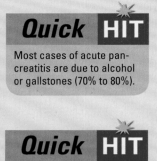

Most cases of acute pancreatitis are due to alcohol or gallstones (70% to 80%).

Quick HIT

Recurrences are common in alcoholic pancreatitis.

Quick HIT

The diagnosis of acute pancreatitis is usually made based on clinical presentation. Laboratory studies are supportive, and CT scan is confirmatory.

Quick HIT

The level of either amylase or lipase does not reliably predict the severity of disease.

Quick HIT

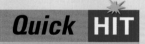

Hypocalcemia that results from acute pancreatitis is due to fat saponification: fat necrosis binds calcium.

5. Drugs—sulfonamides, thiazide diuretics, furosemide, estrogens, HIV medications, and many other drugs have been implicated
6. Postoperative complications (high mortality rate)
7. Scorpion bites
8. Pancreas divisum (controversial)
9. Pancreatic cancer
10. Hypertriglyceridemia, hypercalcemia
11. Uremia
12. Blunt abdominal trauma (most common cause of pancreatitis in children)

C. Clinical features

1. Symptoms
   a. Abdominal pain, usually in the epigastric region
      - May radiate to back (50% of patients)
      - Often steady, dull, and severe; worse when supine and after meals
   b. Nausea and vomiting, anorexia
2. Signs
   a. Low-grade fever, tachycardia, hypotension, leukocytosis
   b. Epigastric tenderness, abdominal distention
   c. Decreased or absent bowel sounds indicate partial ileus
   d. The following signs are seen with hemorrhagic pancreatitis as blood tracks along fascial planes:
      - *Grey Turner sign* (flank ecchymoses)
      - *Cullen sign* (periumbilical ecchymoses)
      - *Fox sign* (ecchymosis of inguinal ligament)

D. Diagnosis

1. Laboratory studies
   a. Serum amylase is the most common test, but many conditions cause hyperamylasemia (nonspecific) and its absence does not rule out acute pancreatitis (nonsensitive). However, if levels are more than five times the upper limit of normal, there is a high specificity for acute pancreatitis.
   b. Serum lipase—more specific for pancreatitis than amylase.
   c. LFTs—to identify cause (gallstone pancreatitis).
   d. Hyperglycemia, hypoxemia, and leukocytosis may also be present.
   e. Order the following for assessment of prognosis (see Table 3-4—Ranson criteria): glucose, calcium, hematocrit, BUN, arterial blood gas (PaO_2, base deficit), LDH, AST, WBC count.
2. Abdominal radiograph
   a. Has a limited role in the diagnosis of acute pancreatitis.
   b. More helpful in ruling out other diagnoses, such as intestinal perforation (free air). The presence of calcifications can suggest chronic pancreatitis.
   c. In some cases, one may see a sentinel loop (area of air-filled bowel usually in LUQ, which is a sign of localized ileus) or a colon cut-off sign (air-filled

TABLE 3-4 Ranson Criteria

Admission Criteria (GA LAW)	Initial 48-hr Criteria (C HOBBS)	Mortality
Glucose >200 mg/dL	**C**alcium <8 mg/dL Decrease in **H**ematocrit >10%	<3 criteria—1%
Age >55 yrs	Pa**O**$_2$ <60 mm Hg	3–4 criteria—15%
LDH >350	**B**UN increase >8 mg/dL	5–6 criteria—40%
AST >250	**B**ase deficit >4 mg/dL	>7 criteria—100%
WBC >16,000	Fluid **s**equestration >6 L	

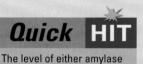

segment of transverse colon abruptly ending or "cutting off" at the region of pancreatic inflammation).
3. Abdominal ultrasound
   a. Can help in identifying cause of pancreatitis (e.g., gallstones)
   b. Useful for following up pseudocysts or abscesses
4. CT scan of the abdomen
   a. Most accurate test for diagnosis of acute pancreatitis and for identifying complications of the disease
   b. Indicated in patients with severe acute pancreatitis
5. ERCP (indications):
   a. Severe gallstone pancreatitis with biliary obstruction
   b. To identify uncommon causes of acute pancreatitis if disease is recurrent

Quick HIT

Pseudocysts may be present at sites distant from the pancreas.

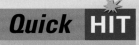

E. Complications

1. Pancreatic necrosis (may be sterile or infected)
   a. Sterile pancreatic necrosis—infection may develop, but half of all cases resolve spontaneously. These patients should be monitored closely in an ICU. Prophylactic antibiotics are controversial but if necrosis involves more than 30% of pancreas, antibiotics should be strongly considered.
   b. Infected pancreatic necrosis—has high mortality rate (results in multiple organ failure in 50% of cases); surgical débridement and antibiotics indicated.
   c. The only way to distinguish sterile from infected necrosis is via CT-guided percutaneous aspiration with Gram stain/culture of the aspirate.
2. Pancreatic pseudocyst
   a. Encapsulated fluid collection that appears 2 to 3 weeks after an acute attack—unlike a true cyst, it lacks an epithelial lining
   b. Complications of untreated pseudocysts include rupture, infection, gastric outlet obstruction, fistula, hemorrhage into cyst, and pancreatic ascites. It may impinge on adjacent abdominal organs (e.g., duodenum, stomach, transverse colon) if large enough; or if located in the head of the pancreas, it may cause compression of the CBD.
   c. Diagnosis: CT scan is the study of choice.
   d. Treatment
      - Cysts <5 cm: observation
      - Cysts >5 cm: drain either percutaneously or surgically
3. Hemorrhagic pancreatitis
   a. Characterized by Cullen sign, Grey Turner sign, and Fox sign
   b. CT scan with IV contrast is the study of choice
4. Adult respiratory distress syndrome—a life-threatening complication with high mortality rate
5. Pancreatic ascites/pleural effusion—the most common cause is inflammation of peritoneal surfaces
6. Ascending cholangitis—due to gallstone in ampulla of Vater, leading to infection of biliary tract; see section on cholangitis
7. Pancreatic abscess (rare)—develops over 4 to 6 weeks and is less life-threatening than infected pancreatic necrosis

Quick HIT

Most patients with acute pancreatitis respond to supportive care of pain control, bowel rest, IV fluids, and correction of electrolyte abnormalities and do not require any further therapy.

F. Treatment

1. Patients with mild acute pancreatitis:
   a. Bowel rest (NPO)—goal is to rest the pancreas.
   b. IV fluids—patients may have severe intravascular volume depletion. Correct electrolyte abnormalities.
   c. Pain control, but be cautious in giving narcotics. Fentanyl and meperidine preferred over morphine which causes an increase in sphincter of Oddi pressure.
   d. Nasogastric tube if severe nausea/vomiting or ileus present; routine use is controversial.
2. Patients with severe pancreatitis should be admitted to the ICU. Early enteral nutrition in the first 72 hours is recommended through a nasojejunal tube. If the

severe acute pancreatitis has not resolved in a few days, supplemental parenteral nutrition should be started. If more than 30% of the pancreas is necrosed, prophylactic antibiotics (imipenem) should be considered to prevent infection (which has high morbidity and mortality).

G. Prognosis

1. Ranson criteria are used to determine prognosis and mortality rates.
2. Patients with more than three or four Ranson criteria should be monitored in an ICU setting.

> **Quick HIT**
>
> The combination of chronic epigastric pain and calcifications on plain abdominal films is diagnostic for chronic pancreatitis. The classic triad of steatorrhea, diabetes mellitus, and pancreatic calcification on plain films or CT scan is also diagnostic.

> **Quick HIT**
>
> Chronic pancreatitis presents as chronic unrelenting pain with episodic flare-ups.

Chronic Pancreatitis

A. General characteristics

1. Persistent or continuing inflammation of the pancreas, with fibrotic tissue replacing pancreatic parenchyma, and alteration of pancreatic ducts (areas of stricture/dilation); eventually results in irreversible destruction of the pancreas
2. The endocrine and exocrine functions of the pancreas are impaired
3. Causes
   a. **Chronic alcoholism is the most common cause (>80% of cases).**
   b. Other causes include hereditary pancreatitis, tropical pancreatitis, and idiopathic chronic pancreatitis.

B. Clinical features

1. Severe pain in the epigastrium; recurrent or persistent abdominal pain
   a. Often accompanied by **nausea and vomiting**
   b. May be aggravated by a drinking episode, or by eating
   c. Radiates to the back (in 50% of cases)
2. Weight loss, due to malabsorption, alcohol abuse, and diabetes; steatorrhea secondary to malabsorption

C. Diagnosis

1. CT scan (Figure 3-4) is the initial study of choice. It may show calcifications not seen on plain films. Mild to moderate cases may not be detectable, so a normal CT scan does not necessarily rule out chronic pancreatitis.
2. Abdominal radiograph—the presence of pancreatic calcifications is 95% specific, but is found in only 30% of cases.
3. ERCP is the gold standard, but is not done routinely because it is invasive.
4. Laboratory studies are not helpful in diagnosis. Serum amylase and lipase levels are not elevated in chronic pancreatitis.

D. Complications

1. Narcotic addiction—probably the most common complication
2. Diabetes mellitus/impaired glucose tolerance
   a. Caused by progressive loss of islets of Langerhans
   b. Eventually appears in up to 70% of patients
3. Malabsorption/steatorrhea
   a. Caused by pancreatic exocrine insufficiency—occurs when pancreatic enzyme secretion decreases significantly
   b. A late manifestation of chronic pancreatitis
4. Pseudocyst formation
5. Pancreatic ductal dilation
6. CBD obstruction (may occur secondary to fibrosis in head of gland)
7. Vitamin B_{12} malabsorption
8. Effusions (e.g., pleural, pericardial, peritoneal)
9. Pancreatic carcinoma—patients with chronic pancreatitis have an increased risk

E. Treatment

1. Nonoperative management
   a. Narcotic analgesics for pain

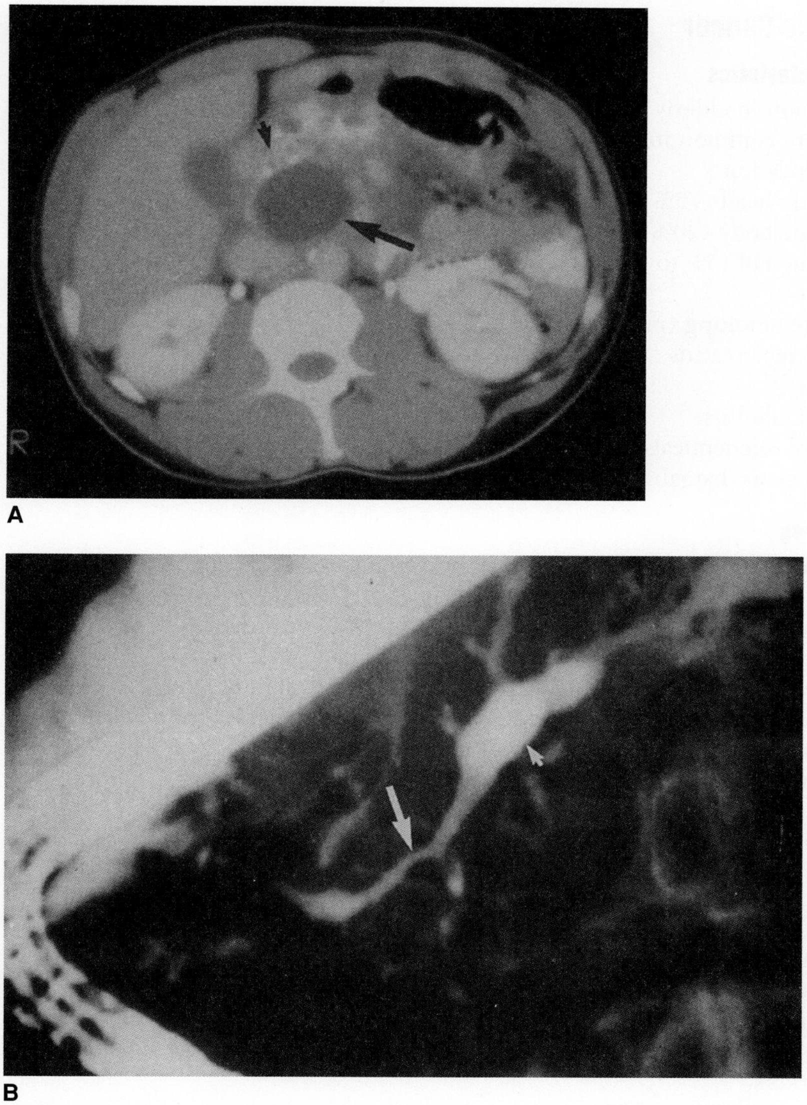

FIGURE 3-4 **A: CT scan of chronic pancreatitis. Note the area of calcification (*small arrow*) and a pseudocyst (*large arrow*) in the head of the pancreas. B: Typical findings on ERCP in chronic pancreatitis. Note the areas of stricture (*large arrow*) and duct dilatation (*small arrow*) throughout the pancreatic duct. This creates a "chain of lakes" appearance.**
(From Humes DH, DuPont HL, Gardner LB, et al. *Kelley's Textbook of Internal Medicine.* 4th ed. Philadelphia, PA: Lippincott Williams & Wilkins, 2000:958, Figures 117.9 and 117.10, respectively.)

b. Bowel rest (NPO)
c. Pancreatic enzymes and H_2 blockers (give simultaneously)
   - Pancreatic enzymes inhibit CCK release and thus decrease pancreatic secretions after meals.
   - H_2 blockers inhibit gastric acid secretion, preventing degradation of the pancreatic enzyme supplements by gastric acid.
d. Insulin—may be necessary due to severe pancreatic endocrine insufficiency
e. Alcohol abstinence
f. Frequent, small-volume, low-fat meals—may improve abdominal pain

2. Surgery—main goal is relief of incapacitating abdominal pain
   a. Pancreaticojejunostomy (pancreatic duct drainage procedure to decompress the dilated pancreatic duct)—most common procedure
   b. Pancreatic resection (distal pancreatectomy, Whipple procedure)

Pancreatic Cancer

A. General characteristics

1. Most common in elderly patients (75% of patients are >60 years old); rare before age 40; more common in African Americans
2. Anatomic location
   a. Pancreatic head (75% of cases)
   b. Pancreatic body (20% of cases)
   c. Pancreatic tail (5% to 10% of cases)
3. Risk factors
   a. **Cigarette smoking** (most clearly established risk)
   b. Chronic pancreatitis
   c. Diabetes
   d. Heavy alcohol use
   e. Exposure to chemicals—benzidine and β-naphthylamine
4. The prognosis is dismal: most patients die within months of diagnosis

Quick HIT

Painless jaundice is **not** common in pancreatic cancer!

Quick HIT

The early clinical findings of pancreatic cancer are very vague and nonspecific. By the time a diagnosis is made, most patients have an incurable level of advanced disease.

Quick HIT

Aortoenteric Fistula is a rare but lethal cause of GI bleeding. The classic presentation is a patient with a history (sometimes distant) of aortic graft surgery who has a small GI bleed involving the duodenum before massive, fatal hemorrhage hours to weeks later. Perform endoscopy or surgery during this small window of opportunity to prevent death.

B. Clinical features

1. Abdominal pain (90% of patients)—may be a vague and dull ache
2. Jaundice
   a. Most common with carcinoma of head of pancreas—less than 10% of patients with cancer involving body and tail of pancreas have jaundice
   b. Indicates obstruction of intrapancreatic CBD and is a sign of advanced disease
3. Weight loss (common due to decreased food intake and malabsorption); anorexia
4. Recent onset of glucose intolerance, but the diabetes is mild
5. Depression, weakness, fatigue
6. Migratory thrombophlebitis—develops in 10% of cases
7. *Courvoisier sign* (palpable gallbladder)—present in 30% of patients with cancer involving head of pancreas; presents without pain

C. Diagnosis

1. ERCP is the most sensitive test for diagnosing pancreatic cancer. It can also distinguish cancer of the head of the pancreas from tumors of the CBD, duodenum, ampulla, and lymphomas, which have a more favorable prognosis.
2. CT scan is the preferred test for diagnosis and assessment of disease spread.
3. Tumor markers.
   a. CA 19-9 (sensitivity of 83% and specificity of 82%).
   b. CEA (sensitivity of 56% and specificity of 75%).

D. Treatment

1. Surgical resection (Whipple procedure) is the only hope for a cure; however, only a minority of tumors are resectable (roughly 10%). **The prognosis is grim even after resection, with a 5-year survival rate of 10%.**
2. If the tumor is unresectable and biliary obstruction is present, perform PTC or ERCP with stent placement across the obstruction for palliation.

Gastrointestinal Bleeding

A. General characteristics

1. Upper GI bleeding refers to a source of bleeding above the ligament of Treitz in the duodenum.
2. Lower GI bleeding is classically defined as bleeding below the ligament of Treitz.

B. Causes

1. Upper GI bleeding
   a. Peptic ulcer disease (PUD)—duodenal ulcer (25% of cases), gastric ulcer (20% of cases), gastritis (25% of cases)
   b. Reflux esophagitis

c. Esophageal varices (10% of cases)—venous bleeding
d. Gastric varices
e. Gastric erosions, duodenitis
f. Mallory–Weiss tear
g. Hemobilia
h. Dieulafoy's vascular malformation—submucosal dilated arterial lesions that can cause massive GI bleeding
i. Aortoenteric fistulas—after aortic surgery (ask about prior aortic aneurysm/graft)
j. Neoplasm—bleeding is not rapid—usually not an emergency

2. Lower GI bleeding
   a. Diverticulosis (40% of cases)—most common source of GI bleeding in patients over age 60; usually painless
   b. Angiodysplasia (40% of cases)—second most common source in patients over age 60
   c. IBD (UC, Crohn disease)
   d. Colorectal carcinoma
   e. Colorectal adenomatous polyps
   f. Ischemic colitis
   g. Hemorrhoids, anal fissures
   h. Small intestinal bleeding—diagnosed by excluding upper GI and colonic bleeding

C. Clinical features

1. Type of bleeding:
   a. Hematemesis—vomiting blood; suggests upper GI bleeding (bleeding proximal to ligament of Treitz). Indicates moderate to severe bleeding that may be ongoing.
   b. "Coffee grounds" emesis—suggests upper GI bleeding as well as a **lower rate of bleeding** (enough time for vomitus to transform into "coffee grounds").
   c. Melena—black, tarry, liquid, foul-smelling stool.
      - Caused by degradation of hemoglobin by bacteria in the colon; presence of melena indicates that blood has remained in GI tract for several hours.
      - The further the bleeding site is from the rectum, the more likely melena will occur.
      - **Note that dark stools can also result from bismuth, iron, spinach, charcoal, and licorice.**
      - Melena suggests upper GI bleeding 90% of the time. Occasionally, the jejunum or ileum is the source. It is unusual for melena to be caused by a colonic lesion, but if it is, the ascending colon is the most likely site.
   d. Hematochezia—bright red blood per rectum.
      - This usually represents a lower GI source (typically **left colon** or **rectum**). Consider diverticulosis, arteriovenous malformations, hemorrhoids, and colon cancers.
      - It may result from massive upper GI bleeding that is bleeding very briskly (so that blood does not remain in colon to turn into melena—see above). This often indicates heavy bleeding, and patient often has some degree of hemodynamic instability. An upper GI source is present in about 5% to 10% of patients with hematochezia.
   e. Occult blood in stool—source of bleeding may be anywhere along GI tract.
2. Signs of volume depletion (depending on rate and severity of blood loss).
3. Symptoms and signs of anemia (e.g., fatigue, pallor, exertional dyspnea).

D. Diagnosis

1. Laboratory tests (see also Clinical Pearl 3-6 and Figure 3-5)
   a. Stool guaiac for occult blood.
   b. Hemoglobin/hematocrit level (may not be decreased in acute bleeds): A hemoglobin level >7 to 8 g/dL is generally acceptable in young, healthy patients without active bleeding. However, most elderly patients (especially those with cardiac disease) should have a hemoglobin level >10 g/dL.

Quick HIT
A lower GI bleed (or positive occult blood test of stool) in patients over 40 is colon cancer until proven otherwise.

Quick HIT
About 80% of episodes of upper GI bleeding stop spontaneously and only need supportive therapy.

Quick HIT
- Bleeding from the small bowel may manifest as melena or hematochezia.
- Colonic sources of bleeding present with either occult blood in the stool or hematochezia.

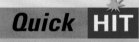

Quick HIT
Always ask patients with GI bleeding if they take any NSAIDs/aspirin, clopidogrel or anticoagulants.

Quick HIT
Hematemesis and melena are the most common presentations of acute upper GI bleed, and patients may have both symptoms. Occasionally, a brisk upper GI bleed presents as hematochezia.

Quick HIT
An elevated PT may be indicative of liver dysfunction, vitamin K deficiency, a consumptive coagulopathy, or warfarin therapy.

CLINICAL PEARL 3-6

Tests to Order in Patients With GI Bleeding

- Hematemesis—An upper GI endoscopy is the initial test.
- Hematochezia—First rule out an anorectal cause (e.g., hemorrhoids). Colonoscopy should be the initial test because colon cancer is the main concern in patients over age 50.
- Melena—Upper endoscopy is usually the initial test because the most likely bleeding site is in the upper GI tract. Order a colonoscopy if no bleeding site is identified from the endoscopy.
- Occult blood—Colonoscopy is the initial test in most cases (colon cancer is the main concern). Order an upper endoscopy if no bleeding site is identified from the colonoscopy.

Quick HIT

If you suspect lower GI bleeding, still exclude upper GI bleeding before attempting to localize the site of the lower GI bleed.

Quick HIT

Initial Steps in any Patient with GI Bleeding

- Vital signs: Decreased BP, tachycardia, or postural changes in BP or HR are signs of significant hemorrhage. However, vital signs may also be normal when significant hemorrhage is present.
- Resuscitation is the first step (e.g., IV fluids, transfusion).
- Perform rectal examination (hemoccult test).

c. A low mean corpuscular volume is suggestive of iron deficiency anemia (chronic blood loss). Patients with acute bleeding have normocytic red blood cells.
d. Coagulation profile (platelet count, PT, PTT, INR).
e. LFTs, renal function.
f. The BUN-creatinine ratio is elevated with upper GI bleeding. This is suggestive of upper GI bleeding if patient has no renal insufficiency. The higher the ratio, the more likely the bleeding is from an upper GI source.

2. Upper endoscopy
   a. Most accurate diagnostic test in evaluation of upper GI bleeding.
   b. Both diagnostic and potentially therapeutic (coagulate bleeding vessel).
   c. Most patients with upper GI bleeding should have upper endoscopy within 24 hours.
3. Nasogastric tube
   a. This is often the initial procedure for determining whether GI bleeding is from an upper or lower GI source.

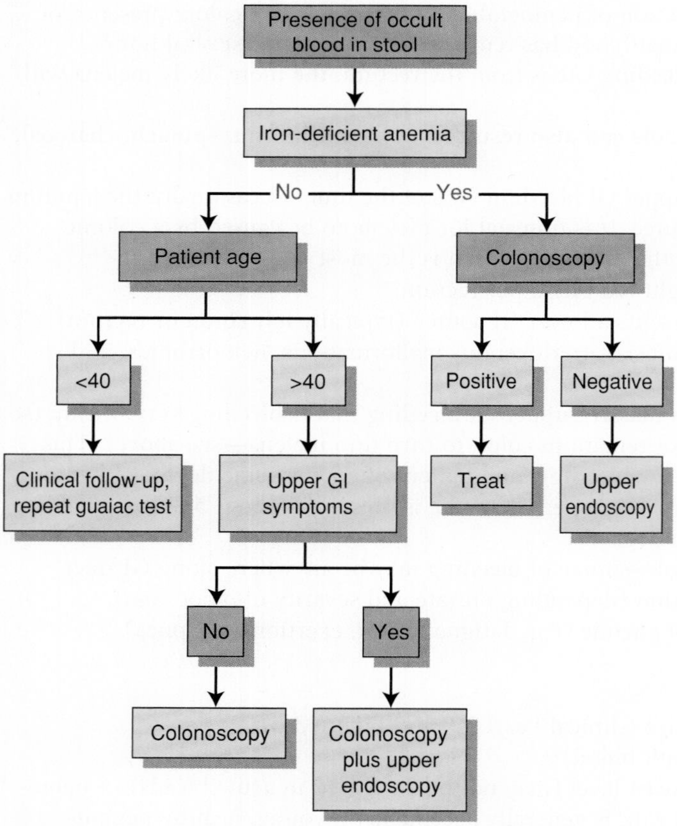

FIGURE 3-5 **Evaluation of occult GI bleeding.**

b. Use the nasogastric tube to empty the stomach to prevent aspiration.
c. False-negative findings are possible if upper GI bleeding is intermittent or from a lesion in the duodenum.
d. Evaluation of aspirate
   - Bile but no blood—upper GI bleeding unlikely; source is probably distal to ligament of Treitz.
   - Bright red blood or "coffee grounds" appearance—upper GI bleeding.
   - Nonbloody aspirate (clear gastric fluid)—upper GI bleeding unlikely, but cannot be ruled out definitively (source may possibly be in the duodenum).

4. Anoscopy or proctosigmoidoscopy can exclude an anal/rectal source. Perform this if there is no obvious bleeding from hemorrhoids.
5. Colonoscopy identifies the site of the lower GI bleed in >70% of cases, and can also be therapeutic (see below).
6. A bleeding scan (radionuclide scanning) reveals bleeding even with a low rate of blood loss. It does not localize the lesion; it only identifies continued bleeding. Its role is controversial, but it may help determine whether arteriography is needed.
7. Arteriography definitively locates the point of bleeding.
   a. Mostly used in patients with lower GI bleeding.
   b. Should be performed during active bleeding.
   c. Potentially therapeutic (embolization or intra-arterial vasopressin infusion).
8. Exploratory laparotomy—last resort.

Quick HIT

In elderly patients and patients with known cardiovascular disease who present with severe bleeding, rule out myocardial infarctions, especially if there has been hemodynamic instability.

E. Treatment

1. If patient is hemodynamically unstable, resuscitation is always top priority. Remember the ABCs. Once the patient is stabilized, obtain a diagnosis (see also Clinical Pearl 3-7).
   a. Supplemental oxygen.
   b. Place two large-bore IV lines. Give IV fluids or blood if patient is volume depleted.
   c. Draw blood for hemoglobin and hematocrit, PT, PTT, and platelet count. Monitor hemoglobin every 4 to 8 hours until the patient is hemoglobin stable for at least 24 hours.
   d. Type and crossmatch adequate blood (PRBCs). Transfuse as the clinical condition demands (e.g., shock, patients with cardiopulmonary disease).
2. Treatment depends on the cause/source of the bleed.
   a. Upper GI bleeding.
      - EGD with coagulation of the bleeding vessel. If bleeding continues, repeat endoscopic therapy or proceed with surgical intervention (ligation of bleeding vessel).
   b. Lower GI bleeding.
      - Colonoscopy—polyp excision, injection, laser, cautery.
      - Arteriographic vasoconstrictor infusion.
      - Surgical resection of involved area—last resort.

CLINICAL PEARL 3-7

Factors That Increase Mortality in GI Bleeding

- Age >65 years
- Severity of initial bleed
- Extensive comorbid illnesses
- Onset or recurrence of bleeding while hospitalized for another condition
- Need for emergency surgery
- Significant transfusion requirements
- Diagnosis (esophageal varices have a 30% mortality rate)
- Endoscopic stigmata of recent hemorrhage

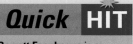

3. Indications for surgery.
   a. Hemodynamically unstable patients who have not responded to IV fluid, transfusion, endoscopic intervention, or correction of coagulopathies.
   b. Severe initial bleed or recurrence of bleed after endoscopic treatment.
   c. Continued bleeding for more than 24 hours.
   d. Visible vessel at base of ulcer (30% to 50% chance of rebleed).
   e. Ongoing transfusion requirement (five units within first 4 to 6 hours).

Diseases of the Esophagus

Esophageal Cancer

A. General characteristics

1. There are two pathologic types. In the past, squamous cell carcinoma (SCC) accounted for up to 90% of cases. However, the incidence of adenocarcinoma has increased dramatically in the United States, and it now accounts for up to 50% of new cases.
   a. SCC
      - Incidence is higher in African-American men than in other groups.
      - Most common locations are the upper- and midthoracic esophagus. About one-third may be in distal 10 cm of esophagus.
      - Risk factors are **alcohol and tobacco use**, diet (nitrosamines, betel nuts, chronic ingestion of hot foods and beverages such as tea), human papillomavirus, achalasia, Plummer–Vinson syndrome, caustic ingestion, and nasopharyngeal carcinoma.
   b. Adenocarcinoma
      - More common in Caucasians and men (5:1 over women).
      - Most common in distal third of the esophagus/gastroesophageal junction (in 80% of cases).
      - Risk factors: **GERD and Barrett esophagus** are main risk factors; alcohol and tobacco may not be as important as in SCC.
2. **The prognosis is poor:** Five-year survival rate is about 30% to 40% if locoregional disease, but only 5% if distant metastasis present at diagnosis.
3. Staging
   a. Stage I—tumor invades lamina propria or submucosa; nodes negative
   b. Stage IIa—tumor invades muscularis propria or adventitia; nodes negative
   c. Stage IIb—tumor invades up to muscularis propria; positive regional nodes
   d. Stage III—tumor invades adventitia (positive regional nodes) **or** tumor invades adjacent structures (positive or negative nodes)
   e. Stage IV—distant metastasis

Quick HIT

Barrett Esophagus is a complication of longstanding acid reflux disease in which there is columnar metaplasia of the squamous epithelium. Patients with Barrett esophagus are at increased risk of developing adenocarcinoma of the esophagus. Monitor these patients with routine endoscopic surveillance.

B. Clinical features

1. Dysphagia—most common symptom (initially solids only, then progression to liquids)
2. Weight loss—second most common symptom
3. Anorexia
4. Odynophagia (pain with swallowing)—a late finding that suggests extraesophageal involvement (mediastinal invasion)
5. Hematemesis, hoarseness of voice (recurrent laryngeal nerve involvement)
6. Aspiration pneumonia, respiratory symptoms due to involvement of tracheobronchial tree
7. Tracheoesophageal or bronchoesophageal fistula
8. Chest pain

C. Diagnosis

1. Barium swallow useful in evaluation of dysphagia. A presumptive diagnosis can be made.
2. Upper endoscopy with biopsy and brush cytology is required for definitive diagnosis. It confirms the diagnosis in 95% of cases.

3. Transesophageal ultrasound helps determine the depth of penetration of the tumor and is the most reliable test for staging local cancer.
4. Full metastatic workup (e.g., CT scan of chest/abdomen, CXR, bone scan).

D. Treatment

1. Palliation is the goal in most patients because the disease is usually advanced at presentation.
2. Surgery (esophagectomy) may be curative for patients with disease in stage 0, 1, or 2A.
3. Chemotherapy plus radiation before surgery has been shown to prolong survival more than surgery alone.

Achalasia

A. General characteristics

1. Acquired motor disorder of esophageal smooth muscle in which the lower esophageal sphincter (LES) fails to completely relax with swallowing, and abnormal peristalsis of esophageal body replaces normal peristalsis of the esophageal body
2. Absolute criteria for diagnosis
   a. Incomplete relaxation of the LES
   b. Aperistalsis of esophagus

B. Causes

1. The majority in the United States are idiopathic.
2. In the United States, adenocarcinoma of proximal stomach is the second most common cause.
3. Worldwide, Chagas disease is an important cause.

C. Clinical features

1. Dysphagia (odynophagia is less common)
   a. Equal difficulty swallowing solids and liquids (in contrast to esophageal cancer, in which dysphagia for solids starts first, than later for liquids).
   b. Patients tend to eat slowly and drink lots of water to wash down food. Also, they may twist their body, extend their neck, or walk about the room in an effort to force food into the stomach.
   c. It is exacerbated by fast eating and by emotional stress.
2. Regurgitation
   a. Food gets "stuck" in the esophagus and then comes back up.
   b. Regurgitation may lead to aspiration.
3. Chest pain
4. Weight loss
5. Recurrent pulmonary complications secondary to aspiration, which may cause lung abscess, bronchiectasis, or hemoptysis

> **Quick HIT**
>
> Patients with achalasia have a sevenfold increase in the risk of esophageal cancer (usually squamous cell)—it occurs in 10% of patients 15 to 25 years after the initial achalasia diagnosis. Often tumors go unnoticed (even when large) due to a dilated esophagus and chronic dysphagia. Therefore, perform surveillance esophagoscopy to detect the tumor at an early stage.

D. Diagnosis

1. Barium swallow (Figure 3-6)—"bird's beak"—beak-like narrowing of distal esophagus and a large, dilated esophagus proximal to the narrowing
2. Upper GI endoscopy—to rule out secondary causes of achalasia (gastric carcinoma) and retention esophagitis or esophageal cancer
3. Manometry—to confirm the diagnosis; reveals failure of LES relaxation and aperistalsis of esophageal body

E. Treatment

1. Instruct patient on adaptive measures: chew food to consistency of pea soup before swallowing; sleep with trunk elevated; avoid eating before sleep.
2. Medical therapy
   a. Antimuscarinic agents (dicyclomine)—usually unsatisfactory
   b. Sublingual nitroglycerin, long-acting nitrates, and calcium channel blockers
      - May improve swallowing in early stages of achalasia (before esophageal dilatation occurs)

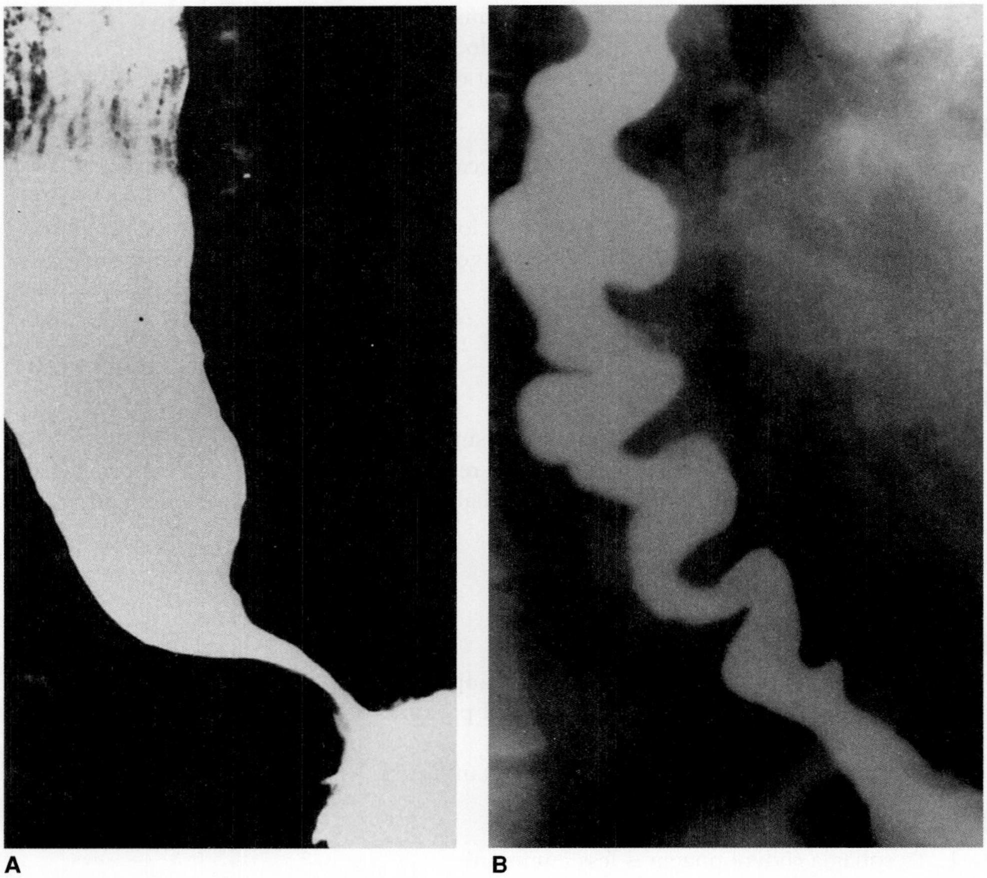

FIGURE 3-6 **Radiographs of achalasia (A) and diffuse esophageal spasm (B).**
(From Humes DH, DuPont HL, Gardner LB, et al. *Kelley's Textbook of Internal Medicine.* 4th ed. Philadelphia, PA: Lippincott Williams & Wilkins, 2000:821, Figure 106.4.)

Quick HIT

There is no Cure for Achalasia. Treatment modalities (including surgery) are only palliative.

Quick HIT

It can be difficult to distinguish the chest pain of diffuse esophageal spasm (DES) from cardiac chest pain. Therefore, many patients undergo a cardiac workup, including cardiac catheterization to rule out ischemic causes of chest pain, before an esophageal cause is investigated.

- Most useful in the short-term treatment of achalasia (before more definitive therapy)

3. Injection of botulinum toxin into the LES during endoscopy
   a. Blocks cholinergic activity in the LES
   b. Can be effective in up to 65% of cases; however, repeat procedure needs to be performed every 2 years
4. Forceful dilatation—mechanical, pneumatic, or hydrostatic
   a. Pneumatic balloon dilatation is most effective
   b. Lowers basal LES tone by disrupting the muscular ring
   c. Can be effective, but there is a 5% risk of perforation
5. Surgical
   a. "Heller myotomy"—circular muscle layer of LES is incised
   b. Usually reserved for patients who do not respond to dilation therapy
6. Early results are promising (80% to 90% of patients experience good to excellent palliation of dysphagia at 1 year)
7. Long-term data are needed

Diffuse Esophageal Spasm

A. General characteristics

1. Nonperistaltic spontaneous contraction of the esophageal body—several segments of the esophagus contract simultaneously and prevent appropriate advancement of food bolus.
2. In contrast to achalasia, **sphincter function is normal** (normal LES pressure).

B. Clinical features

1. There is **noncardiac chest pain** that mimics angina and may radiate to the jaw, arms, and back.
2. Dysphagia is common; however, regurgitation of food is uncommon.

C. Diagnosis

1. Esophageal manometry is diagnostic—simultaneous, multiphasic, repetitive contractions that occur after a swallow; sphincter response is normal
2. Upper GI barium swallow ("corkscrew esophagus")—in 50%, which represents multiple simultaneous contractions

D. Treatment

1. In general there is no completely effective therapy—treatment failure rates are high.
2. Medical treatment involves nitrates and calcium channel blockers (decreases amplitude of contractions). Tricyclic antidepressants may provide symptomatic relief.
3. Esophagomyotomy is usually not performed, and its efficacy is controversial. Some support its use, whereas others only recommend it when a patient is incapacitated by symptoms.

Esophageal Hiatal Hernias

A. General characteristics: There are two types of hiatal hernias: sliding (type 1) and paraesophageal (type 2) (Figure 3-7)

1. Sliding hiatal hernias (type 1) account for >90% of cases. Both the gastroesophageal junction and a portion of the stomach herniate into the thorax through the esophageal hiatus (so that the gastroesophageal junction is above the diaphragm). This is a common and benign finding that is associated with GERD.
2. Paraesophageal hiatal hernia accounts for <5% of cases. The stomach herniates into the thorax through the esophageal hiatus, but the gastroesophageal junction does not; it remains below the diaphragm. This uncommon hernia can become strangulated and should be repaired surgically.

B. Clinical features

1. The majority of cases are asymptomatic and are discovered incidentally.
2. Possible symptoms include heartburn, chest pain, and dysphagia.
3. Complications of sliding hiatal hernias include GERD (most common), reflux esophagitis (with risk of Barrett esophagus/cancer), and aspiration.
4. Complications of paraesophageal hernias are potentially life-threatening and include obstruction, hemorrhage, incarceration, and strangulation.

C. Diagnosis: barium upper GI series and upper endoscopy

D. Treatment

1. Type 1 hernias are treated medically (with antacids, small meals, and elevation of the head after meals); 15% of cases may require surgery (Nissen fundoplication) if there is no response to medical therapy or if there is evidence of esophagitis.
2. Type 2 hernias treated with elective surgery due to risk of above complications.

Mallory–Weiss Syndrome

- This is a mucosal tear at (or just below) the gastroesophageal junction as a result of forceful vomiting or retching. It usually occurs after repeated episodes of vomiting, but it may occur after one episode.
- It is most commonly associated with binge drinking in alcoholics, but any disorder that causes vomiting can induce the mucosal tear.
- Hematemesis is always present—it varies from streaks of blood in vomitus to massive bright red blood.

Quick HIT

- Paraesophageal hernias tend to enlarge with time, and the entire stomach may ultimately move into the thorax.
- Type 3 hernias (combination of type 1 and 2) are treated as type 2 hernias (surgically).

Quick HIT

If a patient with GERD also has a hiatal hernia, the hernia often worsens the symptoms of GERD.

Quick HIT

During forceful vomiting, the marked increase in intra-abdominal pressure is transmitted to the esophagus. This can lead to two conditions, depending on the severity and location of the tear.

- If the tear is mucosal and at the gastroesophageal junction, it is referred to as **Mallory–Weiss syndrome.**
- If a tear is transmural (causing esophageal perforation), it is referred to as **Boerhaave syndrome.**

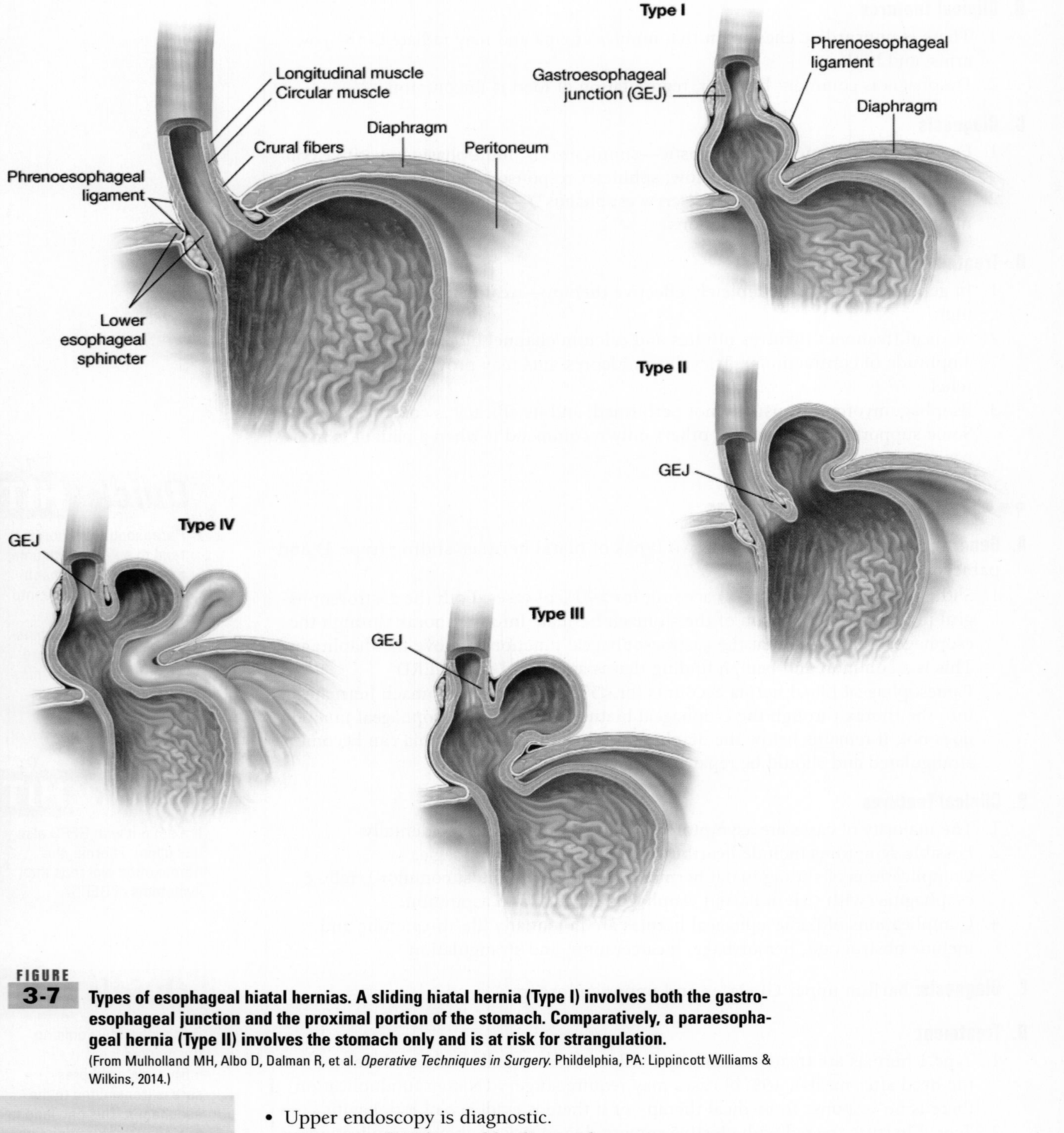

FIGURE 3-7 **Types of esophageal hiatal hernias. A sliding hiatal hernia (Type I) involves both the gastroesophageal junction and the proximal portion of the stomach. Comparatively, a paraesophageal hernia (Type II) involves the stomach only and is at risk for strangulation.**
(From Mulholland MH, Albo D, Dalman R, et al. *Operative Techniques in Surgery.* Phildelphia, PA: Lippincott Williams & Wilkins, 2014.)

- Upper endoscopy is diagnostic.
- Most cases (90%) stop bleeding without any treatment.
- Treatment is surgery (oversewing the tear) or angiographic embolization if bleeding continues, but this is rarely necessary. Acid suppression is used to promote healing.

Plummer–Vinson Syndrome (Upper Esophageal Webs)

- Key features: upper esophageal web (causes dysphagia), iron deficiency anemia, *koilonychia* (spoon-shaped fingernails), and atrophic oral mucosa.
- Ten percent of patients develop SCC of the oral cavity, hypopharynx, or esophagus; therefore, this is considered a premalignant lesion.
- Treatment: esophageal dilatation; correct nutritional deficiency.

Schatzki Ring (Distal Esophageal Webs)

- A circumferential ring in the lower esophagus that is always accompanied by a sliding hiatal hernia.
- It is usually asymptomatic, but mild to moderate dysphagia may be present.
- If the patient is symptomatic (but has no reflux), consider esophageal dilatation. If the patient has reflux, consider antireflux surgery.
- Usually due to ingestion of alkali, acids, bleach, or detergents (e.g., in suicide attempts).
- Ingesting alkali is more dangerous than ingesting acid because it may lead to liquefactive necrosis of the esophagus with full-thickness perforation. Acid ingestion does not cause full-thickness damage (only causes necrosis of esophageal mucosa).
- Complications: stricture formation and risk of esophageal cancer.
- Treatment is esophagectomy if full-thickness necrosis has occurred. Patient should avoid vomiting, gastric lavage, and all oral intake (can compound the original injury). Give the patient steroids and antibiotics as well. Perform bougienage for esophageal stricture.

Esophageal Diverticula

- Most esophageal diverticula are caused by an **underlying motility disorder** of the esophagus (Figure 3-8).
- **Zenker diverticulum** is the most common type; found in upper third of the esophagus.
- Failure of the cricopharyngeal muscle to relax during swallowing leads to increased intraluminal pressure. This causes outpouching of mucosa through an area of weakness in the pharyngeal constrictors.
- Clinical features include dysphagia, regurgitation, halitosis (bad breath), weight loss, and chronic cough.
- It is typically seen in patients >50 years old.
- **Traction diverticula** are located in the midpoint of the esophagus near the tracheal bifurcation. It is due to traction from contiguous mediastinal inflammation and

Quick HIT

An underlying motility disorder is the cause of both proximal **(Zenker)** and distal **(epiphrenic) esophageal diverticula.** Surgical treatment is aimed at correcting the motility disorder (i.e., myotomy). Diverticulectomy is of secondary importance.

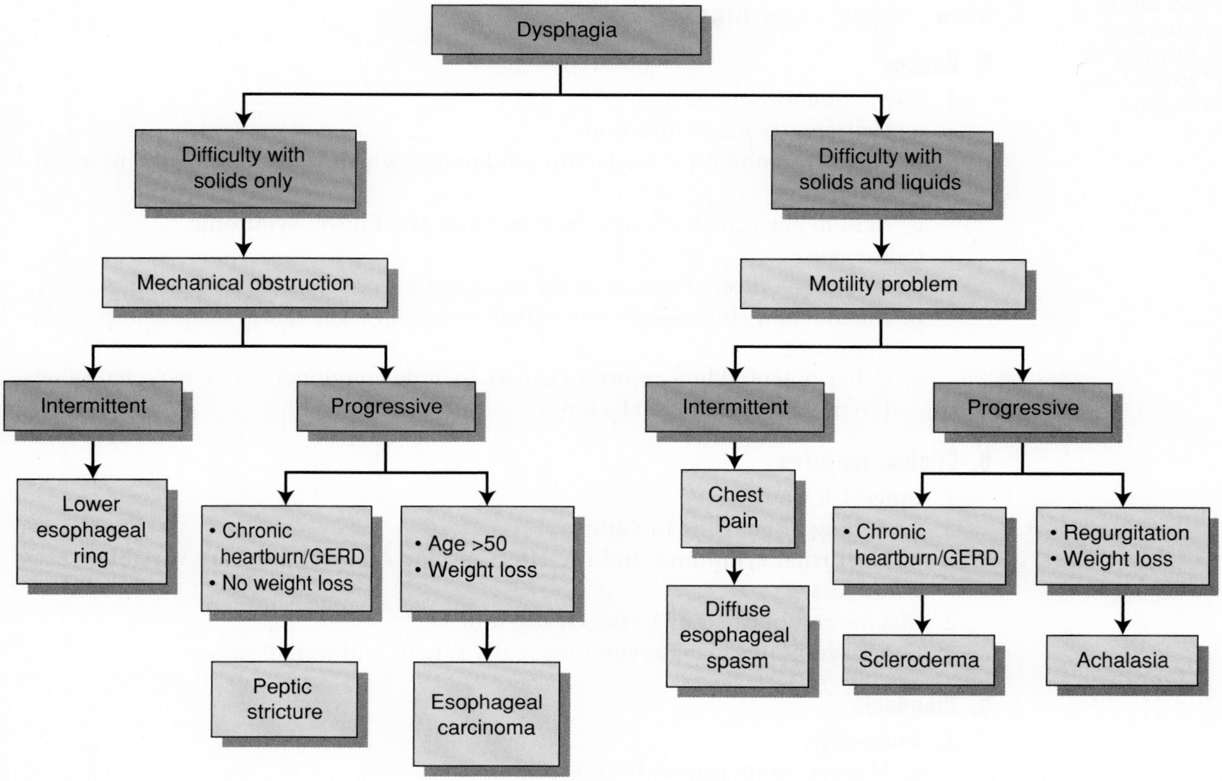

FIGURE 3-8 **Causes of dysphagia.**

adenopathy (pulmonary tuberculosis). Tuberculosis causes hilar node scarring, which causes retraction of esophagus. It is usually asymptomatic and does not require treatment.

- **Epiphrenic diverticula** are found in lower third of esophagus. It is usually associated with spastic esophageal dysmotility or achalasia. Symptoms of dysphagia are more often related to the underlying motility disorder, unless the diverticulum is very large.
- Barium swallow is the best diagnostic test for diverticula.
- Treatment of Zenker diverticula is surgery. Cricopharyngeal myotomy has excellent results. Treatment of epiphrenic diverticula is esophagomyotomy. Diverticulectomy is of secondary importance in both cases.

Quick HIT

If gastric/esophageal contents leak into the mediastinum or pleura, infection and septic sequelae may result.

Esophageal Perforation

- Etiology: blunt trauma, medical tubes and instruments, forceful vomiting **(Boerhaave syndrome)** that is associated with alcoholic binges and bulimia.
- Clinical features: pain (severe retrosternal/chest/shoulder pain), tachycardia, hypotension, tachypnea, dyspnea, fever, *Hamman sign* ("mediastinal crunch" produced by the heart beating against air-filled tissues), pneumothorax, or pleural effusion.
- Contrast esophagram is definitive diagnostic study (soluble Gastrografin swallow preferred).
- CXR usually shows air in the mediastinum.
- If the patient is stable and the perforation is small (draining into lumen), medical management is appropriate: IV fluids, NPO, antibiotics, and H_2 blockers.
- If patient is ill and the perforation is large (or if there is communication into pleural cavity), surgery should be performed within 24 hours of presentation (success rate is higher).

Quick HIT

The time interval between esophageal perforation and surgery is the most important factor in determining survival. **If surgery is delayed beyond 24 hours, the mortality rate and the likelihood of fistulization increase.**

Diseases of the Stomach

Peptic Ulcer Disease

Quick HIT

Most cases of PUD are due to *H. pylori* infection and NSAID use. It can be difficult to determine the cause in a patient with *H. pylori* infection who also uses NSAIDs. Both may be responsible. Therefore, if in doubt, test for *H. pylori.*

A. Causes

1. Most common causes
   a. *Helicobacter pylori* infection
   b. NSAIDs—inhibit prostaglandin production, which leads to impaired mucosal defenses
   c. Acid hypersecretory states, such as Zollinger–Ellison syndrome
2. Other causes
   a. Smoking—ulcers twice as likely in cigarette smokers as in nonsmokers
   b. Alcohol and coffee—may exacerbate symptoms, but causal relationship as yet unproven
   c. Other potential but unproven causes include emotional stress, personality type ("type A"), and dietary factors

B. Clinical features

1. Epigastric pain
   a. Aching or gnawing in nature
   b. **Nocturnal symptoms and the effect of food on symptoms are variable** (see Table 3-5).
2. May be complicated by upper GI bleeding
3. Other symptoms: nausea/vomiting, early satiety, and weight loss

C. Diagnosis

1. Endoscopy
   a. Most accurate test in diagnosing ulcers.
   b. Essential in diagnosis of gastric ulcers because biopsy is necessary to rule out malignancy—duodenal ulcers do not require biopsy.

TABLE 3-5 Duodenal Versus Gastric Ulcers

	Duodenal Ulcers	Gastric Ulcers
Pathogenesis	Caused by an increase in offensive factors (higher rates of basal and stimulated gastric acid secretion)	Caused by a decrease in defensive factors (gastric acid level is normal/low unless ulcer is pyloric or prepyloric)
***Helicobacter pylori* Infection**	70%–90% of patients	60%–70% of patients
Malignant Potential	Low (malignancy is very rare) should undergo biopsy to rule out	High (5%–10% are malignant)—malignancy
Location	Majority are 1–2 cm distal to pylorus (usually on posterior wall)	Type I (most common, 70%): on lesser curvature Type II: gastric and duodenal ulcer Type III: prepyloric (within 2 cm of pylorus) Type IV: near esophagogastric junction
Age Distribution	Occurs in younger patients (<40)	Occurs in older patients (>40)
Associated Blood Type	Type O	Type A
Risk Factors	NSAIDs	Smoking
Other	Eating usually relieves pain Nocturnal pain is more common than in gastric ulcers	Eating does not usually relieve pain Complication rates are higher than those of duodenal ulcers. There is a higher recurrence rate with medical therapy alone

c. Preferred when severe or acute bleeding is present (can perform electrocautery of bleeding ulcers).
d. Can obtain endoscopic biopsy for diagnosis of *H. pylori*.

2. Barium swallow
   a. Sometimes used initially but is less reliable than endoscopy.
   b. Double-contrast techniques preferred due to improved accuracy.
3. Laboratory test—for diagnosis of *H. pylori* infection
   a. Biopsy: Histologic evaluation of endoscopic biopsy is the gold standard.
   b. Urease detection via urea breath test is the most convenient test (sensitivity and specificity >95%). It documents active infection and helps to assess the results of antibiotic therapy.
   c. Serology (lower specificity)—The presence of antibodies to *H. pylori* does not necessarily indicate current infection—Antibodies to *H. pylori* can remain elevated for months or even years after eradication of infection (90% sensitive).
      - The following may lead to false-negative test results: proton pump inhibitors (PPIs), bismuth, many antibiotics and upper GI bleeding.
4. Serum gastrin measurement—if considering Zollinger–Ellison syndrome as a diagnosis

Quick HIT

If a peptic ulcer is uncomplicated, a barium study or endoscopy is not needed initially. Initiate empiric therapy. However, if you suspect any of the complications of PUD, order confirmatory studies.

D. Treatment

1. Medical—Majority of patients with PUD can be successfully treated by curing *H. pylori* infection, avoidance of NSAIDs, and appropriate use of antisecretory drugs.
   a. Supportive (patient directives)
      - Discontinue aspirin/NSAIDs.
      - Restrict alcohol use but do not restrict any foods.
      - Stop smoking, decrease emotional stress.
      - Avoid eating before bedtime (eating stimulates nocturnal gastric acid levels); decrease coffee intake (although no strong link has been established with ulcer disease).

TABLE 3-6 *Helicobacter pylori* Eradication

	Regimen	Advantage	Disadvantage
Triple Therapy	PPI plus amoxicillin and clarithromycin	Twice daily dosing	More expensive than bismuth-based triple therapy
Quadruple Therapy	PPI, bismuth subsalicylate, metronidazole, and tetracycline	Half the time as triple therapy (a 1-week program as opposed to 2 weeks for triple therapy), yet has similar eradication results	Expense of PPI

Quick HIT

Acid Suppression Therapy
- **H_2 blockers**
- Ranitidine
- Famotidine
- Nizatidine
- Cimetidine
- **PPIs**
- Esomeprazole
- Omeprazole
- Lansoprazole
- Pantoprazole
- Rabeprazole

b. Acid suppression therapy
   - H_2 receptor blockers—Cimetidine (Tagamet) and Ranitidine (Zantac). Block histamine–based parietal cell acid secretion. Accelerate healing of ulcers.
   - PPIs—omeprazole (Prilosec), lansoprazole (Prevacid), Block H+/K+ ATPase pump directly in parietal cell membrane. Most effective antisecretory agents (although expensive).
   - Antacids—somewhat outdated for primary therapy and more appropriately used for adjunctive therapy/symptomatic relief. Examples include aluminum hydroxide (Mylanta), calcium carbonate (Tums), Bismuth subsalicylate (Pepto-Bismol).

c. Eradicate *H. pylori* with triple or quadruple therapy (see Table 3-5). Once infection is cleared, the rate of recurrence is very low.
   - For initial therapy, triple therapy (PPI, amoxicillin and clarithromycin) for 10 days to 2 weeks.
   - For retreatment, quadruple therapy (PPI, bismuth, metronidazole, and tetracycline).

d. Cytoprotection
   - Sucralfate—facilitates ulcer healing, must be taken frequently, is costly, and can cause GI upset.
   - Misoprostol—reduces risk for ulcer formation associated with NSAID therapy, is costly, and can cause GI upset (common side effect).

e. Treatment regimens
   - If *H. pylori* test is positive, begin eradication therapy with either triple or quadruple therapy (see Table 3-6). Also begin acid suppression with antacids, an H_2 blocker, or a PPI.
   - If the patient has an active NSAID-induced ulcer, stop NSAID use (may switch to acetaminophen). Also begin with either a PPI or misoprostol. Continue for 4 to 8 weeks, depending on severity. Treat the *H. pylori* infection as above if present.
   - Antisecretory drugs can be discontinued after 4 to 6 weeks in patients with uncomplicated ulcers who are asymptomatic. Patients at increased risk of recurrence (especially if underlying cause of ulcer is not reversed) may benefit from maintenance therapy.
   - *H. pylori*-negative ulcers that are NOT caused by NSAIDs can be treated with antisecretory drugs (either H_2 blockers or PPI).

2. Surgical
   a. Rarely needed electively
   b. Required for the complications of PUD (bleeding, perforation, gastric outlet obstruction) (see Table 3-7 and Figure 3-9)

Acute Gastritis

- Acute gastritis refers to inflammation of the gastric mucosa.
- There are multiple causes: NSAIDs/aspirin; *H. pylori* infection; alcohol, heavy cigarette smoking, or caffeine; extreme physiologic stress (e.g., shock, sepsis, burns).

TABLE 3-7 Complications of Peptic Ulcer Disease

	Clinical Findings	Diagnostic Studies	Management	Other
Perforation	Acute, severe abdominal pain, signs of peritonitis, hemodynamic instability	Upright CXR **(free air under diaphragm)**, CT scan is the most sensitive test for perforation (detects free abdominal air)	Emergency surgery to close perforation and perform definitive ulcer operation (such as highly selective vagotomy or truncal vagotomy/pyloroplasty)	**Can progress to sepsis and death if untreated**
Gastric Outlet Obstruction	Nausea/vomiting (poorly digested food), epigastric fullness/early satiety, weight loss	Barium swallow and upper endoscopy; saline load test (empty stomach with a nasogastric tube, add 750 mL saline, aspirate after 30 min—test is positive if aspirate >400 mL)	Initially, nasogastric suction; replace electrolyte/volume deficits; supplement nutrition if obstruction is longstanding Surgery is eventually necessary in 75% of patients	Most common with duodenal ulcers and type III gastric ulcers
GI Bleeding	Bleeding may be slow (leading to anemic symptoms) or can be rapid and severe (leading to shock)	Stool guaiac, upper GI endoscopy (diagnostic and therapeutic)	Resuscitation; diagnose site of bleed via endoscopy and treat; perform surgery for acute bleeds that require transfusion of ≥6 units of blood	**Peptic ulcer disease is the most common cause of upper GI bleeding**

- It can either be asymptomatic or cause epigastric pain. The relationship between eating and pain is not consistent (i.e., food may either aggravate or relieve the pain).
- If epigastric pain is low or moderate and is not associated with worrisome symptoms/findings, empiric therapy with acid suppression is appropriate. Stop NSAIDs.
- If there is no positive response after 4 to 8 weeks of treatment, consider a diagnostic workup. Include upper GI endoscopy and ultrasound (to rule out gallstones), and test for *H. pylori* infection.
- If *H. pylori* infection is confirmed, antibiotic therapy is indicated (see Table 3-6).

Quick HIT

Upper GI endoscopy is the best test for evaluating a patient with epigastric pain. It can diagnose PUD, gastritis, and esophagitis. It can also rule out cancers of the esophagus and stomach, and *H. pylori* infection with biopsy.

Chronic Gastritis

- The most common cause is *H. pylori* infection (over 80% of cases).
- Autoimmune gastritis leads to chronic atrophic gastritis with serum antiparietal and anti-intrinsic factor antibodies (and possible development of pernicious anemia).

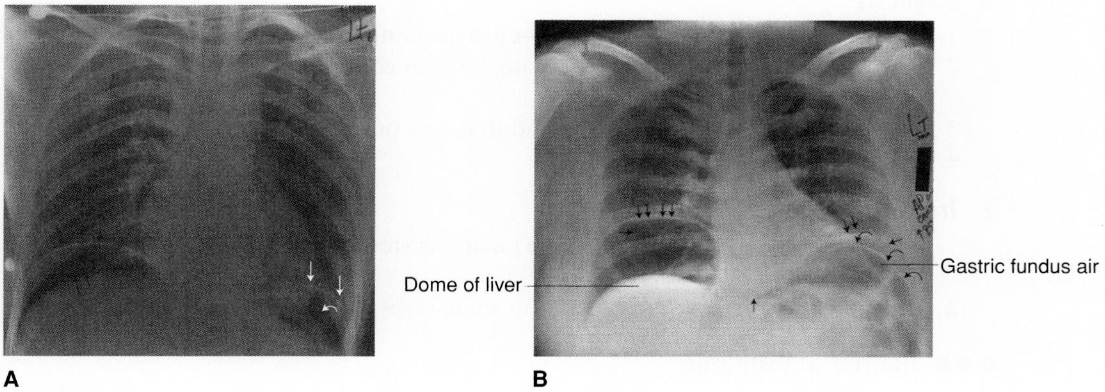

FIGURE 3-9 **A: An AP chest radiograph in a patient with a perforated duodenal ulcer and acute abdomen. The *curved arrow* shows free subdiaphragmatic air due to the perforated ulcer. The *straight arrows* show the diaphragms bilaterally. B: Chest radiograph (upright) showing bilateral subdiaphragmatic intraperitoneal air. *Double arrows* represent right and left hemidiaphragms. Note the bilateral subdiaphragmatic air (*straight arrows*). There is air in the gastric fundus as well as free air surrounding the gastric fundus.**

(From Erkonen WE, Smith WL. *Radiology 101: The Basics and Fundamentals of Imaging.* Philadelphia, PA: Lippincott Williams & Wilkins, 1998:103, Figure 6-46, and 159, Figure 8-22, respectively.)

- Most patients with chronic gastritis due to *H. pylori* are asymptomatic and never develop complications. The condition may manifest as epigastric pain similar to PUD. Other associated symptoms such as nausea/vomiting and anorexia are rare.
- Complications include PUD, gastric carcinoma, and mucosa-associated lymphoid tissue lymphoma.
- Upper GI endoscopy with biopsy is the test of choice for diagnosis of chronic gastritis. Other tests should be used to find the cause (usually *H. pylori*).
- If the patient is symptomatic, treatment involves *H. pylori* eradication with triple or quadruple therapy (see Table 3-6).

Quick HIT

Metastases of Gastric Carcinoma
- **Krukenberg tumor**—metastasis to the ovary
- **Blumer's shelf**—metastasis to the rectum (pelvic cul-de-sac)—can palpate on rectal examination
- **Sister Mary Joseph node**—metastasis to the periumbilical lymph node
- **Virchow node**—metastasis to the supraclavicular fossa nodes
- **Irish node**—metastasis to the left axillary adenopathy

Gastric Cancer

A. General characteristics

1. The majority are adenocarcinomas
2. Gastric cancer is rare in the United States (more common in Japan)
3. Morphology
   a. Ulcerative carcinoma—ulcer through all layers
   b. Polypoid carcinoma—solid mass projects into stomach lumen
   c. Superficial spreading—most favorable prognosis
   d. *Linitis plastica*—"leather bottle"—infiltrates early through all layers, stomach wall is thick and rigid, poor prognosis

B. Risk factors

1. Severe atrophic gastritis, intestinal metaplasia, gastric dysplasia
2. Adenomatous gastric polyps, chronic atrophic gastritis
3. *H. pylori* infection—threefold to sixfold increase in risk
4. Postantrectomy—many cases reported after Billroth II anastomosis (15 to 20 years after surgery)
5. Pernicious anemia—threefold increase in risk
6. Ménétrier disease—10% of these patients develop cancer
7. High intake of preserved foods (high salt, nitrates, nitrites—smoked fish)
8. Blood type A

C. Clinical features

1. Abdominal pain and unexplained weight loss are most common symptoms
2. Reduced appetite, anorexia, dyspepsia, early satiety
3. Nausea and vomiting, anemia, melena, guaiac-positive stool

D. Diagnosis

1. Endoscopy with multiple biopsies—most accurate test
2. Barium upper GI series—less accurate, but can complement upper endoscopy/biopsy findings
3. Abdominal CT scan—for staging and to detect presence of metastases
4. FOBT

E. Treatment

1. Surgical resection with wide (>5 cm) margins (total or subtotal gastrectomy) with extended lymph node dissection.
2. Chemotherapy may be appropriate in some cases.

Gastric Lymphoma

- A type of non-Hodgkin lymphoma that arises in the stomach.
- Clinical features are similar to those of adenocarcinoma of the stomach (e.g., abdominal pain, weight loss, anorexia).
- Complications include bleeding, obstruction, and perforation (possibly presented as an emergency).
- EGD with biopsy is the standard for diagnosis (same as adenocarcinoma of stomach).
- Treatment depends on the stage of the disease and the presence of complications. Options include surgical resection, radiation, and chemotherapy.

Diseases of the Small Intestine

Small Bowel Obstruction

A. General characteristics

1. There are three main points of differentiation to consider in small bowel obstruction (SBO).
   a. Partial versus complete obstruction
      - With partial obstruction, patients are able to pass gas or have bowel movements, as opposed to complete obstruction.
      - However, patients with complete obstruction may occasionally be able to pass gas or stool because they may have residual stool or gas in the colon.
   b. Closed loop versus open loop obstruction
      - With closed loop obstruction, the lumen is occluded at two points by an adhesive band or hernia ring. This can compromise the blood supply, requiring emergent surgery.
   c. Proximal versus distal SBO
      - Distal obstruction causes distention of proximal bowel segments, making diagnosis easier on plain radiograph.
2. Pathophysiology
   a. **Dehydration is a key event in SBO.** Intestinal distention causes reflex vomiting, increased intestinal secretion proximal to the point of obstruction, and decreased absorption. This leads to hypochloremia, hypokalemia, and metabolic alkalosis.
   b. The resulting hypovolemia leads to systemic findings such as tachycardia, hypotension, tachypnea, altered mental status, and oliguria.

B. Causes

1. Adhesions from previous abdominal surgery—most common cause in adults
2. Incarcerated hernias—second most common cause
3. Malignancy, intussusception, Crohn disease, carcinomatosis, and superior mesenteric artery syndrome (compression of third portion of duodenum)

C. Clinical features

1. Cramping abdominal pain—if pain is continuous and severe, strangulation may be present
2. Nausea, vomiting—may be feculent
3. Obstipation (absence of stool and flatus)
4. Abdominal distention

D. Diagnosis

1. Abdominal plain films—dilated loops of small bowel, air–fluid levels proximal to point of obstruction (on upright film), and minimal gas in colon (if complete SBO) (Figure 3-10)
2. Barium enema—to rule out colonic obstruction if plain films do not distinguish small from large bowel obstruction; barium enema identifies site of obstruction
3. Upper GI series—with small bowel follow-through if above are not diagnostic

E. Treatment

1. Nonoperative management—appropriate if bowel obstruction is incomplete and there is no fever, tachycardia, peritoneal signs, or leukocytosis
2. IV fluids to establish adequate urine output; add potassium to fluids to correct hypokalemia (which is typically present)
3. Nasogastric tube to empty stomach (gastric decompression)
4. Antibiotics
5. Surgery is indicated for complete obstruction, for partial obstruction that is persistent and/or associated with constant pain, or if strangulation is suspected. Perform an exploratory laparotomy **with lysis of adhesions and resection of any necrotic bowel**

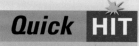

> **Quick HIT**
>
> **SBO**
> - Proximal obstruction: frequent vomiting, severe pain, minimal abdominal distention
> - Distal obstruction: less frequent vomiting and significant abdominal distention

> **Quick HIT**
>
> Excessively high intraluminal pressure may compromise blood supply, leading to strangulation. This can lead to shock, gangrene, peritonitis, or perforation of bowel—all devastating complications.

> **Quick HIT**
>
> **Large Bowel Obstruction**
> - Causes: volvulus, adhesions, hernias, colon cancer (most common cause)
> - Results in less fluid and electrolyte disorder than SBO
> - See Figure 3-11 for radiographic findings

> **Quick HIT**
>
> Manifestations of strangulated bowel in SBO include fever, severe and continuous pain, hematemesis, shock, gas in the bowel wall or portal vein, abdominal free air, peritoneal signs, and acidosis (increased lactic acid).

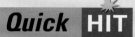

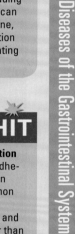

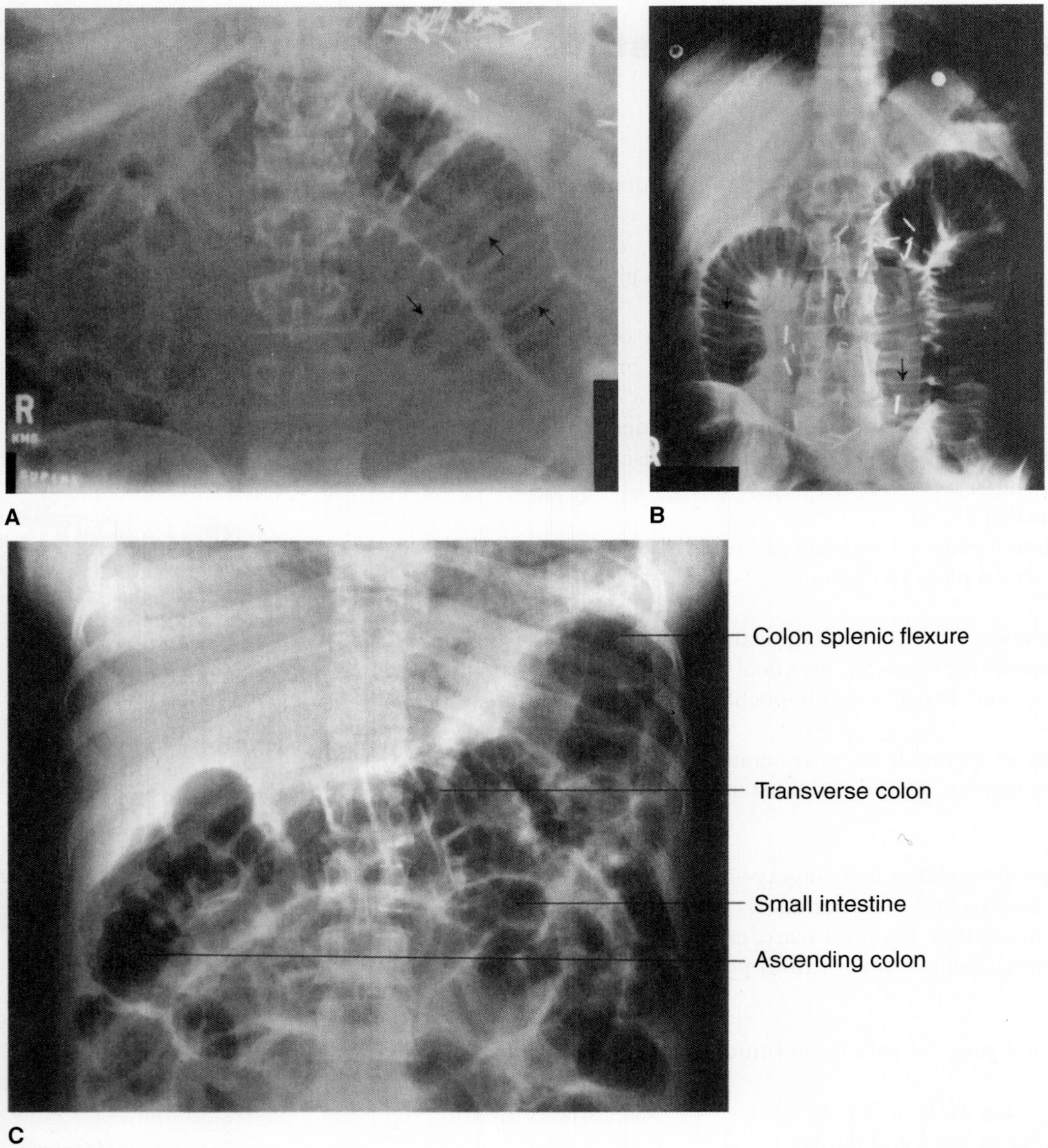

FIGURE 3-10 **A: An AP supine film of small bowel obstruction shows prominent valvulae conniventes. Air is confined to the small bowel, with no obvious air in the colon. Note surgical clips from previous surgery. B: An AP upright film in the same patient as shown in A. Note air–fluid levels in the small bowel (*arrow*) with little or no distal bowel gas. C: An AP supine film of postoperative ileus. Note the presence of air throughout the entire GI tract.**

(From Erkonen WE, Smith WL. *Radiology 101: The Basics and Fundamentals of Imaging.* Philadelphia, PA: Lippincott Williams & Wilkins, 1998:157, Figure 8-20a and c, and 156, Figure 8-19a.)

Paralytic Ileus

- Peristalsis is decreased or absent (no mechanical obstruction is present).
- Causes include medications (e.g., narcotics, drugs with anticholinergic effects), postoperative state (after abdominal surgery), spinal cord injury, shock, metabolic disorders (especially hypokalemia), and peritonitis.
- Abdominal plain films show a uniform distribution of gas in the small bowel, colon, and rectum (in contrast to small bowel or colonic obstruction).
- Failure to pass contrast medium beyond a fixed point is diagnostic.
- Treatment involves IV fluids, NPO, correction of electrolyte imbalances (especially hypokalemia), nasogastric suction if necessary, and placement of a long tube if ileus persists postoperatively.

Quick HIT

Paralytic ileus resolves with time or when the cause is addressed medically. Surgery is usually not needed.

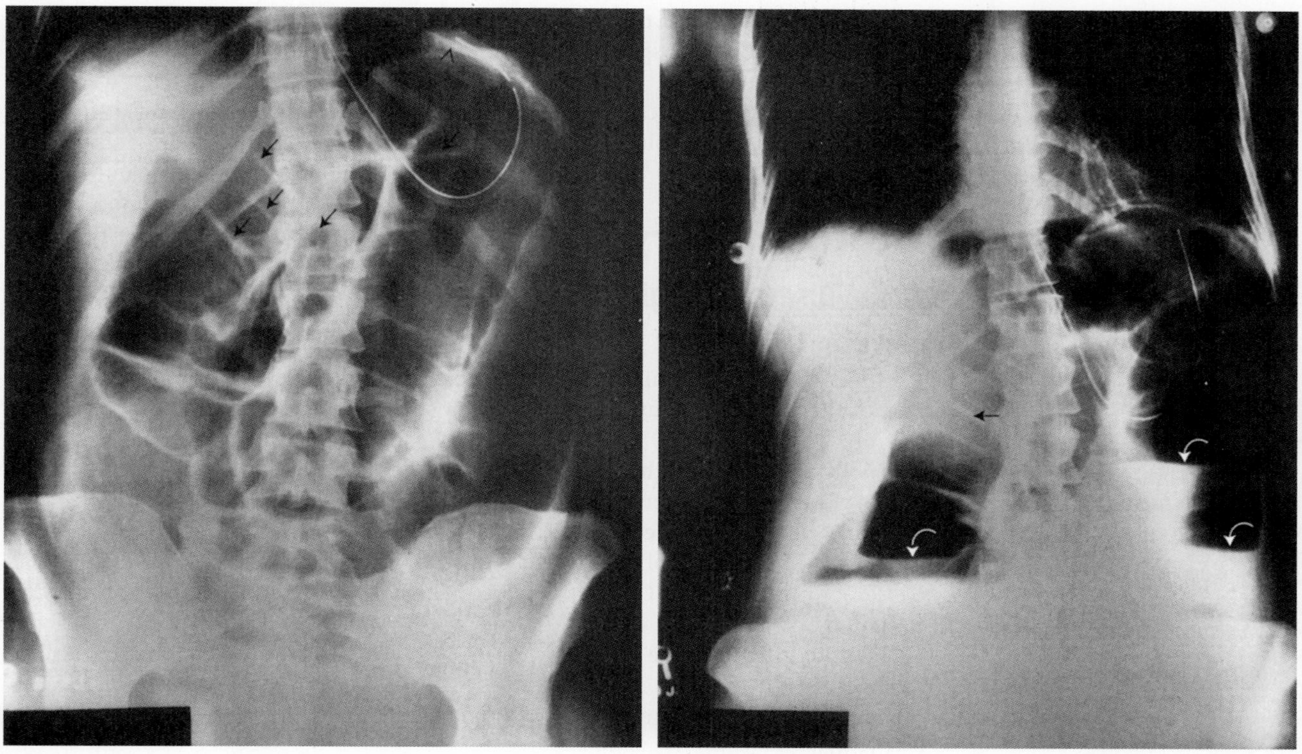

A B

FIGURE **3-11** **A: An AP supine film of large bowel obstruction. Note the dilated air-filled proximal colon with an absence of air in the distal colon. B: An AP upright film of large bowel obstruction. Note multiple colon air–fluid levels (*curved arrows*).**

(From Erkonen WE, Smith WL. *Radiology 101: The Basics and Fundamentals of Imaging.* Philadelphia, PA: Lippincott Williams & Wilkins, 1998:158, Figure 8-21A and B.)

Celiac Sprue

- Characterized by hypersensitivity to gluten (in wheat products).
- Prevalence of the condition in first-degree relatives is approximately 10%
- Results in diarrhea (most common symptom), weight loss, abdominal distention, bloating, weakness, and fatigue.
- Patients may suffer from vitamin deficiency secondary to fat malabsorption, leading to osteoporosis (vitamin D deficiency), easy bleeding (vitamin K deficiency), and megaloblastic anemia (secondary to impaired folate and vitamin B_{12} absorption).
- **Dermatitis herpetiformis (papulovesicular lesion seen on the extensor surfaces), is found in 10% to 20% of patients with celiac disease.**
- Biopsy in proximal small bowel reveals flattening of villi, which causes malabsorption.
- Strict adherence to a gluten-free diet is essential.

Whipple Disease

- Rare disease caused by infection by the bacterium *Tropheryma whipplei*
- Inflammation secondary to the infection damages villi in the small intestine
- Weight loss, diarrhea, joint pain, and arthritis are common symptoms but clinical presentation is extremely variable
- Diagnosis is made by visualization of **periodic acid-Schiff stain (PAS)–positive macrophages in the lamina propria containing non–acid-fast gram-positive bacilli**
- Treatment is with antibiotic therapy for up to 1 to 2 years

Tropical Sprue

- Also known as "environmental enteropathy," occurs in people who live in or visit tropical areas

- Unknown etiology, believed to be casued by overgrowth of bacteria
- Similar symptoms to celiac sprue including weight loss, diarrhea, cramps, fatigue, malabsorption
- Abnormal flattening of villi can be observed during endoscopy
- Treat with antibiotics and folic acid for 6 months or longer

Inflammatory Bowel Disease

Crohn Disease ("Regional Enteritis")

A. General characteristics

1. Crohn disease is a chronic transmural inflammatory disease that can affect any part of the GI tract (mouth to anus) but most commonly involves the small bowel (terminal ileum).
2. Distribution: There are three major patterns of disease.
   a. Forty percent of patients have disease in the terminal ileum and cecum.
   b. Thirty percent of patients have disease confined to the small intestine.
   c. Twenty-five percent of patients have disease confined to the colon.
   d. Rarely, other parts of GI tract may be involved (stomach, mouth, esophagus).
3. Pathology
   a. **Terminal ileum is the hallmark location**, but other sites of GI tract may also be involved
   b. Skip lesions—discontinuous involvement
   c. Fistulae
   d. Luminal strictures
   e. Noncaseating granulomas
   f. Transmural thickening and inflammation (full-thickness wall involvement)—results in narrowing of the lumen
   g. Mesenteric "fat creeping" onto the antimesenteric border of small bowel

Quick HIT

Epidemiology of IBD
- More common in Caucasians than other racial groups
- Particularly common in Jewish populations
- Mean age of onset is 15 to 35 years

Quick HIT

Crohn disease has a chronic, indolent course characterized by unpredictable **flares and remissions.** The effectiveness of medical treatment decreases with advancing disease, and complications eventually develop, requiring surgery. There is no cure, and recurrence is common even after surgery.

B. Clinical features

1. Diarrhea (usually without blood)
2. Malabsorption and weight loss (common)
3. Abdominal pain (usually RLQ), nausea, and vomiting
4. Fever, malaise
5. Extraintestinal manifestations in 15% to 20% of cases (uveitis, arthritis, ankylosing spondylitis, erythema nodosum, pyoderma gangrenosum, aphthous oral ulcers, cholelithiasis, and nephrolithiasis) (see also Clinical Pearl 3-8)

C. Diagnosis

1. Endoscopy (sigmoidoscopy or colonoscopy) with biopsy—typical findings are aphthous ulcers, cobblestone appearance, pseudopolyps, patchy (skip) lesions
2. Barium enema
3. Upper GI with small bowel follow-through

D. Complications

1. Fistulae—between colon and other segments of intestine (enteroenteral), bladder (enterovesical), vagina (enterovaginal), and skin (enterocutaneous)
2. Anorectal disease (in 30% of patients)—fissures, abscesses, perianal fistulas
3. SBO (in 20% to 30% of patients) is the most common indication for surgery. Initially, it is due to edema and spasm of bowel with intermittent signs of obstruction; later, scarring and thickening of bowel cause chronic narrowing of lumen
4. Malignancy—increased risk of colonic and small bowel tumors (but less common than in UC)
5. Malabsorption of vitamin B_{12} and bile acids (both occur in terminal ileum)
6. Cholelithiasis may occur secondary to decreased bile acid absorption

Quick HIT

Patients may have vague abdominal pain and diarrhea for years before a diagnosis of Crohn disease is considered.

CLINICAL PEARL 3-8

Extraintestinal Manifestations of IBD

- Eye lesions
  - Episcleritis—parallels bowel disease activity
  - Anterior uveitis—independent course
- Skin lesions
  - Erythema nodosum—especially in Crohn disease; parallels bowel disease activity
  - Pyoderma gangrenosum—especially in UC; parallels bowel disease activity in 50% of cases
- Arthritis—most common extraintestinal manifestation of IBD
  - Migratory monoarticular arthritis—parallels bowel disease activity (coincides with exacerbation of colitis)
  - Ankylosing spondylitis—patients with UC have a 30 times greater incidence of ankylosing spondylitis than the general population; the course is independent of the colitis
  - Sacroiliitis—does not parallel bowel disease activity
- Thromboembolic-hypercoagulable state—can lead to deep venous thrombosis (DVT), pulmonary embolism (PE), or a cardiovascular accident (CVA)
- Idiopathic thrombocytopenic purpura
- Osteoporosis
- Gallstones in Crohn disease (ileal involvement)
- Sclerosing cholangitis in UC

7. Nephrolithiasis—increased colonic absorption of dietary oxalate can lead to calcium oxalate kidney stones
8. Aphthous ulcers of lips, gingiva, and buccal mucosa (common)
9. Toxic megacolon—less common in Crohn disease than in UC
10. Growth retardation
11. Narcotic abuse, psychosocial issues due to chronicity and often disabling nature of the disease

E. Treatment

1. Medical
   a. Sulfasalazine
      - This is useful if the colon is involved. 5-ASA (mesalamine) is the active compound and is released in the colon—it is more useful in UC than in Crohn disease.
      - 5-ASA compounds block prostaglandin release and serve to reduce inflammation.
      - There are preparations of 5-ASA that are more useful in distal small bowel disease.

   b. Metronidazole—if no response to 5-ASA
   c. Systemic corticosteroids (prednisone)—for acute exacerbations and if no response to metronidazole
   d. Immunosuppressants (azathioprine, 6-mercaptopurine)—in conjunction with steroids if the patient does not respond to above agents
   e. Bile acid sequestrants (cholestyramine or colestipol)—for patients with terminal ileal disease who cannot absorb bile acids
   f. Antidiarrheal agents generally not a good choice (may cause ileus)
2. Surgical (eventually required in most patients)
   a. Reserve for complications of Crohn disease
   b. Involves segmental resection of involved bowel
   c. Disease recurrence after surgery is high—up to 50% of patients experience disease recurrence at 10 years postoperatively
   d. Indications for surgery include SBO, fistulae (especially between bowel and bladder, vagina), disabling disease, and perforation or abscess
3. Nutritional supplementation and support—parenteral nutrition is sometimes necessary

Ulcerative Colitis

A. General characteristics

1. UC is a chronic inflammatory disease of the colon or rectal mucosa (see also Table 3-8).
2. It may occur at any age (usually begins in adolescence or young adulthood).
3. Distribution: UC **involves the rectum in all cases** and can involve the colon either partially or entirely.
   a. Rectum alone (in 10% of cases)
   b. Rectum and left colon (in 40% of cases)
   c. Rectum, left colon, and right colon (in 30% of cases)
   d. Pancolitis (in 30% of cases)
   e. The small bowel is not usually involved in UC, but it may reach the distal ileum in a small percentage of patients ("backwash ileitis" in 10% of cases)
4. The course is unpredictable and variable and is characterized by periodic exacerbations and periods of complete remission. Less than 5% of patients have an initial attack without any recurrence.
5. Pathology
   a. Uninterrupted involvement of rectum and/or colon—**no skip lesions**
   b. Inflammation is not transmural (as it is in Crohn disease). It is limited to the mucosa and submucosa.
   c. PMNs accumulate in the crypts of the colon (crypt abscesses).

B. Clinical features (wide range of presentation)

1. **Hematochezia (bloody diarrhea)**
2. **Abdominal pain**
3. Bowel movements are frequent but small
4. Fever, anorexia, and weight loss (severe cases)
5. Tenesmus (rectal dry heaves)
6. Extraintestinal symptoms (e.g., jaundice, uveitis, arthritis, skin lesions)—see Clinical Pearl 3-8

Quick HIT

Patients with UC may have nonbloody diarrhea at first, with eventual progression to bloody diarrhea.

C. Diagnosis: perform the following initial studies

1. Stool cultures for *C. difficile*, ova, and parasites—to rule out infectious diarrhea
2. Fecal leukocytes
3. WBCs can appear in UC, ischemic colitis, or infectious diarrhea
4. Colonoscopy—to assess the extent of disease and the presence of any complications

D. Complications

1. Iron deficiency anemia
2. Hemorrhage

TABLE 3-8 Crohn Disease Versus Ulcerative Colitis

	Crohn Disease	Ulcerative Colitis
Involvement	Transmural—intestinal wall from mucosa to serosa Discontinuous involvement (skip lesions)	Mucosa and submucosa Continuous involvement (no skip lesions)
Location	Terminal ileum (most common) Can involve any part of the GI tract (resection is not curative—recurrences occur)	Confined to colon and rectum Colectomy is curative
Complications	Fistulae and abscesses are more common than in UC because the entire wall is involved	SC and colorectal cancer are more common than in Crohn disease

3. Electrolyte disturbances and dehydration secondary to diarrhea
4. Strictures, benign and malignant (usually malignant)
5. Colon cancer—The risk correlates with extent and duration of colitis. In distal proctitis there is no increased risk of CRC
6. Sclerosing cholangitis (SC)—The course not parallel with bowel disease and is not prevented by colectomy
7. Cholangiocarcinoma—Half of all bile duct cancers are associated with UC
8. Toxic megacolon is the leading cause of death in UC and affects <5% of patients. It is associated with the risk of colonic perforation
9. Growth retardation
10. Narcotic abuse
11. Psychosocial issues (e.g., depression) due to chronicity and often disabling nature of the disease

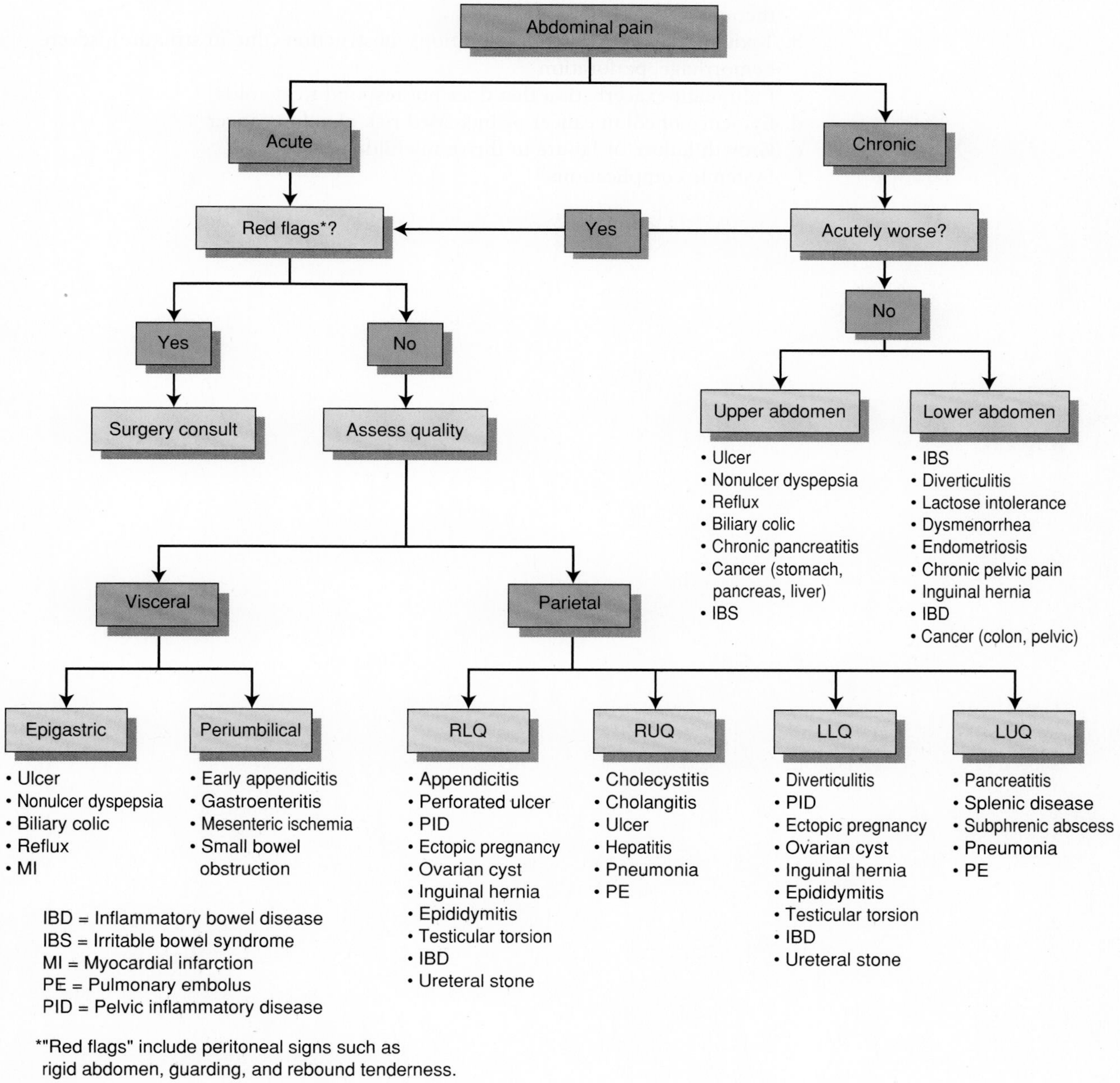

FIGURE 3-12 **Approach to the diagnosis of nontraumatic abdominal pain in adults.**
(Adapted from Sloane PD, Slatt LM, Ebell MH, et al. *Essentials of Family Medicine.* 4th ed. Philadelphia, PA: Lippincott Williams & Wilkins, 2002:245, Figure 16.2.)

Quick HIT

Sulfasalazine is metabolized by bacteria to 5-ASA and sulfapyridine. 5-ASA is the effective moiety of the drug, and sulfapyridine causes the side effects.

E. Treatment

1. Medical (Figure 3-12)
   a. Systemic corticosteroids are used for acute exacerbations.
   b. Sulfasalazine (topical application as a suppository) is the mainstay of treatment. Preferred over topical steroids because they are effective as maintenance therapy. Remission rates as high as 93% have been reported.
      - It is effective in maintaining remissions. 5-ASA (mesalamine) is the active component.
      - 5-ASA enemas can be used for proctitis and distal colitis.
   c. Immunosuppressive agents in patients with refractory disease may prevent relapses but are not effective for acute attacks.
2. Surgical—often curative (unlike Crohn disease) and involves total colectomy. Indications for surgery include:
   a. Severe disease that is debilitating, refractory, and unresponsive to medical therapy
   b. Toxic megacolon (risk of perforation), obstruction (due to stricture), severe hemorrhage, perforation
   c. Fulminant exacerbation that does not respond to steroids
   d. Evidence of colon cancer or increased risk of colon cancer
   e. Growth failure or failure to thrive in children
   f. Systemic complications

ENDOCRINE AND METABOLIC DISEASES

4

Diseases of the Thyroid Gland

Hyperthyroidism

A. Causes

1. **Graves disease (diffuse toxic goiter)** is the most common cause—80% of all cases.
   a. An autoimmune disorder: A thyroid-stimulating immunoglobulin (IgG) antibody binds to the TSH receptors on the surface of thyroid cells and triggers the synthesis of excess thyroid hormone.
   b. Seen most often in younger women. Commonly associated with other autoimmune disorders.
   c. A radioiodide scan shows *diffuse uptake* because every thyroid cell is hyperfunctioning.
2. **Plummer disease (multinodular toxic goiter)**—15% of all cases.
   a. Characterized by hyperfunctioning areas that produce high T_4 and T_3 levels, thereby decreasing TSH levels. As a result, the rest of the thyroid is not functioning (atrophy due to decreased TSH).
   b. Consequently, *patchy uptake* appears on the thyroid scan.
   c. More common in elderly patients, and more common in women than men.
3. Toxic thyroid adenoma (single nodule)—2% of all cases.
4. Hashimoto thyroiditis and subacute (granulomatous) thyroiditis (both can cause **transient** hyperthyroidism).
5. Other causes (rare)
   a. Postpartum thyroiditis (transient hyperthyroidism)
   b. Iodine-induced hyperthyroidism
   c. Excessive doses of levothyroxine (e.g., iatrogenic by health care provider or surreptitious self-administration)

B. Clinical features

1. Symptoms
   a. Nervousness, insomnia, irritability
   b. Hand tremor, hyperactivity, tremulousness
   c. Excessive sweating, heat intolerance
   d. Weight loss despite increased appetite
   e. Diarrhea
   f. Palpitations (due to tachyarrhythmias)
   g. Muscle weakness
2. Signs
   a. Thyroid gland
      - Graves disease: a diffusely enlarged (symmetric), nontender thyroid gland; **a bruit may be present**

Quick HIT

Hyperthyroidism in the Elderly

- In the elderly, classic symptoms of hyperthyroidism (e.g., nervousness, insomnia, hyperactivity) may be absent. The only manifestations may be weight loss, weakness, and/or atrial fibrillation.
- Consider hyperthyroidism before assuming that an elderly patient with unexplained weight loss has depression or occult malignancy.

Quick HIT

There are three signs of hyperthyroidism specific to Graves disease:

- Exophthalmos
- Pretibial myxedema
- Thyroid bruit

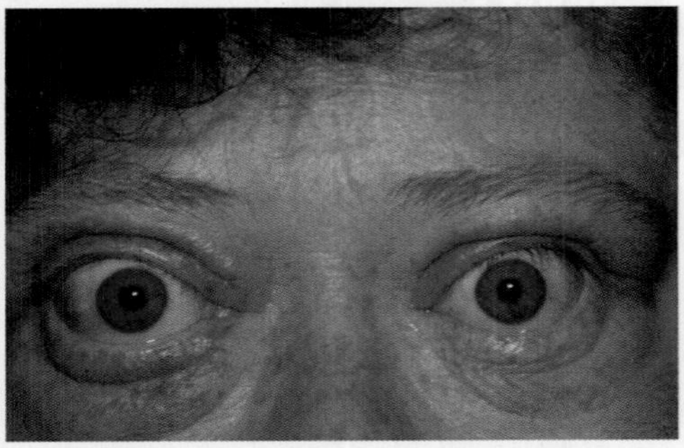

FIGURE 4-1 **Exophthalmos (thyrotoxicosis).**
(From Goodheart HP. *Goodheart's Photoguide of Common Skin Disorders*. 2nd ed. Philadelphia, PA: Lippincott Williams & Wilkins, 2003, Photo 25.9).

- Subacute thyroiditis: an exquisitely tender, diffusely enlarged gland (with a viral illness)
- Plummer disease and Hashimoto thyroiditis (if multinodularity is present): thyroid gland is bumpy, irregular, and asymmetric
- Toxic adenoma: single nodule with an otherwise atrophic gland

b. Extrathyroidal
- Eyes: **Proptosis, due to edema of the extraocular muscles and retro-orbital tissue, is a hallmark of Graves disease** (but not always present). Irritation and excessive tearing are common due to corneal exposure. Lid retraction may be the only sign in milder disease (Figure 4-1). Lid lag may be present
- Cardiovascular effects: arrhythmias (sinus tachycardia, atrial fibrillation, and premature ventricular contractions), elevated BP
- Skin changes: warm and moist, **pretibial myxedema** (edema over tibial surface due to dermal accumulation of mucopolysaccharides)
- Neurologic: brisk deep tendon reflexes, tremor

Quick HIT

Thyroid Hormones and TBG
- T_4 is converted to T_3 by deiodination outside of the thyroid.
- T_3 is more biologically active than T_4.
- Most of T_4 (and T_3) is reversibly bound to TBG and is inactive.
- Factors that increase TBG (and therefore total T_4) include pregnancy, liver disease, oral contraceptives, and aspirin.

C. Diagnosis

1. Serum TSH level (low)—**initial test of choice**: If TSH is normal or high, hyperthyroidism is unlikely. (TSH-induced hyperthyroidism is quite uncommon.)
2. Next order thyroid hormone levels: T_4 level should be elevated. Consider a free T_4 assay.
3. Testing the T_3 level is usually unnecessary but may be helpful if TSH level is low and free T_4 is not elevated, because excess T_3 alone can cause hyperthyroidism.
4. Other tests (less commonly used but often tested).

a. Radioactive T_3 uptake.
- Gives information regarding the status of thyroid-binding globulin (TBG)
- Radioactive T_3 can bind either to TBG or to "resin" that has been given (binds to resin only if there is no "space" on TBG, as in hyperthyroidism when T_4 is bound to TBG). Consequently, you measure how much radioactive T_3 was taken up by the resin.
- **The importance of this test is that it helps differentiate between elevations in thyroid hormones due to increased TBG from true hyperthyroidism (due to an actual increase in free T_4).**
- **Consider hyperthyroidism when the thyroid gland is producing excess T_4.** In this case, all of the binding sites on TBG will be bound by T_4, so radioactive T_3 uptake will increase.
- **Consider pregnancy when there is high TBG.** There are more binding sites for radioactive T_3, so radioactive T_3 uptake decreases. Therefore, high TBG production leads to low radioactive T_3 uptake.

b. Free thyroxine index (FTI).
- FTI 5 (radioactive T_3 uptake 3 serum total T_4)/100.
- FTI 5 (patient's radioactive T_3 uptake/normal radioactive T_3 uptake) 3 total T_4.

- Normal FTI values are 4 to 11. FTI should not change (as T_4 decreases, radioactive T_3 uptake increases and vice versa).
- FTI is proportional to actual free T_4 concentration.

D. Treatment types

1. Pharmacologic
   a. Thionamides—Methimazole and propylthiouracil (PTU) inhibit thyroid hormone synthesis, and PTU also inhibits conversion of T_4 to T_3. Treatment with thionamides results in long-term remission in a minority of patients; a major serious side effect is agranulocytosis. Other side effects shared by both methimazole and PTU include skin rash, arthralgias, and hepatotoxicity.
   b. β-blockers—for acute management of some symptoms such as palpitations, tremors, anxiety, tachycardia, sweating, and muscle weakness.
   c. Sodium ipodate or iopanoic acid—lowers serum T_3 and T_4 levels and causes rapid improvement of hyperthyroidism; appropriate for acute management of severe hyperthyroidism that is not responding to conventional therapy.
2. Radioiodine 131 (^{131}I).
   a. Causes destruction of thyroid follicular cells.
   b. Most common therapy in the United States for Graves hyperthyroidism.
   c. Main complication is hypothyroidism and occurs in majority of patients.
   d. If the first dose does not control the hyperthyroidism within 6 to 12 months, then administer another dose.
   e. Contraindicated during pregnancy and breastfeeding due to risk of cretinism (stunted physical and mental growth from severe hypothyroidism).
3. Surgical—subtotal thyroidectomy.
   a. Very effective, but only 1% of patients with hyperthyroidism are treated with surgery due to the following side effects: permanent hypothyroidism (30%), recurrence of hyperthyroidism (10%), recurrent laryngeal nerve palsy (1%), and permanent hypoparathyroidism (1%).
   b. Often reserved for patients with very large goiters (more common in TMNG), those who are allergic to antithyroid drugs, or patients who prefer surgery over medication.
   c. Watch for clinical manifestations of hypocalcemia after surgery that may not return to normal due to parathyroid inflammation or accidental removal.

Quick HIT

For all patients taking antithyroid medication, consider monitoring the leukocyte count on a regular basis (for agranulocytes).

Quick HIT

Thyroid cells are the only cells in the body that absorb iodine. Therefore, giving radioactive iodine destroys only thyroid cells.

E. Treatment

1. For immediate control of adrenergic symptoms of hyperthyroidism (of any cause): β-blocker (propranolol).
2. For *nonpregnant* patients with Graves disease.
   a. Start methimazole (in addition to the β-blocker).
   b. Taper β-blocker after 4 to 8 weeks (once methimazole starts to take effect).
   c. Continue methimazole for 1 to 2 years. Measure thyroid-stimulating IgG antibody at 12 months. If it is absent, then discontinue therapy. If relapse occurs, then resume methimazole for about 1 more year or consider radioiodine therapy.
3. For *pregnant* patients with Graves disease.
   a. Endocrinology consult is indicated before starting treatment.
   b. **PTU is preferred.**
4. Radioactive iodine ablation therapy.
   a. Leads to hypothyroidism over time in many patients.
   b. Consider therapy with ^{131}I for the following patients:
      - Elderly patients with Graves disease.
      - Patients with a solitary toxic nodule.
      - Patients with Graves disease in whom therapy with antithyroid drugs fails (e.g., due to relapse, agranulocytosis).

Thyroid Storm

- **This is a rare, life-threatening complication of thyrotoxicosis** characterized by an acute exacerbation of the manifestations of hyperthyroidism.

Quick HIT

The terms hyperthyroidism and thyrotoxicosis are interchangeable and refer to hyperfunctioning thyroid disease. **Thyroid storm is a medical emergency with life-threatening sequelae.**

- There is usually a precipitating factor, such as infection, diabetic ketoacidosis (DKA), or stress (e.g., severe trauma, surgery, illness, childbirth).
- **High mortality rate: up to 20% of patients enter a coma or die.**
- Clinical manifestations include marked fever, tachycardia, agitation or psychosis, confusion, and GI symptoms (e.g., nausea, vomiting, diarrhea).
- Provide supportive therapy with IV fluids, cooling blankets, and glucose.
- Give antithyroid agents (PTU every 2 hours). Follow with iodine to inhibit thyroid hormone release.
- Administer β-blockers for control of heart rate. Give dexamethasone to impair peripheral generation of T_3 from T_4 and to provide adrenal support.

Hypothyroidism

A. General characteristics

1. The onset of symptoms is usually insidious, and the condition may go undetected for years (see also Clinical Pearl 4-1).
2. Sometimes a diagnosis is made solely on laboratory evidence in an asymptomatic patient.

Quick HIT

Hashimoto thyroiditis is associated with other autoimmune disorders (e.g., lupus, pernicious anemia).

Patients with Hashimoto thyroiditis are at an increased risk of thyroid carcinoma and thyroid lymphoma.

B. Causes

1. Primary hypothyroidism is the failure of the thyroid to produce sufficient thyroid hormone. This accounts for about 95% of all cases
   a. **Hashimoto disease (chronic thyroiditis)**—most common cause of primary hypothyroidism
   b. Iatrogenic—second most common cause of primary hypothyroidism; results from prior treatments of hyperthyroidism, including:
      - Radioiodine therapy
      - Thyroidectomy
      - Medications (e.g., lithium)
2. Secondary hypothyroidism (due to pituitary disease; i.e., deficiency of TSH) and tertiary hypothyroidism (due to hypothalamic disease; i.e., deficiency of TRH) account for less than 5% of cases. **Both are associated with a low free T_4 and a low TSH level.**

C. Clinical features

1. Symptoms
   a. Fatigue, weakness, lethargy
   b. Heavy menstrual periods (menorrhagia), slight weight gain (10 to 30 lb)—patients are **not** typically obese
   c. Cold intolerance
   d. Constipation
   e. Slow mentation, inability to concentrate (mild at first, in later stages dementia can occur), dull expression
   f. Muscle weakness, arthralgias
   g. Depression
   h. Diminished hearing

CLINICAL PEARL 4-1

Myxedema Coma

- A rare condition that presents with a depressed state of consciousness, profound hypothermia, and respiratory depression
- May develop after years of severe untreated hypothyroidism
- Precipitating factors are trauma, infection, cold exposure, and narcotics.
- **A medical emergency, with a high mortality rate (50% to 75%) even with treatment**
- Provide supportive therapy to maintain BP and respiration. Give IV thyroxine and hydrocortisone while carefully monitoring the hemodynamic state.

CLINICAL PEARL 4-2

Subclinical Hypothyroidism

- Thyroid function is inadequate, but increased TSH production maintains T_4 level within the reference range of normalcy; therefore, TSH level is elevated and T_4 level is normal.
- Look for nonspecific or mild symptoms of hypothyroidism, as well as elevated serum LDL levels.
- Treat with thyroxine if patients develop goiter, hypercholesterolemia, symptoms of hypothyroidism, or significantly elevated TSH level (>20 μU/mL).

2. Signs
   a. Dry skin, coarse hair; thickened, puffy features
   b. Hoarseness
   c. Nonpitting edema (edema due to glycosaminoglycan in interstitial tissues, not water and salt)
   d. Carpal tunnel syndrome
   e. Slow relaxation of deep tendon reflexes
   f. Loss of lateral portion of eyebrows
   g. Bradycardia
   h. Goiter (Hashimoto disease—goiter is rubbery, nontender, and even nodular; subacute thyroiditis—goiter is very tender and enlarged, although not always symmetrically.)
   i. History of upper respiratory infection and fever (subacute thyroiditis)

Quick HIT

TSH is the primary test in screening for thyroid dysfunction. Also, order a lipid profile and a CBC.

D. Diagnosis

1. **High TSH level—most sensitive indicator of hypothyroidism** (see also Clinical Pearl 4-2).
2. Low TSH level (secondary hypothyroidism).
3. Low free T_4 level (or free T_4 index) in patients with clinically overt hypothyroidism. Free T_4 may be normal in subclinical cases.
4. **Increased antimicrosomal antibodies (Hashimoto thyroiditis).**
5. Other laboratory value abnormalities that may be present:
   a. Elevated LDL and decreased HDL levels.
   b. Anemia—mild normocytic anemia is the most common.

E. Treatment: levothyroxine (T_4)—treatment of choice

1. Effect is evident in 2 to 4 weeks; highly effective in achieving euthyroid state.
2. Convenient once—daily morning dose.
3. Treatment is continued indefinitely.
4. Monitor TSH level and clinical state periodically.

Thyroiditis

A. Subacute (viral) thyroiditis (subacute granulomatous thyroiditis)

1. Causes—usually follows a viral illness; associated with HLA-B35
2. Clinical features
   a. Prodromal phase of a few weeks (fever, flu-like illness)
   b. It can cause transient hyperthyroidism due to leakage of hormone from inflamed thyroid gland. This is followed by a euthyroid state and then a hypothyroid state (as hormones are depleted)
   c. **Painful**, tender thyroid gland (may be enlarged)
3. Diagnosis
   a. **Radioiodine uptake is low** because thyroid follicular cells are damaged and cannot trap iodine.
   b. Low TSH level secondary to suppression by increased T_4 and T_3 levels; high erythrocyte sedimentation rate (ESR).

4. Treatment
   a. Use NSAIDs and aspirin for mild symptoms; corticosteroids, if the pain is more severe.
   b. Most patients have recovery of thyroid function within a few months to 1 year.

B. Subacute lymphocytic thyroiditis (painless thyroiditis, silent thyroiditis)

1. A transient thyrotoxic phase of 2 to 5 months may be followed by a hypothyroid phase. The hypothyroid phase is usually self-limited and may be the only manifestation of this disease if the hyperthyroid phase is brief.
2. Low radioactive iodine uptake—differentiates it from Graves disease during thyrotoxic phase.
3. Similar to subacute (viral) thyroiditis, only *without the pain or tenderness* of the thyroid gland.

C. Chronic lymphocytic thyroiditis (Hashimoto thyroiditis, lymphocytic thyroiditis)

1. Most common cause of autoimmune thyroid disorder; more common in women
2. Causes
   a. Genetic component—family history is common.
   b. Antithyroid antibodies are present in the majority of patients.
3. Clinical manifestations (see also Clinical Pearl 4-3)
   a. Goiter is the most common feature.
   b. Slow decline in thyroid function is common. Hypothyroidism is present in 20% of cases when first diagnosed but often occurs later in disease.
4. Diagnosis
   a. Thyroid function studies are normal (unless hypothyroidism is present).
   b. Antithyroid antibodies: antiperoxidase antibodies (present in 90% of patients), antithyroglobulin antibodies (present in 50%).
   c. Irregular distribution of ^{131}I on thyroid scan—not required for diagnosis.
5. Treatment—thyroid hormone (to achieve euthyroid state)

D. Fibrous thyroiditis (Riedel thyroiditis)

1. Fibrous tissue replaces thyroid tissue, leading to a firm thyroid.
2. Surgery may be necessary if complications occur.
3. Patient may be hypothyroid as well, in which case thyroid hormone should be prescribed.

Thyroid Nodules

A. General characteristics

1. Cancer is found in 4% to 10% of nodules that are investigated.
2. A solitary nodule can be either thyroid cancer or a benign adenoma. However, multinodular conditions may cause confusion because only one of these nodules may be palpable.
3. The most important function of the physical examination is the detection of the thyroid nodule, rather than the determination of its benign or malignant status.
4. To be detectable on palpation, a nodule must be at least 1 cm in diameter.

CLINICAL PEARL 4-3

Thyroid-associated Ophthalmopathy (TAO)

- TAO is an autoimmune attack on the periorbital connective tissue and extraocular muscles.
- Clinical findings include lid retraction ("thyroid stare"), proptosis, eyelid edema, lagophthalmos (inability to close eyelids completely), and diplopia.
- Patients may be hypothyroid, hyperthyroid (Graves disease), or euthyroid when TAO presents. Most euthyroid patients will go on to develop thyroid dysfunction within 2 years of developing TAO.
- Treatment of thyroid dysfunction has little effect on the course of TAO. TAO is usually self-limited, but surgery may be required if disease is severe. Oral steroids may also be helpful.

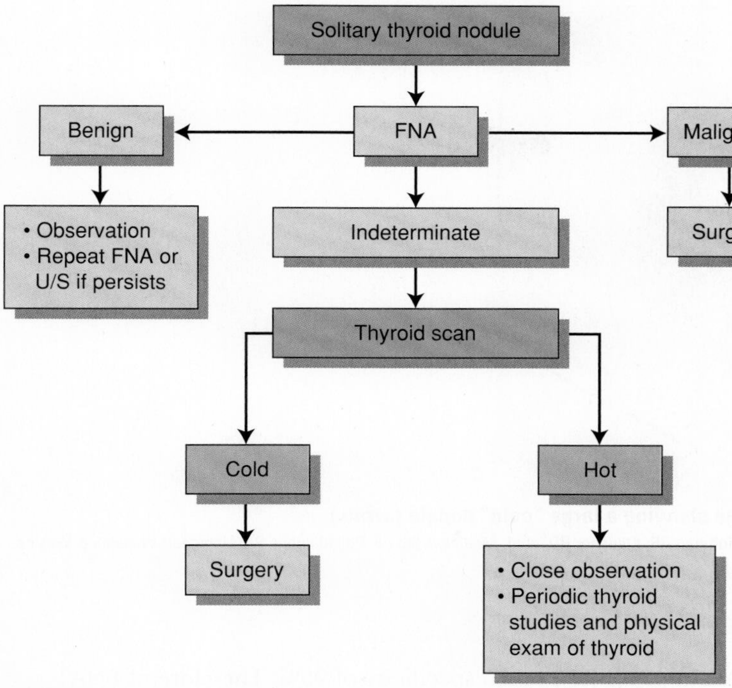

FIGURE 4-2 **Algorithm for the evaluation of a solitary thyroid nodule. Once a thyroid nodule is detected on physical examination, FNA is the initial study of choice.**

5. Malignancy is suggested by the following:
   a. If the nodule is fixed in place and no movement occurs on swallowing
   b. Unusually firm consistency or irregularity of the nodule
   c. If the nodule is solitary
   d. History of radiation therapy to the neck
   e. History of rapid development
   f. Vocal cord paralysis (recurrent laryngeal nerve paralysis)
   g. Cervical adenopathy
   h. Elevated serum calcitonin
   i. Family history of thyroid cancer

B. Diagnosis

1. Fine-needle aspiration (FNA) biopsy (see also Clinical Pearl 4-4) (Figure 4-2).
   a. **Test of choice for initial evaluation of a thyroid nodule**—often combined with ultrasound guidance for better diagnostic utility.

CLINICAL PEARL 4-4

Fine-needle Aspiration

- A needle is inserted into the nodule, and cells are aspirated and then examined under a microscope.
- False-positive and false-negative rates approach 5%.
- **This is the only test that can reliably differentiate between benign and malignant nodules.**
  - Ultrasound differentiates between solid and cystic nodules, but either may be malignant.
  - On the thyroid scan, "cold" nodules are more likely to be malignant than "hot," but this is not reliable.
- FNA findings:
  - Probable cancer (15%): Most of these are really cancers. Surgery is indicated.
  - Indeterminate (19%): A thyroid scan should be performed, and if the lesion is "cold" by the scan, surgical resection is indicated because about 20% of these lesions are found to be malignant.
  - Benign (66%): Most of these are benign. Observe for 1 year, then follow up with an ultrasound.
  - Follicular neoplasm: Surgery is recommended because it is difficult to distinguish between benign and malignant follicular cells on histology.

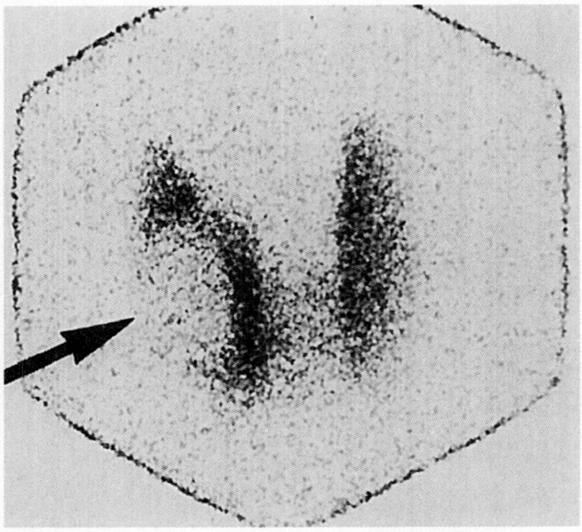

FIGURE 4-3 A ^{123}I thyroid scan showing a large "cold" nodule (*arrow*).
(From Fishman MC, Hoffman AR, Klausner RD, et al. *Medicine.* 5th ed. Philadelphia, PA: Lippincott Williams & Wilkins, 2004:185, Figure 22-1.)

b. Accuracy.
   - FNA has a sensitivity of 95% and a specificity of 95%. Therefore, if FNA shows a benign nodule, the nodule is likely to be benign.
   - However, FNA biopsies have 5% false-negative results, so follow up with periodic FNA if thyroid nodularity persists. Benign lesions should continue to show consistently benign cytology.
   - FNA is reliable for all cancers (papillary, medullary, anaplastic) **except follicular.**

2. Thyroid scan (radioactive iodine) (Figure 4-3)
   a. Thyroid scan plays a supplemental role. It is performed if the FNA biopsy is indeterminate. It is also performed in patients with a low TSH, as these patients are more likely to have a hyperfunctioning nodule.
   b. It gives graphic representations of the distribution of radioactive iodine in the gland—useful in identifying whether thyroid nodules show decreased ("cold") or increased ("hot") accumulation of radioactive iodine compared with normal paranodular tissue. Nodules are classified as "cold" (hypofunctional), "warm" (normally functioning), or "hot" (hyperfunctional).
   c. It should be limited to patients whose FNA biopsy results suggest neoplasm. (It is not cost effective to scan all patients with thyroid nodules.) When such lesions are "cold" on scan, thyroid lobectomy is recommended.
3. Thyroid ultrasound
   a. Differentiates a solid from a cystic nodule; most cancers are solid.
   b. Can identify nodules 1 to 3 mm in diameter.
   c. Cystic masses larger than 4 cm in diameter are not malignant.
   d. Cannot distinguish between benign and malignant thyroid nodules.

Quick HIT

In general, most patients with thyroid cancer do not die of thyroid cancer (although this depends on the type of thyroid cancer).

Thyroid Cancer

A. General characteristics

1. Risk factors
   a. Head and neck radiation (during childhood)
   b. Gardner syndrome and Cowden syndrome for papillary cancer
   c. **MEN type II** for medullary cancer
2. Types (see also Clinical Pearl 4-5)
   a. Papillary carcinoma
      - Accounts for 70% to 80% of all thyroid cancers
      - Least aggressive thyroid cancer—slow growth and slow spreading with excellent prognosis
      - Most important risk factor is a history of radiation to the head/neck

CLINICAL PEARL 4-5

Nodules

"Cold" Nodules

- Decreased iodine uptake = hypofunctioning nodule
- Significant risk of malignancy—approximately 20% of cold nodules are malignant
- Of all nodules, 70% to 90% are cold and most of these are benign. Therefore, scanning may indicate a greatly reduced risk of malignancy in a nodule that is warm or hot, but it does not yield much additional information in a nodule that is cold

"Hot" Nodules

- Increased iodine uptake = hyperfunctioning nodule
- Rarely associated with malignancy

- Spreads via lymphatics in neck; frequently metastasizes to cervical lymph nodes (cervical lymphadenopathy); distant metastasis is rare
- Positive iodine uptake

b. Follicular carcinoma
- Accounts for 15% of all thyroid cancers; avidly absorbs iodine
- Prognosis is worse than for papillary cancer—it spreads early via a hematogenous route (brain, lung, bone, liver). Distant metastasis occurs in 20% of patients; lymph node involvement is uncommon
- May be associated with iodine deficiency
- Tumor extension through the tumor capsule or vascular invasion distinguishes it from a benign adenoma. A tissue sample is therefore needed for diagnosis
- More malignant than papillary cancer, but these are also slow growing
- One variant is the Hürthle cell carcinoma—characteristic cells contain abundant cytoplasm, tightly packed mitochondria, and oval nuclei with prominent nucleoli. These tumors are radioiodine resistant.

c. Medullary carcinoma
- Accounts for 2% to 3% of all thyroid cancers
- One-third sporadic, one-third familial, one-third associated with MEN II (always screen for pheochromocytoma)
- Arises from the parafollicular cells (C cells)—**produces calcitonin**
- More malignant than follicular cancer but less so than anaplastic cancer—survival of approximately 10 years

d. Anaplastic carcinoma
- Accounts for 5% of all thyroid cancers; mostly seen in elderly patients
- Highly malignant
- May arise from a longstanding follicular or papillary thyroid carcinoma
- Prognosis (grim)—death typically occurs within a few months. Mortality is usually due to invasion of adjacent organs (trachea, neck vessels)

Quick HIT

Hürthle Cell Tumor
- A variant of follicular cancer but more aggressive
- Spread by lymphatics; does not take up iodine
- Treatment: total thyroidectomy

Quick HIT

Papillary carcinoma is the most common type of thyroid cancer to develop after radiation exposure (accounts for 80% to 90% of postradiation cancers of the thyroid).

B. Diagnosis

1. Thyroid hormone level (frequently normal)
2. Calcitonin level (if medullary carcinoma)
3. Refer to the section on thyroid nodules for diagnostic approach

C. Treatment

1. Papillary carcinoma
   a. Lobectomy with isthmusectomy.
   b. Total thyroidectomy if tumor is >3 cm, tumor is bilateral, tumor is advanced, or distant metastases are present.
   c. Adjuvant treatment: TSH suppression therapy; radioiodine therapy for larger tumors.
2. Follicular carcinoma—total thyroidectomy with postoperative iodine ablation.

3. Medullary carcinoma—total thyroidectomy; radioiodine therapy usually unsuccessful. Modified radical neck dissection is also indicated when there is lymph node involvement (most cases).
4. Anaplastic carcinoma—chemotherapy and radiation may provide a modest improvement in survival. Palliative surgery for airway compromise may be needed.

Diseases of the Pituitary Gland

Pituitary Adenomas

A. General characteristics

1. Pituitary adenomas account for about 10% of all intracranial neoplasms.
2. Almost all pituitary tumors are benign. They may grow in any direction causing "parasellar" signs and symptoms.
3. Size: microadenoma (diameter ≤10 mm); macroadenoma (diameter >10 mm).

B. Clinical features

1. Hormonal effects occur due to hypersecretion of one or more of the following hormones:
   a. Prolactin—see the following section on hyperprolactinemia
   b. GH—results in acromegaly (or gigantism if epiphyseal closure has not occurred; seen in the pediatric population)
   c. Adrenocorticotropic hormone (ACTH)—results in Cushing disease
   d. TSH—results in hyperthyroidism
2. Hypopituitarism—compression of hypothalamic-pituitary stalk; GH deficiency and hypogonadotropic hypogonadism are the most common problems
3. Mass effects
   a. Headache
   b. Visual defects—Bitemporal hemianopsia (due to compression of optic chiasm) is the most common finding, but it depends on the size and symmetry of the tumor

C. Diagnosis

1. **MRI** is the imaging study of choice
2. Pituitary hormone levels

D. Treatment

1. Transsphenoidal surgery is indicated in most patients (except patients with prolactinomas, for which medical management can be tried first).
2. Radiation therapy and medical therapy are adjuncts in most patients.

Quick HIT

High levels of prolactin inhibit secretion of GnRH. This leads to decreased secretion of LH and FSH, which in turn leads to decreased production of estrogen and testosterone (see **clinical features**).

Hyperprolactinemia

A. Causes

1. Prolactinoma
   a. Most common cause of hyperprolactinemia
   b. Most common type of pituitary adenoma (up to 40%)
2. Medications (e.g., psychiatric medications, H_2 blockers, metoclopramide, verapamil, estrogen)
3. Pregnancy
4. Renal failure
5. Suprasellar mass lesions (can compress hypothalamus or pituitary stalk)
6. Hypothyroidism
7. Idiopathic

B. Clinical features

1. Men
   a. Hypogonadism, decreased libido, infertility, impotence
   b. Galactorrhea or gynecomastia (uncommon)
   c. Parasellar signs and symptoms (visual field defects and headaches)

2. Women
   a. Premenopausal: menstrual irregularities, oligomenorrhea or amenorrhea, anovulation and infertility, decreased libido, dyspareunia, vaginal dryness, risk of osteoporosis, galactorrhea
   b. Postmenopausal: parasellar signs and symptoms (less common than in men)

C. Diagnosis

1. Elevated serum prolactin level.
2. Order a pregnancy test and TSH level, because both pregnancy and primary hypothyroidism are on the differential diagnosis for hyperprolactinemia.
3. CT scan or MRI to identify any mass lesions.

D. Treatment

1. Treat the underlying cause (e.g., stop medication, treat hypothyroidism).
2. If prolactinoma is the cause and the patient is symptomatic, treat with **bromocriptine**, a dopamine agonist that secondarily diminishes the production and release of prolactin. Continue treatment for approximately 2 years before attempting cessation. **Cabergoline** (another dopamine agonist) may be better tolerated than bromocriptine and is often chosen as first-line therapy.
3. Consider surgical intervention if symptoms progress despite appropriate medical therapy. However, the recurrence rate after surgery is high.

Acromegaly

A. General characteristics

1. Acromegaly is broadening of the skeleton, which results from excess secretion of pituitary GH after epiphyseal closure (if before epiphyseal closure, gigantism [excessive height] results).
2. It is almost always caused by a GH-secreting pituitary adenoma (represents 10% of pituitary adenomas).

B. Clinical features

1. Growth promotion
   a. Soft tissue and skeleton overgrowth
   b. Coarsening of facial features
   c. Abnormally large hand and foot size (ask about increasing glove/ring size)
   d. Organomegaly
   e. Arthralgia due to joint tissue overgrowth
   f. Hypertrophic cardiomyopathy
   g. Enlarged jaw (macrognathia)
2. Metabolic disturbances
   a. Glucose intolerance and DM in 10% to 25% of patients
   b. Hyperhidrosis
3. Parasellar manifestations
   a. Headache
   b. Superior growth leads to compression of the optic chiasm, which results in visual loss (**bitemporal hemianopsia**)
   c. Lateral growth leads to cavernous sinus compression
   d. Inferior growth leads to sphenoid sinus invasion
   e. HTN, sleep apnea

C. Diagnosis

1. IGF-1, also known as somatomedin C, should be significantly elevated in acromegaly.
2. Oral glucose suppression test—glucose load fails to suppress GH (as it should in healthy individuals). This confirms the diagnosis if the IGF-1 level is equivocal.
3. MRI of the pituitary.
4. A random GH level is not useful because there is wide physiologic fluctuation of GH levels.

> **Quick HIT**
> Parasellar signs and symptoms (mass effects of the tumor) are more prevalent in men than in women. This is largely because the early symptoms in men (e.g., impotence) are often attributed to psychological causes and medical evaluation is delayed, allowing for larger tumor growth.

> **Quick HIT**
> Microadenomas (<10 mm diameter) tend to either remain the same size or regress with time. Only 10% to 20% continue to grow.

> **Quick HIT**
> Cardiovascular disease (cardiomyopathy) is the most common cause of death in patients with acromegaly.

> **Quick HIT**
> **Other Laboratory Abnormalities in Patients with Acromegaly**
> - Hyperprolactinemia (tumor secretes prolactin and growth hormone)—30% of patients
> - Elevations in serum glucose, triglycerides, and phosphate levels

D. Treatment

1. Transsphenoidal resection of pituitary adenoma—treatment of choice
2. Radiation therapy if IGF-1 levels stay elevated after surgery
3. Octreotide or other somatostatin analog to suppress GH secretion

Craniopharyngioma

- Tumors of the suprasellar region arising from embryologic remnants of Rathke pouch.
- These tumors comprise 20% to 25% of all pituitary mass lesions (**pituitary adenoma is most common**).
- They result in visual field defects (bitemporal hemianopsia) due to compression of the optic chiasm and may also cause headaches, papilledema, and changes in mentation.
- They are diagnosed by brain MRI.
- They may cause hyperprolactinemia, diabetes insipidus, or panhypopituitarism.
- Treatment is surgical excision (total or partial resection) with or without radiation therapy.

Quick HIT

Calcification of the suprasellar region seen on brain imaging is nearly diagnostic of craniopharyngioma.

Hypopituitarism

A. General characteristics

1. All or some of the hormones released from the anterior pituitary may be absent.
2. Loss of hormones is unpredictable, but LH, FSH, and GH are usually lost before TSH and ACTH.
3. Clinical manifestations depend on which hormones are lost.

B. Causes

1. Hypothalamic or pituitary tumor is the most common cause.
2. Other causes: radiation therapy, Sheehan syndrome, infiltrative processes (e.g., sarcoidosis, hemochromatosis), head trauma, cavernous sinus thrombosis, surgery.

C. Clinical features

1. Reduced GH: growth failure (decreased muscle mass in adults), increased LDL, increased risk of heart disease, increased LDL
2. Reduced prolactin: failure to lactate
3. Reduced ACTH: adrenal insufficiency
4. Reduced TSH: hypothyroidism
5. Reduced gonadotropins (LH and FSH): infertility, amenorrhea, loss of secondary sex characteristics, diminished libido
6. Reduced antidiuretic hormone (ADH) (if hypothalamic lesion): diabetes insipidus
7. Reduced melanocyte-stimulating hormone (MSH): decreased skin and hair pigmentation

D. Diagnosis

1. Low levels of target hormones with low or normal levels of trophic hormones (it is the suppression of the trophic hormone that is important, although the absolute level may be in the normal reference range)
2. MRI of the brain (may miss microadenomas)

E. Treatment

1. Replacement of appropriate hormones
2. Women who want to conceive should be referred to an endocrinologist

Diabetes Insipidus

A. General characteristics

1. Two forms
   a. Central DI is the most common form—due to low ADH secretion by posterior pituitary
   b. Nephrogenic DI—ADH secretion is normal but tubules cannot respond to ADH

2. Causes
   a. Central DI
      - Idiopathic—50% of all cases
      - Trauma—surgery, head trauma
      - Other destructive processes involving the hypothalamus, including tumors, sarcoidosis, tuberculosis, syphilis, Hand–Schüller–Christian disease, eosinophilic granuloma, and encephalitis
   b. Nephrogenic DI—the most common cause in adults is *chronic lithium use.* Other causes include hypercalcemia, pyelonephritis, and demeclocycline use. It may also be congenital—caused by mutations in the ADH receptor gene or the aquaporin-2 gene

Quick HIT

If a patient presents with polyuria and polydipsia, consider the following first in the differential diagnosis:
- Diabetes mellitus
- Diuretic use
- Diabetes insipidus
- Primary polydipsia

B. Clinical features

1. Polyuria is a hallmark finding: 5 to 15 L daily; urine is colorless (because it is so dilute).
2. Thirst and polydipsia—hydration is maintained if the patient is conscious and has access to water.
3. Hypernatremia is usually mild unless the patient has an impaired thirst drive.

Quick HIT

- Primary polydipsia is usually seen in patients with psychiatric disturbances.
- If the patient is deprived of water, urine osmolarity will increase appropriately.

C. Diagnosis

1. Urine—low specific gravity and low osmolality indicate DI
2. Plasma osmolality
   a. Normal: 250 to 290 mOsm/kg
   b. Primary polydipsia: 255 to 280 mOsm/kg
   c. DI: 280 to 310 mOsm/kg
3. A water deprivation test (dehydration test) is required to make the diagnosis (see Table 4-1)
   a. Procedure
      - Withhold fluids, and measure urine osmolality every hour
      - When urine osmolality is stable (<30 mOsm/kg hourly increase for 3 hours), inject 2 g desmopressin subcutaneously. Measure urine osmolality 1 hour later
   b. Response—see Table 4-1
4. ADH level (not the test of choice; takes a long time to get results)
   a. Low in central DI
   b. Normal or elevated in nephrogenic DI

D. Treatment

1. Central DI
   a. Desmopressin (DDAVP) is the primary therapy and can be given by nasal spray, orally, or by injection.
   b. Chlorpropamide increases ADH secretion and enhances the effect of ADH.
   c. Treat the underlying cause.

TABLE 4-1 Response to the Water Deprivation Test

	Increase in Urine Osmolality Above 280 mOsm/kg with Dehydration	Further Response to ADH
Normal Patients	+	−
Diabetes Insipidus Patients	−	+
Nephrogenic Diabetes Insipidus Patients	−	−

2. Nephrogenic DI—treat with sodium restriction and thiazide diuretics.
   a. These deplete the body of sodium, which leads to increased reabsorption of sodium and water in the proximal tubules.
   b. The reabsorption of sodium and water in the proximal tubules means that less water reaches the distal tubules, leading to decreased urine volume.

Syndrome of Inappropriate Secretion of Antidiuretic Hormone

Quick HIT

In SIADH, volume expansion occurs (due to water retention), but edema is prevented (due to natriuresis).

A. General characteristics

1. Pathophysiology
   a. Excess ADH is secreted from the posterior pituitary or an ectopic source. Elevated levels lead to water retention and excretion of concentrated urine. This has two major effects: hyponatremia and volume expansion.
   b. **Despite volume expansion, edema is not seen in syndrome of inappropriate secretion of antidiuretic hormone (SIADH).** This is because natriuresis (excretion of excessive sodium in urine) occurs despite hyponatremia.
   c. Reasons for natriuresis
      - Volume expansion causes an increase in atrial natriuretic peptide (increases urine sodium excretion).
      - Volume expansion leads to a decrease in proximal tubular sodium absorption.
      - The renin–angiotensin–aldosterone system is inhibited.

Quick HIT

Hyponatremia Pearls
- Hypovolemic hyponatremia—volume contracted
- Hypervolemic hyponatremia—volume expanded with edema
- SIADH—volume expanded without edema

B. Causes

1. Neoplasms (e.g., in lung, pancreas, prostate, bladder), lymphomas, leukemia
2. CNS disorders (e.g., stroke, head trauma, infection)
3. Pulmonary disorders (e.g., pneumonia, tuberculosis)
4. Ventilators with positive pressure
5. Medication (e.g., vincristine, selective serotonin reuptake inhibitors [SSRIs], chlorpropamide, oxytocin, morphine, desmopressin)
6. Postoperative state (e.g., as a result of anesthesia, pain)

C. Clinical features

1. Acute hyponatremia—Signs and symptoms are secondary to brain swelling (osmotic water shifts, leading to increased ICF volume) and are primarily neurologic
   a. Lethargy, somnolence, weakness
   b. **Can lead to seizures, coma, or death if untreated**
2. Chronic hyponatremia
   a. May be asymptomatic
   b. Anorexia, nausea, and vomiting
   c. CNS symptoms are less common because chronic loss of sodium and potassium from brain cells decreases brain edema (due to secondary water shifts from ICF to ECF)

Quick HIT

Major characteristics of SIADH
- Hyponatremia
- Volume expansion without edema
- Natriuresis
- Hypouricemia and low BUN
- Normal or reduced serum creatinine level because of dilution
- Normal thyroid and adrenal function

D. Diagnosis

1. **SIADH is a diagnosis of exclusion** (after other causes of hyponatremia have been ruled out). The following help in supporting the diagnosis:
   a. Hyponatremia and inappropriately concentrated urine; plasma osmolality, 270 mmol/kg
   b. Low serum uric acid level
   c. Low BUN and creatinine
   d. Normal thyroid and adrenal function, as well as renal, cardiac, and liver function
   e. Measurement of plasma and urine ADH level
   f. Absence of significant hypervolemia

E. Treatment

1. Correct the underlying cause, if known.
2. For asymptomatic patients
   a. Water restriction is usually sufficient.

b. Use normal saline in combination with a loop diuretic if faster results are desired.
c. Lithium carbonate or demeclocycline are other options (with side effects)—both inhibit the effect of ADH in the kidney.

3. For symptomatic patients
   a. Restrict water intake.
   b. Give isotonic saline. Hypertonic saline may occasionally be indicated in severe cases.
4. Do not raise the serum sodium concentration too quickly. Rapid flux of water into the ECF can result in **central pontine myelinolysis** (demyelination syndrome may result). A general guideline is that the rate of sodium replacement should not exceed 0.5 mEq/L per hour.

Diseases of the Parathyroid Glands

Hypoparathyroidism

A. Causes

1. Head and neck surgery account for the majority of cases—thyroidectomy, parathyroidectomy, radical surgery for head and neck malignancies.
2. Nonsurgical hypoparathyroidism is rare.

> **Quick HIT**
> **Pseudohypoparathyroidism**
> - End-organ resistance to action of PTH
> - Laboratory value findings: hypocalcemia, hyperphosphatemia, high PTH, low urinary cAMP

B. Clinical features

1. Cardiac arrhythmias
2. Rickets and osteomalacia
3. Increased neuromuscular irritability due to hypocalcemia
   a. Numbness/tingling—circumoral, fingers, toes
   b. Tetany
      - Hyperactive deep tendon reflexes
      - *Chvostek sign*—Tapping the facial nerve elicits contraction of facial muscles
      - *Trousseau sign*—Inflating the BP cuff to a pressure higher than the patient's systolic BP for 3 minutes elicits carpal spasms
   c. Grand mal seizures
4. Basal ganglia calcifications
5. **Prolonged QT interval** on ECG—Hypocalcemia should always be in the differential diagnosis of a prolonged QT interval
6. Cataracts

C. Diagnosis

1. Low serum calcium
2. High serum phosphate
3. Serum PTH inappropriately low
4. Low urine cAMP

D. Treatment

1. IV calcium gluconate in severe cases, oral calcium in mild to moderate cases.
2. Vitamin D supplementation (calcitriol).
3. Note that both vitamin D and calcium replacement can increase urinary calcium excretion, precipitating kidney stones. Therefore, administer with caution to avoid hypercalciuria (the goal is to keep serum calcium at 8.0 to 8.5 mg/dL).

Primary Hyperparathyroidism

A. General characteristics

1. One or more glands produce inappropriately high amounts of PTH relative to the serum calcium level.
2. Most common cause of hypercalcemia in the outpatient setting.

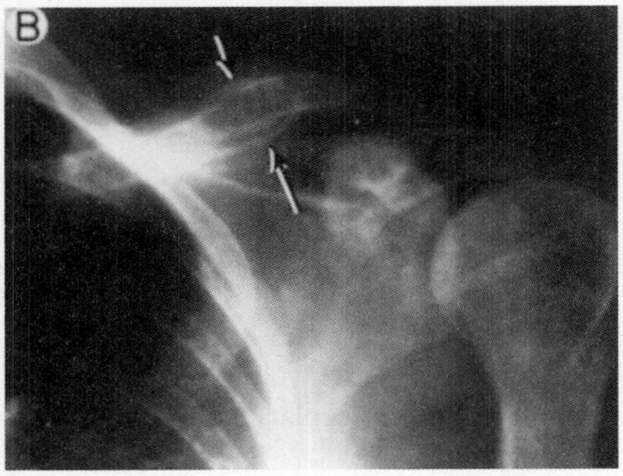

FIGURE **4-4** **X-ray of the clavicle in a patient with osteitis fibrosa cystica ("brown tumors"), a disease in which cystic bone spaces are filled with brown fibrous tissue. Brown tumors predispose patients to pathologic fractures.**
(From Becker KL, Bilezikian JP, Brenner WJ, et al. *Principles and Practice of Endocrinology and Metabolism*, 3rd ed. Philadelphia, PA: Lippincott Williams & Wilkins, 2001.)

B. Causes

1. Adenoma (80% of cases)—majority involve only one gland
2. Hyperplasia (15% to 20% of cases)—all four glands usually affected
3. Carcinoma (<1% of cases)

C. Clinical features

1. *"Stones"*
   a. Nephrolithiasis
   b. Nephrocalcinosis
2. *"Bones"*
   a. Bone aches and pains
   b. **Osteitis fibrosa cystica** ("**brown tumors**")—predisposes patient to pathologic fractures (Figure 4-4)
3. *"Groans"*
   a. Muscle pain and weakness
   b. Pancreatitis
   c. Peptic ulcer disease
   d. Gout
   e. Constipation
4. *"Psychiatric overtones"*—depression, fatigue, anorexia, sleep disturbances, anxiety, lethargy
5. Other symptoms:
   a. Polydipsia, polyuria
   b. HTN, shortened QT interval
   c. Weight loss

D. Diagnosis

1. Laboratory (see also Clinical Pearl 4-6)
   a. Calcium levels (hypercalcemia)—when calculating calcium levels, be aware of albumin levels. Calculate the ionized fraction or get an ionized calcium level

CLINICAL PEARL 4-6

Secondary Hyperparathyroidism

- Characterized by an elevated concentration of PTH and a low or low-normal serum calcium level.
- Caused by chronic renal failure (most common cause), as well as vitamin D deficiency and renal hypercalciuria.
- Treatment depends on the cause: if vitamin D deficiency, give vitamin D; if renal failure, give calcitriol and oral calcium supplements plus dietary phosphorus restriction.

b. PTH levels
   - Should be elevated relative to serum calcium level
   - Note that in the presence of hypercalcemia, a normal PTH level is "abnormal" (i.e., high) because high calcium levels suppress PTH secretion

c. Hypophosphatemia
d. Hypercalciuria
e. Urine cAMP is elevated
f. Chloride/phosphorus ratio of >33 is diagnostic of primary hyperparathyroidism (33-to-1 rule). Chloride is high secondary to renal bicarbonate wasting (direct effect of PTH).

2. Radiographs
   a. Subperiosteal bone resorption (usually on radial aspect of second and third phalanges), but can appear in any location (see Figure 4-4)
   b. Osteopenia

Quick HIT

Relative Indications for Surgery in Primary Hyperparathyroidism
- Age <50 years
- Marked decrease in bone mass
- Nephrolithiasis, renal insufficiency
- Markedly elevated serum calcium level or episode of severe hypercalcemia
- Urine calcium >400 mg in 24 hours

E. Treatment

1. Surgery is the only definitive treatment, but not all patients require it. If the patient is over 50 years of age and is asymptomatic (with normal bone mass and renal function), surgery may not be needed.
   a. Primary hyperparathyroidism due to hyperplasia—All the four glands are removed. A small amount of parathyroid tissue is placed in the forearm muscle (prevents the need for reexploration of the neck if hyperplasia recurs postoperatively) to retain parathyroid function.
   b. Primary hyperparathyroidism due to adenoma—Surgical removal of the adenoma is curative.
   c. Primary hyperparathyroidism due to carcinoma—Remove the tumor, ipsilateral thyroid lobe, and all enlarged lymph nodes.
2. Medical—Encourage fluids. Give diuretics (furosemide) to enhance calcium excretion if hypercalcemia is severe. (Do not give thiazide diuretics!)

Diseases of the Adrenal Glands

Cushing Syndrome

Quick HIT

Effects of cortisol (Generally Catabolic)
- Impaired collagen production, enhanced protein catabolism
- Anti-insulin effects (leading to glucose intolerance)
- Impaired immunity (has inhibitory effects on PMNs, T cells)
- Enhances catecholamine activity (HTN)

A. General characteristics

1. Cushing **syndrome** results from excessive levels of glucocorticoids (cortisol is the principal glucocorticoid) due to any cause.
2. Cushing **disease** results from pituitary Cushing syndrome (pituitary adenoma).

B. Causes

1. Iatrogenic Cushing syndrome is the most common cause, and is due to prescribed prednisone or other steroids. Androgen excess is absent (because the exogenous steroid suppresses androgen production by the adrenals).
2. ACTH-secreting adenoma of the pituitary (Cushing disease) is the second most common cause and leads to bilateral adrenal hyperplasia. Androgen excess is common.
3. Adrenal adenomas and carcinomas (10% to 15%).
4. Ectopic ACTH production (10% to 15%).
   a. ACTH-secreting tumor stimulates the cortisol release from the adrenal glands without the normal negative feedback loop (because the source of the ACTH is outside the pituitary gland).
   b. More than two-thirds are small cell carcinomas of the lung. Bronchial carcinoid and thymoma may be the cause.

Quick HIT

Some signs and symptoms in patients with high cortisol (e.g., obesity, HTN, osteoporosis, DM) are nonspecific and less helpful in diagnosing the patient. On the other hand, easy bruising, typical striae, myopathy, and virilizing signs are more helpful in diagnosis.

C. Clinical features

1. Changes in appearance: central obesity, hirsutism, moon facies, "buffalo hump," purple striae on abdomen, lanugo hair, acne, easy bruising
2. HTN
3. Decreased glucose tolerance (diabetes)

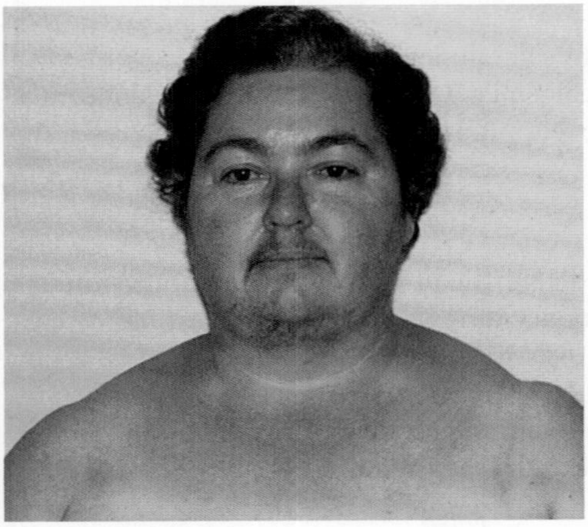

FIGURE 4-5 **Androgen excess manifesting as masculinization in females, only seen in ACTH-dependent forms of Cushing syndrome.**
(From Rubin E. *Essential Pathology*, 3rd ed. Philadelphia, PA: Lippincott Williams & Wilkins, 2000.)

4. Hypogonadism—menstrual irregularity and infertility
5. Masculinization in females (androgen excess, see Figure 4-5)—only seen in ACTH-dependent forms
6. Musculoskeletal—proximal muscle wasting and weakness (due to protein catabolism), osteoporosis, aseptic necrosis of femoral head may occur (especially with exogenous steroid use)
7. Psychiatric disturbances—depression, mania
8. Increased likelihood of infections (due to impaired immunity)

Quick HIT

Patients with **Cushing disease** may have hyperpigmentation due to elevated ACTH levels, whereas patients with Cushing syndrome due to other causes will not have **hyperpigmentation.**

D. Diagnosis

1. Initial screening (Figure 4-6 and Table 4-2).
   a. An overnight (low-dose) dexamethasone suppression test is the initial screening test. Give the patient 1 mg of dexamethasone at 11 pm. Measure the serum cortisol level at 8 am.
      - If the serum cortisol is <5, Cushing syndrome can be excluded (this test is very sensitive).
      - If the serum cortisol is >5 (and often >10), the patient has Cushing syndrome. Order a high-dose dexamethasone suppression test to determine the cause (Cushing disease vs. adrenal tumor vs. ectopic ACTH tumor).
   b. The 24-hour urinary free cortisol level is another excellent screening test; values greater than four times normal are rare except in Cushing syndrome.
2. ACTH level—Once you establish a diagnosis of Cushing syndrome, measure the ACTH level. If it is low, the cause of high cortisol levels is likely an adrenal tumor or hyperplasia, not a pituitary disease or an ectopic ACTH-producing tumor.
3. High-dose dexamethasone suppression test.
   a. In Cushing disease, the result is a decrease in cortisol levels (greater than 50% suppression occurs).
   b. If cortisol suppression does **not** occur and plasma ACTH levels are high, an ectopic ACTH-producing tumor is likely the diagnosis.
4. CRH stimulation test—CRH is administered intravenously.
   a. If ACTH/cortisol levels increase (deemed a "response"), then Cushing disease is the diagnosis.
   b. If ACTH/cortisol levels do not increase (deemed "no response"), then the patient has either ectopic ACTH secretion or an adrenal tumor.
5. Imaging tests (once hormonal studies have established the site of disease, e.g., pituitary or adrenal)—CT scan or MRI of the appropriate area.

E. Treatment

1. Iatrogenic Cushing syndrome: tapering of glucocorticoid

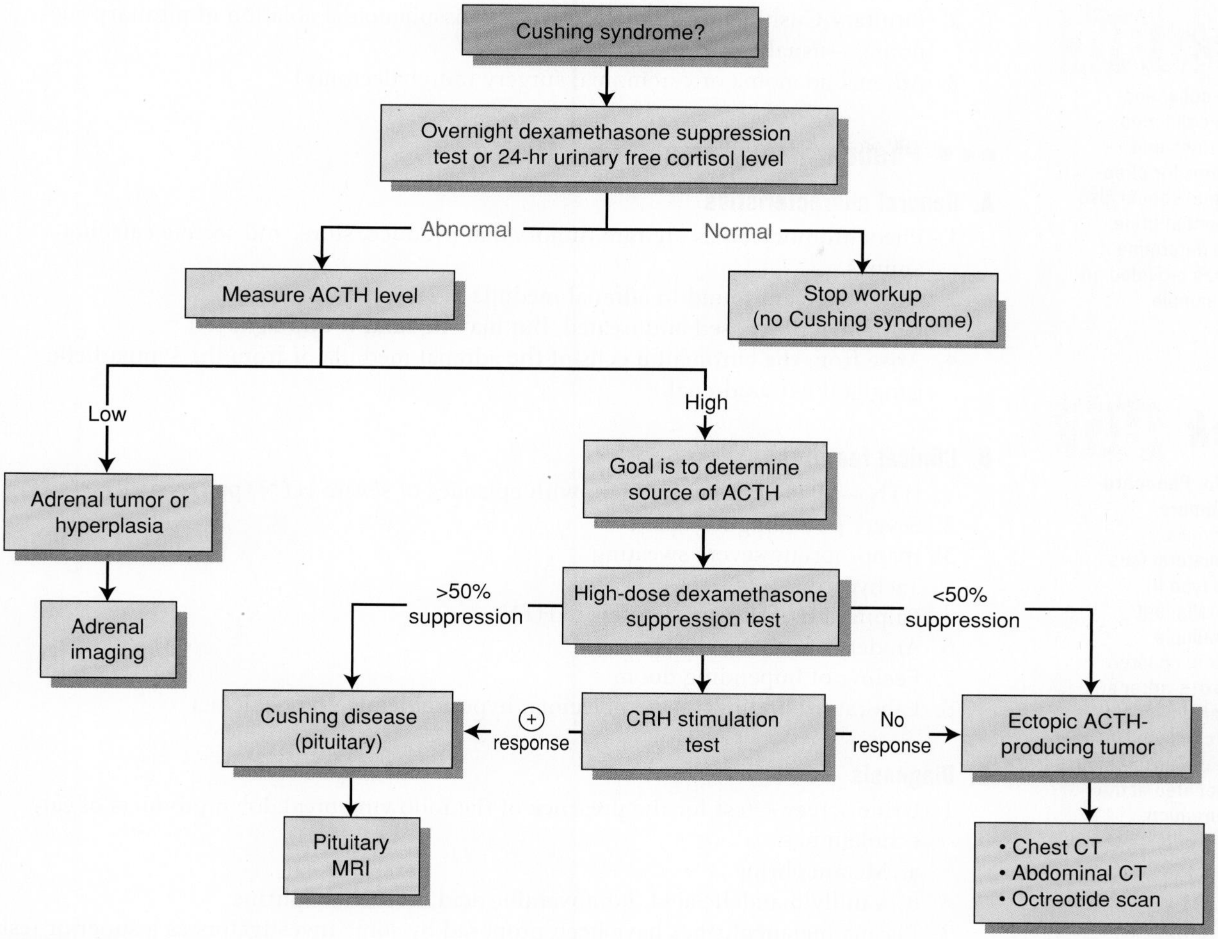

FIGURE 4-6 **Algorithm for the diagnosis of Cushing syndrome and its cause.**
(Adapted from Humes DH, DuPont HL, Gardner LB, et al. *Kelley's Textbook of Internal Medicine*. 4th ed. Philadelphia, PA: Lippincott Williams & Wilkins, 2000:2725, Figure 407-3.)

TABLE 4-2 Response to Diagnostic Tests in Cushing Syndrome

Healthy Patient	• Normal cortisol/normal ACTH • Suppression with low-dose dexamethasone • Suppression with high-dose dexamethasone • Mild increase with CRH test
Cushing Disease	• High cortisol/high ACTH • No suppression with low-dose dexamethasone • Suppression with high-dose dexamethasone • Great increase in cortisol with CRH test
Adrenal Tumor	• High cortisol/low ACTH • No suppression with low-dose dexamethasone • No suppression with high-dose dexamethasone • No change after CRH test
Ectopic ACTH-producing Tumor	• High cortisol/high ACTH • No suppression with low-dose dexamethasone • No suppression with high-dose dexamethasone • No change after CRH test

Quick HIT

Any 24 urine collection (i.e., 24 urine collection of metanephrines and catecholamines for pheochromocytoma) should also test the amount of urine creatinine to determine if the patient has provided an appropriate sample.

Quick HIT

Rule of 10s for Pheochromocytoma Tumors
- 10% are familial
- 10% are bilateral (suspect MEN type II)
- 10% are malignant
- 10% are multiple
- 10% occur in children
- 10% are extra-adrenal (more often malignant)—The most common site is the organ of Zuckerkandl, which is located at the aortic bifurcation.

Quick HIT

If the following are all present, pheochromocytoma is the diagnosis until proven otherwise.
- Headache
- Profuse sweating
- Palpitations
- Tachycardia
- Apprehension or sense of impending doom

Quick HIT

Always suspect hyperaldosteronism in a hypertensive patient with hypokalemia who is not on a diuretic.

2. Pituitary Cushing syndrome: surgery (transsphenoidal ablation of pituitary adenoma)—usually safe and effective
3. Adrenal adenoma or carcinoma: surgery (adrenalectomy)

Pheochromocytoma

A. General characteristics

1. Pheochromocytomas are rare tumors that produce, store, and secrete catecholamines.
2. Ninety percent found in adrenal medulla (10% extra-adrenal).
3. Curable if diagnosed and treated, but **may be fatal if undiagnosed.**
4. Arise from the chromaffin cells of the adrenal medulla or from the sympathetic ganglia if extra-adrenal.

B. Clinical features

1. HTN—BP is persistently high, with episodes of severe HTN (paroxysmal).
2. Severe pounding headache
3. Inappropriate severe sweating
4. Tachycardia
5. Palpitations, with sudden severe HTN
6. Anxiety
7. Feeling of impending doom
8. Laboratory findings: hyperglycemia, hyperlipidemia, hypokalemia

C. Diagnosis

1. Urine screen—test for the presence of the following breakdown products of catecholamines:
   a. Metanephrine
   b. Vanillylmandelic acid, homovanillic acid, normetanephrine
2. Plasma metanephrines have been proposed by some investigators as a superior test to urine metanephrines, especially when clinical suspicion is high
3. Urine/serum epinephrine and norepinephrine levels—if the epinephrine level is elevated, the tumor must be adrenal or near the adrenal gland (organ of Zuckerkandl) because nonadrenal tumors cannot methylate norepinephrine to epinephrine
4. Tumor localization tests—CT, MRI

D. Treatment

1. Surgical tumor resection with early ligation of venous drainage is the treatment of choice. Ligation lowers the possibility of catecholamine release/crisis by tying off drainage. Patients should be treated with α-blockade (typically **phenoxybenzamine**) for 10 to 14 days prior to surgery as well as β-blockade (i.e., propranolol) for 2 to 3 days prior to surgery. The α-blockade is used to control BP, and the β-blockade is used to decrease tachycardia. Laparoscopic adrenalectomy can be safely performed for most small- to medium-sized pheochromocytomas.

Primary Hyperaldosteronism

A. General characteristics

1. Excessive production of aldosterone by the adrenal glands independent of any regulation by the renin–angiotensin system (see also Clinical Pearl 4-7)
2. Excessive mineralocorticoids increase the activity of the Na^+/K^+ pumps in the cortical collecting tubules
   a. Sodium retention, causing ECF volume expansion and HTN
   b. Potassium loss—results in hypokalemia
3. Excess aldosterone also increases the secretion of hydrogen ions into the lumen of the medullary collecting tubules; results in metabolic alkalosis

CLINICAL PEARL 4-7

Multiple Endocrine Neoplasia (MEN) Syndrome

- Inherited condition: propensity to develop multiple endocrine tumors
- Autosomal dominant inheritance with incomplete penetrance
- Types
  - **MEN type I** (Wermer syndrome)—"3 Ps"
    - **P**arathyroid hyperplasia (in 90% of the patients with MEN I)
    - **P**ancreatic islet cell tumors (in two-thirds of the patients with MEN I)—ZES (50%), insulinoma (20%)
    - **P**ituitary tumors (in two-thirds of the patients with MEN I)
  - **MEN** type IIA (Sipple syndrome)—"MPH"
    - **M**edullary thyroid carcinoma (in 100% of the patients with MEN IIA)
    - **P**heochromocytoma (in more than one-third of the patients with MEN IIA)
    - **H**yperparathyroidism (in 50% of the patients with MEN IIA)
  - **MEN type IIB**—"MMMP"
    - **M**ucosal neuromas (in 100% of the patients with MEN IIB)—in the nasopharynx, oropharynx, larynx, and conjunctiva
    - **M**edullary thyroid carcinoma (in 85% of the patients with MEN IIB)—more aggressive than in MEN IIA
    - **M**arfanoid body habitus (long/lanky)
    - **P**heochromocytoma

B. Causes

1. Adrenal adenoma (in two-thirds of the cases)—aldosterone producing adenoma (**Conn syndrome**)
2. Adrenal hyperplasia (in one-third of the cases)—almost always bilateral
3. Adrenal carcinoma (in <1% of the cases)

C. Clinical features

1. HTN (most common clinical feature); may otherwise be asymptomatic
2. Headache, fatigue, weakness
3. Polydipsia, nocturnal polyuria (due to hypokalemia)
4. **Absence of peripheral edema**

D. Diagnosis

1. Ratio of the plasma aldosterone level to plasma renin—A screening test in primary hyperaldosteronism reveals inappropriately elevated levels of plasma aldosterone with coexistent decreased plasma renin activity. Therefore, if the plasma aldosterone-to-renin ratio is >30, evaluate further.
2. For definitive diagnosis, one of the two tests is usually performed.
   a. Saline infusion test
      - Infusion of saline will decrease aldosterone levels in normal patients but not in those with primary aldosteronism.
      - If aldosterone levels are <8.5 ng/dL after saline infusion, primary aldosteronism may be ruled out.

   b. Oral sodium loading
      - The patient is given a high salt diet for 3 days. Serum and urine electrolytes, aldosterone, and creatinine are measured on the third day. High urine aldosterone in the setting of high urine sodium (to document appropriate sodium loading) confirms the diagnosis.
3. To diagnose the cause of primary aldosteronism:
   a. Adrenal venous sampling for aldosterone levels—A high level of aldosterone on one side indicates an adenoma. High levels on both sides indicate bilateral hyperplasia.
   b. Renin–aldosterone stimulation test—Recumbency or upright positions are assumed, followed by measurement of serum aldosterone.

Quick HIT

The prevalence of **adrenal incidentaloma** is on the rise with the more widespread use of imaging techniques. An adrenal incidentaloma is a nonfunctioning adrenal tumor. Most are benign, but the risk of malignancy increases with increasing size. Treat by first ruling out a functioning tumor and then resect any tumor greater than 6 cm (high risk of malignant disease).

Quick HIT

It is important to distinguish adenoma from hyperplasia because HTN associated with hyperplasia is **not** benefited by bilateral adrenalectomy, whereas HTN associated with adenoma is usually improved/cured by removal of the adenoma.

CLINICAL PEARL 4-8

Adrenal Crisis

- An acute and severely symptomatic stage of adrenal insufficiency that can include severe hypotension and cardiovascular collapse, abdominal pain (can mimic an acute abdomen), acute renal failure, and death.
- Any stress (e.g., trauma, infection, surgery) can precipitate an adrenal crisis.
- Can be fatal if untreated.
- Treat with IV hydrocortisone, IV fluids (several liters of normal saline with 5% dextrose), and a search for the underlying condition that precipitated the crisis.

Quick HIT

The most common cause of Addison disease worldwide is tuberculosis (autoimmune disease is the most common cause in the Western world). However, the most common cause of adrenal insufficiency overall (99% of all cases) is abrupt cessation of exogenous glucocorticoids.

c. Imaging tests
   - CT scan/MRI of adrenals—may demonstrate adenoma or hyperplasia anatomically.
   - Iodocholesterol scanning—a functional approach to differentiating between adenoma and hyperplasia.
   - Arteriography/venography (retrograde).

E. Treatment

1. For adenoma—Surgical resection (adrenalectomy) is often curative.
2. For bilateral hyperplasia
   a. Spironolactone inhibits the action of aldosterone.
   b. Surgery is not indicated.

Quick HIT

Most Common Clinical Findings of Adrenal Insufficiency
- Weight loss
- Weakness
- Pigmentation
- Anorexia
- Nausea
- Postural hypotension
- Abdominal pain
- Hypoglycemia

Adrenal Insufficiency

A. Causes

1. Primary adrenal insufficiency (**Addison disease**) (see also Clinical Pearl 4-8).
   a. Idiopathic (thought to be autoimmune disease) is the most common type in the industrialized world.
   b. Infectious diseases—these include tuberculosis (most common cause worldwide) and fungal infections. Causes also include cytomegalovirus, cryptococcus, toxoplasmosis, and pneumocystis.
   c. Iatrogenic—for example, a bilateral adrenalectomy.
   d. Metastatic disease—from lung or breast cancer.
2. Secondary adrenal insufficiency
   a. Patients on long-term steroid therapy—**This is the most common cause of secondary adrenal insufficiency today.** When these patients develop a serious illness or undergo trauma, they cannot release an appropriate amount of cortisol because of chronic suppression of CRH and ACTH by the exogenous steroids. Therefore, symptoms of adrenal insufficiency result.
   b. Hypopituitarism (rare)—due to a variety of insults.
3. Tertiary adrenal insufficiency—hypothalamic disease.

Quick HIT

Hyperpigmentation and hyperkalemia appear in **primary**, not secondary, adrenal insufficiency.

B. Clinical features

1. Lack of cortisol
   a. GI symptoms—anorexia, nausea and vomiting, vague abdominal pain, weight loss
   b. Mental symptoms—lethargy, confusion, psychosis.
   c. **Hypoglycemia**—Cortisol is a gluconeogenic hormone.
   d. **Hyperpigmentation**
      - This is a common finding in primary adrenal insufficiency; not seen in secondary adrenal insufficiency because in secondary adrenal insufficiency ACTH levels are low, not high.
      - Low cortisol stimulates ACTH and MSH secretion.
   e. Intolerance to physiologic stress is a feared complication.
2. Low aldosterone (only seen in primary adrenal insufficiency because aldosterone depends on the renin–angiotensin system, not ACTH). Results in:

Quick HIT

The most common presentation of secondary adrenal insufficiency is a patient who has been on long-term steroids who stops them suddenly (i.e., for surgery) or who has an increased need (infection). Treatment is easy—give corticosteroids until the patient is stable clinically.

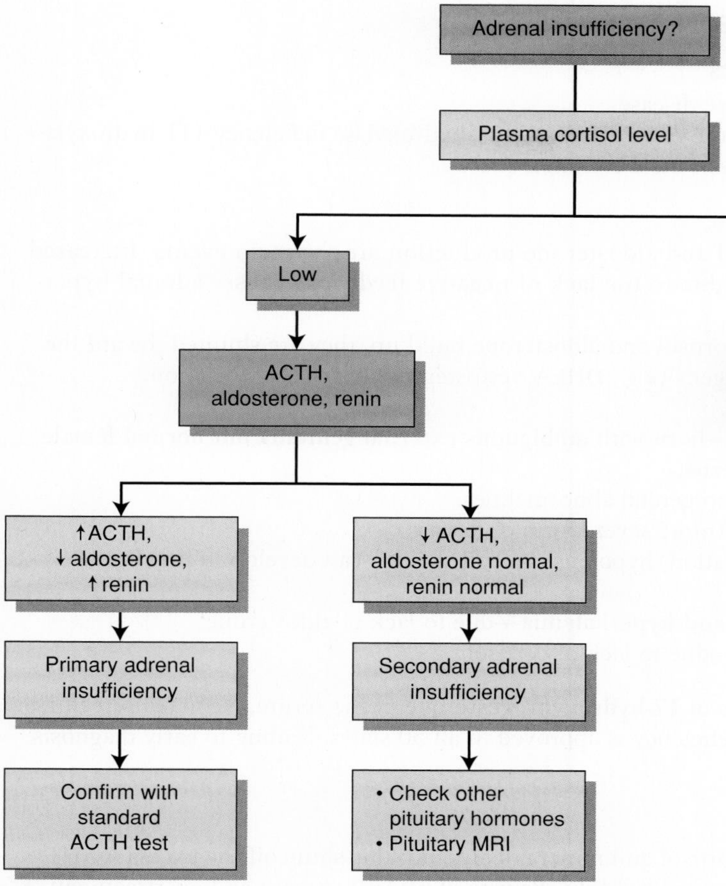

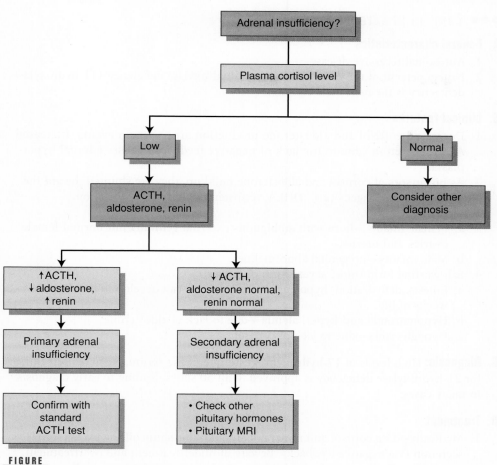

FIGURE **4-7** **Algorithm for the diagnosis of adrenal insufficiency.**
(Adapted from Humes DH, DuPont HL, Gardner LB, et al. *Kelley's Textbook of Internal Medicine.* 4th ed. Philadelphia, PA: Lippincott Williams & Wilkins, 2000:2730, Figure 407-5.)

a. Sodium loss, causing hyponatremia and hypovolemia, which may lead to:
   - **Hypotension**, decreased cardiac output, and decreased renal perfusion.
   - Weakness, **shock**, and syncope.

b. Hyperkalemia (due to retention of potassium).

C. Diagnosis

1. Decreased plasma cortisol level (Figure 4-7).
2. Plasma ACTH level—if low, this implies a secondary adrenal insufficiency (ACTH-dependent cause).
3. Standard ACTH test.
   a. This is a definitive test for primary adrenal insufficiency; give an IV infusion of synthetic ACTH, and measure plasma cortisol at the end of the infusion.
   b. In primary adrenal insufficiency, cortisol does not increase sufficiently.
   c. In secondary adrenal insufficiency, cortisol fails to respond to ACTH infusion, as in primary adrenal insufficiency (the adrenals are not used to being stimulated, so they do not respond right away). If the test is repeated for 4 or 5 days, the adrenals eventually respond normally.
4. Perform imaging tests (MRI of brain—pituitary/hypothalamus) if secondary or tertiary adrenal insufficiency is diagnosed.

D. Treatment

1. Primary adrenal insufficiency: daily oral glucocorticoid (hydrocortisone or prednisone) and daily fludrocortisone (mineralocorticoid).
2. Secondary adrenal insufficiency: same as in primary adrenal insufficiency, except that mineralocorticoid replacement is not necessary.

Quick HIT

Congenital adrenal hyperplasia (CAH) is a very treatable condition. Affected female patients will develop normally and will be fertile if treated early.

Congenital Adrenal Hyperplasia

A. General characteristics

1. Autosomal recessive disease.
2. Ninety percent of the cases are due to 21-hydroxylase deficiency. (11-hydroxylase deficiency is the next most common cause.)

B. Clinical features

1. Decreased cortisol and aldosterone production are the main events. Increased ACTH secretion (due to the lack of negative feedback) causes adrenal hyperplasia.
2. As precursors of cortisol and aldosterone build up, they are shunted toward the synthesis of androgens (e.g., DHEA, testosterone), causing virilization.
3. Virilizing features.
   a. Female infants—born with **ambiguous external genitalia but normal female ovaries and uterus.**
   b. Male infants—no genital abnormalities.
4. Salt wasting form (more severe form of disease).
   a. Emesis, dehydration, hypotension, and shock—can develop in first 2 to 4 weeks of life.
   b. **Hyponatremia and hyperkalemia**—due to lack of aldosterone.
   c. Hypoglycemia—due to lack of cortisol.

C. Diagnosis: High levels of **17-hydroxyprogesterone** in the serum. Neonatal screening for 21-hydroxylase deficiency is approved in all 50 states, leading to early diagnosis in many cases.

D. Treatment

1. Medically—Use cortisol and mineralocorticoid; this shuts off the excess ACTH secretion (via negative feedback). Beware of undertreatment and overtreatment.
2. Surgically—Early correction of female genital abnormalities is generally recommended.

Diseases of the Pancreas

Diabetes Mellitus

A. General characteristics

1. Classification (see also Table 4-3).
   a. Type I IDDM—approximately 5% of all diabetic patients.
      - This is characterized by a severe deficiency of insulin. **Patients require insulin to live.**
      - The onset is typically in youth (before age 20), but can occur at any age.
      - Not related to obesity.
   b. Type II NIDDM—90% or more of all diabetic patients.
      - Insulin levels are usually normal to high but may diminish over many years of having diabetes.
      - Insulin resistance (due to obesity) plays a major role.
      - It often goes undiagnosed for many years.
   c. Impaired glucose tolerance.
      - Fasting glucose between 110 and 125 mg/dL or a 2-hour postprandial glucose between 140 and 199 mg/dL.
      - One percent to five percent annual increase in risk of developing type II diabetes.
      - Increased risk for cardiovascular disease.
2. Pathogenesis of type I diabetes (see also Clinical Pearls 4-9 and 4-10)
   a. An autoimmune disease—The immune system mediates the destruction of β-cells.

Endocrine and Metabolic Diseases

TABLE 4-3 **Comparison of Type I and II Diabetes Mellitus**

	Type I	Type II
Onset	Sudden	Gradual
Age at Onset	Any age (typically young)	Mostly in adults
Body Habitus	Usually thin	Frequently obese
Ketosis	Common	Rare
Autoantibodies	Present in most cases	Absent
Endogenous Insulin	Low or absent	Can be normal, decreased, or increased
HLA Association	**Yes (HLA-DQ/DR)**	**No**
Genetic Factors	Concordance rate between identical twins is 50%	Concordance rate between identical twins is 90%. Therefore, type II demonstrates a much stronger genetic component than type I.

b. It develops in genetically susceptible individuals who are exposed to an environmental factor that triggers the autoimmune response; β-cell destruction ensues.
c. Overt IDDM does not appear until about 90% of β-cells are destroyed.

3. Pathogenesis of type II diabetes.
   a. Risk factors
      - Obesity (greatest risk factor)
      - Genetics
      - Age (insulin production decreases with age)
   b. Obesity (plays a major role)
      - Obesity is associated with increased plasma levels of free fatty acids, which make muscles more insulin resistant, reducing glucose uptake. **Therefore, obesity exacerbates insulin resistance.**
      - In the liver, free fatty acids increase the production of glucose.
   c. Lack of compensation in type II diabetic patients
      - In normal individuals, the pancreas secretes more insulin in response to free fatty acids, thus neutralizing the excess glucose.
      - In type II diabetic patients, free fatty acids fail to stimulate pancreatic insulin secretion. Therefore, compensation does not occur and hyperglycemia develops; β-cells become desensitized to glucose, leading to decreased insulin secretion.

Quick HIT

Hypertriglyceridemia with HDL depletion is the characteristic lipid profile of insulin resistance and poorly controlled diabetes.

Quick HIT

Diabetes is diagnosed by **one** of the following:
1. Two fasting glucose measurements greater than 125 mg/dL
2. Single glucose level of 200 mg/dL with symptoms
3. Increased glucose level on oral glucose tolerance testing
4. Hemoglobin A1c >6.5%

CLINICAL PEARL 4-9

Dawn Phenomenon and Somogyi Effect

- Both cause morning hyperglycemia.
- The dawn phenomenon is probably due to an increase in the nocturnal secretion of growth hormone. This phenomenon is independent of the Somogyi effect.
- The Somogyi effect is a rebound response to nocturnal hypoglycemia—that is, counterregulatory systems are activated in response to hypoglycemia, leading to morning hyperglycemia.
- If morning hyperglycemia is present, check the glucose level at 3:00 am. If the glucose level is elevated, the patient has the dawn phenomenon and his or her evening insulin should be increased to provide additional coverage in the overnight hours. If the glucose level is low, the patient has the Somogyi effect and his or her evening insulin should be decreased to avoid nocturnal hypoglycemia.

CLINICAL PEARL 4-10

General Principles in Outpatient Management and Monitoring of All Diabetic Patients

- Monitor HbA_{1c} level every 3 months. Keeping HbA_{1c} <7 is the objective (although difficult to achieve) because it is associated with a marked reduction in risk for microvascular complications.
- All diabetic patients should monitor daily glycemic levels with home blood glucose determinations. Patients on insulin therapy should check blood glucose levels before meals and at bedtime. Monitoring blood glucose 90 to 120 minutes after meals enables the patient to control postprandial hyperglycemia and should be strongly encouraged.
- Screen for microalbuminuria at least once per year in diabetic patients with no evidence of nephropathy. Prescribe ACE inhibitor or ARB if urine test is positive for microalbuminuria.
- Check BUN and creatinine level at least once per year.
- Order eye screening yearly by an ophthalmologist to screen for diabetic retinopathy.
- Check the feet at every visit. Refer high-risk patients to a foot care specialist (e.g., podiatrist). Patients should check their feet regularly for ulcers and neuropathy.
- Check cholesterol levels at least once per year. Give statin medication if LDL is above 100 mg/dL.
- Take BP at every visit. Give ACE inhibitor or ARB if BP is greater than 130/80 mm Hg.
- Daily aspirin in all diabetics over age 30.
- Pneumococcal vaccine.

B. Diagnosis

1. Testing recommendations (see also Table 4-4).
   a. Screen all adults over age 45 every 3 years.
   b. For those with risk factors for diabetes (obesity, family history, history of gestational diabetes), start screening earlier. Some recommend early screening for African Americans and Native Americans.
   c. Test anyone with signs or symptoms of diabetes.
2. Perform any one of the following tests on *two separate days* (see Table 4-4).
   a. Fasting plasma glucose—criteria for DM: glucose >126 mg/dL.
      - Preferred test for screening.
      - If between 100 and 126 mg/dL, perform a 75 g oral glucose tolerance test (although this is rarely done) or recheck fasting glucose.
   b. Random plasma glucose—criteria for DM: glucose >200 mg/dL in a person with diabetic symptoms.
   c. Two-hour postprandial plasma glucose level—criteria for DM: glucose >200 mg/dL after administration of the equivalent of a 75 g glucose load (more sensitive than fasting glucose level, but less convenient).
   d. Hemoglobin A1c—criteria for DM: A1c >6.5% (repeat test should occur several months later as opposed to the next day).

TABLE 4-4 Diagnostic Criteria for Diabetes Mellitus

Glucose Test	Impaired Glucose Tolerance (mg/dL)	Diabetes Mellitus (mg/dL)
Random plasma	—	>200 with diabetic symptoms
Fasting	110–126	>126 on two occasions
2-hr postprandial	140–200	>200
Hemoglobin A1c (%)	5.7–6.4	>6.5

TABLE 4-5 Symptoms of Diabetes Mellitus

Symptom	Cause
Polyuria	Glucose in renal tubule causes osmotic retention of water, causing a diuresis
Polydipsia	A physiologic response to diuresis to maintain plasma volume
Fatigue	Mechanism unknown, but probably due to increased glucose in plasma
Weight loss	Due to loss of anabolic effects of insulin
Blurred vision	Swelling of lens due to osmosis (caused by increased glucose)
Fungal infections	Fungal infections of mouth and vagina common—*Candida albicans* thrives under increased glucose conditions
Numbness, tingling of hands and feet	Neuropathy Mononeuropathy: due to microscopic vasculitis leading to axonal ischemia Polyneuropathy: etiology is probably multifactorial

Quick HIT

While evaluating a diabetic patient, focus on:
- The feet
- Vascular disease (CAD, PVD)
- Neurologic disease (neuropathies)
- Eyes (retinopathy)
- Renal disease
- Infectious disease

Quick HIT

Optimal Treatment for Type II Diabetic Patients
- Glycemic control
- BP control—goal is <130/85 (the lower the better, as long as tolerated by the patient)
- Optimization of serum lipids—goals: LDL ≤100, HDL ≥40. Check lipids annually
- Smoking cessation
- Daily aspirin (if not contraindicated)
- Inspect feet at every visit
- Dilated eye examination yearly
- Urine albumin–creatinine ratio annually
- Measure A1C every 3 to 6 months.

C. Clinical presentation

1. Type I (see Table 4-5 and Figure 4-8)
   a. Symptoms develop quickly over days to weeks.
   b. Sometimes symptoms appear after an illness.
   c. Patients often present with acute DKA.
2. Type II
   a. This is usually discovered on screening urinalysis or blood sugar measurement. Sometimes the diagnosis is made during evaluation for other diseases (e.g., heart, kidney, neurologic, infection).
   b. Symptomatic patients may present with polyuria, polydipsia, polyphagia, fatigue, blurred vision, weight loss, and/or candidal vaginitis. These symptoms are usually noted in retrospect, after elevated blood glucose has been documented.
   c. Patients who have not routinely sought medical attention may present with complications such as myocardial ischemia, stroke, intermittent claudication, impotence, peripheral neuropathy, proteinuria, or retinopathy.

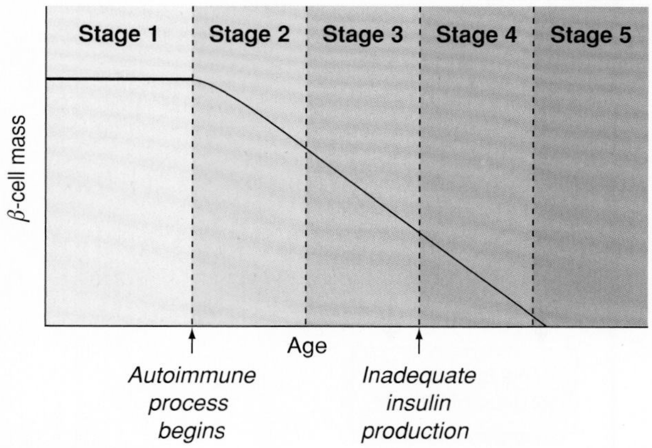

Stage 1: Genetic susceptibility
Stage 2: Autoimmune process of β-cell destruction begins. Normal insulin is released.
Stage 3: As β-cell destruction continues, insulin release is decreased. Glucose level is still normal.
Stage 4: Overt diabetes mellitus. Patient is insulin dependent at this point. C-peptide is still present.
Stage 5: No C-peptide present

FIGURE 4-8 Progression of type I diabetes mellitus.

TABLE 4-6 Oral Hypoglycemic Drugs

Medication	Mechanism	Site of Action	Advantages	Side Effects
Sulfonylureas (e.g., glyburide, glipizide, glimepiride)	Stimulate pancreas to produce more insulin	Pancreas	Effective Inexpensive	Hypoglycemia, weight gain
Metformin[a]	Enhances insulin sensitivity	Liver	May cause mild weight loss Does not cause hypoglycemia (insulin levels do not increase)	GI upset (diarrhea, nausea, abdominal pain), lactic acidosis, metallic taste
Acarbose	Reduces glucose absorption from the gut, thereby reducing calorie intake	GI tract	Low risk (does not have significant toxicity)	GI upset (diarrhea, abdominal cramping, flatulence)
Thiazolidinediones (e.g., rosiglitazone, pioglitazone)	Reduce insulin resistance	Fat, muscle	Reduce insulin levels	Hepatotoxicity (monitor LFTs)

Note: Most oral hypoglycemic drugs are contraindicated in pregnancy (potentially teratogenic). Treat with insulin.

[a]Serum creatinine ≥1.5 (≥1.4 in women) is a contraindication to metformin.

Quick HIT

Insulin Versus Oral Hypoglycemic Agents in Type II Diabetes

- If the patient has severe hyperglycemia (fasting glucose >240 mg/dL), insulin typically is the agent of choice (whether type I or type II disease).
- Oral hypoglycemic agents are effective in type II disease with moderate hyperglycemia (fasting glucose between 140 and 240 mg/dL).

D. Treatment

1. Diet and exercise should ideally be the only interventions in most type II diabetic patients.
   a. Diet and exercise are especially effective in obese and sedentary patients (who constitute the majority of type II diabetic patients).
   b. Most patients, however, do not lose enough weight to control glucose levels through diet and exercise alone, and will require pharmacologic treatment.
   c. Glycemic control minimizes risks for nephropathy, neuropathy, and retinopathy in both Type 1 and 2 DM, and decreases risk for cardiovascular disease for Type 1 DM.
2. Oral hypoglycemic drugs (see Table 4-6; Figures 4-9 and 4-10)
   a. Use these in type II diabetic patients when conservative therapy (diet and exercise) fails.

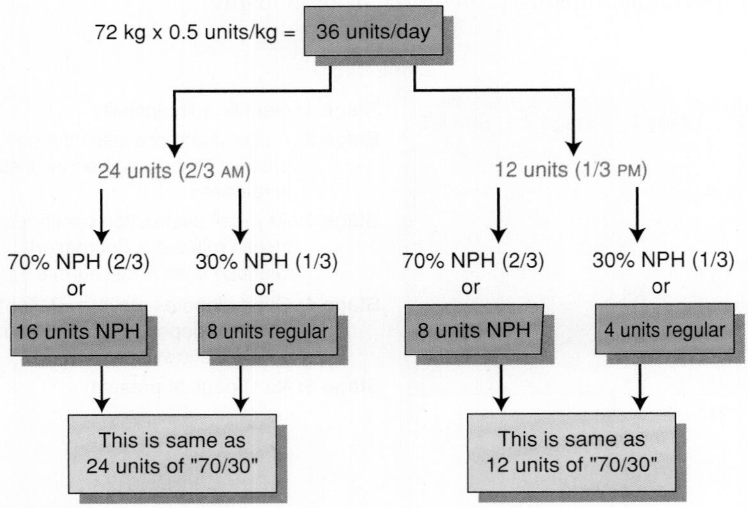

FIGURE 4-9 A typical two-third to one-third insulin dosing regimen in a 72 kg patient.

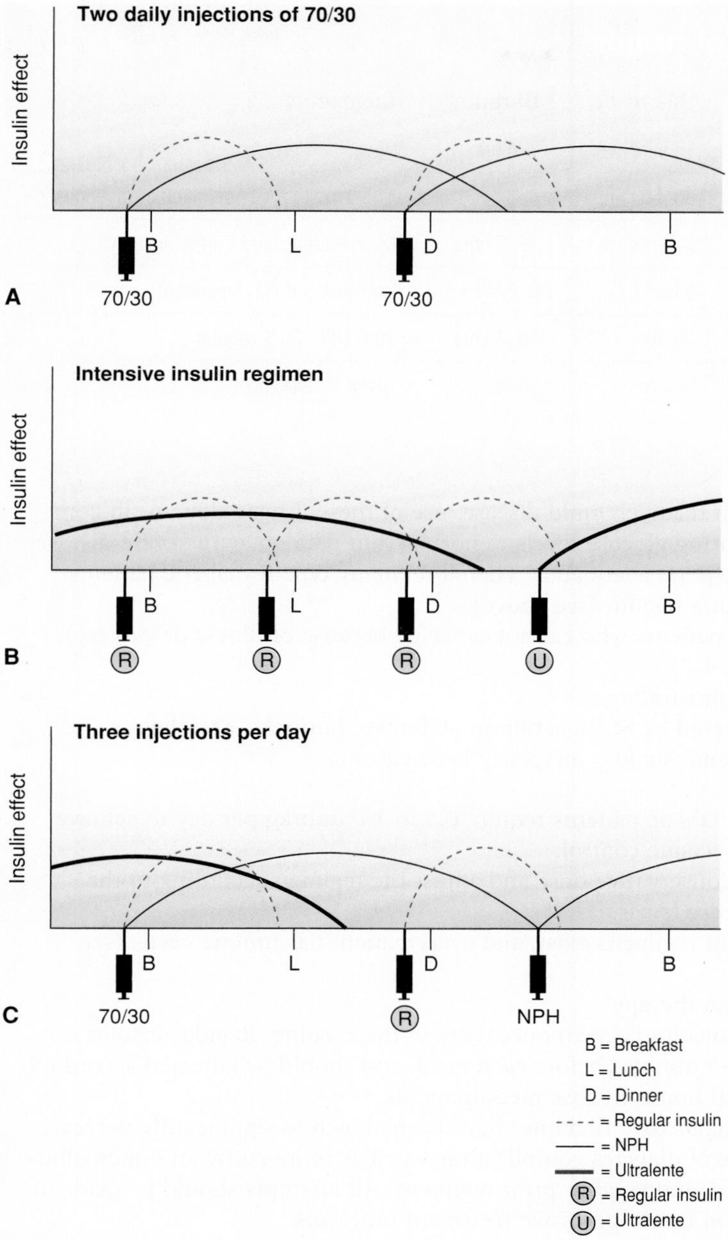

FIGURE 4-10 **Graphic depiction of three different insulin dosing regimens, illustrating time of injection (30 minutes before each meal) and insulin effect. Note that many different regimens exist and each patient has unique needs.**

b. Start with one agent (metformin is best initial drug therapy). If monotherapy fails, use two agents from different classes in combination. Each agent has advantages and disadvantages, so clinical judgment is required in selecting the initial agent.

c. Metformin blocks gluconeogenesis. It is contraindicated in patients with renal failure.

d. Other oral hypoglycemics include:
- Sulfonylureas
- Thiazolidinediones (glitazones)
- Alpha glucosidase inhibitors (acarbose, miglitol)
- Incretins
- Pramlintide
- Repaglinide/nateglinide

Quick HIT

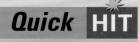

Treatment of Diabetes
- Type I diabetic patients require insulin to live.
- Type II diabetic patients require exercise and diet (initial steps) as well as oral hypoglycemic drugs. The current emphasis is to treat aggressively and move quickly to insulin if needed to optimize hga_{1c}.

TABLE 4-7 Types of Insulin

Type	Onset	Duration	Comments
Human insulin lispro	15 min	2–4 hrs	
Regular insulin	30–60 min	4–6 hrs	Only type that can be given intravenously
NPH insulin/lente insulin	2–4 hrs	18–28 hrs	Most widely used form of insulin
Insulin Detemir	2 hrs	6–24 hrs	Duration is dose-dependent
70/30 mixture	30 min	10–16 hrs	70% NPH, 30% regular
Glargine (lantus)	3–4 hrs	24 hrs	Given at bedtime

e. In patients with relatively mild disease, use of these drugs (alone or in combination) can bring glucose levels to normal, but patients with severe disease often do not respond adequately. Therefore, many type II diabetic patients eventually require insulin (see above).

f. Do not give to patients who cannot eat (e.g., because of illness or surgery).

3. Insulin (see Table 4-7).
   a. Method of administration.
      - Self-administered by SC injection in abdomen, buttocks, arm, leg.
      - Given intravenously for emergency ketoacidosis.
   b. Regimens
      - Most type I diabetic patients require 0.5 to 1.0 unit/kg per day to achieve acceptable glycemic control.
      - Start with a conservative dose and adjust the regimen according to the patient's glucose levels.
      - Many different regimens exist, and every patient has unique needs (see Table 4-7).
   c. Intensive insulin therapy
      - Long-acting insulin is given once daily in the evening. Regular insulin is given 30 to 45 minutes before each meal, and should be adjusted according to preprandial home glucose measurements.
      - These more aggressive therapies have been shown to significantly decrease the incidence of diabetes complications such as retinopathy and microalbuminuria when compared to prior regimens. All attempts should be made to get patients on more aggressive treatment protocols.
      - With intensive insulin therapy, the risk for hypoglycemia is a serious concern.
      - Alternatively, a continuous SC infusion of insulin can be given via an insulin pump. Preprandial boluses are given in addition to the basal infusion.
   d. If the patient is unable/unwilling to carry out an intensive insulin program:
      - Give 70/30 units before breakfast and before the evening meal for basal coverage.
      - Give a short-acting insulin (regular) for prandial control if necessary.
      - Adjust doses according to fasting and 4 pm glucose determinations.
   e. Inpatient management of diabetic patients (sliding scale).
      - An insulin sliding scale (SSI) of regular insulin doses given according to bedside finger-stick glucose determinations is helpful in controlling blood glucose levels in the hospital setting.
      - In general, SSI should be used in addition to a regimen of intermediate-acting insulin. If given alone, hyperglycemia usually results.
      - Monitor blood glucose four times per day: before meals and at bedtime.
      - If the home insulin dose is unclear, or if the patient anticipates greater requirements of insulin due to an illness, use the following approach to adjust appropriate insulin doses:

CLINICAL PEARL 4-11

Monitoring Glucose Levels in DM

- HbA_{1c} gives an estimate of the degree of glucose control over 2 to 3 months.
- The American Diabetes Association recommends a treatment goal of HbA_{1c} <7.0%. In general, HbA_{1c} >10% is poor control, 8.5% to 10% is fair control, 7.0% to 8.5% is good control, and <7.0% is ideal.
- The American Diabetes Association recommends keeping fasting blood glucose level <130 mg/dL and peak postprandial blood glucose <180 mg/dL.

- Take the total number of units of regular insulin that the patient required in 1 day (while on the sliding scale).
- Add two-thirds of this to the prebreakfast dose and one-third before dinner. It should be given as 70/30 (i.e., 70% NPH/30% regular).

f. Modifying insulin doses (see also Clinical Pearl 4-11)
- Physical activity—depending on the intensity of the activity, decrease insulin dosage 1 to 2 units per 20 to 30 minutes of activity.
- During illness, administer all of the routine insulin. **Many episodes of DKA occur during episodes of illness.**
- Stress and changes in diet require dosing adjustments.
- Patients undergoing surgery should get one-third to one-half of the usual daily insulin requirement that day, with frequent monitoring and adjustments as necessary.

4. Surgical treatment—Surgical weight loss therapy (i.e., gastric bypass) is an effective treatment for some patients, including adolescents. Additionally, islet cell transplantation offers definitive treatment for selected qualified patients.

Chronic Complications of Diabetes Mellitus

A. Macrovascular complications

1. The main problem is accelerated atherosclerosis, which puts patients at increased risk of stroke, MI, and CHF (Figure 4-11). The accelerated atherosclerosis in diabetics is the reason the target BP is lower in diabetics (130/80) than in general population (140/90), and the reason the target LDL is lower in diabetics is less than 100 mg/dL. The cause of accelerated atherosclerosis is not known, although glycation of lipoproteins and increased platelet adhesiveness/aggregation are thought to be two potential causes. In addition, the process of fibrinolysis may be impaired in diabetic patients.
2. The manifestations of atherosclerosis include the following:
   a. Coronary artery disease (CAD).
   - Risk of CAD is two to four times greater in diabetic than in nondiabetic persons.
   - **Most common cause of death in diabetic patients.**
   - Silent myocardial infarctions are common.

   b. Peripheral vascular disease—in up to 60% of diabetic patients.
   c. Cerebrovascular disease (strokes).

Quick HIT

The risk of coronary events is greatly reduced if the patient can eliminate or reduce other major cardiovascular risk factors (smoking, HTN, hyperlipidemia, obesity).

Quick HIT

Definition of Microalbuminuria
- 30 to 300 mg/day
- Albumin–creatinine ratio of 0.02 to 0.20

B. Microvascular complications—risk can be markedly reduced by achieving tight glucose control (see also Clinical Pearl 4-12)

1. **Diabetic nephropathy**—most important cause of end-stage renal disease (ESRD)
   a. Pathologic types
   - Nodular glomerular sclerosis (Kimmelstiel–Wilson syndrome)—hyaline deposition in **one** area of glomerulus—pathognomonic for DM
   - Diffuse glomerular sclerosis—hyaline deposition is global—also occurs in HTN
   - Isolated glomerular basement membrane thickening

   b. Microalbuminuria/proteinuria
   - If microalbuminuria is present, strict glycemic control is critical (has been shown to limit progression from microalbuminuria to clinical proteinuria).

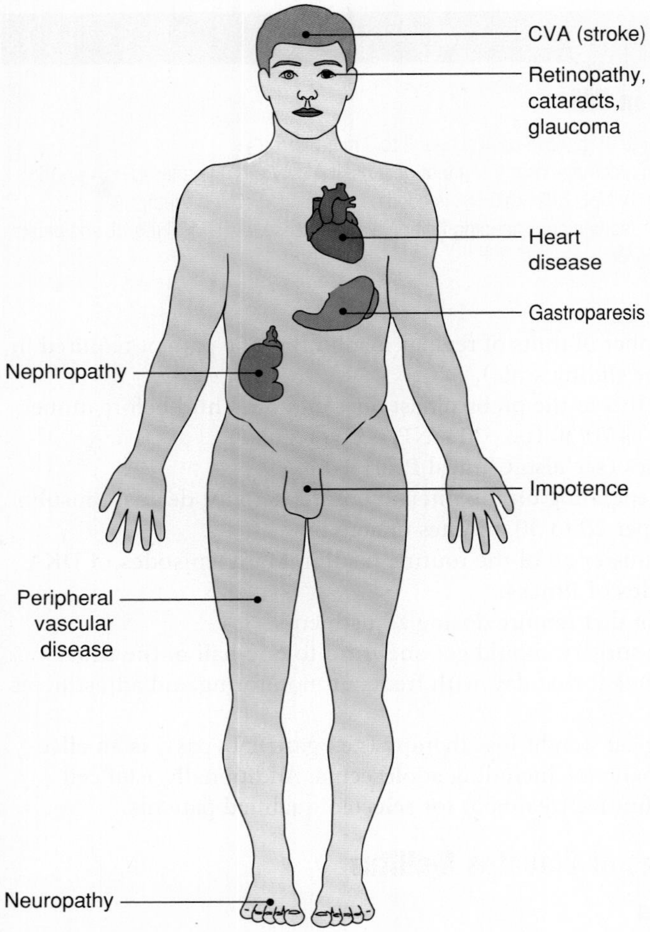

FIGURE 4-11 **Chronic complications of diabetes mellitus.**

- Without effective treatment, the albuminuria gradually worsens—HTN usually develops during the transition between microalbuminuria and progressive proteinuria. Persistent HTN and proteinuria cause a decrease in glomerular filtration rate (GFR), leading to renal insufficiency and eventually ESRD.
- **HTN increases the risk of progression of diabetic nephropathy to ESRD. Control BP aggressively.**
- **Initiate ACE inhibitors or ARB immediately. These agents are proven to decrease the rate of progression of nephropathy.**
- **Microalbuminuria is the screening test!** If you wait for the dipstick to be positive for protein, you have waited too long. Remember that microalbuminuria means levels of albumin are between 30 and 300 mg per 24 hours. But the dipstick for urine becomes trace positive at 300 mg of protein per 24 hours.

CLINICAL PEARL 4-12

Radiocontrast Agents in Diabetic Patients

- Patients with diabetes are particularly susceptible to developing radiocontrast-induced acute renal failure.
- If IV contrast is necessary, give generous hydration before administering the contrast agent to avoid precipitating acute renal failure.
- Hold metformin for 48 hours after radiocontrast is given to prevent renal damage, and make sure renal function has returned to baseline before resuming it.

- It usually takes 1 to 5 years for microalbuminuria to advance to full-blown proteinuria. However, with proper treatment (i.e., using ACE inhibitors to control BP) this can be prolonged.

c. Once diabetic nephropathy has progressed to the stage of proteinuria or early renal failure, glycemic control does not significantly influence its course. ACE inhibitors and dietary restriction of protein are recommended.

2. **Diabetic retinopathy**
   a. Prevalence is approximately 75% after 20 years of diabetes. **Annual screening of all diabetic patients by an ophthalmologist is recommended.**
   b. Background (nonproliferative) retinopathy accounts for the majority of cases.
      - Funduscopic examination shows hemorrhages, exudates, microaneurysms, and venous dilatation.
      - These patients are usually asymptomatic unless retinal edema or ischemia involves the central macula.
      - Edema of the macula is the leading cause of visual loss in diabetic patients.
      - HTN and fluid retention exacerbate this condition.
   c. Proliferative retinopathy
      - Key characteristics are new vessel formation (neovascularization) and scarring.
      - Two serious complications are vitreal hemorrhage and retinal detachment.
      - **Can lead to blindness. Laser photocoagulation is the treatment.**

> **Quick HIT**
> - Ocular problems in diabetic patients include cataracts, retinopathy, and glaucoma.
> - Diabetic retinopathy is the leading cause of blindness in the United States.

3. **Diabetic neuropathy** (Figure 4-12)
   a. Peripheral neuropathy (distal symmetric neuropathy)
      - Usually affects sensory nerves in a "stocking/glove pattern"—Usually begins in feet, later involves hands (longest nerves affected first). Numbness and paresthesias are common.
      - Loss of sensation leads to the following: ulcer formation (patients do not shift their weight) with subsequent ischemia of pressure point areas; *Charcot joints*.
      - Painful diabetic neuropathy—hypersensitivity to light touch; severe "burning" pain (especially at night) that can be difficult to tolerate. Treatment is with gabapentin, tricyclic antidepressants, or pregabalin.
   b. CN complications—secondary to nerve infarction.
      - Most often involves CN III, but may also involve CN VI and IV.
      - Diabetic third nerve palsy: eye pain, diplopia, ptosis, inability to adduct the eye; **pupils are spared.**
   c. Mononeuropathies—secondary to nerve infarction.
      - Median nerve neuropathy, ulnar neuropathy, common peroneal neuropathy.
      - Diabetic lumbosacral plexopathy—severe, deep pain in the thigh; atrophy and weakness in thigh and hip muscles; recovery takes weeks to months.
      - Diabetic truncal neuropathy—pain in distribution of one of the intercostal nerves.
   d. Autonomic neuropathy
      - Impotence in men (most common presentation)
      - Neurogenic bladder—retention, incontinence
      - Gastroparesis—chronic nausea and vomiting, early satiety
      - Constipation and diarrhea (alternating)
      - Postural hypotension

> **Quick HIT**
> The Diabetes Control and Complications Trial showed that tight glucose control reduces the risk of microvascular disease by 50% to 60%. However, whether it can reduce the risk of macrovascular disease remains to be proven. It is the macrovascular complications that cause death in the majority of type II diabetic patients.

4. **Diabetic foot**
   a. Caused by a combination of artery disease (ischemia) and nerve disease (neuropathy)—can lead to ulcers/infections and may require amputation.

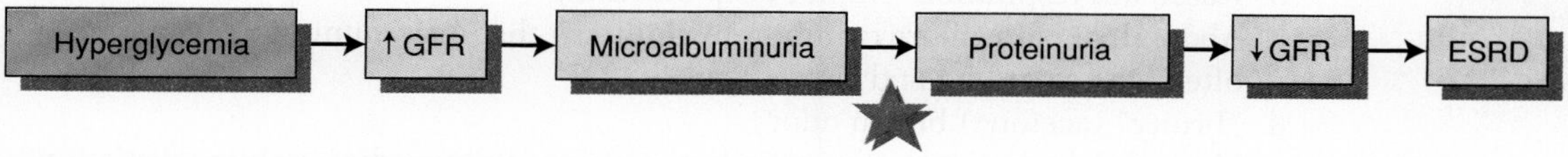

FIGURE 4-12 **Progression in diabetic nephropathy. Strict glycemic control has been shown to slow or prevent progression from microalbuminuria to proteinuria. This is the critical stage (marked by *star*)—once proteinuria develops, glycemic control does little to control the course and will eventually lead to ESRD.**

b. With neuropathy, the patient does not feel pain, so repetitive injuries go unnoticed and ultimately lead to nonhealing.
c. In addition, neuropathy may mask symptoms of PVD (claudication/rest pain). Also, calcific medial arterial disease is common and can cause erroneously high BP readings in lower extremities.

5. Increased susceptibility to infection
   a. This results from impaired WBC function, reduced blood supply, and neuropathy. Wound healing is impaired in diabetic patients, and this can be problematic postoperatively.
   b. Diabetic patients are at increased risk for the following infections: cellulitis, candidiasis, pneumonia, osteomyelitis, and polymicrobial foot ulcers.
   c. Infections of ischemic foot ulcers may lead to osteomyelitis and may require amputation.

C. Specific treatment of chronic diabetic complications

1. Macrovascular disease—treatment involves reduction of risk factors (e.g., BP reduction, lipid-lowering agents, smoking cessation, exercise), a daily aspirin (if not contraindicated), and strict glycemic control.
2. Nephropathy—ACE inhibitors, benefits of which include:
   a. Slow progression of microalbuminuria to proteinuria.
   b. Slow decline of GFR.
3. Retinopathy—Treatment involves referral to an ophthalmologist and possible photocoagulation.
4. Neuropathy—Treatment is complex. Pharmacologic agents that may be helpful include NSAIDs, tricyclic antidepressants, and gabapentin. For gastroparesis, a promotility agent such as metoclopramide can be helpful, in addition to exercise and a low-fat diet.
5. Diabetic foot—The best treatment is prevention: regular foot care, **regular podiatrist visits.** Amputation is a last resort.

Acute Complications of Diabetes Mellitus

A. Diabetic ketoacidosis

1. **General characteristics**
   a. DKA is an acute, life-threatening medical emergency that can occur in both type I and type II diabetic patients (more common in type I).
   b. Pathogenesis
      - This is secondary to insulin deficiency and glucagons excess, both of which contribute to accelerated severe hyperglycemia and accelerated ketogenesis.
      - Severe hyperglycemia leads to an osmotic diuresis, which causes dehydration and volume depletion.

   c. Consequences of DKA include hyperglycemia, ketonemia, metabolic acidosis, and volume depletion.
2. **Precipitating factors**
   a. Any type of stress or illness (e.g., infectious process, trauma, myocardial infarction, stroke, recent surgery, sepsis, GI bleeding)
   b. Inadequate administration of insulin
3. **Clinical features**
   a. Nausea and vomiting
   b. Kussmaul respiration—rapid, deep breathing
   c. Abdominal pain (more common in children) that may mimic acute abdomen–often with guarding and rigidity
   d. "Fruity" (acetone) breath odor
   e. Marked dehydration, orthostatic hypotension, tachycardia—volume depletion is always present
   f. Polydipsia, polyuria, polyphagia, weakness
   g. Altered consciousness, drowsiness, and frank coma may occur if not treated
   h. Symptoms usually occur rapidly, typically in less than 24 hours

Quick HIT

Key Features of DKA
- Hyperglycemia
- Positive serum or urine ketones
- Metabolic acidosis

Quick HIT

Differential Diagnosis of DKA
- Alcoholic ketoacidosis
- Hyperosmolar hyperglycemic nonketotic syndrome (HHNS)
- Hypoglycemia (altered mental status, abdominal pain, and acidosis are possible)
- Sepsis
- Intoxication (e.g., methanol, ethanol, salicylates, isopropyl alcohol, paraldehyde, ethylene glycol)

4. **Diagnosis**
   a. Hyperglycemia: serum glucose typically >450 mg/dL and <850 mg/dL (in certain conditions, e.g., alcohol ingestion, the patient may be euglycemic)
   b. Metabolic acidosis
      - Blood pH <7.3 and serum HCO_3^- <15 mEq/L
      - Increased anion gap—due to production of ketones (acetoacetate and β-hydroxybutyrate)
   c. Ketonemia (serum positive for ketones) and ketonuria
      - Serum levels of acetoacetate, acetone, and β-hydroxybutyrate are greatly increased.
      - When DKA is accompanied by circulatory collapse, serum and urine may be **falsely negative** for ketones. This is because lactate production results in less acetoacetate and more β-hydroxybutyrate production, and acetoacetate is the only ketoacid that can be measured by nitroprusside agents.
   d. Ketonemia and acidosis are required for the diagnosis of DKA.
5. **Other laboratory value abnormalities**
   a. Hyperosmolarity
   b. Hyponatremia—Serum sodium decreases 1.6 mEq/L for every 100 mg/dL increase in glucose level because of the osmotic shift of fluid from the ICF to the ECF space. Total body sodium level is normal. This generally does not require treatment
   c. Other electrolyte disturbances
      - Potassium—Because of the acidosis, hyperkalemia may be present initially, although total body potassium is low. As insulin is given, it causes a shift of potassium into cells, resulting in a hypokalemia, and this can happen very rapidly.
      - Phosphate and magnesium levels may also be low.
6. **Treatment**
   a. Insulin
      - Give insulin immediately after the diagnosis is established.
      - Give a priming dose of 0.1 units/kg of regular insulin (IV) followed by an infusion of 0.1 units/kg per hour. This is sufficient to replace the insulin deficit in most patients. **Be certain that the patient is not hypokalemic before giving insulin.**
      - Continue the insulin until the anion gap closes and metabolic acidosis is corrected, then begin to decrease the insulin. Give SC insulin when the patient starts eating again.
   b. Fluid replacement (normal saline)
      - Give fluids immediately after the diagnosis is established.
      - Add 5% glucose once the blood glucose reaches **250 mg/dL** to prevent hypoglycemia.
   c. Replace potassium prophylactically with IV fluids.
      - Initiate within 1 to 2 hours of starting insulin.
      - Ensure adequate renal function (urine output) before administering these.
      - Monitor potassium, magnesium, and phosphate levels **very closely** and replace as necessary.
   d. HCO_3^- replacement is controversial and is not necessary in most cases.

Quick HIT

If a patient presents with DKA:
- Take a history and perform a physical examination.
- Order laboratory tests: blood glucose, arterial blood gas, CBC, electrolytes, BUN, creatinine, and urinary analysis.
- Order ECG, CXR, and cultures.
- Initiate IV fluids.
- Give insulin and start potassium soon thereafter.
- Admit to the ICU or a very closely monitored floor bed.

Quick HIT

Treatment of DKA: **insulin, fluids, potassium.**

Quick HIT

Complications of Treatment of DKA
- Cerebral edema—if glucose levels decrease too rapidly
- Hyperchloremic nongap metabolic acidosis—due to rapid infusion of a large amount of saline

B. Hyperosmolar hyperglycemic nonketotic syndrome

1. **General characteristics** (see also Table 4-8)
   a. A state of severe hyperglycemia, hyperosmolarity, and dehydration is typically seen in elderly type II diabetic patients.
   b. Pathogenesis
      - Low insulin levels lead to hyperglycemia. Severe hyperglycemia causes an osmotic diuresis, leading to dehydration.
      - Ketogenesis is minimal because a small amount of insulin is released to blunt counterregulatory hormone release (glucagons).
      - Ketosis and acidosis are typically absent or minimal.

Quick HIT

A number of names have been used for this clinical entity, including HHNS, hyperosmolar nonketotic coma (HHNC), and hyperosmolar nonacidotic diabetes.

TABLE 4-8 **Diabetic Ketoacidosis Versus Hyperosmolar Hyperglycemic Nonketotic Syndrome**

	DKA	HHNS
Pathophysiology	Insulin deficiency → ketosis, acidosis, dehydration	Insulin deficiency → hyperosmolarity, osmotic diuresis, profound dehydration
Laboratory Findings	• Hyperglycemia (>450) • Metabolic acidosis (anion gap)—serum pH <7.3 • Ketosis	• Hyperglycemia (>900 mg/dL) • Hyperosmolarity (>320 mOsm/L) • Serum pH >7.3 (no acidosis)
Treatment	Insulin, IV fluids, potassium	Aggressive IV fluids, low-dose insulin infusion
Mortality Rate	5%–10%	10%–20%

Quick HIT

HHNS has a higher mortality rate than DKA, but it is less common than DKA. This may be because many HHNS patients are elderly with other comorbid conditions (e.g., heart, renal, or pulmonary disease).

Quick HIT

Key Features of HHNS
- Severe hyperosmolarity (>320 mOsm/L)
- Hyperglycemia (>600 mg/dL)
- Dehydration
- Acidosis and ketosis are absent (unlike in DKA)

- Severe dehydration is due to continued hyperglycemic (osmotic) diuresis. The patient's inability to drink enough fluids (either due to lack of access in elderly/bedridden patients or to inadequate thirst drive) to keep up with urinary fluid losses exacerbates the condition.

c. Precipitating events are similar to those of DKA.

2. **Clinical features**
   a. Thirst, polyuria
   b. Signs of extreme dehydration and volume depletion—hypotension, tachycardia
   c. **CNS findings and focal neurologic signs are common** (e.g., seizures)—secondary to hyperosmolarity.
   d. Lethargy and confusion may develop, leading to convulsions and coma.
3. **Diagnosis**
   a. Hyperglycemia: serum glucose typically **higher than DKA** and frequently **>900 mg/dL.**
   b. Hyperosmolarity: serum osmolarity >320 mOsm/L.
   c. Serum pH >7.3 (no acidosis); serum HCO_3^- > 15.
   d. BUN is usually elevated. Prerenal azotemia is common.
4. **Treatment**
   a. **Fluid replacement** is most important (normal saline): 1 L in the first hour, another liter in the next 2 hours. Most patients respond well. Switch to half normal saline once the patient stabilizes.
      - Glucose levels are lowered as the patient is rehydrated (but the patient still requires insulin).
      - When glucose levels reach 250 mg/dL, add 5% glucose ($D_5$1/2NS) as in DKA.
      - Very rapid lowering of blood glucose can lead to cerebral edema in children (just as in DKA).
      - In patients with cardiac disease or renal insufficiency, avoid volume overload (can lead to CHF), but generous fluids are still needed.

   b. Insulin: An initial bolus of 5 to 10 units intravenously, followed by a continuous low-dose infusion (2 to 4 units/hr) is usually appropriate.

Obesity

A. General characteristics

1. **BMI ≥30 kg/m²**
2. About one-third of US population is obese (increasing prevalence in adults, adolescents, and children)
3. Obesity is associated with an increased risk of hypertension, dyslipidemia, diabetes mellitus, cardiovascular disease, and osteoarthritis.

B. Causes

1. Result of chronic mismatches in energy balance (energy intake > energy expenditure)
2. Energy balance determined by several variables, including **metabolic rate, appetite, diet, and physical activity.**
3. These factors that determine energy balance are influenced by **both** genetic traits and environmental behaviors (excessive food intake, decreased physical activity.)
4. Drug-induced (less common)—glucocorticoids, antipsychotics, antidepressants, oral hypoglycemics, and antiepileptics
5. Neuroendocrine disorders such as Cushing syndrome and polycystic ovarian syndrome (PCOS)

C. Diagnosis

1. All adults should be screened by measuring height, weight, and calculating body mass index (BMI)
2. BMI = body weight (kg)/height^2 (meters)
3. Overweight and obese patient should be further screened with waist circumference to assess **abdominal obesity.**
4. Waist circumference of ≥40 in in men and ≥35 in in women is considered elevated and corresponds with an increased **cardiometabolic risk.**
5. Patients with abdominal obesity are at increased risk for heart disease, diabetes, hypertension, dyslipidemia, and nonalcoholic fatty liver disease.

D. Treatment

1. The main treatment for obesity is **dieting** and **physical exercise.**
2. Medications if dieting and physical exercise fail. **Orlistat** (pancreatic lipase inhibitor), **lorcaserin** (selective 5-HT_{2C} receptor agonist), and combination **phentermine and topiramate** (exact mechanism of action unknown), have shown some benefit.
3. **Bariatric surgery** remains the most effective treatment for obesity. It has been ... -term weight loss, improvement in obesity-related complica- ... mortality.
   ... ould **only** be attempted in patients with a BMI of 40 kg/m^2 or ... iled a sufficient exercise and diet regimen (regardless of use ... on) **and** who present with obesity-related comorbid conditions ... ion, diabetes mellitus, and hyperlipidemia).

A. ... cs

1. **The primary organ at risk in hypoglycemia is the brain**—The brain uses glucose as its main energy source (except when using ketone bodies during fasting) (see also Clinical Pearl 4-13).
2. Unlike other tissues, the brain cannot use free fatty acids as an energy source.
3. Hypoglycemia is really due to an imbalance between glucagon and insulin.
4. If there is no correlation between the symptoms and low glucose levels (e.g., patient has symptoms when glucose levels are normal), an underlying disorder of glucose metabolism is unlikely (i.e., the patient does not have true hypoglycemia).

Quick HIT

BMI Classification:
- Underweight—BMI <18.5 kg/m^2
- Normal weight—BMI ≥18.5 kg/m^2 and <25 kg/m^2
- Overweight—BMI ≥25 kg/m^2 and <30 kg/m^2
- Obese—BMI ≥30 kg/m^2
- Severe obesity—BMI ≥40 kg/m^2

CLINICAL PEARL 4-13

Physiologic Responses to Hypoglycemia

- When glucose levels approach the low 80s, insulin levels decrease—This decrease is normally enough to prevent hypoglycemia.
- As glucose levels decrease further, glucagon levels increase (glucagon is the first line of defense against more severe hypoglycemia).
- Epinephrine is the next hormone to combat hypoglycemia. Cortisol and other catecholamines also play a role.
- As glucose levels decrease into the 50s and below, symptoms begin.

Quick HIT

If a patient presents with hypoglycemia of unknown cause, measure:
- Plasma insulin level
- C-peptide
- Anti-insulin antibodies
- Plasma and urine sulfonylurea levels

Quick HIT

Hypoglycemic Unawareness
- In diabetic patients, if severe neuropathy is present, the autonomic response (epinephrine) to hypoglycemia is not activated. This leads to neuroglycopenic symptoms.
- It is common for diabetic patients to become hypoglycemic with conventional therapy (insulin or oral hypoglycemics). With longstanding disease in which they lose their neurogenic symptom response to hypoglycemia, patients do not recognize the impending hypoglycemia and may even have a seizure or enter a coma.

B. Causes

1. Drug-induced—taking too much insulin is a common problem in diabetic patients attempting tight control of their disease.
2. Factitious hypoglycemia
   a. If the patient took insulin surreptitiously, there will be a high blood insulin level and a low blood C-peptide level (because exogenous insulin does not contain C-peptide).
   b. Patients taking exogenous insulin will also develop anti-insulin antibodies, which can be measured.
   c. If the patient took sulfonylurea, check urine or serum for levels of this drug.
3. Insulinoma
4. Ethanol ingestion—due to:
   a. Poor nutrition that leads to decreased glycogen (and loss of glycogenolysis)
   b. Metabolism of alcohol that lowers nicotinamide adenine dinucleotide levels and decreases gluconeogenesis
5. Postoperative complications after gastric surgery (due to rapid gastric emptying)
6. Reactive (idiopathic) hypoglycemia—symptoms occur 2 to 4 hours after a meal; rarely indicates a serious underlying disorder
7. Adrenal insufficiency
8. Liver failure
9. Critical illness
10. Disorders of carbohydrate metabolism (e.g., glycogen storage diseases)—usually diagnosed at a much younger age

C. Clinical features

1. Symptoms occur at a blood glucose level of 40 to 50 mg/dL.
2. Elevated epinephrine levels cause sweating, tremors, increased BP and pulse, anxiety, and palpitations.
3. Neuroglycopenic symptoms—decreased glucose for the brain (CNS dysfunction), resulting in irritability, behavioral changes, weakness, drowsiness, headache, confusion, convulsions, coma, and even death.

D. Diagnosis

1. Blood glucose level—Symptoms generally begin when levels drop below 50. However, there is no cutoff value to define hypoglycemia.
2. **Whipple triad** is used to diagnose true hypoglycemia (i.e., hypoglycemia due to underlying disease). (See the **Insulinoma section**).
3. Laboratory tests—for measurement of serum insulin, C-peptide, and glucose when symptoms occur (an overnight fast may be sufficient to produce symptoms).
4. 72-hour fast (24 hours is usually sufficient)—used to diagnose insulinoma (if suspected).

E. Treatment

1. Acute treatment of hypoglycemia.
   a. If the patient can eat, give sugar-containing foods; if not, give 1/2 to 2 ampules of D50W intravenously.
   b. Repeat administration of D50W as necessary, but switch to D10W as clinical condition improves and glucose level is approximately >100 mg/dL.
2. Appropriate management of underlying cause (e.g., diabetes, insulinoma)
3. If reactive hypoglycemia is suspected, dietary interventions are appropriate.
4. If the patient is an alcoholic (or suspected alcoholic), give thiamine before administering glucose to avoid Wernicke encephalopathy.

●●● Insulinoma

A. General characteristics

1. Insulin-producing tumor arising from the β-cells of the pancreas
2. Associated with MEN I syndrome
3. Usually benign (in up to 90% of the cases)

TABLE 4-9 Laboratory Values in Hyperinsulinemic Hypoglycemia

Diagnosis	Laboratory Value			
	Insulin Level	Glucose Level	C-peptide Level	Proinsulin Level
Insulinoma	↑	↓	↑	↑
Surreptitious insulin	↑↑	↓	↓	↓
Sulfonylurea abuse	↑	↓	↑	Normal

B. Clinical features: Hypoglycemia, which leads to:

1. Sympathetic activation—diaphoresis, palpitations, tremors, high blood pressure, anxiety
2. Neuroglycopenic symptoms—headache, visual disturbances, confusion, seizures, coma

C. Diagnosis

1. 72-hour fast (see also Table 4-9).
   a. The patient becomes hypoglycemic. Normally, the insulin level should decrease as hypoglycemia develops.
   b. In persons with insulinoma, insulin does not respond appropriately to hypoglycemia. It may decrease or increase, or it may not change. Nevertheless, the insulin levels are still higher than they would be in a normal individual for any given glucose concentration.
2. Whipple triad.
   a. Hypoglycemic symptoms brought on by fasting.
   b. Blood glucose <50 mg/dL during symptomatic attack.
   c. Glucose administration brings relief of symptoms.
3. Elevated fasting serum insulin level. C-peptide levels should also be elevated, which distinguishes insulinoma from exogenous insulin administration.

D. Treatment: Surgical resection of tumor (up to 80% to 90% cure rate)

Zollinger–Ellison Syndrome (Gastrinoma)

- A pancreatic islet cell tumor that secretes high gastrin, which leads to profound gastric acid hypersecretion, resulting in ulcers.
- Up to 60% are malignant; 20% associated with MEN I (80% are sporadic); 90% located in the "gastrinoma triangle" (formed by the following points: cystic duct superiorly, junction of second and third portions of the duodenum inferiorly, and neck of pancreas medially).
- Possible complications: GI hemorrhage, GI perforation, gastric outlet obstruction/stricture, and metastatic disease (liver is the most common site).
- Clinical features: peptic ulcers, diarrhea, weight loss, abdominal pain.
- Secretin injection test is diagnostic test of choice. Normally, secretin inhibits gastrin secretion. In patients with Zollinger–Ellison Syndrome (ZES), gastrin levels increase substantially after being given secretin.
- Fasting gastrin level is elevated in patients with ZES.
- Normal basal acid output is <10 mEq/hr; in patients with ZES, it is >15 mEq/hr.
- Treatment consists of high-dose proton pump inhibitors.
- All patients with ZES should undergo exploration to attempt curative resection (20% of patients are cured with complete resection). If there is widely metastatic or incurable gastrinoma, debulking surgery and chemotherapy are indicated.

Glucagonoma

- A glucagon-producing tumor located in the pancreas.

- Clinical manifestations include **necrotizing migratory erythema** (usually below the waist), glossitis, stomatitis, DM (mild), and hyperglycemia (with low amino acid levels and high glucagon levels).
- Treatment is surgical resection.

••• Somatostatinoma

- A rare, malignant pancreatic tumor (metastases usually present by diagnosis)
- Poor prognosis
- Classic triad of gallstones, diabetes, and steatorrhea

••• VIPoma (Verner-Morrison or Watery Diarrhea, Hypokalemia, Achlorhydria Syndrome)

- A rare pancreatic tumor (>50% are malignant).
- Clinical features include watery diarrhea (leading to dehydration, hypokalemia, acidosis), achlorhydria (VIP inhibits gastric acid secretion), hyperglycemia, and hypercalcemia.
- Treatment is surgical resection.

DISEASES OF THE CENTRAL AND PERIPHERAL NERVOUS SYSTEMS 5

Cerebrovascular Disease (Stroke)

Ischemic Stroke (Cerebral Infarction)

A. General characteristics

1. Epidemiology
   a. Stroke, or cerebrovascular accident (CVA), is the third most common cause of death in the United States.
   b. It is the **leading cause of neurologic disability.**
2. Classes of ischemic stroke
   a. Transient ischemic attack (TIA)—see below
   b. **Reversible ischemic neurologic deficit** is the same as TIA except for the duration of symptoms. It lasts longer than 24 hours, but resolves in less than 2 weeks. This term is not commonly used.
   c. **Evolving stroke** is a stroke that is worsening.
   d. **Completed stroke** is one in which the maximal deficit has occurred.
3. TIAs (see Clinical Pearl 5-1)
   a. A TIA is a neurologic deficit that lasts from a few minutes to no more than 24 hours (but usually lasts less than 30 minutes).
      - Stroke may be indistinguishable from a TIA at the time of presentation: **Duration of symptoms** is the determining difference.
      - Symptoms are transient with a TIA because reperfusion occurs, either because of collateral circulation or because of the breaking up of an embolus.
   b. **The blockage in blood flow does not last long enough to cause permanent infarction.**
   c. A TIA is usually embolic. However, transient hypotension in the presence of severe carotid stenosis (>75% occlusion) can lead to a TIA.
   d. **Once a patient has a TIA, there is a high risk of stroke in subsequent months.** The risk of a stroke in a patient with a history of TIA is about 10% per year. TIAs carry a **30% 5-year risk of stroke.** Therefore, cardiac risk factors should be closely investigated and, if possible, eliminated in a patient who has had a TIA.
4. Risk factors
   a. The most important risk factors are **age** and **HTN.** Others include smoking, DM, hyperlipidemia, atrial fibrillation, coronary artery disease (CAD), family history of stroke, previous stroke/TIA, and carotid bruits.
   b. In younger patients, risk factors include oral contraceptive use, hypercoagulable states (e.g., protein C and S deficiencies, antiphospholipid antibody syndrome), vasoconstrictive drug use (e.g., cocaine, amphetamines), polycythemia vera, and sickle cell disease.

Quick HIT

Types of strokes
- Ischemic strokes (85% of cases)
- Hemorrhagic strokes (15% of cases)

CLINICAL PEARL 5-1

TIAs Can Involve Either the Carotid or the Vertebrobasilar System

Carotid System

- Temporary loss of speech; paralysis or paresthesias of contralateral extremity; clumsiness of one limb
- **Amaurosis fugax** (an example of a TIA): transient, curtain-like loss of sight in ipsilateral eye due to microemboli to the retina

Vertebrobasilar System (i.e., Vertebrobasilar TIAs)

- Decreased perfusion of the posterior fossa
- Dizziness, double vision, vertigo, numbness of ipsilateral face and contralateral limbs, dysarthria, hoarseness, dysphagia, projectile vomiting, headaches, and drop attacks

Quick HIT

Remember these causes of stroke:
- Ischemia due to atherosclerosis
- Atrial fibrillation with clot emboli to brain
- Septic emboli from endocarditis

Quick HIT

The source of an embolic stroke is evaluated by:
1. Echocardiogram
2. Carotid Dopplers
3. ECG, Holter monitoring

B. Causes

1. **Emboli are** the most common etiology of TIA/CVA (Figure 5-1). Possible origins of an embolus include:
   a. **Heart** (most common): Typically due to embolization of mural thrombus in patients with atrial fibrillation
   b. Internal carotid artery
   c. Aorta
   d. Paradoxical: Emboli arise from blood clots in the peripheral veins, pass through septal defects (atrial septal defect, a patent foramen ovale, or a pulmonary AV fistula), and reach the brain.
2. Thrombotic stroke—Atherosclerotic plaques may be in the large arteries of the neck (carotid artery disease, which most commonly involves the bifurcation of the common carotid artery), or in medium-sized arteries in the brain (especially the middle cerebral artery [MCA]).
3. Lacunar stroke—**small vessel** thrombotic disease
   a. Causes approximately 20% of all strokes; usually affects subcortical structures (basal ganglia, thalamus, internal capsule, brainstem) and not the cerebral cortex

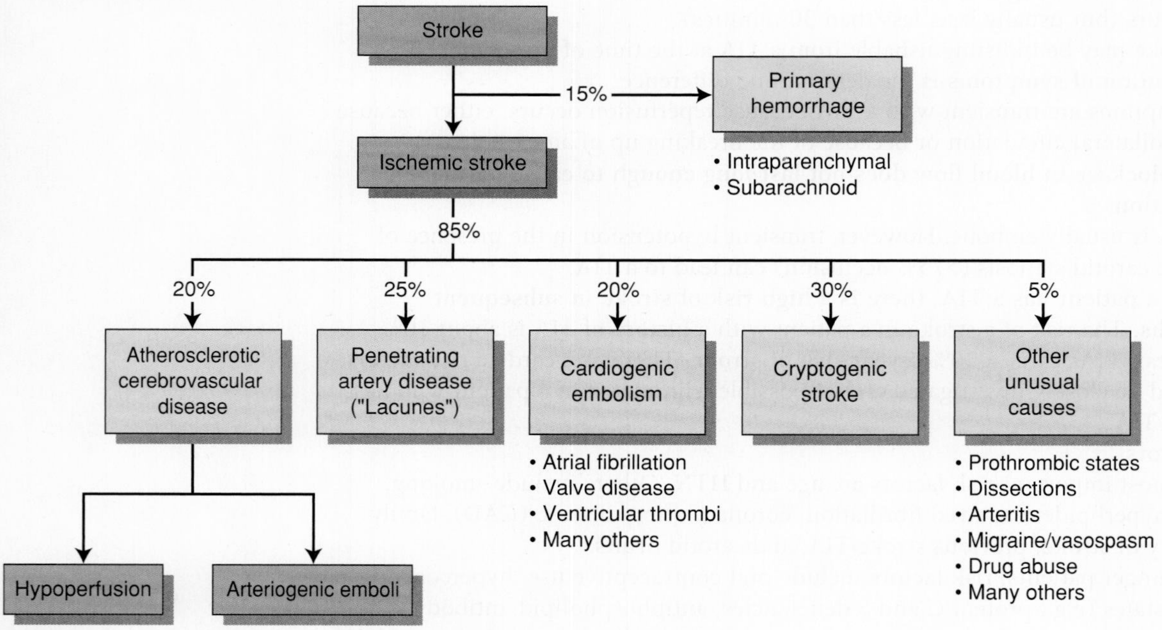

FIGURE 5-1 **Etiology of stroke.**
(Redrawn from Verstraete M, Fuster V, Topol EJ, eds. *Cardiovascular Thrombosis-Thrombocardiology and Thromboneurology.* 2nd ed. Philadelphia, PA: Lippincott Williams & Wilkins, 1998:586, Figure 34-2.)

Diseases of the Central and Peripheral Nervous Systems

CLINICAL PEARL 5-2

Subclavian Steal Syndrome

- Caused by stenosis of subclavian artery proximal to origin of vertebral artery—exercise of left arm causes reversal of blood flow down the ipsilateral vertebral artery to fill the subclavian artery distal to the stenosis because it cannot supply adequate blood to left arm
- Leads to decreased cerebral blood flow (blood "stolen" from basilar system)
- Causes symptoms of vertebrobasilar arterial insufficiency (see Clinical Pearl 5-1)
- BP in left arm is less than in right arm; decrease in pulse in left arm
- Upper extremity claudication
- Treatment: surgical bypass

b. Predisposing factor: A history of **HTN** is present in 80% to 90% of lacunar infarctions. Diabetes is another important risk factor.
c. Narrowing of the arterial lumen is due to **thickening of vessel wall** (not by thrombosis).
d. The arteries affected include small branches of the MCA, the arteries that make up the circle of Willis, and the basilar and vertebral arteries (see Clinical Pearl 5-2).
e. When these small vessels occlude, small infarcts result; when they heal, they are called lacunes.

4. Nonvascular causes—Examples include low cardiac output and anoxia (may cause global ischemia and infarction).

Quick HIT

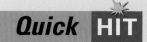

Most common location involves the MCA—results in contralateral weakness, sensory loss, and hyperreflexia.

C. Clinical features

1. Thrombotic stroke—The onset of symptoms may be rapid or stepwise. **Classically the patient awakens from sleep with the neurologic deficits** (see Table 5-1).
2. Embolic stroke
   a. The onset of symptoms is **very rapid** (within seconds), and deficits are maximal initially.
   b. Clinical features depend on the artery that is occluded. The MCA is most commonly affected, and neurologic deficits seen in MCA involvement include:
      - Contralateral hemiparesis and hemisensory loss.
      - Aphasia (if dominant hemisphere is involved)—for 90% of population this is left cerebral dominance.
      - Apraxia, contralateral body neglect, confusion (if nondominant hemisphere is involved).
3. Lacunar stroke—Clinical features are focal and usually contralateral pure motor or pure sensory deficits. Lacunar stroke includes four major syndromes:
   a. Pure **motor** lacunar stroke—if lesion involves the **internal capsule.**
   b. Pure **sensory** lacunar stroke—if lesion involves the **thalamus.**

Quick HIT

A carotid bruit has two causes:
- Murmur referred from the heart
- Turbulence in the internal carotid artery (serious stroke risk)

TABLE 5-1 Deficits Seen in Stroke

Distribution	Location and/or Type of Deficiency
Anterior cerebral artery	Contralateral lower extremity and face
Middle cerebral artery	Aphasia, contralateral hemiparesis
Vertebral/basilar	Ipsilateral: ataxia, diplopia, dysphagia, dysarthria, and vertigo Contralateral: homonymous hemianopsia with basilar—PCA lesions
Lacunar	
Internal capsule	Pure motor hemiparesis
Pons	Dysarthria, clumsy hand
Thalamus	Pure sensory deficit

PCA, posterior cerebral artery

Quick HIT

Uses of CT Scan of the Head in the ED
- To differentiate ischemic from hemorrhagic infarction
- Identifies 95% of SAHs (and all bleeds >1 cm)
- Identifies abscess, tumor
- Identifies subdural or epidural hematoma

Quick HIT

Most common location involves the MCA—results in contralateral weakness, sensory loss, and hyperreflexia.

Quick HIT

Screen all patients with a carotid duplex ultrasound who have the following conditions:
- Carotid bruit
- Peripheral vascular disease (PVD)
- CAD

Quick HIT

If a young patient (<50) presents with stroke, look for vasculitis, hypercoagulable state, and thrombophilia. Order the following:
- Protein C, Protein S, antiphospholipid antibodies
- Factor V Leiden mutation
- ANA, ESR, rheumatoid factor
- VDRL/RPR, Lyme serology
- Transesophageal echocardiogram (TEE)

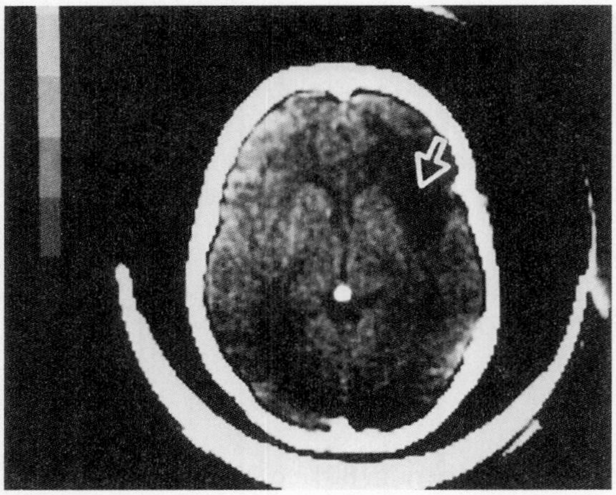

FIGURE **5-2** **CT scan of a patient with a stroke from a nonhemorrhagic infarct (*arrow*).**
(From Fishman MC, Hoffman AR, Klausner RD, et al. *Medicine.* 5th ed. Philadelphia, PA: Lippincott Williams & Wilkins, 2004:593, Figure 64-7.)

c. Ataxic hemiparesis—incoordination ipsilaterally.
d. Clumsy hand dysarthria.

D. Diagnosis

1. CT scan (without contrast) of head.
   a. This differentiates an ischemic from a hemorrhagic infarction and **is the first imaging study that you should obtain.** Contrast should not be used because a hemorrhagic CVA has not been excluded yet. Ischemic strokes appear as dark areas on the CT scan (hemorrhagic strokes appear white—Figure 5-2).
   b. It may take 24 to 48 hours to visualize an infarct on CT, but it is immediately useful in excluding an intracerebral hemorrhage (ICH).
   c. Smaller infarcts (<1 cm) may be missed.
2. MRI of brain—more sensitive than CT scan
   a. Identifies all infarcts, and does so earlier than CT scan. 95% of infarcts identified on MRI within 24 hours.
   b. Not preferred in an emergency setting because it takes longer to perform and is not suitable for potentially unstable patients.
3. ECG—Acute MI or atrial fibrillation may be the cause of embolic strokes.
4. Carotid duplex ultrasound estimates the degree of carotid stenosis, if present.
5. Magnetic resonance arteriogram (MRA) is the definitive test for identifying stenosis of vessels of the head and neck, and for aneurysms. Evaluates carotids, vertebrobasilar circulation, the circle of Willis, and the anterior, middle, and posterior cerebral arteries.

E. Complications

1. Progression of neurologic insult.
2. Cerebral edema occurs within 1 to 2 days and can cause **mass effects** for up to 10 days. Hyperventilation and mannitol may be needed to lower intracranial pressure (ICP).
3. Hemorrhage into the infarction—rare.
4. Seizures—fewer than 5% of patients.

F. Treatment

1. Acute—Supportive treatment (airway protection, oxygen, IV fluids) is initiated. Early recognition of the cause of stroke is unreliable, and early treatment is critical. Therefore, choose therapies that have broad efficacy and safety.
   a. Thrombolytic therapy (t-PA)
      - If administered **within 3 hours** of the onset of an acute ischemic stroke, improved clinical outcome is seen at 3 months.

Diseases of the Central and Peripheral Nervous Systems

- Do not give t-PA if the time of stroke is unknown, if more than 3 hours have passed, or if the patient has any of the following: uncontrolled HTN, bleeding disorder, is taking anticoagulants or has a history of recent trauma or surgery. These patients are at increased risk for hemorrhagic transformation.
- If t-PA is given, there is risk of **intracranial hemorrhage.** Therefore, do not give aspirin for the first 24 hours, perform frequent neurologic checks (every hour), and carefully monitor BP. (Keep BP <185/110 mm Hg.)

b. Aspirin is best if given within 24 hours of symptom onset. Do not give aspirin if the patient received t-PA (due to an increased risk of ICH). **If patient presents within 3 hours of stroke onset, thrombolytics are indicated. If after 3 hours, give aspirin only. If patient cannot take aspirin, give clopidogrel. If patient cannot take either aspirin or clopidogrel (allergy, intolerance), next option is ticlopidine.**

c. Anticoagulants (heparin or warfarin) **have not been proven to have efficacy in acute stroke.** They are generally **not** given in the acute setting.

d. Assess the patient's ability to protect his or her airway, keep NPO, and elevate the head of the bed 30 degrees to prevent aspiration.

2. BP control—In general, do not give antihypertensive agents unless one of the following three conditions is present:
   a. The patient's BP is very high (systolic >220, diastolic >120, or mean arterial pressure >130 mm Hg).
   b. The patient has a significant medical indication for antihypertensive therapy. Examples include:
      - Acute MI
      - Aortic dissection
      - Severe heart failure
      - Hypertensive encephalopathy
   c. The patient is receiving t-PA—aggressive blood pressure control is necessary to reduce the likelihood of bleeding.
3. Prevention—specific recommendations for the prevention of strokes depend on the underlying etiology of the stroke.
   a. Prevention of strokes due to atherosclerosis of the carotid arteries.
      - Control of risk factors—HTN, DM, smoking, hypercholesterolemia, obesity
      - Aspirin
      - Surgery (carotid endarterectomy) (Figure 5-3)

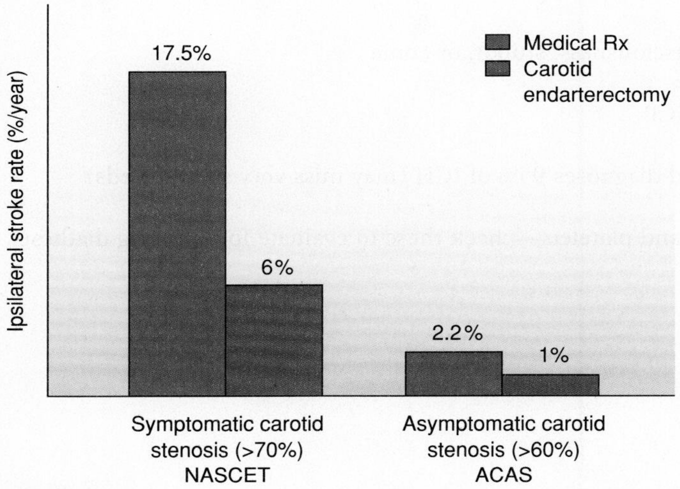

FIGURE 5-3 **Effect of carotid endarterectomy in carotid stenosis. NASCET, North American Symptomatic Carotid Endarterectomy Trial; ACAS, asymptomatic carotid atherosclerosis study.**
(Redrawn from Verstraete M, Fuster V, Topol EJ, eds. *Cardiovascular Thrombosis-Thrombocardiology and Thromboneurology.* 2nd ed. Philadelphia, PA: Lippincott Williams & Wilkins, 1998:590, Figure 34-4.)

Quick HIT

If a patient presents to the ED with findings suggestive of an acute stroke, order the following:
- Noncontrast CT scan of the brain
- ECG, chest radiograph
- CBC, platelet count
- PT, PTT
- Serum electrolytes
- Glucose level
- Bilateral carotid ultrasound
- Echocardiogram

Quick HIT

If stroke is caused by emboli from a cardiac source, anticoagulation is the treatment.

Quick HIT

Treatment of strokes is prophylactic. Once a stroke has occurred, there is nothing that can be done to salvage the dead brain tissue. The goal is to prevent ischemic events in the future.

Quick HIT

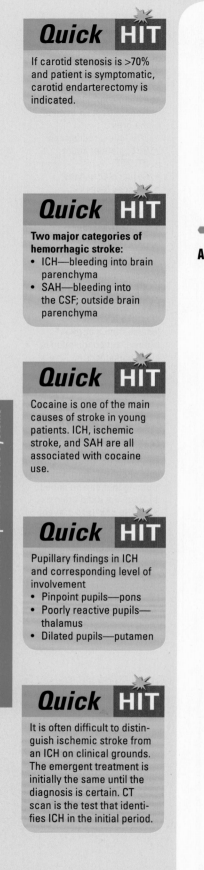

If carotid stenosis is >70% and patient is symptomatic, carotid endarterectomy is indicated.

- **Symptomatic patients**—three major studies have established the benefit of carotid endarterectomy in symptomatic patients with carotid artery stenosis of >70%. (The NASCET trial was the most influential.)
- **Asymptomatic patients**—four major studies have investigated the benefit of carotid endarterectomy in asymptomatic patients. Three found no benefit. One study (ACAS) found that in asymptomatic patients who have a carotid artery stenosis of >60%, the benefits of surgery are very small. **Therefore, in asymptomatic patients, reduction of atherosclerotic risk factors and use of aspirin are recommended.**

b. Prevention of strokes due to embolic disease—anticoagulation (aspirin), reduction of atherosclerotic risk factors.

c. Prevention of lacunar strokes—control of hypertension.

Quick HIT

Two major categories of hemorrhagic stroke:
- ICH—bleeding into brain parenchyma
- SAH—bleeding into the CSF; outside brain parenchyma

Hemorrhagic Stroke

A. Intracerebral hemorrhage

1. **General characteristics**
   a. ICH is associated with a high mortality rate (50% at 30 days). For those who survive, there is significant morbidity.
   b. Hematoma formation and enlargement may lead to local injury and increase in intracerebral pressure.
2. **Causes**
   a. HTN **(particularly a sudden increase in BP)** is the most common cause (50% to 60% of cases).
   - HTN causes a rupture of small vessels deep within the brain parenchyma. Chronic HTN causes degeneration of small arteries, leading to microaneurysms, which can rupture easily.
   - It is typically seen in older patients; risk increases with age.

   b. Ischemic stroke may convert to a hemorrhagic stroke.
   c. Other causes include amyloid angiopathy (10%), anticoagulant/antithrombolytic use (10%), brain tumors (5%), and AV malformations (5%).

Quick HIT

Cocaine is one of the main causes of stroke in young patients. ICH, ischemic stroke, and SAH are all associated with cocaine use.

3. **Locations**
   a. Basal ganglia (66%)
   b. Pons (10%)
   c. Cerebellum (10%)
   d. Other cortical areas
4. **Clinical features**
   a. Abrupt onset of a focal neurologic deficit that worsens steadily over 30 to 90 minutes
   b. Altered level of consciousness, stupor, or coma
   c. Headache, vomiting
   d. Signs of increased ICP

Quick HIT

Pupillary findings in ICH and corresponding level of involvement
- Pinpoint pupils—pons
- Poorly reactive pupils—thalamus
- Dilated pupils—putamen

5. **Diagnosis**
   a. CT scan of the head diagnoses 95% of ICH (may miss very small bleeds) (Figure 5-4).
   b. Coagulation panel and platelets—check these to evaluate for bleeding diathesis.
6. **Complications**
   a. Increased ICP
   b. Seizures
   c. Rebleeding
   d. Vasospasm
   e. Hydrocephalus
   f. SIADH
7. **Treatment**
   a. Admission to the ICU
   b. ABC's (airway, breathing, and circulation)—airway management is important due to altered mental status and decreased respiratory drive. Patients often require intubation

Quick HIT

It is often difficult to distinguish ischemic stroke from an ICH on clinical grounds. The emergent treatment is initially the same until the diagnosis is certain. CT scan is the test that identifies ICH in the initial period.

Diseases of the Central and Peripheral Nervous Systems

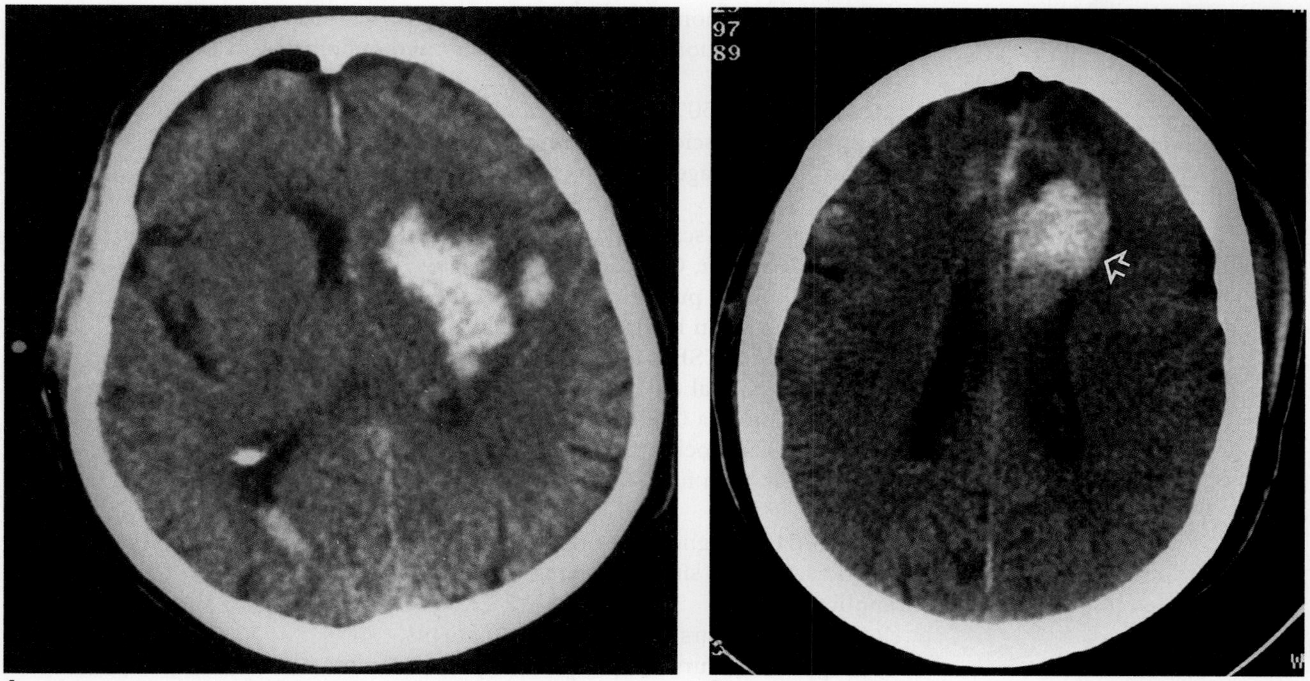

FIGURE 5-4 **A: Spontaneous ICH hemorrhage in a hypertensive patient. B: On CT scan, ischemic stroke appears dark, whereas hemorrhagic stroke appears white.**
(**A** from Daffner RH, ed. *Clinical Radiology: The Essentials.* 2nd ed. Philadelphia, PA: Lippincott Williams & Wilkins, 1999:526, Figure 12.37A.) (**B** from Daffner RH, ed. *Clinical Radiology: The Essentials.* 2nd ed. Philadelphia, PA: Lippincott Williams & Wilkins, 1999:528, Figure 12.40B.)

c. BP reduction
   - Elevated BP increases ICP and can cause further bleeding. However, hypotension can lower cerebral blood flow, worsening the neurologic deficits. Therefore, **BP reduction must be gradual so as to not induce hypotension.**
   - Treatment is indicated if systolic BP is >160 to 180 or diastolic BP is >105. Treatment for BP lower than these values is controversial.
   - Nitroprusside is often the agent of choice.

d. Mannitol (osmotic agent) and diuretics can be given to reduce ICP. Use these agents only if ICP is elevated; do not give them prophylactically.
e. Use of steroids is harmful and is **not** recommended.
f. Rapid surgical evacuation of **cerebellar** hematomas can be lifesaving. However, surgery is **not** helpful in most cases of ICH.

B. Subarachnoid hemorrhage

1. **General characteristics**
   a. Mortality rate can be as high as 40% to 50% at 30 days.
   b. Locations—Saccular (berry) aneurysms occur at bifurcations of arteries of the circle of Willis.
2. **Causes**
   a. Ruptured saccular (berry) aneurysms are the most common cause—has higher morbidity and mortality than other causes.
   b. Trauma is also a common cause.
   c. AV malformation.
3. **Clinical features**
   a. Sudden, severe (**often excruciating**) headache in the absence of focal neurologic symptoms; classic description is "**the worst headache of my life**" but may also be more subtle.
   b. Sudden, transient loss of consciousness—in approximately 50% of patients.

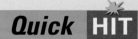

Quick HIT
Treatment of intraparenchymal hemorrhagic stroke is supportive. There is generally no specific therapy.

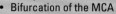

Quick HIT
Common Sites of SAH
- Junction of anterior communicating artery with anterior cerebral artery
- Junction of posterior communicating artery with the internal carotid artery
- Bifurcation of the MCA

Quick HIT
Polycystic kidney disease is associated with berry aneurysms.

Quick HIT

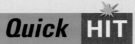

Caution: Ophthalmologic examination is mandatory to rule out papilledema. If **papilledema** is present, do not perform an LP—you may cause a herniation. Repeat the CT scan first.

c. Vomiting (common).
d. Meningeal irritation, nuchal rigidity, and photophobia—can take several hours to develop.
e. Death—25% to 50% of patients die with the first rupture. Those who survive will recover consciousness within minutes.
f. Retinal hemorrhages—in up to 30% of patients.

4. **Diagnosis**
   a. Noncontrast CT scan—identifies the majority of subarachnoid hemorrhages (SAHs). However, CT scan may be negative in up to 10% of cases.
   b. **Perform lumbar puncture (LP) if the CT scan is unrevealing or negative and clinical suspicion is high. LP is diagnostic.**
      - **Blood in the CSF** is a hallmark of SAH. (Be certain that it is not blood from a traumatic spinal tap)
      - **Xanthochromia** (yellow color of the CSF) is the gold standard for diagnosis of SAH. Xanthochromia results from RBC lysis. Xanthochromia implies that blood has been in CSF for several hours and that it is not due to a traumatic tap.
   c. Once SAH is diagnosed, order a cerebral angiogram. It is the definitive study for detecting the site of bleeding (for surgical clipping).
5. **Complications**
   a. Rerupture—occurs in up to 30% of patients.
   b. Vasospasm—occurs in up to 50% of patients (more often with aneurysmal SAH); can cause ischemia/infarction and therefore stroke.
   c. Hydrocephalus (communicating)—secondary to blood within the subarachnoid space hindering normal CSF flow.
   d. Seizures may occur (blood acts as an irritant).
   e. SIADH
6. **Treatment**
   a. Surgical—consult neurosurgery. Berry aneurysms are usually treated surgically: Surgically clip the aneurysm to prevent rebleeding.
   b. Medical—therapy reduces the risks of rebleeding and cerebral vasospasm.
      - Bed rest in a quiet, dark room.
      - Stool softeners to avoid straining (increases ICP and risk of rerupture).
      - Analgesia for headache (acetaminophen).
      - IV fluids for hydration.
      - Control of HTN—lower the BP gradually because the elevation in BP may be a compensation for the decrease in cerebral perfusion pressure (secondary to increased ICP or cerebral arterial narrowing).
      - Calcium channel blocker (nifedipine) for vasospasm—lowers the incidence of cerebral infarction by one-third.

Movement Disorders

Parkinson Disease

Quick HIT

The basal ganglia/striatal region normally operates as a balanced system comprising the dopaminergic system and the cholinergic system. In Parkinson disease, the dopaminergic pathway is compromised, and the cholinergic system operates unopposed. Therefore, the goal of treatment is either to enhance dopamine's influence or to inhibit acetylcholine's influence.

A. General characteristics

1. Results from a loss of dopamine-containing neurons—nerve cells that are located in the pigmented **substantia nigra** and the **locus ceruleus** in the midbrain.
2. Onset is usually after age 50 years.
3. Parkinsonism refers to symptoms and signs of Parkinson disease and can result from many conditions (e.g., medications).
4. **Parkinson disease is essentially a clinical diagnosis.** Laboratory studies play no role in diagnosis.

B. Clinical features

1. Pill-rolling tremor at **rest** (worsens with emotional stress) (see Clinical Pearl 5-3). Tremor goes away when performing routine tasks.
2. Bradykinesia—slowness of voluntary movements.

CLINICAL PEARL 5-3

Progressive Supranuclear Palsy (PSP)

- PSP is a degenerative condition of the brainstem, basal ganglia, and cerebellum, most commonly affecting middle-aged and elderly men.
- Like Parkinson disease, PSP causes bradykinesia, limb rigidity, cognitive decline, and follows a progressive course.
- Unlike Parkinson disease, PSP
  - Does **not cause tremor**
  - Does cause ophthalmoplegia

3. Rigidity is characteristic. "Cogwheel rigidity" refers to a ratchet-like jerking, which can be elicited by testing the tone in one limb while the patient clenches the opposite fist.
4. Poor postural reflexes; difficulty initiating the first step, and walking with small shuffling steps; stooped posture.
5. Masked (expressionless) facies; decreased blinking.
6. Dysarthria and dysphagia, micrographia (small handwriting).
7. Impairment of cognitive function (dementia) in advanced disease.
8. Autonomic dysfunction can lead to orthostatic hypotension, constipation, increased sweating, and oily skin.
9. Personality changes present in early stages. Patients become withdrawn, apathetic, and dependent on others. Depression is common and can be significant—causes worsening of parkinsonian symptoms.
10. Follows progressive course—significant disability usually presents within 5 to 10 years; indirectly leads to increased mortality.

Quick HIT

Shy–Drager syndrome = parkinsonian symptoms + autonomic insufficiency

Quick HIT

Lewy bodies (hyaline inclusion bodies) are a key neuronal finding in the brains of patients with Parkinson disease.

C. Treatment

1. No cure—goals are to delay disease progression and relieve symptoms.
2. Carbidopa-levodopa (Sinemet)—drug of choice for treating parkinsonian symptoms.
   a. As the name implies, it is a combination of levodopa (l-Dopa) and carbidopa.
   b. It ameliorates all the symptoms of Parkinson disease. It is the most effective of all the antiparkinsonian drugs.
   c. Side effects.
      - Dyskinesias (involuntary, often choreic movements) can occur after 5 to 7 years of therapy. This is a major concern, and may warrant delay in initiating carbidopa-levodopa for as long as possible.
      - Nausea/vomiting, anorexia, HTN, hallucinations.
   d. Levodopa does show an "on–off" phenomenon (over the course of the day) during treatment, which leads to fluctuations in symptoms. This is due to dose–response relationships. It often occurs in advanced disease.
3. Dopamine-receptor agonists (bromocriptine, pramipexole).
   a. May control symptoms and delay need for levodopa for several years.
   b. Initiate one of these agents when you have established the diagnosis. You may use levodopa and one of these agents at the same time.
   c. Pramipexole is the most commonly used.
   d. These can be useful for sudden episodes of hesitancy or immobility (described as "freezing").
4. Selegiline—it inhibits monoamine oxidase B activity (increases dopamine activity) and reduces metabolism of levodopa. It is an adjunctive agent, and is often used in early disease. It has mild symptomatic benefit.
5. Amantadine (antiviral agent)—mild benefit, mostly for early or mild disease.
6. Anticholinergic drugs.
   a. Trihexyphenidyl and benztropine.
   b. These may be particularly helpful in patients with tremor as a major finding. Do not use in older patients or demented patients.

Quick HIT

Medications that Cause Parkinsonian Side Effects
- Neuroleptic drugs (chlorpromazine, haloperidol, perphenazine)
- Metoclopramide
- Reserpine

Quick HIT

Patients with tremor as a major symptom of Parkinson disease have a better prognosis than those who have bradykinesia as a predominant finding.

7. Amitriptyline—useful in the treatment of Parkinson disease both as an anticholinergic agent and as an antidepressant.
8. Surgery (deep brain stimulation)—if patient does not respond to medications or in patients who develop severe disease before age 40 years.

Huntington Chorea

A. General characteristics

1. **Autosomal dominant**, so lack of family history makes this diagnosis unlikely.
2. Onset is between 30 and 50 years of age. Symptoms worsen steadily, with 15 years being the typical duration from onset to death.
3. It is caused by a mutation on chromosome 4 (expanded triplet repeat sequence)—CAG leads to a loss of GABA-producing neurons in the striatum.

B. Clinical features

1. Chorea—involving the face, head and neck, tongue, trunk, and extremities.
2. Altered behavior—irritability, personality changes, antisocial behavior, depression, obsessive-compulsive features, and/or psychosis.
3. Impaired mentation—progressive dementia is a key feature; 90% of patients are demented before age 50 years.
4. Gait is unsteady and irregular. Ultimately bradykinesia and rigidity prevail.
5. Incontinence.

Quick HIT

Always keep Wilson disease in mind in a **young patient** with movement disorders (see Chapter 3).

C. Diagnosis

1. MRI shows atrophy of the head of caudate nuclei.
2. DNA testing confirms the diagnosis. Genetic counseling plays an important role.

D. Treatment

Treatment is symptomatic—there is no curative treatment. Dopamine blockers may help with the psychosis and improve chorea. Anxiolytic and antidepressant therapy may be necessary.

Tremor

A. Physiologic tremor

1. **Causes** (see Table 5-2)
   a. Fear, anxiety, fatigue
   b. Metabolic causes: hypoglycemia, hyperthyroidism, pheochromocytoma
   c. Toxic causes (e.g., alcohol withdrawal, valproic acid, lithium, methylxanthines—caffeine and theophylline)
2. **Treatment:** Treat the underlying cause, if known; otherwise, no treatment is necessary

TABLE 5-2 Common Tremors and Associated Features

Feature	Parkinsonian	Cerebellar	Essential
Characteristic Setting	Rest	With action—"intention tremor"	With certain postures (e.g., arms outstretched) or certain tasks (e.g., handwriting)
Description	Pill-rolling	Coarse	Fine
Etiology	Idiopathic or adverse effect of neuroleptic	Multiple possible etiologies	Often familiar
Associated Features	Rigidity, bradykinesia, shuffling gait	Ataxia, nystagmus, dysarthria	Head tremor, vocal tremulousness
Improved By	Action	Rest (no tremor at rest)	Alcohol

B. Essential tremor

1. Common; inherited (autosomal dominant) in up to one-third of patients.
2. It is induced or exacerbated by intentional activity, such as drinking from a cup or use of utensils, and is **markedly decreased by alcohol use** (useful in diagnosis).
3. Distorted handwriting is often present. Note that bradykinesia, rigidity, shuffling gait, or postural instability are all absent.
4. Treat with propranolol.

C. Neurologic diseases (e.g., Parkinson disease, cerebellar disease, Wilson disease)

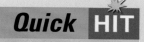

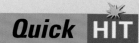

> **Quick HIT**
> There is no known association between essential tremor and Parkinson disease.

Ataxia

A. General characteristics

1. Gait instability
2. Loss of balance
3. Impaired limb coordination

B. Causes

1. Acquired causes: alcohol intoxication, vitamin B_{12} or thiamine deficiency, cerebellar infarction or neoplasm, demyelinating disease (multiple sclerosis [MS], AIDS), and tertiary syphilis **(tabes dorsalis)**
2. Inherited causes
   a. Friedreich ataxia
      - Autosomal recessive inheritance, onset by young adulthood
      - Presents with ataxia, nystagmus, impaired vibratory sense, and proprioception
   b. Ataxia telangiectasia
      - Autosomal recessive inheritance, childhood onset
      - Symptoms similar to those of Friedreich ataxia plus telangiectases
      - Increased incidence of cancer

C. Treatment: Treat underlying cause if possible.

Tourette Syndrome

A. General characteristics

1. Associated with obsessive-compulsive disorder.
2. Onset before age 21 years.
3. Thought to have autosomal dominant inheritance pattern.
4. Not all patients with tics have Tourette syndrome.
5. Not all patients with Tourette syndrome experience coprolalia (involuntary swearing).

B. Clinical features (occur frequently and regularly). Must have both motor and phonic tics.

1. Motor tics (multiple)
2. Phonic tics (at least one kind)

C. Treatment (if symptoms are affecting the patient's quality of life; patient education is important)

1. Clonidine
2. Pimozide
3. Haloperidol

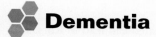

> **Quick HIT**
> **Tics**
> - Motor tics (e.g., facial grimace, blinking, head jerking, shoulder shrugging)
> - Phonic tics (e.g., grunting, sniffing, clearing throat, coprolalia, repetition of words)
> - Conditions that must be ruled out include seizures, tardive dyskinesias, and Huntington disease.

Dementia

Overview

A. General characteristics

1. Dementia is a progressive deterioration of intellectual function, typically characterized by **preservation of consciousness.**
2. The most important risk factor for dementia is **increasing age.**

> **Quick HIT**
> **Forgetfulness Versus Dementia**
> - Some degree of memory loss is accepted as a normal part of aging. It may be difficult to distinguish this condition, sometimes referred to as benign forgetfulness of elderly patients, from true dementia.
> - In general, benign forgetfulness does not adversely affect normal day-to-day living or baseline functioning, but it may be a risk factor for progressive dementias such as **Alzheimer disease.**

CLINICAL PEARL 5-4

Causes of Dementia

Potentially Reversible Causes of Dementia

- Hypothyroidism
- Neurosyphilis
- Vitamin B_{12}/folate deficiency/thiamine deficiency
- Medications
- Normal pressure hydrocephalus
- Depression
- Subdural hematoma

Irreversible Causes of Dementia

- Alzheimer disease
- Parkinson, Huntington
- Multi-infarct dementia
- Dementia with Lewy bodies, Pick disease
- Unresectable brain mass
- HIV dementia
- Korsakoff syndrome
- Progressive multifocal leukoencephalopathy
- Creutzfeldt–Jakob disease

B. Differential diagnosis of dementia

1. Primary neurologic disorders (see Clinical Pearl 5-4)
   a. Alzheimer disease—accounts for 66% of all cases of dementia (see the section on Alzheimer disease below)
   b. Vascular dementia
      - **Multi-infarct dementia** is a stepwise decline due to a series of cerebral infarctions
      - Binswanger disease—insidious onset, due to diffuse subcortical white matter degeneration, most commonly seen in patients with long-standing HTN and atherosclerosis
   c. Space-occupying lesions, such as brain tumor or chronic subdural hematoma
   d. Normal pressure hydrocephalus—triad of dementia, gait disturbance, and urinary incontinence; normal CSF pressure and dilated ventricles
   e. Dementia with Lewy bodies (see section below)
   f. Pick disease (Frontotemporal Dementia)—clinically identical to Alzheimer disease
   g. Other neurologic conditions: MS, Parkinson disease, Huntington disease, Wilson disease
2. Infections
   a. HIV infection (AIDS-related dementia)
   b. Neurosyphilis
   c. Cryptococcal infection of CNS
   d. Creutzfeldt–Jakob disease (spongiform encephalopathy)
   e. Progressive multifocal leukoencephalopathy
3. Metabolic disorders
   a. Thyroid disease (hypothyroidism or hyperthyroidism)
   b. Vitamin B_{12} deficiency
   c. Thiamine deficiency—common in alcoholics; if untreated can lead to Korsakoff dementia (irreversible)
   d. Niacin deficiency
4. Drugs and toxins
   a. Drug abuse; chronic alcoholism (may cause dementia independent from thiamine malnutrition)
   b. Toxic substances: aniline dyes, metals (e.g., lead)

5. Pseudodementia (depression)—severe depression may cause a decline in cognition that is difficult to distinguish clinically from Alzheimer disease, but is responsive to antidepressant therapy

C. Clinical approach to dementia

1. Patient history—Ask patients and their family members about the nature of onset, specific deficits, physical symptoms, and comorbid conditions. Review all medications, as well as family and social history.
2. Physical examination.
   a. Focus on a thorough neurologic examination and mental status examination.
   b. Gait analysis often sheds light on movement disorders, mass lesions, and non-pressure hydrocephalus.
3. Laboratory and imaging studies—Consider the following when investigating the cause of dementia: CBC with differential, chemistry panel, thyroid function tests (TSH), vitamin B_{12}, folate level, VDRL (syphilis), HIV screening, and CT scan or MRI of the head.

D. Treatment and management: general principles

1. Treat reversible causes.
2. Avoid and/or monitor doses of medications with adverse cognitive side effects (glucocorticoids, opiates, sedative hypnotics, anxiolytics, anticholinergics, lithium).
3. Treat/control comorbid medical conditions; for example, diabetes, HTN, depression, visual and hearing impairment.
4. Pharmacologic therapy may include vitamin E, tacrine, and donepezil. The evidence supporting the efficacy of many pharmacologic treatments is inconclusive.
5. A multidisciplinary approach includes support groups for caregivers/families of patients with irreversible dementias.

Alzheimer Disease

A. General characteristics

1. Epidemiology
   a. Alzheimer disease is the fourth most common cause of death in the United States.
   b. Prevalence increases with age—Approximately 10% to 15% of individuals over age 65, and 15% to 30% of individuals over age 80 have Alzheimer disease. However, many will die of other causes first.
2. Risk factors
   a. **Age**
   b. Family history (especially for early-onset Alzheimer disease)
   c. Down syndrome
3. Etiology is unknown, but a heritable component may be present. Chromosomes 21, 14, and 19 have been linked to Alzheimer disease
4. Pathology (noted at autopsy)
   a. Quantity of senile plaques (age-specific)—focal collections of dilated, tortuous neuritic processes surrounding a central amyloid core (amyloid beta-protein)
   b. Quantity of neurofibrillary tangles (age-specific)
      - Bundles of neurofilaments in cytoplasm of neurons
      - Denote neuronal degeneration

B. Clinical features

1. Begins insidiously but tends to progress at a steady rate.
2. The average time from onset to death is 5 to 10 years (with some variability).
3. Stages
   a. Early stages—mild forgetfulness, impaired ability to learn new material, poor performance at work, poor concentration, changes in personality, impaired judgment (e.g., inappropriate humor).
   b. Intermediate stages—memory is progressively impaired. Patients may be aware of the condition, yet denial is often present. Visuospatial disturbances are

Quick HIT

Most important risk factor for Alzheimer disease is age.

Quick HIT

Patients with Alzheimer disease often have **cerebral atrophy** secondary to neuronal loss. Ventricles will correspondingly be enlarged.

Quick HIT

Alzheimer Disease: Treatment/Prevention
- No treatment has been found to have a significant effect on cognitive effects.
- Hormone replacement therapy is associated with a lower risk of developing Alzheimer disease.

Quick HIT

Patients with AD have decreased acetylcholine synthesis and thus impaired cortical cholinergic function. Cholinesterase inhibitors increase cholinergic transmission by inhibiting cholinesterase.

Quick HIT

AChE medications (e.g., donepezil) are only indicated for Alzheimer dementia and Lewy body dementia. No specific therapy for other causes of dementia.

common (getting lost in a familiar place and difficulty following directions). Patients may repeat questions over and over.

c. Later stages—assistance is needed for activities of daily living. Patients have difficulty remembering the names of relatives/friends or major aspects of their lives. Paranoid delusions (e.g., victim of theft) and hallucinations are common.

d. Advanced disease—complete debilitation and dependence on others, incontinence (bowel/bladder); patient may even forget his or her own name.

e. Death is usually secondary to infection or other complications of a debilitated state.

C. Diagnosis

1. Alzheimer disease is essentially a **clinical diagnosis**; exclude other causes first.
2. CT scan or MRI showing diffuse cortical atrophy with enlargement of the ventricles strengthens the diagnosis.

D. Treatment

1. Cholinesterase Inhibitors—brains of patients with Alzheimer disease have lower levels of acetylcholine. **Avoid anticholinergic medications!** Options include donepezil, rivastigmine, and galantamine.
   a. Currently the first-line agent.
2. Certain dietary supplements (ginkgo, lecithin) have not been proven to be beneficial.
3. Vitamin E.
   a. In one study, megadoses of vitamin E (2,000 IU/day) slowed disease progression and preserved function in people with moderately severe Alzheimer disease.
   b. Full benefit remains to be defined.

Dementia With Lewy Bodies

- Dementia with Lewy bodies has features of both Alzheimer disease and Parkinson disease, but progression may be more rapid than in Alzheimer disease.
- Initially, visual hallucinations predominate. Other symptoms include extrapyramidal features and fluctuating mental status.
- These patients are sensitive to the adverse effects of neuroleptic agents, which often exacerbate symptoms.
- Treatment is similar to that for Alzheimer disease, with neuroleptic agents (for hallucinations and psychotic features). Selegiline may slow the progression of disease.

Altered Mental Status

Acute Confusional State (Delirium)

A. General characteristics

1. Delirium is an acute period of cognitive dysfunction due to a medical disturbance or condition (See Clinical Pearl 5-5) (see Table 5-3).
2. Elderly patients are especially prone to delirium.

CLINICAL PEARL 5-5

Altered Mental Status

- Consciousness relies on arousal and cognition. Arousal is dependent on an intact brainstem (reticular activating system in brainstem). Cognition is dependent on an intact cerebral cortex.
- Altered mental status, diminished level of consciousness (drowsiness, stupor, coma), and confusion are caused by many of the same conditions and are often variations of the same theme.
- Depressed level of consciousness and coma can be caused by a variety of disorders. To help in classification and to organize one's thinking, it is useful to organize these causes into two categories:
  - Diffuse injury to the brain due to any metabolic, systemic, or toxic disorder
  - Focal intracranial structural lesions—for example, hemorrhage, infarction, tumor

TABLE 5-3 Delirium Versus Dementia

Feature	Delirium	Dementia
Causes	• Infections (UTI, systemic infection) • Medications (narcotics, benzodiazepines) • Postoperative delirium (in elderly patients) • Alcoholism • Electrolyte imbalances • Medical conditions (stroke, heart disease, seizures, hepatic and renal disorders)	• Alzheimer disease • Multi-infarct dementia • Pick disease (Frontotemporal dementia)
Level of Consciousness	Altered, fluctuating	Preserved
Hallucinations	Frequently present (visual)	Rarely present
Presence of Tremor	Sometimes present (e.g., asterixis)	Usually absent unless dementia is due to Parkinson disease
Course	• Rapid onset, **waxing and waning** • **"Sundowning"** (worsening at night) may be present	Insidious, progressive
Reversibility	Almost always reversible	Typically irreversible

B. Causes: Causes of delirium include those of coma (see Clinical Pearl 5-6, "SMASHED"), plus the following: "P. DIMM WIT."

1. P = postoperative state (compounded by narcotic pain medications)
2. D = dehydration and malnutrition
3. I = infection (sepsis, meningitis, encephalitis, urinary tract infection, and so on)
4. M = medications and drug intoxications—tricyclic antidepressants, corticosteroids, anticholinergics, hallucinogens, cocaine
5. M = metals (heavy metal exposure)
6. W = withdrawal states (from alcohol, benzodiazepines)
7. I = inflammation, fever
8. T = trauma, burns

C. Clinical features

1. In contrast to both dementia and psychosis, delirium is characterized by a rapid deterioration in mental status (over hours to days), a fluctuating level of awareness, disorientation, and, frequently, abnormal vital signs.

CLINICAL PEARL 5-6

Differential Diagnosis of Coma or Stupor: SMASHED

- **S** = **s**tructural brain pathology: stroke, subdural or epidural hematoma, tumor, hydrocephalus, herniation, abscess
- **M** = **m**eningitis, mental illness (e.g., conversion disorder, catatonia—mimic coma)
- **A** = **a**lcohol, acidosis
- **S** = **s**eizures (postictal state), substrate deficiency (e.g., thiamine)
- **H** = **h**ypercapnia, hyperglycemia, hyperthermia; hyponatremia, hypoglycemia, hypoxia, hypotension/cerebral hypoperfusion, hypothermia
- **E** = **e**ndocrine causes (Addisonian crisis, thyrotoxicosis, hypothyroidism); encephalitis, encephalopathy (hypertensive, hepatic, or uremic); extreme disturbances in calcium, magnesium, phosphate
- **D** = **d**rugs (opiates, barbiturates, benzodiazepines, other sedatives); dangerous compounds (carbon monoxide, cyanide, methanol)

2. Delirium may often be accompanied by acute abnormalities of perception, such as hallucinations.
3. Patients may not necessarily be agitated, but may have a slow, blunted responsiveness.

D. Diagnosis

1. Mental status examination—Mini-Mental Status Examination
2. Laboratory—for example, chemistry panel, vitamin B_{12}, thiamine
3. LP—Perform in any febrile, delirious patient unless there are contraindications (e.g., cerebral edema).

E. Treatment

1. Treat the underlying cause
2. Haloperidol—for agitation/psychotic-like delirious behavior
3. Supportive treatment

Coma

A. General characteristics

1. A coma is a depressed level of consciousness to the extent that the patient is completely unresponsive to any stimuli.
2. Causes
   a. Structural brain lesions that cause a coma are usually bilateral unless they produce enough mass effect to compress the brainstem or the opposite cerebral hemisphere (see Clinical Pearl 5-6).
   b. Global brain dysfunction (e.g., metabolic or systemic disorders)
   c. Psychiatric causes—conversion disorders and malingering may be difficult to differentiate from a true coma.

B. Approach

1. Initial steps
   a. Assess vital signs. ABC's take priority.
   b. Always assume underlying trauma (stabilize cervical spine) and assess the patient for signs of underlying causes of trauma.
   c. Assess the level of consciousness using the Glasgow Coma Scale (see Table 5-4). Repeat this serially because it can change.
2. Approach to diagnosing the cause of coma.
   a. Rapid motor examination—if asymmetry is noted in movements, a mass lesion is the likely cause. Metabolic or systemic causes of coma do not produce asymmetric motor abnormalities.

TABLE 5-4 Glasgow Coma Scale

Eye Opening (E)	Does not open eyes	1
	Opens to painful stimulus	2
	Opens to voice (command)	3
	Opens spontaneously	4
Motor Response (M)	No movement	1
	Decerebrate posture	2
	Decorticate posture	3
	Withdraws from pain	4
	Localizes pain stimulus	5
	Obeys commands	6
Verbal Response (V)	No sounds	1
	Incomprehensible sounds	2
	Inappropriate words	3
	Appropriate but confused	4
	Appropriate and oriented	5

CLINICAL PEARL 5-7

Brain Death Versus Persistent Vegetative State

- Criteria for diagnosing brain death:
  - **Irreversible** absence of brain and brainstem function—unresponsiveness, apnea despite adequate oxygenation and ventilation, no brainstem reflexes (pupils, calorics, gag, cornea, doll's eyes).
  - No drug intoxication or metabolic condition that can reversibly inhibit brain function.
  - Core body temperature >32°C/89.6°F. Brain death cannot be established in the presence of hypothermia.
  - Clinical evidence or imaging study that provides a causative explanation for brain death.
  - Examinations must be repeated or EEG performed. EEG shows isoelectric activity (electrical silence).
- In most US states, **if a patient is proven to be brain dead,** the physician has the right to disconnect life support—the patient is **legally dead.** (Obviously, sensitivity and consideration must be demonstrated to the family. They must be informed and given a chance to say good-bye to their loved one.)
- Patients in a "vegetative state" are completely unresponsive (comatose), but eyes are open and they appear awake. May have random head or limb movements. Patient **may** have no hope of meaningful recovery but do not meet brain death criteria. Ethical and legal issues surrounding supportive measures are much more complicated.

b. Brainstem reflexes (see Clinical Pearl 5-7).
  - Pupillary light reflex—If the pupils are round and symmetrically reactive (constrict to bright light), the midbrain is intact and not the cause of coma. Anisocoria (asymmetric pupils) may be a sign of uncal herniation. Keep in mind that certain eye drops or systemic medications may alter pupil size.
  - Eye movements—if the cervical spine is uninjured, perform the oculocephalic test ("doll's eyes"). When the head is turned to one side, the eyes should move conjugately to the opposite direction if the brainstem is intact.
  - If the patient is breathing on her or his own, the brainstem is functioning.

c. Laboratory tests—CBC, electrolytes, calcium BUN, creatinine, glucose, plasma osmolarity, arterial blood gas, ECG.
d. Toxicologic analysis of blood and urine.
e. CT or MRI of the brain.
f. LP—if meningitis or SAH is suspected.

C. Treatment

1. Correct reversible causes and treat the underlying problem (if identified)—control airway; give supplemental oxygen, naloxone (for narcotic overdose), dextrose (for hypoglycemia). Give thiamine before a glucose load. Correct any abnormalities in BP, electrolytes, or body temperature.
2. Identify and treat herniation—lowering the ICP is critical.

Quick HIT

Assessing the Cause of a Coma
- Abnormal pupillary light reflex—structural intracranial lesions (hemorrhage, mass); drugs that affect the pupil (morphine, atropine-like agents); anoxic encephalopathy; recent eye drops
- Bilateral fixed, dilated pupils—severe anoxia
- Unilateral fixed, dilated pupil—herniation with CN III compression
- Pinpoint pupils—narcotics, ICH

Quick HIT

"Locked in" Syndrome
- Mimics coma, because patients are completely paralyzed (with sparing of muscles required for respiration, blinking, and vertical eye movement).
- Patients are **fully aware** of their surroundings and capable of feeling pain.
- This is usually caused by infarction or hemorrhage of the ventral pons.

Demyelinating Disease

Multiple Sclerosis

A. General characteristics

1. Pathology
   a. Selective **demyelination of CNS**—multifocal zones of demyelination (plaques) are scattered throughout the white matter. Classic location of plaques is at the angles of the lateral ventricles.
   b. Demyelination primarily involves **white matter** of the brain and spinal cord; tends to spare the gray matter/axons and the peripheral nervous system. However, improved imaging techniques are showing that cortical demyelination may be more prevalent than previously appreciated.
   c. Commonly involved tracts: pyramidal and cerebellar pathways, medial longitudinal fasciculus, optic nerve, posterior columns.

CLINICAL PEARL 5-8

Diagnosis of MS

Clinically Definite MS

- Two episodes of symptoms
- Evidence of two white matter lesions (imaging or clinical)

Laboratory-supported Definite MS

- Two episodes of symptoms
- Evidence of at least one white matter lesion on MRI
- Abnormal CSF (**oligoclonal bands** in CSF)

Probable MS

- Two episodes of symptoms and either one white matter lesion or oligoclonal bands in CSF

Quick HIT

There are a variety of presenting symptoms in MS that involve many different areas of the CNS, and the inability to attribute them all to one localizing lesion is a characteristic feature of the disease.

Quick HIT

Relapses of MS produce symptoms for longer than 24 hours. They average one per year, but usually decrease in frequency over time.

2. Women are two to three times more likely than men to have MS.
3. Etiology is unknown, but is probably secondary to the interplay of environmental, immunologic, and genetic factors.

B. Clinical features

1. Transient sensory deficits (see Clinical Pearl 5-8)
   a. Most common initial presentation
   b. Decreased sensation or paresthesias in upper or lower limbs
2. Fatigue—one of the most common complaints
3. Motor symptoms—mainly weakness or spasticity
   a. May appear insidiously or acutely
   b. Caused by pyramidal tract involvement (upper motor neuron involvement)
   c. Spasticity (such as leg stiffness) can impair the patient's ability to walk and maintain balance
   d. Can lead to weakness with progression to paraparesis, hemiparesis, or quadriparesis
4. Visual disturbances
   a. **Optic neuritis**
      - Monocular visual loss (in up to 20% of patients)
      - Pain on movement of eyes
      - Central scotoma (black spot in center of vision)
      - Decreased pupillary reaction to light
   b. **Internuclear ophthalmoplegia**—strongly suggests the diagnosis
      - A lesion in the medial longitudinal fasciculus results in ipsilateral medial rectus palsy on attempted lateral gaze (adduction defect) and horizontal nystagmus of abducting eye (contralateral to side of lesion)
      - Diplopia can occur
5. Cerebellar involvement—can cause ataxia, intention tremor, dysarthria
6. Loss of bladder control—consequence of upper motor neuron injury in spinal cord
7. Autonomic involvement—may present as impotence and/or constipation
8. Cerebral involvement—may occur in advanced illness and manifests as memory loss, personality change, and emotional lability; anxiety and depression are common
9. Neuropathic pain—a frustrating but common complaint that manifests as hyperesthesias and trigeminal neuralgia

C. Course

1. Most patients at initial presentation are in their 20s to 30s and present with a localizing deficit such as optic neuritis, one-sided weakness, or numbness. Patients may or may not go on to develop MS.
2. Attacks average up to one per year. No one precipitant has been proven to cause attacks.

3. Prognosis is highly variable, with normal life spans in most patients.
   a. Although quality of life is diminished, many patients never develop debilitating disease.
   b. Approximately one-third of patients eventually progress to severe disability.
   c. The following increase the chances of severe disability: frequent attacks early in the disease course, onset at an older age, progressive course, and early cerebellar or pyramidal involvement.

D. Diagnosis

1. The diagnosis is essentially clinical—suspect it in young adults with relapsing and remitting neurologic signs and symptoms that are difficult to explain (due to involvement of different areas of CNS white matter). Nevertheless, on suspicion, order the MRI and consider LP (discussed below), because it is important to diagnose MS with as much certainty as possible due to the implications surrounding the management approach.
2. MRI is the most sensitive test and is diagnostic in the majority of cases.
   a. Now considered standard of care.
   b. Sensitive in identifying demyelinating lesions in CNS.
   c. The number of lesions on the MRI is **not** necessarily proportional to disease severity or speed of progression.
3. LP and CSF analysis—Although no laboratory tests are specific for MS, **oligoclonal bands** of immunoglobulin G are present in 90% of MS patients.
4. Evoked potentials can suggest demyelination of certain areas by measuring the speed of nerve conduction within the brain: Newly remyelinated nerves will conduct sensory impulses more slowly.

E. Treatment

1. Treatment of acute attacks.
   a. **High-dose IV corticosteroids can shorten an acute attack.** Oral steroids have not shown the same efficacy.
   b. Studies have shown that treatment of **acute** exacerbations does **not** alter the outcome or course of MS.
   c. Most acute attacks resolve within 6 weeks with or without treatment.
2. Disease-modifying therapy.
   a. Interferon therapy.
      - Recombinant interferon β-1a, recombinant interferon β-1b, and glatiramer acetate have shown a reduction in relapse rates of 37%, 33%, and 29%, respectively.
      - The interferons can cause flu-like symptoms, which can be severe and persistent.
      - Interferon therapy should be started early in the course of disease before the disability becomes irreversible.
      - Present studies have lasted less than 5 years, so long-term benefits are unknown.
   b. Nonspecific immunosuppressive therapy such as cyclophosphamide should be reserved for rapidly progressive disease, because there are many toxic side effects of these drugs.
3. Symptomatic therapy:
   a. Baclofen or dantrolene for muscle spasticity.
   b. Carbamazepine or gabapentin for neuropathic pain.
   c. Treat depression if indicated.

Guillain–Barré Syndrome

A. General characteristics

1. Inflammatory demyelinating polyneuropathy that primarily affects motor nerves.
2. Usually preceded by a viral or mycoplasmal infection of upper respiratory or GI tract. Common infections include *Campylobacter jejuni,* CMV, hepatitis, and HIV.
3. May also occur in Hodgkin disease, lupus, after surgery, or after HIV seroconversion.

Quick HIT

Diagnostic Tests for MS (helpful hints)
- MRI is abnormal in 90% of MS patients.
- CSF is abnormal in 90% of MS patients.
- Evoked potentials are abnormal in 90% of MS patients.

Quick HIT

There is no cure for MS. There are two primary goals:
- Prevent relapses
- Relieve symptoms of acute exacerbations

Quick HIT

IV steroids help hasten recovery of the acute episode in MS but do not result in any improvement in long-term outcome.

Quick HIT

Prognosis for Guillain–Barré Syndrome
- Signs of recovery within 1 to 3 weeks after onset favor a good prognosis. If illness continues for a longer period (e.g., beyond 6 weeks), a chronic relapsing course is more likely and prognosis is less favorable.
- It may take months before the patient recovers. A minority of patients experience recurrent attacks, and about 5% die due to respiratory failure, pneumonia, or arrhythmias.

Quick HIT

Diagnosis made by a combination of CSF fluid analysis, clinical findings, and nerve conduction velocities.

Quick HIT

In Guillain–Barré syndrome, rapid progression to respiratory failure can occur within hours. Therefore, a timely and accurate diagnosis is critical. If you suspect Guillain–Barré syndrome, immediately admit the patient to the hospital for monitoring.

Quick HIT

Myasthenia gravis may be limited to extraocular muscles, especially in elderly patients.

B. Clinical features

1. Abrupt onset with rapidly **ascending weakness/paralysis** of all four extremities; frequently progresses to involve respiratory, facial, and bulbar muscles.
   a. Usually symmetric (but not always).
   b. Weakness may be mild or severe.
   c. Weakness usually progresses from distal to central muscles.
   d. **If generalized paralysis is present, it can lead to respiratory arrest.**
2. Extremities may be painful, but sensory loss is not typical.
3. Sphincter control and mentation are typically spared.
4. Autonomic features (e.g., arrhythmias, tachycardia, postural hypotension) are dangerous complications.

C. Diagnosis

1. CSF analysis—elevated protein, but normal cell count.
2. Electrodiagnostic studies—decreased motor nerve conduction velocity.

D. Treatment

1. Carefully monitor pulmonary function. Mechanical ventilation may be necessary.
2. Administer IV immunoglobulin if the patient has significant weakness. If progression continues, plasmapheresis may reduce severity of disease.
3. Do **not** give steroids. They are usually harmful and never helpful in Guillain–Barré syndrome.

Neuromuscular Diseases

Myasthenia Gravis

A. General characteristics

1. **Autoimmune disorder**—Autoantibodies are directed against the nicotinic acetylcholine receptors of the neuromuscular junction, which leads to a reduced postsynaptic response to acetylcholine and results in significant muscle fatigue.
2. Muscles that are stimulated repeatedly (e.g., extraocular muscles) are prone to fatigue.
3. The peak incidence in women is age 20 to 30; in men, 50 to 70. It is more common in women.

B. Clinical features

1. **Skeletal muscle weakness**—with preservation of sensation and reflexes.
   a. Weakness is exacerbated by continued use of muscle and improved by rest (see Clinical Pearl 5-9). Symptoms worsen toward the end of the day (due to fatigue).
   b. Involved muscles vary and may include the following:
      - Cranial muscles: extraocular muscles, eyelids (ptosis), facial muscles (facial weakness, difficulty in chewing, slurred speech).
      - Limb muscles (proximal and asymmetric).
2. Ptosis, diplopia, and blurred vision—most common initial symptoms.
3. Generalized weakness, dysarthria, and dysphagia.

CLINICAL PEARL 5-9

Lambert–Eaton Myasthenic Syndrome

- Associated with small cell lung cancer
- Caused by autoantibodies directed against **presynaptic** calcium channels
- Clinical features include proximal muscle weakness and hyporeflexia
- Distinguished from myasthenia gravis in that symptoms **improve** with repeated muscle stimulation

4. The condition progresses slowly with periodic exacerbations. **Myasthenic crisis is a medical emergency that occurs in 15% of patients.** Diaphragm and intercostal fatigue result in respiratory failure, often requiring mechanical ventilation.

C. Diagnosis

1. Acetylcholine receptor antibody test is the test of choice (most specific). Nevertheless, 20% of patients with clinical manifestations of myasthenia gravis may be "antibody negative."
2. EMG shows a decremental response to repetitive stimulation of motor nerves.
3. A CT scan of the thorax can rule out **thymoma.** Thymoma is present in only 10% to 15% of patients, but the thymus is histologically abnormal in 75% of patients.
4. Edrophonium (Tensilon) test—anticholinesterase (AChE) medications cause marked improvement of symptoms, but a high false-positive rate limits utility.

D. Treatment

1. AChE inhibitors—for example, pyridostigmine.
   a. Inhibiting AChE increases concentration of acetylcholine at the synapse by decreasing the breakdown of acetylcholine.
   b. This is a symptomatic benefit only.
2. Thymectomy.
   a. This provides a symptomatic benefit and complete remission in many patients, even in the absence of a thymoma.
   b. Although usually benign, thymoma is an absolute indication for thymectomy.
3. Immunosuppressive drugs.
   a. Use corticosteroids for patients with a poor response to AChE inhibitors.
   b. Azathioprine and cyclosporine are alternative third-line agents.
4. Plasmapheresis removes antibodies to acetylcholine receptors. Use it if all else fails or if the patient is in respiratory failure.
5. IV immunoglobulin therapy is now sometimes used for acute exacerbations.
6. Monitor serial forced vital capacities. A forced vital capacity of 15 mL/kg (about 1 L) is generally an indication for intubation. **Patients in myasthenic crisis have a low threshold for intubation—do not wait until the patient is hypoxic.**

Quick HIT

Medications that exacerbate symptoms of myasthenia gravis
- Antibiotics—aminoglycosides and tetracyclines
- β-blockers
- Antiarrhythmics—quinidine, procainamide, and lidocaine

Duchenne Muscular Dystrophy

A. General characteristics

1. **X-linked recessive** (almost exclusively in **males**) disease involving a mutation on a gene that codes for the dystrophin protein (dystrophin is absent causing muscle cells to die).
2. Characteristically, there is **no inflammation.**

B. Clinical features

1. Muscle weakness is progressive, symmetric, and starts in childhood. Proximal muscles primarily affected (pelvic girdle). Eventually involves the respiratory muscles.
2. *Gowers maneuver*—patient uses hands to get up from floor because the weakness in the proximal lower extremity muscles makes it difficult to arise without support.
3. Enlarged calf muscles—true muscle hypertrophy at first, followed by **pseudohypertrophy** as fat replaces muscle.
4. Ultimately results in wheelchair confinement, respiratory failure, and death in third decade.

C. Diagnosis

1. Serum creatine phosphokinase—levels are markedly elevated.
2. DNA testing has now replaced muscle biopsy for diagnosis.

D. Treatment

1. Prednisone is beneficial and is associated with a significant increase in strength, muscle function, and pulmonary function and may reduce risk of scoliosis.

Chronic steroid treatment does have side effects, but it is recommended for boys 5 years of age and older whose motor skills are declining.
2. Surgery to correct progressive scoliosis is often necessary once patient becomes wheelchair dependent.

Becker Muscular Dystrophy

- Less common than Duchenne muscular dystrophy
- Also X-linked recessive
- Similar to Duchenne muscular dystrophy, but there is **later onset and a less severe course.** Some dystrophin is present.

Quick HIT

Other Hereditary Causes of Muscle Weakness
- Mitochondrial disorders: associated with maternal inheritance and ragged red muscle fibers
- Glycogen storage diseases such as McArdle disease (autosomal recessive, muscle cramping after exercise due to glycogen phosphorylase deficiency)

Neurocutaneous Syndromes

Neurofibromatosis Type I (von Recklinghausen Disease)

- **Autosomal dominant** disease characterized by café au lait spots, neurofibromas, CNS tumors (gliomas, meningiomas), axillary or inguinal freckling, iris hamartomas (*Lisch nodules*), bony lesions.
- Cutaneous neurofibromas—may be disfiguring.
- Complications include scoliosis, pheochromocytomas, optic nerve gliomas, renal artery stenosis, and erosive bone defects. Musculoskeletal manifestations include spinal deformity and congenital tibial dysplasia.
- Complications may require treatment. Surgically excise any symptomatic neurofibromas.

Quick HIT

Other features that may be present in neurofibromatosis patients (both types)
- Seizures
- Mental retardation, learning disabilities
- Short height
- Macrocephalic

Neurofibromatosis Type II

- **Autosomal dominant** disease; less common than type I neurofibromatosis.
- Clinical features include bilateral (sometimes unilateral) acoustic neuromas (classic finding), multiple meningiomas, café au lait spots, neurofibromas (much less common than type I), and cataracts.

Quick HIT

In patients with neurofibromatosis, prognosis depends on the type and number of tumors and their location. Most patients can function well.

Tuberous Sclerosis

- Usually autosomal dominant.
- Presents with cognitive impairment, epilepsy, and skin lesions (including facial angiofibromas, adenoma sebaceum).
- Retinal hamartomas, renal angiomyolipomas, and rhabdomyomas of the heart may also be present.
- Treat complications.

Sturge–Weber Syndrome

- Acquired disease.
- Key pathologic feature is the presence of capillary angiomatoses of the pia mater.
- Classic feature is facial vascular nevi (port-wine stain).
- Epilepsy and mental retardation are usually present.
- Treatment of epilepsy is often the mainstay of treatment.

Von Hippel–Lindau Disease

- Autosomal dominant.
- Important features are cavernous hemangiomas of the brain or brainstem, renal angiomas, and cysts in multiple organs.
- Associated with renal cell carcinoma.
- Associated with pheochromocytomas.

Spinal Cord Diseases

Syringomyelia

- Central cavitation of the cervical cord due to abnormal collection of fluid within the spinal cord parenchyma (Figure 5-5).
- Most commonly associated with Arnold–Chiari malformation. Other causes are posttraumatic, postinfectious, tethered cord, intramedullary tumors.
- Clinical features—most often asymptomatic and discovered incidentally on MRI obtained for other reasons. Symptoms may include **bilateral loss of pain** and temperature sensation over the shoulders in a **"cape-like" distribution** (lateral spinothalamic tract involvement), preservation of touch, thoracic scoliosis and muscle atrophy of the hands may occur.
- Diagnosed by MRI.
- Treatment depends on size of syrinx, symptoms, and associated findings (Chiari, tethered cord). Evaluation by neurosurgery recommended.

Brown-Séquard Syndrome

- Spinal cord hemisection (i.e., lesion involving either the right or the left half of the spinal cord), usually at the cervical levels (where spinal cord enlarges) (see Figure 5-5).
- Causes include trauma (e.g., fracture, stab wound) that causes hemisection of spinal cord or most commonly, a crush injury to one side of spinal cord, tumors, and abscesses (less common).
- Clinical features: **contralateral loss of pain and temperature** (spinothalamic tract), **ipsilateral hemiparesis** (corticospinal tract), and **ipsilateral loss** of position/vibration (dorsal columns).
- Prognosis for neurologic recovery is very good.

Transverse Myelitis

- This is a rare condition that specifically affects the tracts across the horizontal aspect of the spinal cord at a given level. The thoracic spine is the most commonly involved.
- The cause is usually unknown, but it can occur after viral infections. Progression is usually rapid.
- Clinical features include lower extremity weakness or plegia, back pain, sensory deficits below the level of the lesion, and sphincter disturbance (especially urinary retention).
- MRI with contrast is the imaging study of choice.
- High-dose steroid therapy is often used, but evidence supporting its use is equivocal.
- The prognosis is highly variable and unpredictable, ranging from full recovery to death.

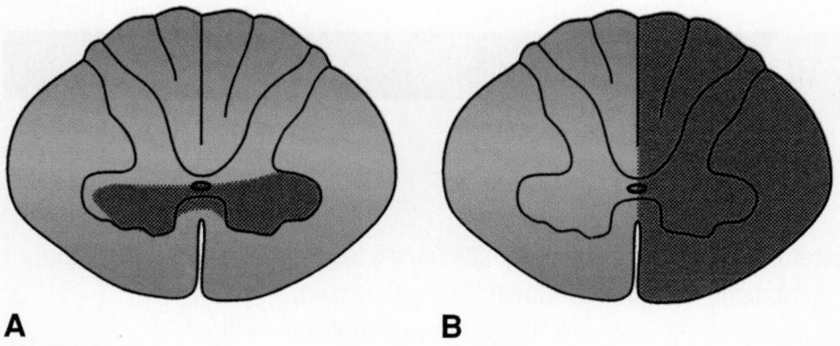

FIGURE 5-5 Classic lesions of the spinal cord. A: Syringomyelia. B: Hemisection of the spinal cord (Brown-Séquard syndrome).

(From Fix JD. *High-Yield Neuroanatomy.* 2nd ed. Philadelphia, PA: Lippincott Williams & Wilkins, 2000:46, Figure 8-2H and E, respectively.)

Horner Syndrome

A. General characteristics

1. Results from the interruption of cervical sympathetic nerves
2. Can be preganglionic (central lesions) or postganglionic (distal to superior cervical ganglion); the former is more worrisome and requires more thorough evaluation

B. Clinical features

1. Ipsilateral **ptosis**—mild drooping of lid (levator palpebrae still intact)
2. Ipsilateral **miosis**—"pinpoint pupil"
3. Ipsilateral **anhidrosis** (decreased sweating on forehead)—may be difficult to detect

C. Causes

1. Idiopathic (most cases)
2. Pancoast tumor (pulmonary neoplasm of the superior sulcus at lung apex)
3. Internal carotid dissection
4. Brainstem stroke
5. Neck trauma (cervical spine injury)

Poliomyelitis

- Poliovirus affects the anterior horn cells and motor neurons of spinal cord and brainstem. Causes lower motor neuron involvement.
- Characteristic features include asymmetric muscle weakness (legs more commonly involved); absent deep tendon reflexes; flaccid, atrophic muscles; and **normal sensation.**
- Bulbar involvement (of CN IX and CN X) in 10% to 15% of cases can lead to respiratory and cardiovascular impairment.
- No treatment is available, although poliomyelitis is entirely preventable by vaccination.

Miscellaneous Conditions

Dizziness

A. General characteristics

1. There are three major causes of dizziness.
   a. Presyncope (lightheadedness).
   b. Vertigo (see Clinical Pearl 5-10 and Vertigo section below).
   c. Multisensory stimuli—This happens in times of profound shock or overwhelming sensory overload (e.g., standing over the Grand Canyon or hearing shocking news).
2. Many conditions cause a sensation of "dizziness": cerebellar disease, cerebrovascular disease, TIAs, hyperventilation, anxiety, panic attacks, and phobias.

CLINICAL PEARL 5-10

Vertigo

Central Vertigo

- Gradual onset; other neurologic (brainstem) findings are present in most cases (e.g., weakness, hemiplegia, diplopia, dysphagia, dysarthria, facial numbness). Look for cardiovascular risk factors.
- Accompanying nystagmus can be bidirectional or vertical (does not occur in peripheral vertigo).

Peripheral Vertigo

- Lesions are cochlear or retrocochlear.
- Abrupt onset, nausea/vomiting, head position has strong effect on symptoms. Other brainstem deficits are absent, except for tinnitus/hearing loss.

B. Diagnosis

1. Audiogram—if vestibular symptoms present
2. CT scan/MRA—if TIA is suspected
3. MRI of posterior fossa—if structural lesion is suspected

C. Treatment: Treat the underlying cause.

Vertigo

A. General characteristics

1. Vertigo refers to a disturbance of the vestibular system characterized by a sensation of spinning or hallucination of movement.
2. The initial goal is to determine whether the cause of the vertigo is peripheral (inner ear) or central (e.g., tumor, CVA).
3. Peripheral vertigo is usually benign, but central vertigo can have serious consequences.

B. Types of peripheral vertigo

1. Benign positional vertigo (BPV).
   a. Vertigo is experienced only in specific positions or during change in position and lasts for a few moments. It has an abrupt onset as soon as the particular position is assumed.
   b. Usually presents in patients over 60 years old. Treat with meclizine.
   c. Recovery is usually complete (resolves within 6 months).
2. Ménière disease.
   a. Triad of **vertigo, tinnitus, and hearing loss.**
   b. Attacks may last for hours to days and recur several months or years later.
   c. The hearing loss eventually becomes permanent.
   d. Treat with sodium restriction and diuretics.
3. Acute labyrinthitis—due to viral infection of the cochlea and labyrinth; may last for several days.
4. Ototoxic drugs (aminoglycosides, some loop diuretics).
5. Acoustic neuroma (schwannoma) of the 8th cranial nerve—ataxia, gait unsteadiness, nystagmus, hearing loss, tinnitus.

Quick HIT

In a patient with vertigo, goal is to differentiate between peripheral (benign) and central (worrisome) vertigo (see Table 5-5). If in doubt, an MRI of the brainstem is the best imaging study to rule out an ischemic event.

Quick HIT

Hearing loss and tinnitus only occur with peripheral vertigo. Focal neurologic problems only occur with central vertigo.

Quick HIT

BPV is vertigo and nystagmus without hearing loss or tinnitus.

Quick HIT

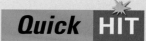

Meclizine is useful for vertigo and as an antiemetic. It has anticholinergic and antihistamine effects.

TABLE 5-5 Central Versus Peripheral Vertigo

Central Vertigo	Peripheral Vertigo
Gradual onset	Sudden onset
Mild intensity	Severe intensity
Mild nausea/vomiting	Intense nausea/vomiting
Associated neurologic findings typically present	No associated neurologic findings
Mild nystagmus	Relatively intense nystagmus
Position change has mild effect	Position change has intense effect
No refractoriness—can repeat the "tilt" test and patient responds every time	Rapidly refractory—cannot repeat the "tilt" test; patient will not respond again
Patient falls to same side as lesion	Patient falls to same side as lesion
Direction of nystagmus: multidirectional and even vertical	Direction of nystagmus: unilateral vertical; nystagmus is never peripheral

C. Causes of central vertigo

1. MS—demyelination of vestibular pathways of brainstem
2. Vertebrobasilar insufficiency
3. Migraine-associated vertigo—headache may or may not be present

Syncope

A. General characteristics

1. Syncope refers to a transient loss of consciousness/postural tone secondary to acute decrease in cerebral blood flow.
2. It is characterized by rapid recovery of consciousness without resuscitation.

B. Causes

1. Seizure disorder
2. Cardiac
   a. Cardiac syncope is usually sudden and without prodromal symptoms—for example, the patient's face hits the floor
   b. Syncope may be the first manifestation of a life-threatening cardiac condition
   c. Causes
      - Arrhythmias (e.g., sick sinus syndrome, ventricular tachycardia, AV block, rapid supraventricular tachycardia)
      - Obstruction of blood flow (e.g., aortic stenosis, hypertrophic cardiomyopathy, pulmonary HTN, atrial myxoma, prolapsed mitral valve, severe asymmetric septal hypertrophy)
      - Massive MI
3. Vasovagal syncope ("neurocardiogenic," "vasodepressor," "simple faints")
   a. Most **common cause of syncope**; may account for up to 50% of all cases of syncope
   b. Most people have one episode, but for some it is a recurrent problem
   c. Clues to diagnosis
      - Emotional stress, pain, fear, extreme fatigue, or claustrophobic situations as precipitating factors
      - Premonitory symptoms (pallor, diaphoresis, lightheadedness, nausea, dimming of vision, roaring in the ears)
      - Can occur at any age, but if the first episode is after age 40, be reluctant to make this diagnosis
      - **Tilt-table study can reproduce the symptoms in susceptible people**
   d. Pathophysiology
      - Normally, standing up causes blood to pool in the lower extremities (leading to a decrease in cardiac output, stroke volume, and BP). These changes are compensated for by increased sympathetic tone (leading to vasoconstriction and tachycardia), and decreased parasympathetic tone
      - In patients with vasovagal syncope, the compensatory response is interrupted in a few minutes by a paradoxical withdrawal of sympathetic stimulation and a replacement by enhanced parasympathetic (vagal) activity. This leads to an inappropriate bradycardia, vasodilation, marked decrease in BP, and cerebral perfusion
   e. Treatment
      - Can usually be reversed by assuming the supine posture and elevating the legs
      - β-blockers and disopyramide
      - Prognosis is excellent (there is no heart disease or arrhythmias)
   f. Prevention—avoid circumstances that precipitate attack
4. Orthostatic hypotension (ganglionic-blocking agents, diabetes, old age, prolonged bed rest)
   a. Caused by defect in vasomotor reflexes; overlaps with vasovagal syncope
   b. Common in elderly people; diabetics (autonomic neuropathy); patients taking ganglionic-blocking agents, vasodilators, diuretics

Quick HIT

Prognosis of syncope is generally good, unless cardiac disease is the underlying cause.

Quick HIT

Two ways to differentiate between seizures and syncope
- In seizures, duration of unconsciousness tends to be longer. In syncope, loss of consciousness is momentary.
- In syncope, bladder control is usually retained, but in seizures it is often lost.

Quick HIT

Vasovagal and orthostatic syncope occur when the patient is upright (sitting up or standing). They do not occur when the patient is recumbent.

Quick HIT

If syncope occurs with exertion, assess for potentially life-threatening causes such as hypertrophic cardiomyopathy or aortic stenosis.

   c. Posture is the main cause here. Sudden standing and prolonged standing are the precipitating causes. A positive tilt-table test result is expected
   d. It is also associated with premonitory symptoms (lightheadedness, nausea, and so on)
   e. Treat with increased sodium intake and fluids. Consider fludrocortisone
5. Severe cerebrovascular disease
   a. A rare cause of syncope
   b. A TIA involving the **vertebrobasilar** circulation may lead to syncope ("drop attacks")
   c. One practically never sees dizziness (or vertigo) in isolation with vertebrobasilar insufficiency—there will always be other deficits as well
6. Other noncardiogenic causes include metabolic causes (e.g., hypoglycemia, hyperventilation), hypovolemia (e.g., hemorrhage), hypersensitivity (syncope precipitated by wearing a tight collar or turning the head), mechanical reduction of venous return (e.g., Valsalva maneuver, postmicturition), and various medications (e.g., β-blockers, nitrates, antiarrhythmic agents)

Quick HIT

Syncope is uncommon in setting of a stroke, unless the vertebrobasilar system is involved.

C. Diagnosis

1. First, attempt to rule out conditions that are life-threatening (e.g., MI, hemorrhage, and arrhythmias) (Figure 5-6)

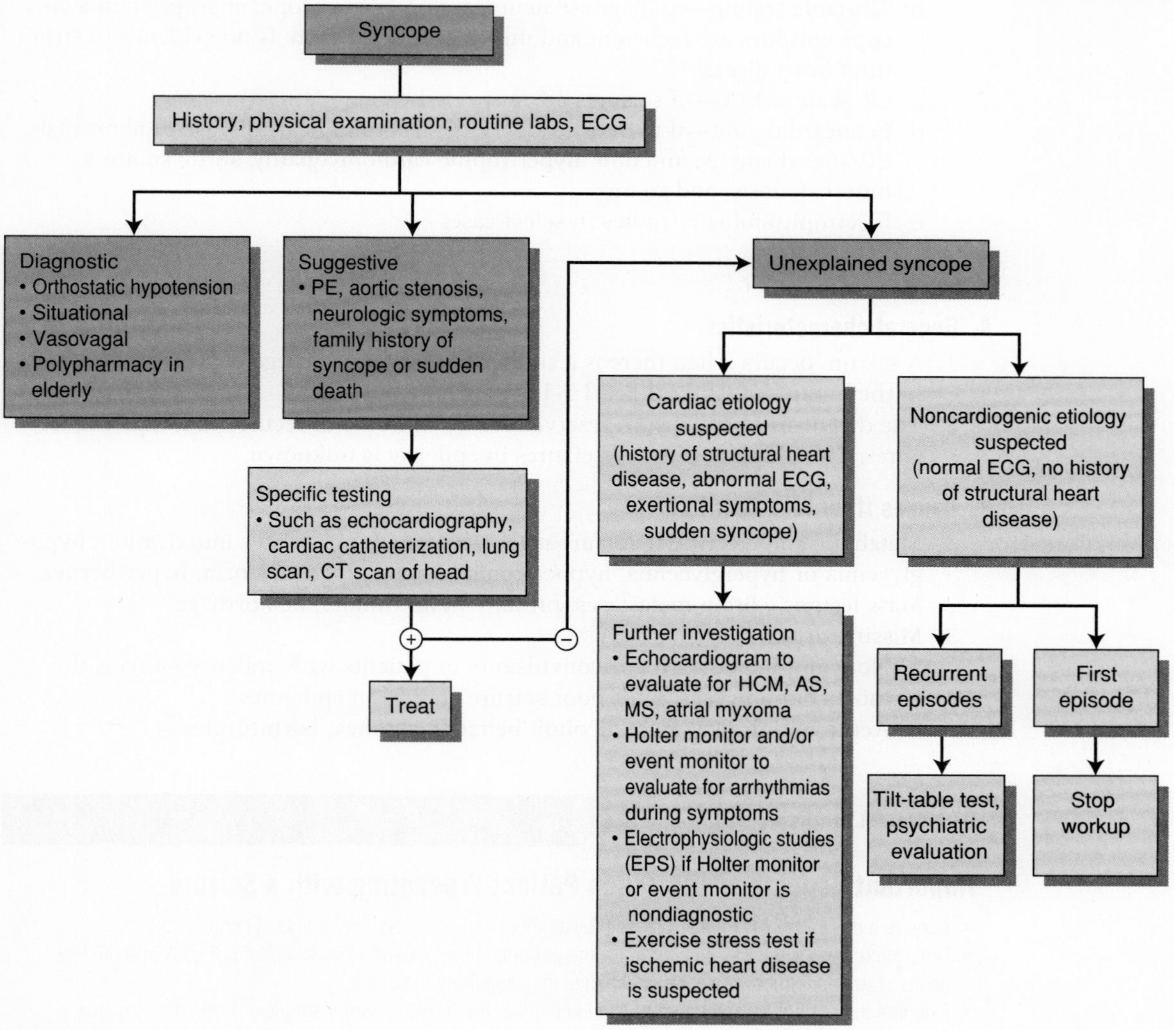

FIGURE 5-6 Syncope flowchart.

(Adapted from Heaven DJ, Sutton R. Syncope. *Crit Care Med.* 2000;28(10 Suppl):118, Fig. 1. Copyright © 2000 Lippincott Williams & Wilkins.)

Quick HIT

Evaluating syncope
- The most important factors in decision making in syncope patients are presence/absence of structural heart disease and abnormal ECG.
- If the patient has no heart disease and syncope is unexplained, the most important test is tilt-table testing for evaluation of vasovagal syncope.

2. The main goal is to **differentiate between cardiac and noncardiac etiologies**, because the prognosis is poorest for those with underlying heart disease
3. History
   a. Three key elements need to be determined: events before, during, and after the syncopal episode
   b. Check the patient's medications—this is especially important in elderly patients
   c. Seek reports from witnesses of the syncopal event
4. Physical examination (priority given to cardiovascular system)
   a. BP and pulse measurements in supine, sitting, and standing positions
   b. Mental status (postictal state)
   c. Murmurs (aortic stenosis, hypertrophic cardiomyopathy)
   d. Carotid pulses—auscultated for bruits
   e. Apply pressure to the carotid sinus—observe for reflex bradycardia and hypotension
5. Diagnosis
   a. **ECG** can identify life-threatening causes (ventricular tachycardia, other arrhythmias, ischemia). **Obtain ECG for all patients**
   b. CBC, metabolic panel, may be appropriate
6. Additional diagnostic tests
   a. Twenty-four–hour ambulatory ECG recording (Holter monitoring) and/or event monitor—if arrhythmia is suspected and H&P and ECG are nondiagnostic
   b. Tilt-table testing—to diagnose neurocardiogenic syncope; appropriate if syncope episodes are recurrent and unexplained and there is no evidence of structural heart disease
   c. CT scan or EEG—if seizures are suspected
   d. Echocardiogram—if there is evidence of structural heart disease or abnormal ECG; evaluate LV function, hypertrophic cardiomyopathy, aortic stenosis, mitral stenosis, and so on
   e. Electrophysiologic studies in select cases

Seizures

A. General characteristics

1. A seizure occurs when there is a sudden abnormal discharge of electrical activity in the brain (see Clinical Pearl 5-11).
2. The diagnosis of epilepsy is reserved for a syndrome of recurrent, idiopathic seizures. The ultimate cause of seizures in epilepsy is unknown.

B. Causes (four M's, four I's)

1. Metabolic and electrolyte disturbances—hyponatremia, water intoxication, hypoglycemia or hyperglycemia, hypocalcemia, uremia, thyroid storm, hyperthermia
2. Mass lesions—brain metastases, primary brain tumors, hemorrhage
3. Missing drugs
   a. **Noncompliance with anticonvulsants** in patients with epilepsy—this is the most common reason for poor seizure control in epileptics
   b. **Acute withdrawal from alcohol, benzodiazepines, barbiturates**

CLINICAL PEARL 5-11

Important Aspects of H & P in a Patient Presenting with a Seizure

- Acquire a description of the seizure from bystanders (e.g., postictal state, loss of continence).
- Determine what is the baseline state for the patient. Is the patient a known epileptic? Look into missed doses of antiepileptics, or any recent change in dosages/medications.
- Examine the patient for any injuries—head or spine, fractures, posterior shoulder dislocation, tongue lacerations, bowel/bladder incontinence.
- Look for signs of increased ICP.
- Perform a complete neurologic examination.

4. Miscellaneous
   a. Pseudoseizures—not true seizures but are psychiatric in origin; are often difficult to distinguish from true seizures without an EEG
   b. Eclampsia—A preeclamptic pregnant woman seizing no longer has preeclampsia! The only definitive treatment for eclampsia is delivery, but a magnesium infusion is the pharmacologic treatment of choice
   c. Hypertensive encephalopathy—severe hypertension can cause cerebral edema
5. Intoxications—cocaine, lithium, lidocaine, theophylline, metal poisoning (e.g., mercury, lead), carbon monoxide poisoning
6. Infections—septic shock, bacterial or viral meningitis, brain abscess
7. Ischemia—stroke, TIA (common cause of seizure in elderly patients)
8. Increased ICP—for example, due to trauma

Quick HIT

Partial seizures may evolve into generalized seizures. When this happens, it is called **secondary generalization.**

C. Types of epileptic seizures

1. Partial seizure—accounts for 70% of patients with epilepsy older than 18 years of age (Figure 5-7). It begins in one part of the brain (typically the temporal lobe) and initially produces symptoms that are referable to the region of the cortex involved.
   a. Simple partial seizure.
      - **Consciousness remains intact.** The seizure remains localized but may evolve into a complex partial seizure.
      - May involve transient unilateral clonic–tonic movement.
   b. Complex partial seizure.
      - **Consciousness is impaired**; postictal confusion.
      - Automatisms (last 1 to 3 minutes)—purposeless, involuntary, repetitive movements (such as lip smacking or chewing); patients may become aggressive if restraint is attempted.
      - Olfactory or gustatory hallucinations.
2. Generalized seizure—characterized by **loss of consciousness.** Involves disruption of electrical activity in the entire brain.
   a. Tonic–clonic (grand mal) seizure—bilaterally symmetric and without focal onset
      - Begins with sudden loss of consciousness—a fall to the ground

Quick HIT

It is important (although sometimes difficult) to differentiate between absence (petit mal) and complex partial seizures because their treatments are different. Also, absence seizures disappear in adulthood, whereas complex partial seizures do not.

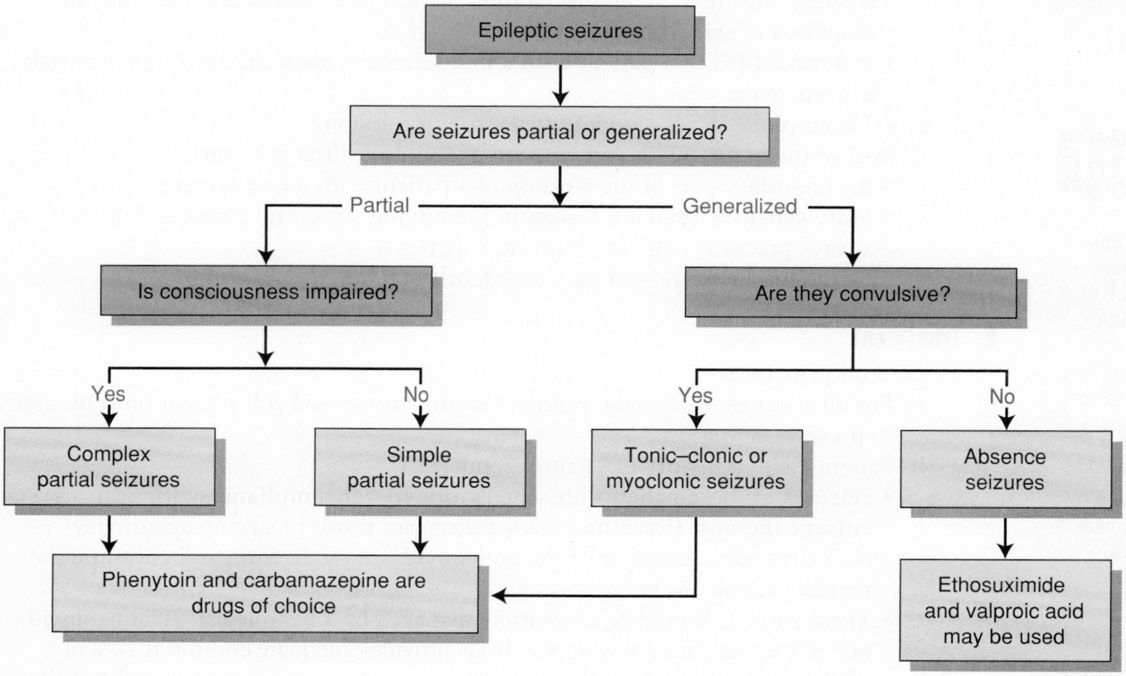

FIGURE 5-7 **Epileptic seizure flowchart.**
(Adapted from Humes DH, DuPont HL, Gardner LB, et al. *Kelley's Textbook of Internal Medicine.* 4th ed. Philadelphia, PA: Lippincott Williams & Wilkins, 2000:2866, Figure 426.1.)

- Tonic phase—The patient becomes rigid; trunk and limb extension occurs. The patient may become apneic during this phase.
- Clonic phase—This is musculature jerking of the limbs and body for at least 30 seconds.
- The patient then becomes flaccid and comatose before regaining consciousness.
- Postictal confusion and drowsiness are characteristic and can last for hours, although 10 to 30 minutes is more typical.
- Other features may include tongue biting, vomiting, apnea, and incontinence (urine and/or feces).

b. Absence (petit mal) seizure.
- Typically involves school-age children—usually resolves as child grows older.
- Patient seems to disengage from current activity and "stare into space"—then returns to the activity several seconds later; patient looks "absent minded" during these episodes, which are often confused with "daydreaming."
- Episodes are brief (lasting a few seconds) but may be quite frequent (up to 100 times per day).
- Impairment of consciousness but **no** loss of postural tone or continence, and no postictal confusion.
- Minor clonic activity (eye blinks or head nodding) in up to 45% of cases.

D. Diagnosis

1. If the patient has a known seizure disorder (epileptic), check anticonvulsant levels—This is usually the only test that is needed. Because therapeutic anticonvulsant levels are variable, **one dose may be toxic for one patient and therapeutic for another.** Therefore, take the range given in laboratory reports as a general guideline.
2. If the patient history is unclear or if this is the patient's first seizure:
   a. CBC, electrolytes, blood glucose, LFTs, renal function tests, serum calcium, urinalysis.
   b. EEG
   - Although the EEG is the most helpful diagnostic test in the diagnosis of a seizure disorder, an abnormal EEG pattern alone is not adequate for the diagnosis of seizures.
   - A normal EEG in a patient with a first seizure is associated with a lower risk of recurrence.

   c. CT scan of the head—to identify a structural lesion.
   d. MRI of the brain—with and without gadolinium (first without).
   - An important part of the workup of a patient with a first seizure.
   - **More sensitive than a CT scan** in identifying structural changes, but not always practical (e.g., in an unstable patient).

   e. LP and blood cultures—if patient is febrile.

E. Treatment

1. General principles.
   a. For all seizures, ABCs take priority: Secure airway and roll patient onto his side to prevent aspiration.
   b. Patients with a history of seizures (epilepsy).
   - Seizures in these patients are usually due to **noncompliance with anticonvulsant therapy.** (Even one missed dose can result in subtherapeutic levels.) Give a loading dose of the anticonvulsant medication and continue the regular regimen as before.
   - These patients should be chronically managed by a neurologist. Treatment with one of the standard antiepileptic drugs provides adequate control in 70% of adult patients. In another 15% to 20%, a combination regimen controls seizures.
   - If seizures persist, increase the dosage of the first anticonvulsant until signs of toxicity appear. Add a second drug if the seizures cannot be controlled with the drug of first choice.

Quick HIT

Laboratory values to check immediately in an unfamiliar, seizing patient
- Serum calcium
- Serum sodium
- Serum glucose or Accu-Chek
- BUN

Quick HIT

Status Epilepticus
- Refers to prolonged, sustained unconsciousness with persistent convulsive activity in a seizing patient
- A medical emergency, with a mortality rate of up to 20%
- May be caused by poor compliance with medication, alcohol withdrawal, intracranial infection, neoplasm, a metabolic disorder, or a drug overdose
- Management involves establishing an airway, and **giving IV diazepam,** IV phenytoin, and 50 mg dextrose. Treat resistant cases with IV phenobarbital.

- If the seizures are controlled, have the patient continue the medication for at least 2 years. If the patient remains seizure free, taper the medication(s) cautiously. Confirm this decision with a lack of seizure activity on the EEG.

c. Patient with a first seizure.
- EEG and neurology consult—first steps.
- Anticonvulsant therapy—weigh risks and benefits of treatment and the risk of recurrence before initiating.
- With a normal EEG, the risk of recurrence is relatively low (15% in the first year), compared to the risk with an abnormal EEG (41% in the first year).
- Do not treat patients with a single seizure. Antiepileptic drugs are started if EEG is abnormal, brain MRI is abnormal, patient is in status epilepticus.

2. Anticonvulsant agents.
   a. For generalized tonic–clonic seizures and partial seizures:
   - **Phenytoin and carbamazepine are the drugs of choice.** They are equally effective, and side-effect profiles are similar.
   - Other options include phenobarbital, valproate, and primidone.

   b. For petit mal (absence) seizures, ethosuximide and valproic acid are the drugs of choice.

Quick HIT

Remember that anticonvulsants are teratogenic. (Do a pregnancy test before prescribing!)

Amyotrophic Lateral Sclerosis or "Lou Gehrig Disease"

A. General characteristics

1. A disorder affecting the anterior horn cells and corticospinal tracts at many levels. Corticobulbar involvement is common as well. **The presence of upper and lower motor neuron signs is a hallmark of amyotrophic lateral sclerosis (ALS).** Note that only the motor system is involved.
2. Onset is usually between 50 and 70 years of age. (Lou Gehrig was unusually young [in his 30s] when the disease developed.) Occurrence of ALS before age 40 is uncommon.
3. Only 10% of cases are familial, with the remainder being sporadic.
4. Prognosis is dismal: 80% mortality rate at 5 years; 100% mortality rate at 10 years.

Quick HIT

Initially ALS can involve virtually any muscle, but as the disease progresses, every region of the body becomes symmetrically involved.

B. Clinical features

1. **Progressive muscle weakness is the hallmark feature**
   a. Usually first noted in the legs or arms, but then spreads to other muscle groups
   b. No associated pain
   c. Muscle atrophy
2. Muscle cramps and spasticity
3. Fasciculations (unnoticed by patient)
4. Impaired speech and swallowing; dysphagia can lead to aspiration
5. Respiratory muscle weakness—dyspnea on exertion, and later, at rest; orthopnea; sleep apnea; end-stage ALS is characterized by respiratory failure
6. Weight loss and fatigue
7. The following are normal and unaffected, even in late stages:
   a. Bowel and bladder control
   b. Sensation
   c. Cognitive function
   d. Extraocular muscles
   e. Sexual function

C. Diagnosis

1. There is no specific diagnostic test for ALS. EMG and nerve conduction studies can confirm degeneration of lower motor neurons and can rule out neuromuscular junction disorders
2. Clinical or electrical evidence
   a. Involvement of two regions (probable ALS)
   b. Involvement of three to four regions (definite ALS)—affected regions include bulbar (face, larynx, tongue, jaw), cervical, thoracic, and lumbosacral

Quick HIT

EMG and Nerve Conduction Studies
- EMG measures the contractile properties of skeletal muscles
- Lower motor neuron lesions: fibrillations and fasciculations at rest
- Myopathy: No electrical activity at rest (as expected), but amplitude decreases with muscle contraction.
- Nerve conduction studies
- Demyelination decreases nerve conduction velocity (MS, Guillain–Barré syndrome)
- Repetitive stimulation causes fatigue (myasthenia gravis)

Quick HIT

The most common cause of aphasia is cerebrovascular disease. In aphasia, when speech is fluent, the lesion is posterior to the central sulcus. When speech is nonfluent, the lesion is anterior to the central sulcus.

D. Treatment
1. Treatment has been very disappointing and is mainly supportive.
2. Riluzole is a glutamate-blocking agent—it may delay death by only 3 to 5 months.

Aphasia

A. General characteristics
1. Aphasia is the **loss or defect of language** (e.g., in speaking, fluency, reading, writing, comprehension of written or spoken material).
2. Most lesions that cause aphasia involve the **dominant hemisphere.**
   a. In 95% of right-handed people, the left cerebral hemisphere is dominant for language.
   b. In 50% of left-handed people, the left hemisphere is dominant for language (however, the right hemisphere also has language functions in most left-handed people).
3. There are four types of aphasia (described below): Wernicke aphasia, Broca aphasia, conduction aphasia, and global aphasia.

B. Causes
1. Stroke (most common cause)
2. Trauma to brain
3. Brain tumor
4. Alzheimer disease

C. Types of aphasia
1. Wernicke aphasia
   a. Receptive, fluent aphasia
   b. **Impaired comprehension of written or spoken language (key feature)**
   c. **Speech is grammatically correct and is fluid but does not make much sense.** Patients articulate well but often use the wrong words because they cannot understand their own words
2. Broca aphasia
   a. Expressive, nonfluent aphasia
   b. Speech is slow and requires effort
   c. The patient uses short sentences (as few words as possible) without grammatical construction. The content is appropriate and meaningful
   d. Good comprehension of language (written and spoken)
   e. Often associated with a right hemiparesis and hemisensory loss
3. Conduction aphasia
   a. Disturbance in repetition
   b. Pathology involves the connections between Wernicke and Broca areas
4. Global aphasia
   a. Disturbance in all areas of language function (e.g., comprehension, speaking, reading, fluency)
   b. Often associated with a right hemiparesis

D. Treatment of aphasia
1. Most patients spontaneously recover or improve within the first month.
2. Speech therapy is helpful, but is unlikely to be of much benefit after the first few months.

Bell Palsy

A. General characteristics
1. This refers to hemifacial weakness/paralysis of muscles innervated by **CN VII** due to swelling of the cranial nerve.
2. The prognosis is very good; 80% of patients recover fully within weeks to months.

B. Causes
1. Cause is uncertain.

2. Possible viral etiology (herpes simplex)—immunologic and ischemic factors implicated as well.
3. Upper respiratory infection is a common preceding event.

C. Clinical features: There is acute onset of unilateral facial weakness/paralysis. Both upper and lower parts of the face are affected.

D. Diagnosis

1. Diagnosis is clinical, but consider Lyme disease in endemic areas as the treatment approach is different.
2. **Do not use steroids if Lyme is suspected!**
3. Consider EMG testing if paresis fails to resolve within 10 days.

E. Treatment

1. Usually none is required, as most cases resolve in 1 month.
2. Short course of steroid therapy (prednisone) and acyclovir, if necessary.
3. Patient should wear eye patch at night to prevent corneal abrasion (cornea is exposed due to weakness of orbicularis oculi muscle).
4. Surgical decompression of CN VII is indicated if the paralysis progresses or if tests indicate deterioration.

> **Quick HIT**
>
> **Differential Diagnosis for Facial Nerve Palsy**
> - Trauma (e.g., temporal bone, forceps delivery)
> - Lyme disease
> - Tumor (acoustic neuroma, cholesteatoma, neurofibroma)
> - Guillain–Barré syndrome (palsy is usually bilateral)
> - Herpes zoster

Trigeminal Neuralgia (Tic Douloureux)

A. General characteristics

1. **Trigeminal neuralgia is one of the most painful conditions known to mankind.**
2. Usually idiopathic in origin.

B. Clinical features

1. Brief (seconds to minutes) but frequent attacks of severe, lancinating facial pain
2. Involves the jaw, lips, gums, and maxillary area (ophthalmic division is less commonly affected)
3. Recurrent attacks may continue for weeks at a time.
4. No motor or sensory paralysis

> **Quick HIT**
>
> **Trigeminal Neuralgia**
> - Complete, spontaneous resolution in 85% of cases
> - Mild residual disease in 10% of cases
> - No resolution in 5% of cases

C. Diagnosis

1. Clinical diagnosis
2. MRI—to rule out cerebellopontine angle tumor

D. Treatment

1. Drug of choice is **carbamazepine** (usually effective in relieving pain); other choices are baclofen and phenytoin, either alone or in combination with carbamazepine.
2. Consider surgical decompression if medical therapy fails.
3. Patients typically experience a remitting/relapsing course. Over time, pain may become more refractory to treatment.

How to Localize a Neurologic Lesion

A. Introduction

1. Generally, neurologic deficits can be localized to one of the following 10 sites:
   a. Cerebral cortex
   b. Subcortical area
   c. Cerebellum
   d. Brainstem
   e. Spinal cord
   f. Plexus (plexopathy)
   g. Roots (radiculopathy)
   h. Peripheral nerve (peripheral neuropathy)
   i. Neuromuscular junction
   j. Muscle (myopathy)

2. Lesions in each of the above sites present with different neurologic findings. A good understanding of the deficits that accompany each lesion can help with localization.

B. Cerebral cortex

1. Lesions in the cerebral cortex often cause two main deficits:
   a. **Contralateral** motor or sensory deficits (depending on which region of the cortex is involved)
   b. Aphasia
2. The hemiparesis seen with cortical lesions primarily affects the face, arms, and trunk. The legs may be affected, but typically that deficit is not as severe. This is because the neurons that control the lower extremities are in the interhemispheric fissure (see homunculus in Figure 5-8)

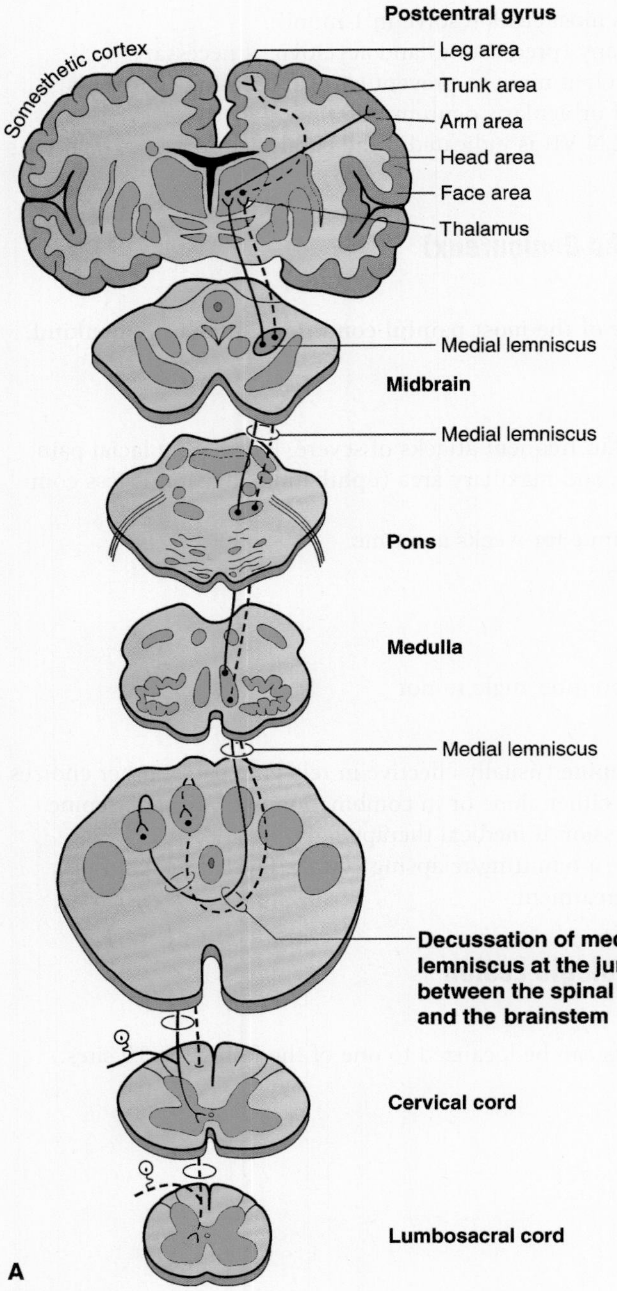

FIGURE 5-8 **A: Dorsal column–medial lemniscus pathway.** ***(continued)***
(**A** from Fix JD. *High-Yield Neuroanatomy.* 2nd ed. Philadelphia, PA: Lippincott Williams & Wilkins, 2000:39, Figure 7-2.)

3. Aphasia is common when the left hemisphere is involved. Visual-spatial deficits are more common when the right hemisphere is involved.

C. Subcortical lesions

1. These involve the internal capsule, cerebral peduncles, thalamus, and pons.
2. The hemiparesis is usually **complete** (face, arm, leg) because the neurons controlling these structures all merge together subcortically and are very close together.

D. Cerebellum: incoordination, intention tremor, ataxia

E. Brainstem

1. Cranial nerve and spinal cord findings.
2. There is a **crossed** hemiplegia (deficit on ipsilateral face and contralateral body) because the corticospinal tract, dorsal columns, and spinothalamic tracts cross but the cranial nerves do not.

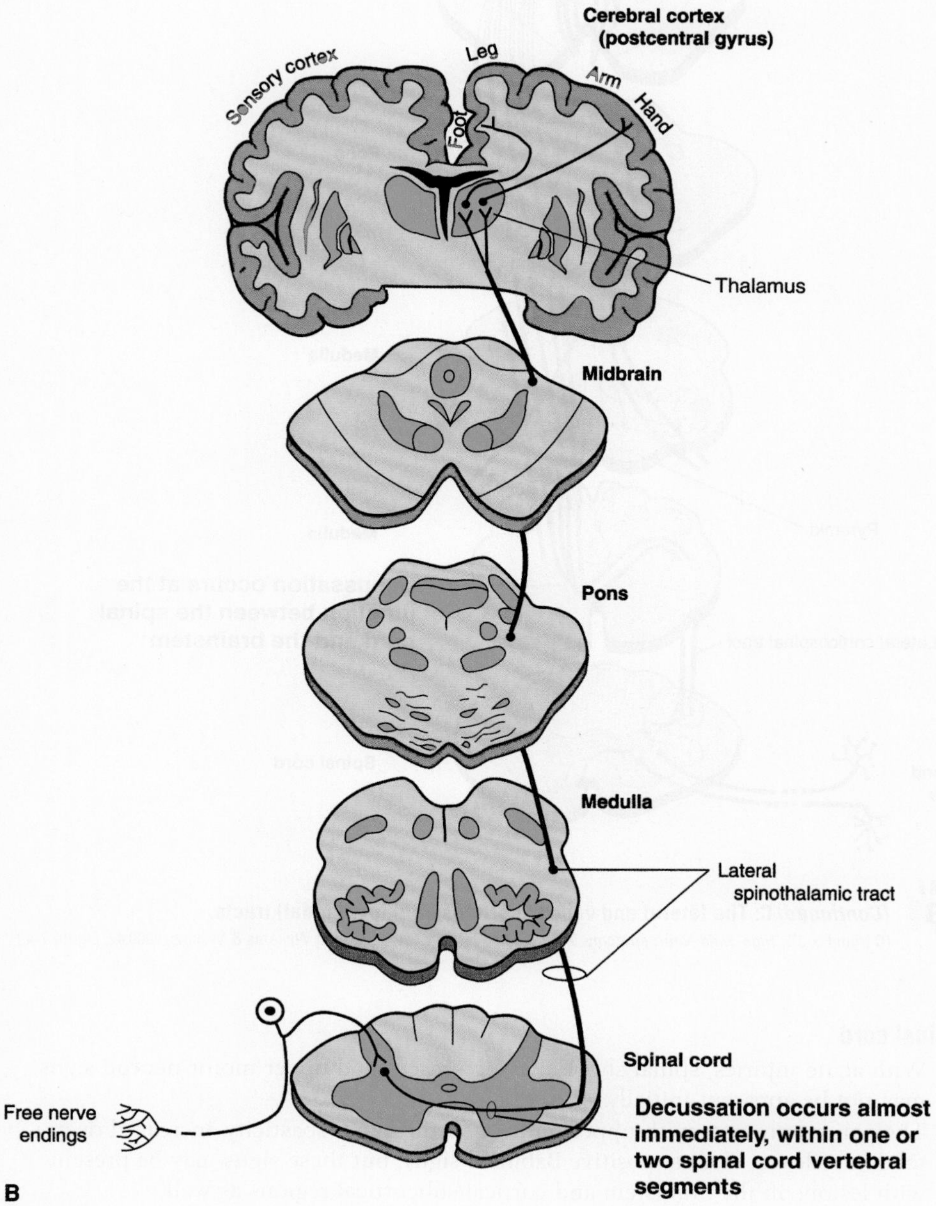

FIGURE 5-8 ***(Continued)*** **B: The lateral spinothalamic tract.**
(**B** from Fix JD. *High-Yield Neuroanatomy.* 2nd ed. Philadelphia, PA: Lippincott Williams & Wilkins, 2000:41, Figure 7-3.)

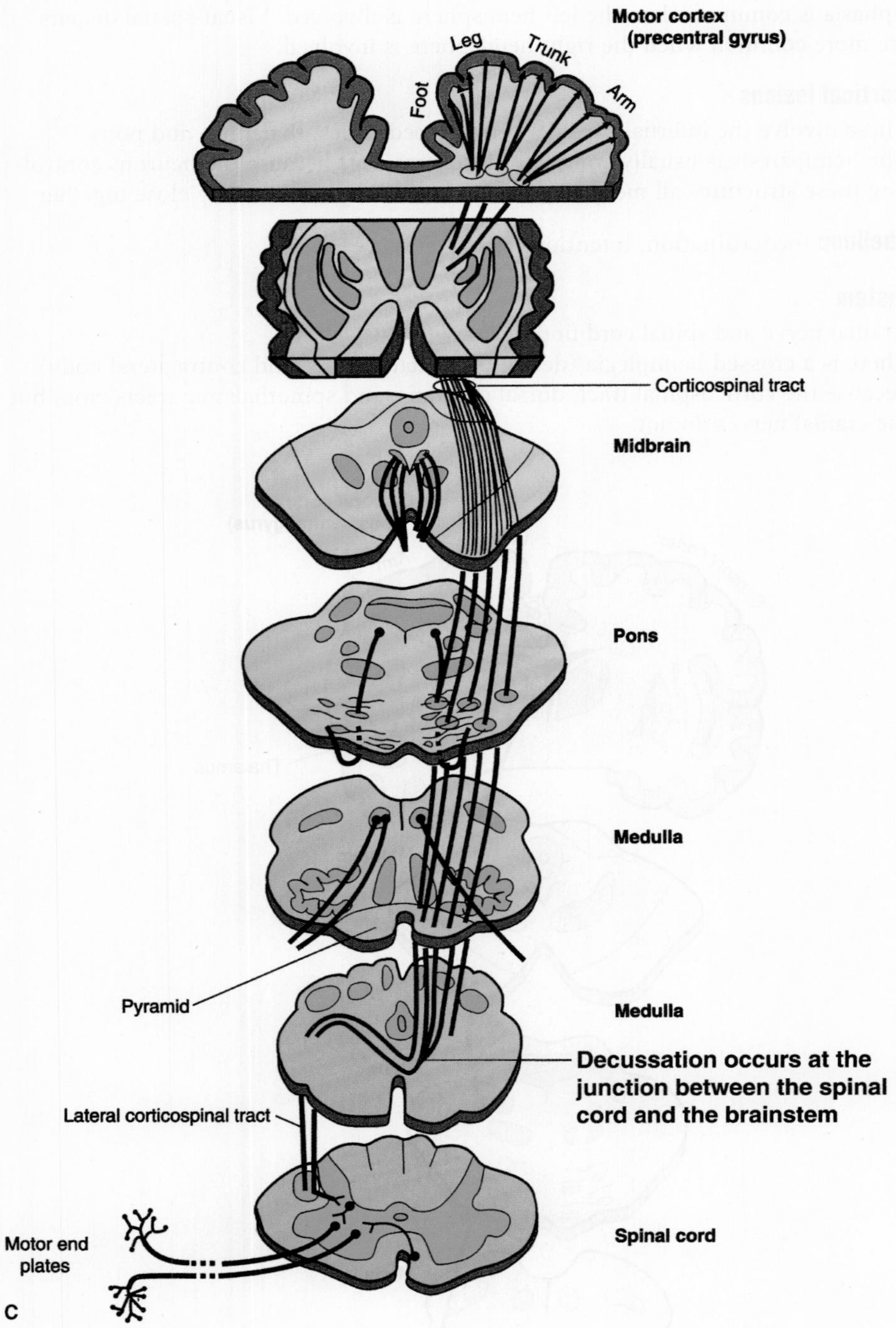

FIGURE 5-8 ***(Continued)*** **C: The lateral and ventral corticospinal (pyramidal) tracts.**
(**C** from Fix JD. *High-Yield Neuroanatomy.* 2nd ed. Philadelphia, PA: Lippincott Williams & Wilkins, 2000:42, Figure 7-4.)

F. Spinal cord

1. With acute injuries, spinal shock may be present and upper motor neuron signs may not be apparent initially.
2. The patient presents with upper motor neuron signs (spasticity, increased deep tendon reflexes, clonus, positive Babinski sign), but these signs may be present with lesions in the brainstem and cortical/subcortical regions as well.
3. There is a decrease in sensation below a sharp band in the abdomen/trunk. A pinprick is felt above this level but not below it. This is pathognomonic for spinal cord disease—the level of the lesion corresponds to the sensory level.

G. Plexus (plexopathy)

1. Deficits (motor and sensory) involve **more than one nerve.** Findings are variable depending on which part of the plexus is involved.
2. Trauma is the most common cause overall, especially for the brachial plexus. A postsurgical hematoma in the pelvis is a more common cause in lumbosacral plexopathy.
3. Plexuses that are commonly involved include:
   a. Brachial plexus—Erb–Duchenne type is the more common (upper trunk—C5-6 roots). Lower trunk (C8-T1) is less common.
   b. Lumbosacral plexus (L5-S3).

H. Roots (radiculopathy)

1. Pain is a key finding.
2. This affects a group of muscles supplied by a spinal root (myotome) and a sensory area supplied by a spinal root (dermatome). Therefore, the distribution of affected areas can help differentiate this from a peripheral neuropathy or a plexopathy.
3. Patients may present with weakness, atrophy, and sensory deficits in a dermatomal pattern; may include fasciculations and diminished deep tendon reflexes.

I. Peripheral nerve (peripheral neuropathy)

1. Weakness is more prominent distally at the outset (as opposed to muscle myopathy [see below])—**usually asymmetric.**
2. Presents with diminished deep tendon reflexes; may include sensory changes (numbness, paresthesias, tingling), muscle atrophy, and fasciculations.
3. Can be due to **diabetes** (nerve infarction), trauma, entrapment, or vasculitis.
4. Common neuropathies include radial/ulnar/median/musculocutaneous nerves, long thoracic nerve, axillary nerve, common peroneal nerve, and femoral nerve.

J. Neuromuscular junction

1. Fatigability is the key finding. Muscles become weaker with use and recover with rest.
2. Normal sensation, no atrophy

K. Muscle (myopathy)

1. Myopathy refers to acquired disease (dystrophy to inherited conditions).
2. Symmetric weakness affects proximal muscles more than distal muscles (shoulders and hip muscles).
3. Presents with normal reflexes, but these may diminish late in the disease in comparison to muscle weakness.
4. **Normal sensation**, no fasciculations.
5. Muscle atrophy may occur late due to disuse (in contrast to rapid atrophy in motor neuron disease).

6 CONNECTIVE TISSUE AND JOINT DISEASES

Connective Tissue Diseases

Systemic Lupus Erythematosus

A. General characteristics

1. An autoimmune disorder leading to inflammation and tissue damage involving multiple organ systems.
2. Systemic lupus erythematosus (SLE) is an idiopathic chronic inflammatory disease with **genetic**, **environmental**, and **hormonal** factors involved.
3. The pathophysiology involves autoantibody production, deposition of immune complexes, complement activation, and accompanying tissue destruction/vasculitis.
4. Types
   a. Spontaneous SLE.
   b. Discoid lupus (skin lesions without systemic disease)
   c. Drug-induced lupus
   d. ANA-negative lupus—associated findings
      - Arthritis, Raynaud phenomenon, subacute cutaneous lupus
      - Serology: Ro (anti-SS-A) antibody-positive, ANA negative
      - Risk of neonatal lupus in infants of affected women

> **Quick HIT**
> **Epidemiology of SLE**
> - **Women** of childbearing age account for 90% of cases.
> - **African-American patients** are more frequently affected than Caucasian patients.
> - Very mild in elderly patients; more severe in children.
> - Usually appears in late childhood or adolescence.

B. Clinical features

1. Constitutional symptoms: Fatigue (often the sign of an impending exacerbation and a prominent finding in most patients), malaise, fever, weight loss
2. Cutaneous: Butterfly rash (erythematous rash over cheeks and bridge of nose—found in one-third of patients) (Figure 6-1), photosensitivity, discoid lesions (erythematous raised patches with keratotic scaling), oral or nasopharyngeal ulcers, alopecia, **Raynaud phenomenon** (vasospasm of small vessels when exposed to cold, usually in fingers—found in about 20% of cases)
3. Musculoskeletal: Joint pain (may be the first symptom of the disease—found in 90% of patients), arthritis (inflammatory and symmetric, not erosive as in rheumatoid arthritis [RA]), arthralgias, myalgia with or without myositis
4. Cardiac: Pericarditis, endocarditis (**Libman–Sacks endocarditis** is a serious complication), myocarditis
5. Pulmonary: Pleuritis (most common pulmonary finding), pleural effusion, pneumonitis (may lead to fibrosis), pulmonary HTN (rare)
6. Hematologic: Hemolytic anemia with anemia or reticulocytosis of chronic disease, leukopenia, lymphopenia, thrombocytopenia
7. Renal: Proteinuria >0.5 g/day (may have nephrotic syndrome), cellular casts, glomerulonephritis (may have hematuria), azotemia, pyuria, uremia, HTN
8. Immunologic: Impaired immune response due to many factors, including autoantibodies to lymphocytes, abnormal T-cell function, and immunosuppressive medications; often associated with antiphospholipid syndrome

> **Quick HIT**
> Clinical findings associated with ***neonatal lupus***
> - Skin lesions
> - Cardiac abnormalities (AV block, transposition of the great vessels)
> - Valvular and septal defects

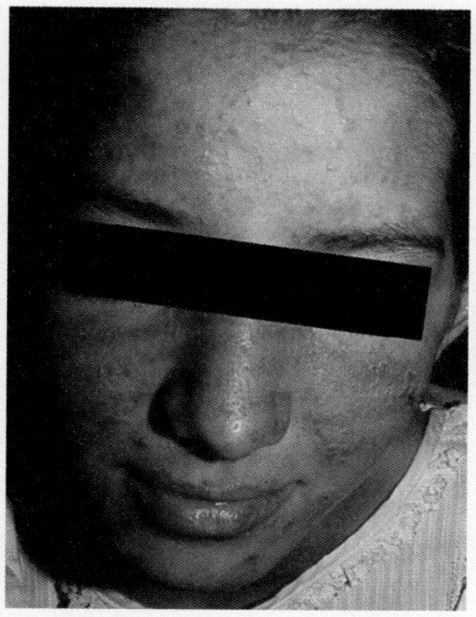

FIGURE 6-1 **SLE butterfly rash.**
(From Goodheart HP. *Goodheart's Photoguide of Common Skin Disorders.* 2nd ed. Philadelphia, PA: Lippincott Williams & Wilkins, 2003, Figure 25.24.)

9. GI: Nausea/vomiting, dyspepsia, dysphagia, peptic ulcer disease
10. CNS: Seizures, psychosis (may be subtle), depression, headaches, TIA, cerebrovascular accident
11. Other findings include conjunctivitis and an increased incidence of Raynaud phenomenon and Sjögren syndrome

C. Diagnosis

1. **Positive ANA screening test:** Sensitive but not specific; almost all patients with SLE have elevated serum ANA levels (see Clinical Pearl 6-1, Figure 6-2, and Table 6-1)
2. Anti-ds DNA (in 40%) and anti-Sm Ab (in 30%): The presence of either of these is diagnostic of SLE—very specific (but obviously not sensitive) (see Table 6-2)
3. Anti-ss DNA (in 70%)
4. **Antihistone Abs** (in 70%) are present in 100% of cases of **drug-induced lupus** (see Clinical Pearl 6-2). If negative, drug-induced lupus can be excluded.
5. **Ro (SS-A)** and **La (SS-B)** are found in 15% to 35%. Associated with:
    a. Sjögren syndrome
    b. Subacute cutaneous SLE
    c. Neonatal lupus (with congenital heart block)
    d. Complement deficiency (C2 and C4)
    e. ANA-negative lupus

Quick HIT

Clinical Course of SLE
- A chronic disease characterized by exacerbations and remissions
- Malar rash, joint pain, and fatigue are the most common initial findings. With more advanced disease, renal, pulmonary, cardiovascular, and nervous systems are affected.

Quick HIT

Conditions in which ANAs are Elevated
- SLE
- RA
- Scleroderma
- Sjögren syndrome
- Mixed connective tissue disease
- Polymyositis and dermatomyositis
- Drug-induced lupus

CLINICAL PEARL 6-1

Useful Criteria for Diagnosing SLE

A patient has SLE if four or more of these 11 criteria are present at any time.

1. Mucocutaneous signs (each counts as one)
    - Butterfly rash
    - Photosensitivity
    - Oral or nasopharyngeal ulcers
    - Discoid rash
2. Arthritis
3. Pericarditis, pleuritic
4. Hematologic disease—hemolytic anemia with reticulocytosis, leukopenia, lymphopenia, thrombocytopenia
5. Renal disease: Proteinuria >0.5 g/day, cellular casts
6. CNS—seizures, psychosis
7. Immunologic manifestations—positive LE preparation, false-positive test result for syphilis, anti-ds DNA, anti-Sm Ab
8. ANAs

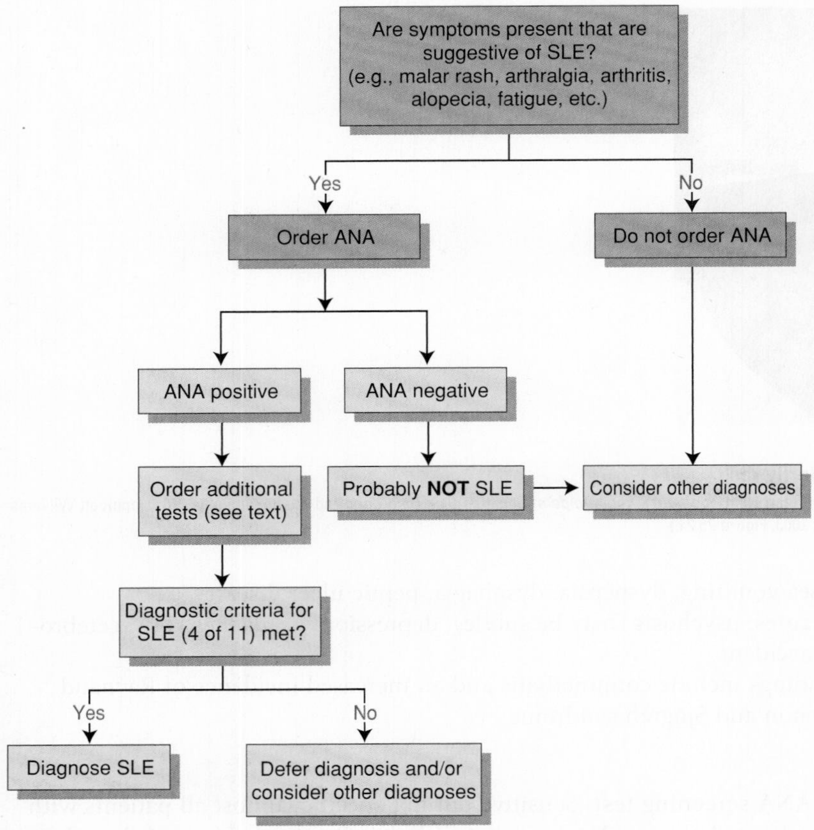

FIGURE 6-2 Diagnosis of SLE.
(Adapted from Humes DH, DuPont HL, Gardner LB, et al. *Kelley's Textbook of Internal Medicine.* 4th ed. Philadelphia, PA: Lippincott Williams & Wilkins, 2000:1387, Figure 178-3.)

TABLE 6-1 Common Laboratory Markers in Rheumatologic Diseases

Laboratory Marker	Conditions	Comments
ANAs	• SLE (almost all patients) • Scleroderma • Sjögren syndrome • Polymyositis	Highly sensitive for SLE but not for the others
RF	• RA (70% of patients) • Healthy populations (up to 3%)	Neither sensitive nor specific for RA
C-ANCA	Wegener granulomatosis	Sensitive and specific Can vary with disease activity
P-ANCA	Polyarteritis nodosa	70%–80% sensitive for microscopic PAN Not specific
Lupus anticoagulant	Antiphospholipid syndrome	
ESR	• Infection (acute or chronic) • Malignancy • Rheumatologic diseases • Miscellaneous (tissue necrosis, pregnancy)	• Low sensitivity and specificity • Major uses: Diagnose/rule out inflammatory process and monitor course of inflammatory conditions
C-reactive protein	• Inflammatory states and infection • Miscellaneous conditions (e.g., MI, vasculitis, trauma, malignancy, pancreatitis)	• Primarily used for infection—much more sensitive and specific than ESR • If levels are markedly elevated (>15), bacterial infection is likely present

TABLE 6-2 HLA Associations with Rheumatic Diseases

Disease	Associated HLA
SLE	HLA-DR2 and HLA-DR3
Sjögren syndrome	HLA-DR3
RA	HLA-DR4
Ankylosing spondylitis, Reiter syndrome, psoriatic arthritis	HLA-B27

6. Positive LE preparation: ANAs bind to nuclei of damaged cells, producing LE bodies
7. **False-positive test result for syphilis**
8. Complement levels are usually decreased
9. CBC, renal function tests (BUN, creatinine), urinalysis, serum electrolytes
10. Anticardiolipin and lupus anticoagulant (see Clinical Pearl 6-3)

D. Treatment

1. Avoid sun exposure because it can exacerbate cutaneous rashes
2. NSAIDs—for less severe symptoms
3. Either local or systemic **corticosteroids—for acute exacerbations**
4. Systemic steroids for severe manifestations
5. Best long-term therapy is antimalarial agents such as hydroxychloroquine—for constitutional, cutaneous, and articular manifestations. **Hydroxychloroquine** is continued as a preventative measure even after resolution of symptoms. Annual eye examination is needed because of **retinal toxicity**
6. Cytotoxic agents such as cyclophosphamide—for active glomerulonephritis
7. Monitor the following and treat appropriately:
   a. Renal disease, which produces the most significant morbidity
   b. HTN

Quick HIT

Steroids are the best treatment for SLE patients with acute flare.

Hydroxychloroquine for long-term treatment for SLE can cause retinal toxicity.

Quick HIT

The most common causes of death in SLE are opportunistic infections and renal failure.

Scleroderma (Systemic Sclerosis)

A. General characteristics

1. A chronic connective tissue disorder that can lead to widespread fibrosis.
2. Pathophysiology: Cytokines stimulate fibroblasts, causing an abnormal amount of collagen deposition. It is the high **quantity** of collagen that causes the problems associated with this disease (composition of the collagen is normal).
3. Scleroderma is more common in women. Average age of onset is 35 to 50 years.
4. There are two types of scleroderma: Diffuse (20%) and limited (80%) (see Table 6-3)

Quick HIT

Only **diffuse scleroderma** form has renal, lung, and heart involvement.

CLINICAL PEARL 6-2

Drug-induced Lupus

- Certain drugs may produce a lupus-like syndrome that is similar to SLE except that it **does not affect the CNS or kidneys.**
- If renal or CNS involvement is present, it is **not** drug-induced lupus. In addition, the classic butterfly rash, alopecia, and ulcers are typically not seen in drug-induced lupus.
- Most patients improve after withdrawal of the offending drug. Therefore, the prognosis is obviously more favorable.
- Commonly implicated agents include hydralazine, procainamide, isoniazid, chlorpromazine, methyldopa, and quinidine.
- Laboratory findings in drug-induced lupus: **Antihistone antibodies** are always present; there is an absence of anti-ds DNA and anti-Sm Ab.

CLINICAL PEARL 6-3

Antiphospholipid Antibody Syndrome

- A hypercoagulable state that can be idiopathic or associated with SLE (or other collagen vascular diseases such as scleroderma)
- Typical findings
  - Recurrent venous thrombosis—pulmonary embolism is a risk
  - Recurrent arterial thrombosis
  - Recurrent fetal loss (abortions)
  - Thrombocytopenia
  - Livedo reticularis
- Laboratory findings: Presence of lupus anticoagulant, anticardiolipin antibody, or both. Prolonged PTT or PT is not corrected by adding normal plasma
- Treatment is long-term anticoagulation (INR of 2.5 to 3.5)
- APA antibodies react with cardiolipin, a reagent in VRDL and RPR tests leading to false positives

B. Clinical features

1. **Raynaud phenomenon**
   a. Present in almost all patients; usually appears before other findings
   b. Caused by vasospasm and thickening of vessel walls in the digits
   c. Can lead to digital ischemia, with ulceration and infarction/gangrene
   d. Cold temperature and stress bring about color changes of fingers—blanching first, then cyanotic, and then red from reactive hyperemia
2. Cutaneous fibrosis
   a. Tightening of skin of the face and extremities (**sclerodactyly** refers to a claw-like appearance of the hand)
   b. Can lead to contractures, disability, and disfigurement
3. GI involvement
   a. Occurs in most patients (both diffuse and limited)

TABLE 6-3 **Diffuse Versus Limited Scleroderma**

Diffuse	Limited
Widespread skin involvement	Skin involvement limited to distal extremities (and face, neck)—sparing of the trunk
Rapid onset of symptoms (skin and other complications occur rapidly after onset of Raynaud phenomenon)	Delayed onset: Skin involvement occurs slowly after the onset of Raynaud phenomenon. Therefore, the patient has a long history or Raynaud phenomenon before other symptoms begin
Significant visceral involvement (i.e., fibrosis of internal organs)—lung, heart, GI tract, kidneys	Visceral involvement occurs late—pulmonary HTN and ischemic vascular disease; minimal constitutional symptoms
Associated with ANAs but absence of anticentromere antibody	Anticentromere antibody is found in most patients
Poorer prognosis—10-yr survival is 40%–65%	Better prognosis than diffuse form. Normal life span is expected in most cases, unless severe pulmonary HTN develops
• Peripheral edema (of hands and legs), polyarthritis, fatigue and weakness (muscle involvement), carpal tunnel syndrome • Renal failure can occur, but now rare • Interstitial lung disease more common	CREST syndrome is a variant **C**alcinosis of the digits **R**aynaud phenomenon **E**sophageal motility dysfunction **S**clerodactyly of the fingers **T**elangiectases (over the digits and under the nails)

b. Findings include dysphagia/reflux from esophageal immobility (up to 90% of patients), delayed gastric emptying, constipation/diarrhea, abdominal distention, and pseudo-obstruction. Prolonged acid reflux may eventually lead to esophageal strictures.

4. Pulmonary involvement
   a. Most common cause of death from scleroderma
   b. Interstitial fibrosis and/or pulmonary HTN may also be present
5. Cardiac involvement: pericardial effusions, myocardial involvement that can lead to CHF, arrhythmias
6. Renal involvement (renal crisis—rapid malignant hypertension) occurs in patients with diffuse disease (rare today)

C. Diagnosis

1. Diagnostic tests are of limited utility. Almost all patients have elevated ANAs (high sensitivity, low specificity).
2. **Anticentromere antibody** is very specific for the limited form.
3. **Antitopoisomerase I** (antiscleroderma-70) Ab is very specific for the diffuse form.
4. Barium swallow (esophageal dysmotility) and pulmonary function test are used to detect complications.

D. Treatment

1. No effective cure, and treatment is symptomatic
2. NSAIDs for musculoskeletal pains
3. H_2 blockers or proton pump inhibitors for esophageal reflux
4. Raynaud phenomenon—avoid cold and smoking, keep hands warm; if severe, use calcium-channel blockers
5. Pulmonary complications—for pulmonary hypertension, treat with bosentan. For pulmonary fibrosis, cyclophosphamide is used
6. ACE inhibitors are used to prevent and treat renal hypertensive crisis

Sjögren Syndrome

A. General characteristics

1. Sjögren's syndrome is an autoimmune disease most common in women. Lymphocytes infiltrate and destroy the lacrimal and salivary glands.
2. A multiorgan disease (can also involve the skin, lungs, thyroid, vessels, and liver)
3. Primary versus secondary Sjögren syndrome
   a. Primary Sjögren syndrome: Dry eyes and dry mouth, along with lymphocytic infiltration of the minor salivary glands (on histology); patients do not have another rheumatologic disease
   b. Secondary Sjögren syndrome: Dry eyes and dry mouth along with a **connective tissue disease** (RA, systemic sclerosis, SLE, polymyositis)
4. Patients have increased risk of non-Hodgkin lymphoma. Malignancy is the most common cause of death.

B. Clinical features

1. Dry eyes—burning, redness, blurred vision, keratoconjunctivitis sicca
2. Dry mouth and tooth decay
3. Arthralgias, arthritis, fatigue
4. Interstitial nephritis and vasculitis

C. Diagnosis

1. ANAs are present in 95% of patients. Rheumatoid factor (RF) is present in 50% to 75% of patients with secondary disease.
2. **Ro (SS-A)** is present in 55% of patients, and **La (SS-B)** Abs is present in 40% of patients.
3. **Schirmer test**: Filter paper inserted in eye to measure lacrimal gland output (degree of wetting in a specified time period)—high sensitivity and specificity.
4. Salivary gland biopsy (lip or parotid) is the most accurate but not needed for diagnosis.

Quick HIT

Differential diagnosis of Raynaud phenomenon
- Primary—no other disorder exists
- Scleroderma
- SLE
- Mixed connective tissue disease
- Vasculitis (e.g., Buerger disease)
- Certain medications (e.g., β-blockers, nicotine, bleomycin)
- Disorders that disrupt blood flow or vessels, such as thromboangiitis obliterans

Quick HIT

The **degree of skin involvement** predicts prognosis: Diffuse scleroderma has a worse prognosis than limited scleroderma.

Quick HIT

- Twenty percent of patients with scleroderma have Sjögren syndrome.
- In patients with Sjögren syndrome, search for **occult lymphoma** (look for lymphadenopathy and hepatosplenomegaly).

Quick HIT

Patients with antibodies to Ro (SS-A) are at increased risk of having a child with neonatal SLE (with congenital heart block).

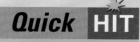

D. Treatment

1. Pilocarpine or Cevimeline (enhance oral and ocular secretions via acytelcholine)
2. Artificial tears for dry eyes
3. Good oral hygiene
4. NSAIDs, steroids for arthralgias, arthritis
5. Patients with secondary Sjögren syndrome—therapy for connective tissue disease

●●● Mixed Connective Tissue Disease

- Mixed connective tissue disease is an "overlap" syndrome with clinical features similar to those of SLE, RA, systemic sclerosis, and polymyositis. Findings consistent with each of these diseases do not necessarily occur simultaneously. It usually takes some time for a pattern to be identified and a diagnosis of mixed connective tissue disease to be made.
- Clinical findings include pulmonary involvement, esophageal dysfunction, polyarthritis, sclerodactyly, cutaneous manifestations, myopathy, and Raynaud phenomenon.
- The presence of **anti-U1-RNP Abs** is a key laboratory finding. High ANA and RF may be present.
- Treatment varies according to which specific disease predominates.

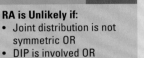

> **Quick HIT**
>
> **RA is Unlikely if:**
> - Joint distribution is not symmetric OR
> - DIP is involved OR
> - Constitutional symptoms (especially morning stiffness) are absent

●●● Rheumatoid Arthritis

A. General characteristics

1. RA is a chronic **inflammatory** autoimmune disease involving the **synovium of joints.** The inflamed synovium can cause damage to cartilage and bone.
2. It is a systemic disease that has many extra-articular manifestations (see below).
3. The usual age of onset is 20 to 40 years; it is more common in women than in men (3:1).
4. Etiology is uncertain. It may be caused by an infection or a series of infections (most likely viral), but genetic predisposition is necessary.

> **Quick HIT**
>
> Much of the joint damage that ultimately leads to disability occurs early in the course of the disease, so early treatment with DMARDs is critical.

B. Clinical features

1. Inflammatory polyarthritis (joint swelling is the most common sign)—can involve every joint in the body **except the DIP joints** (Figure 6-3).
   a. Pain on motion of joints/tenderness in joints.
   b. Joints commonly involved include **joints of the hands (PIP, MCP) and wrists,** knees, ankles, elbows, hips, and shoulders.
   c. Characteristic hand deformities.
      - Ulnar deviation of the MCP joints (Figure 6-4A).
      - *Boutonnière deformities* of the PIP joints (PIP flexed, DIP hyperextended) (Figure 6-4C).
      - *Swan-neck contractures* of the fingers (MCP flexed, PIP hyperextended, DIP flexed) (Figure 6-4B).
2. Constitutional symptoms can be prominent (see Table 6-4).
   a. **Morning stiffness** (present in all patients)—improves as the day progresses.
   b. Low-grade fever, weight loss.
   c. Fatigue can be prominent because this is a systemic disease.
3. Cervical spine involvement is common at **C1-C2 (subluxation and instability),** but it is less common in the lower cervical spine.
   a. Instability of the cervical spine is a potentially life-threatening complication of RA. Most patients do not have neurologic involvement, but if they do, it can be progressive and fatal if not treated surgically.
   b. This is seen in 30% to 40% of patients. All patients with RA should have cervical spine **radiographs before undergoing any surgery** (due to risk of neurologic injury during intubation). However, disease-modifying antirheumatic drugs (DMARDs) have dramatically reduced the need for cervical spine surgery in RA patients.
4. Cardiac involvement may include pericarditis, pericardial effusions, conduction abnormalities, and valvular incompetence.

> **Quick HIT**
>
> **Poor Prognostic Indicators in RA**
> - High RF titers
> - Subcutaneous nodules
> - Erosive arthritis
> - Autoantibodies to RF

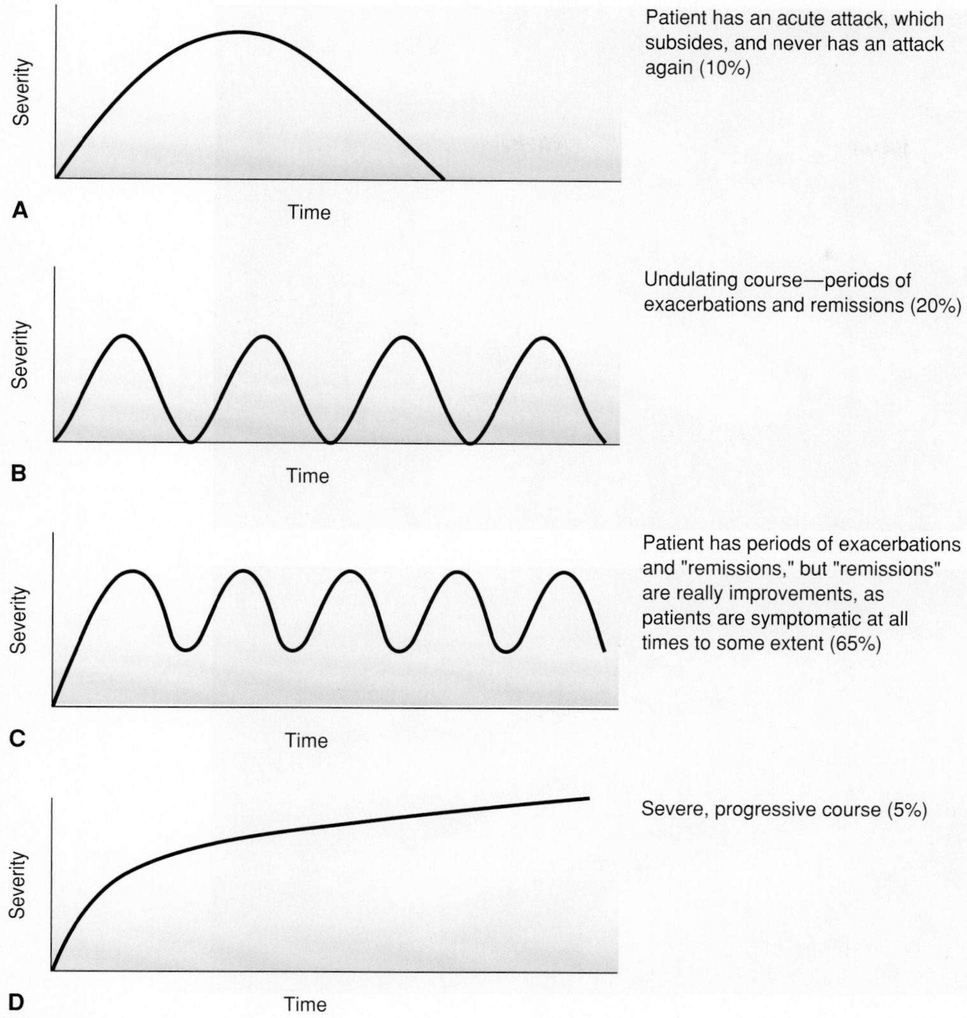
Patient has an acute attack, which subsides, and never has an attack again (10%)
Severity
Time
A
Undulating course—periods of exacerbations and remissions (20%)
Severity
Time
B
Patient has periods of exacerbations and "remissions," but "remissions" are really improvements, as patients are symptomatic at all times to some extent (65%)
Severity
Time
C
Severe, progressive course (5%)
Severity
Time
D

FIGURE 6-3 **The clinical course of RA can be grouped into four classes of patients.**

5. Pulmonary involvement—usually pleural effusions; interstitial fibrosis may occur.
6. Ocular involvement—episcleritis or scleritis.
7. Soft tissue swelling (rather than bony enlargement).
8. Drying of mucous membranes: Sjögren xerostomia.
9. Subcutaneous **rheumatoid nodules** over extensor surfaces may also occur in visceral structures—for example, lungs, pleura, pericardium (Figure 6-5).
   a. Pathognomonic for RA.
   b. Nearly always occurs in seropositive patients (i.e., those with RF).

C. Diagnosis

1. Laboratory findings (see Clinical Pearl 6-4)
   a. High titers of RF are associated with more severe disease and are generally nonspecific. RF is eventually present in 80% of patients with RA (may be absent early in the disease), but is also present in up to 3% of the healthy population.
      - RF titers rarely change with disease activity and are not useful for following patients.
      - Helpful in determining prognosis. High titers → more severe disease.
   b. Anticitrullinated peptide/protein antibodies (ACPA)—sensitivity is 50% to 75%, specificity is over 90%.
   c. Elevated ESR, C-reactive protein.
   d. Anemia of chronic disease.

Quick HIT

In RA, changes in joints are usually more extensive than in OA because the entire synovium is involved in RA. Note that osteophytes (characteristic of OA) are not present in RA.

Quick HIT

Patients with diagnosis of RA who have a positive RF, ACPA, or both are at a higher risk of developing erosive joint damage—early treatment with DMARDs is indicated.

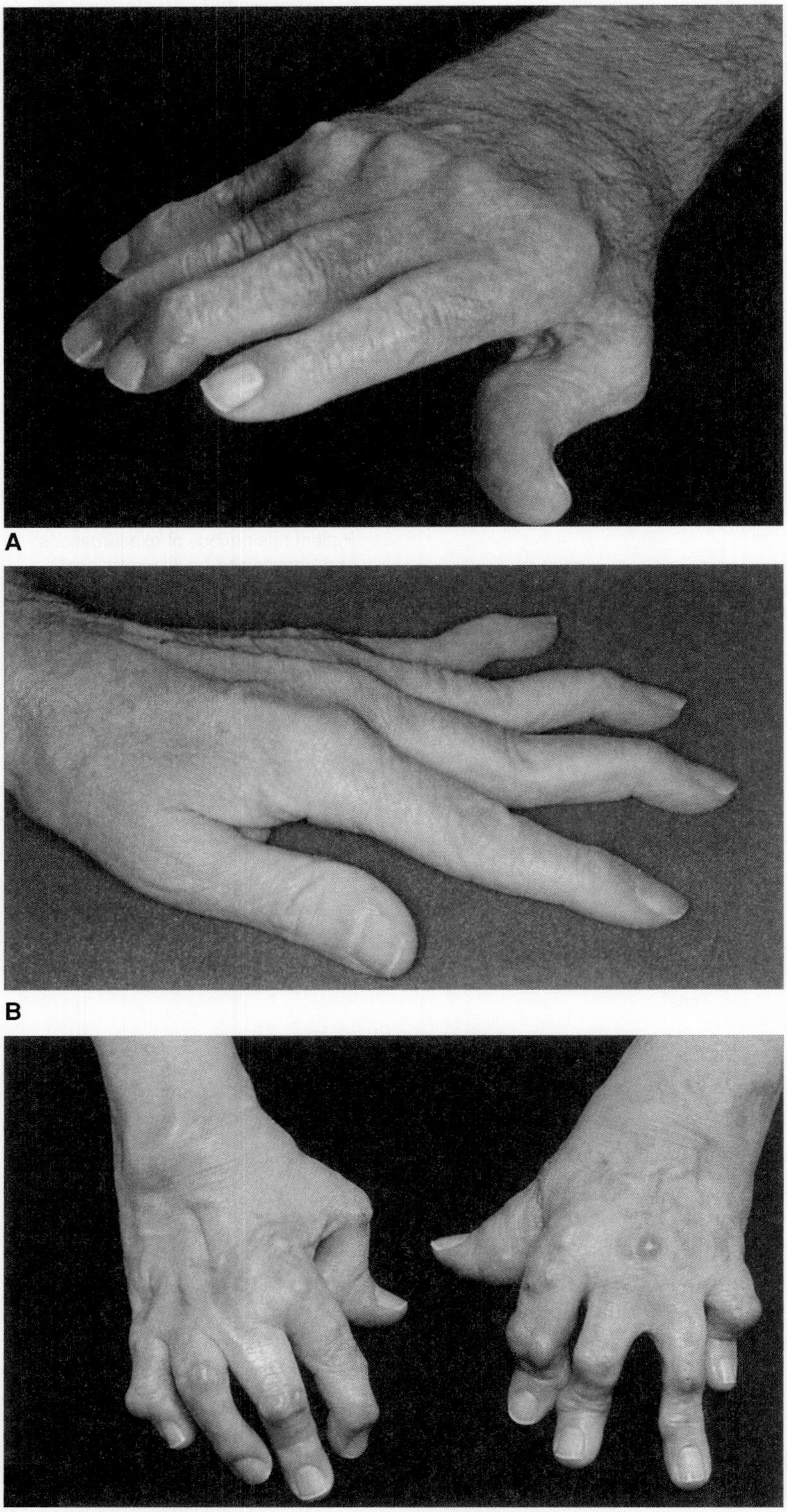

A

B

C

FIGURE 6-4

Rheumatoid arthritis. A: Ulnar deviation at metacarpophalangeal joints. B: Swan-neck deformity. C: Boutonnière deformity.

(From Hunder GG. *Atlas of Rheumatology.* 3rd ed. Philadelphia, PA: Lippincott Williams & Wilkins, 2000:11, Figures 1-27, 1-28, and 1-29A, respectively; and *Curr Med.* 2002:11.)

TABLE 6-4 **Extra-articular Manifestations in Rheumatoid Arthritis**

Constitutional Symptoms	Malaise, Anorexia, Some Weight Loss, Fever
Cutaneous	• Skin becomes thin and atrophic and bruises easily • Vasculitic changes/ulcerations involving fingers, nail folds • Subcutaneous **rheumatoid nodules** (elbows, sacrum, occiput)—**pathognomonic for RA**
Pulmonary	• Pleural effusions (very common)—**pleural fluid characteristically has very low glucose** and low complement • Pulmonary fibrosis—with a restrictive pattern on pulmonary function tests and a honeycomb pattern on CXR • Pulmonary infiltrates • Rheumatic nodules in lungs (similar to those on skin)—can cavitate or become infected
Cardiac	• Rheumatic nodules in heart—can lead to conduction disturbances (heart block and bundle branch block) • Pericarditis—in 40% of patients with RA • Pericardial effusion
Eyes	• Scleritis • Scleromalacia—softening of the sclera; if not treated may perforate, leading to blindness • Dry eyes (and dry mucous membranes in general); may develop Sjögren syndrome
Nervous System	Mononeuritic multiplex—infarction of nerve trunk Patient cannot move the arm or leg; implies systemic vasculitis, which is a bad sign
Felty Syndrome	• Triad of RA, neutropenia, and splenomegaly • Also anemia, thrombocytopenia, and lymphadenopathy • Associated with high titers of RF and extra-articular disease • Increased susceptibility to infection • Usually occurs fairly late in the disease process
Blood	• Anemia of chronic disease: Mild, normocytic, normochromic anemia • Thrombocytosis
Vasculitis	A microvascular vasculitis—can progress to mesenteric vasculitis, PAN, or other vascular syndromes

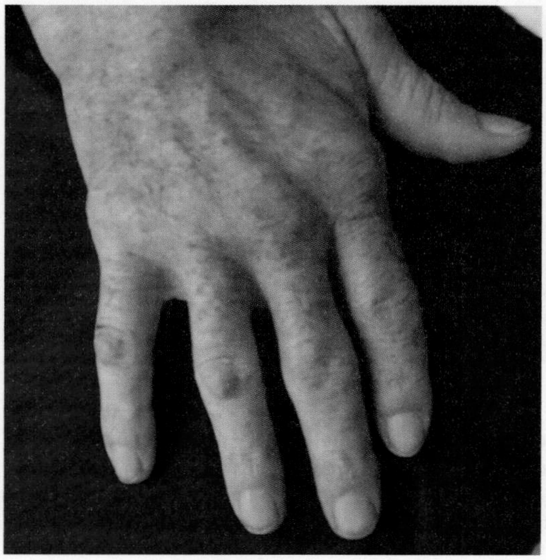

FIGURE 6-5 **Rheumatoid nodules of the hand.**
(Image provided by Stedman's.)

CLINICAL PEARL 6-4

Diagnosis of RA

1. Inflammatory arthritis of three or more joints—MCP, PIP, wrist, elbow, knee, ankle, MIP joints
2. Symptoms lasting at least 6 weeks
3. Elevated CRP and ESR
4. Positive serum RF or ACPA
5. Radiographic changes consistent with RA (erosions and periarticular decalcification)

Quick HIT

Radiographs have become less important in diagnosis of RA, as joint abnormalities occur very late. DMARDs started well before radiographs indicate abnormality.

2. Radiographs (Figure 6-6).
   a. Loss of juxta-articular bone mass (periarticular osteoporosis) near the finger joints.
   b. **Narrowing of the joint space** (due to thinning of the articular cartilage) is usually seen late in the disease.
   c. **Bony erosions** at the margins of the joint.
3. Synovial fluid analysis (see Table 6-5) is nonspecific.

D. Treatment

Quick HIT

NSAIDs and DMARDs are the two main classes of medications used in RA.

1. Goal is to minimize pain and swelling, prevent disease progression, and help patient remain as functional as possible.
2. Exercise helps to maintain range of motion and muscle strength.
3. Symptomatic treatment.
   a. NSAIDs are the drugs of choice for pain control.
   b. Corticosteroids (low dose)—use these if NSAIDs do not provide adequate relief. Short-term treatment may be appropriate but avoid long-term use.

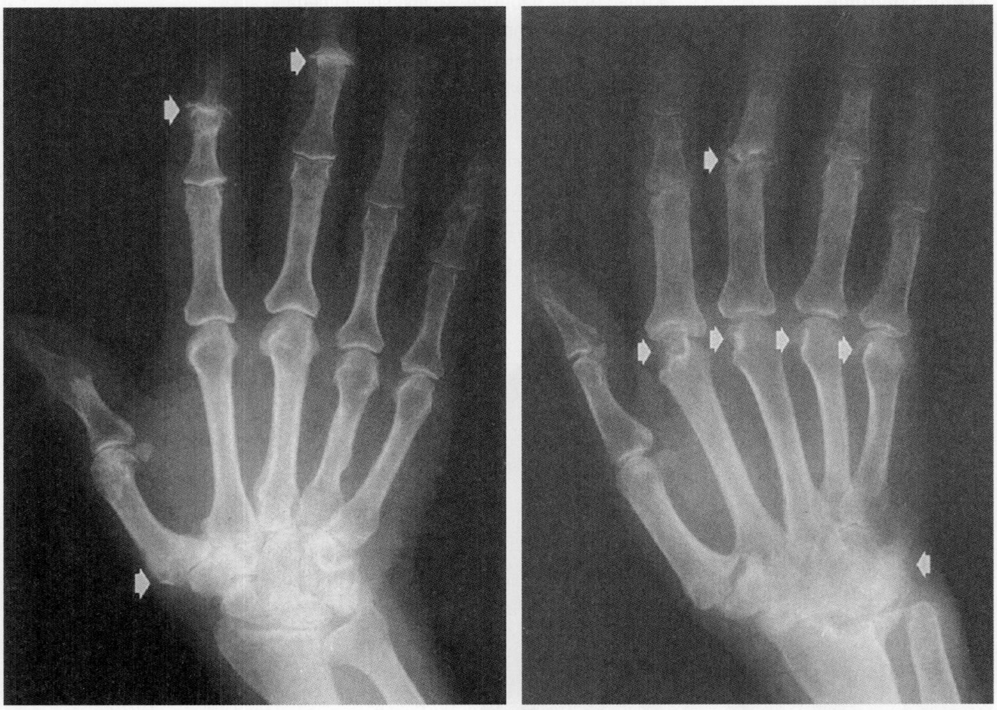

A B

FIGURE 6-6 **Posteroanterior radiographs of the hand showing the typical pattern of involvement for (A) osteoarthritis (osteophytes, subchondral sclerosis, joint space narrowing) (*arrows*) and (B) rheumatoid arthritis (periarticular erosions, osteopenia) (*arrows*).**

(**A** and **B** from Humes DH, DuPont HL, Gardner LB, et al. *Kelley's Textbook of Internal Medicine.* 4th ed. Philadelphia, PA: Lippincott Williams & Wilkins, 2000:1463, Figures 190.4A and B.)

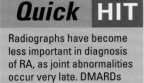

TABLE 6-5 Synovial Fluid Analysis

Condition	Appearance of Fluid	WBC/mm^3	PMNs	Other Findings
Normal	Clear	<200	<25%	
Noninflammatory arthritis (OA/trauma)	Clear, yellow: Possibly red if traumatic	<2,000	<25%	RBCs for trauma
Inflammatory arthritis (RA, gout, pseudogout, Reiter syndrome)	Cloudy yellow	>5,000	50%–70%	Positively birefringent crystals with pseudogout; negatively birefringent crystals with gout
Septic arthritis (bacterial, tuberculosis)	Turbid, purulent	Usually >50,000	>70%	Synovial fluid culture positive for most cases of bacterial arthritis except gonococcal (only 25% are positive)

4. DMARDs
   a. General principles
      - Can reduce morbidity and mortality (by nearly 30%)—by limiting complications, slowing progression of disease, and preserving joint function
      - **Should be initiated early** (at the time of diagnosis)
      - They have a slow onset of action (6 weeks or longer for effect to be seen), so begin treating RA while waiting for the disease-modifying therapy to take effect. Gradually taper and discontinue NSAIDs and corticosteroids once effects are evident
   b. First-line agents
      - Methotrexate—best initial DMARD
      - Initial improvement is seen in 4 to 6 weeks.
      - Side effects include GI upset, oral ulcers (stomatitis), mild alopecia, **bone marrow suppression** (coadminister with folinic acid), hepatocellular injury, and idiosyncratic interstitial pneumonitis, which may lead to pulmonary fibrosis. It increases liver enzymes in some patients
      - Closely monitor liver and renal function
      - Supplement with folate.
      - Leflunomide is an alternative to methotrexate or can be used as an adjunct to therapy with a DMARD.
      - Hydroxychloroquine
      - This is an alternative first-line DMARD, but usually not as effective as methotrexate and is typically used in less severe cases
      - It requires eye examinations every 6 months because of the risk of visual loss due to retinopathy
      - Sulfasalazine—alternate first-line agent, but less effective than methotrexate
      - Antitumor necrosis factor (anti-TNF) inhibiting agents (etanercept, infliximab, etc.)—used if methotrexate does not fully control the disease
      - Requires PPD screening because of risk of reactivation of TB
5. Surgery (in severe cases)
   a. Synovectomy (arthroscopic) decreases joint pain and swelling but does not prevent x-ray progression and does not improve joint range of motion
   b. Joint replacement surgery for severe pain unresponsive to conservative measures

Quick HIT

Variants of RA
- **Felty syndrome:** anemia, neutropenia, splenomegaly, and RA.
- **Juvenile RA:** begins before 18 years of age. Extra-articular manifestations may predominate (***Still disease***) or arthritis may predominate.
- **Caplan syndrome:** RA associated with pneumoconiosis.

Quick HIT

Combination therapy with first-line drugs (methotrexate, hydroxychloroquine, and sulfasalazine) produces higher remission rates.

Quick HIT

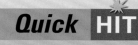

Methotrexate is the mainstay of therapy in RA.

Crystal-induced Arthritides

Gout

A. General characteristics

1. Gout is an inflammatory monoarticular arthritis caused by the crystallization of monosodium urate in joints (Figure 6-7) (see Table 6-6). Hyperuricemia is a hallmark of the disease, but it does not by itself indicate gout.
2. Ninety percent of patients are men over 30 years of age. Women are not affected until after menopause.
3. Pathogenesis
   a. Increased production of uric acid.
      - Hypoxanthine-guanine phosphoribosyltransferase deficiency—for example, in Lesch–Nyhan syndrome
      - **Phosphoribosyl pyrophosphate synthetase** overactivity
      - **Increased cell turnover** associated with a number of conditions, including cancer chemotherapy, chronic hemolysis, and hematologic malignancies

   b. Decreased excretion of uric acid (accounts for 90% of cases)
      - Renal disease
      - NSAIDs, diuretics
      - Acidosis
4. Pathophysiology of inflammation
   a. PMNs play a key role in the acute inflammation of gout
   b. It develops when uric acid crystals collect in the synovial fluid as the extracellular fluid becomes saturated with uric acid
   c. IgGs coat monosodium urate crystals, which are phagocytized by PMNs, leading to the release of inflammatory mediators and proteolytic enzymes from the PMNs, which then result in inflammation.

Quick HIT

Precipitants of an Acute Gouty Attack
- Decrease in temperature
- Dehydration
- Stress (emotional or physical)
- Excessive alcohol intake
- Starvation

B. Clinical features (four stages)

1. Asymptomatic hyperuricemia.
   a. Increased serum uric acid level in the absence of clinical findings of gout, may be present without symptoms for 10 to 20 years or longer.
   b. Should not be treated because over 95% of patients remain asymptomatic.
2. Acute gouty arthritis.
   a. Peak age of onset is 40 to 60 years of age for men.
   b. Initial attack usually involves sudden onset of exquisite pain. Pain often wakes the patient from sleep.

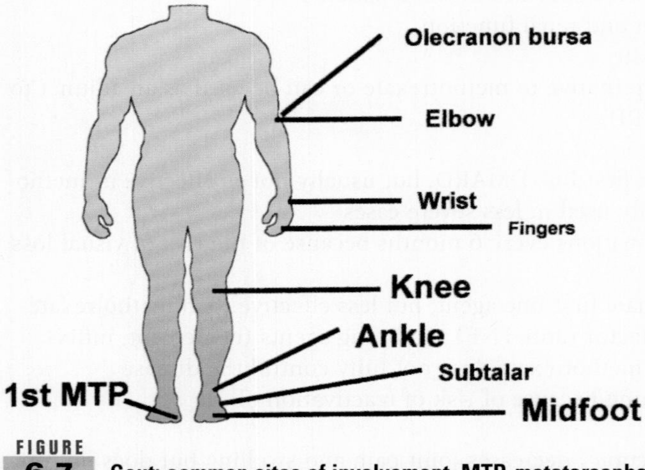

FIGURE 6-7 **Gout: common sites of involvement. MTP, metatarsophalangeal joint.**
(From Stoller JK, Ahmad M, Longworth DL. *The Cleveland Clinic Intensive Review of Internal Medicine*. 3rd ed. Philadelphia, PA: Lippincott Williams & Wilkins, 2002:374, Figure 30.6.)

TABLE 6-6 Major Arthritides

	Osteoarthritis	Rheumatoid Arthritis	Gouty Arthritis
Onset	Insidious	Insidious	Sudden
Common locations	Weight-bearing joints (knees, hips, lumbar/cervical spine), hands	Hands (PIP, MCP), wrists, ankles, knees	Great toe, ankles, knees, elbows
Presence of inflammation	No	Yes	Yes
Radiographic changes	Narrowed joint space, osteophytes, subchondral sclerosis, subchondral cysts	Narrowed joint space, bony erosions	Punched-out erosions with overhanging rim of cortical bone
Laboratory findings	None	Elevated ESR, RF, anemia	Crystals
Other features	• No systemic findings • Bouchard nodes and Heberden nodes in hands	• Systemic findings—extra-articular manifestations common • Ulnar deviation, swan-neck, and boutonnière deformity	• Tophi • Nephrolithiasis

- Most often affects the big toe—the first metatarsophalangeal joint (**podagra**). Other common joints affected are ankles and knees.

c. Pain and cellulitic changes—erythema, swelling, tenderness, and warmth.
d. Fever may or may not be present.
e. As it resolves, the patient may have desquamation of overlying skin.

3. Intercritical gout.
   a. An asymptomatic period after the initial attack. The patient may not have another attack for years.
   b. Sixty percent of patients have a recurrence within 1 year. Some patients (fewer than 10%) never have another attack of gout.
   c. There is a 75% likelihood of a second attack within the first 2 years.
   d. Attacks tend to become polyarticular with increased severity over time.
4. Chronic tophaceous gout.
   a. Occurs in people who have had poorly controlled gout for more than 10 to 20 years.
   b. Tophi
      - Aggregations of urate crystals surrounded by giant cells in an inflammatory reaction.
      - Tophi cause deformity and destruction of hard and soft tissues. In joints, they lead to destruction of cartilage and bone, triggering secondary degeneration and development of arthritis. They may be extra-articular.
   c. Common locations of tophi: Extensor surface of forearms, elbows, knees, Achilles tendons, and pinna of external ear.

Quick HIT

Do a Gram stain and culture of the synovial fluid to **rule out septic arthritis,** which is the most worrisome diagnosis on the differential list.

C. Diagnosis

1. Joint aspiration and synovial fluid analysis (under a polarizing microscope) is the only way to make a definitive diagnosis—**needle-shaped and negatively birefringent urate crystals** appear in synovial fluid.
2. Serum uric acid is **not** helpful in diagnosis because it can be normal even during an acute gouty attack.
3. Radiographs reveal punched-out erosions with an overhanging rim of cortical bone in advanced disease.

> **Quick HIT**
> **Complications of Gout**
> - Nephrolithiasis—risk is small (less than 1% per year)
> - Degenerative arthritis occurs in less than 15% of patients.

> **Quick HIT**
> In acute gout, avoid aspirin (can aggravate the problem) and acetaminophen (has no anti-inflammatory properties).

> **Quick HIT**
> Presentation of pseudogout is similar to gout, but typically occurs in larger joints (knee).

D. Treatment

1. In all stages, avoid secondary causes of hyperuricemia.
   a. Medications that increase uric acid levels (thiazide and loop diuretics).
   b. Obesity
   c. Reduce alcohol intake.
   d. Reduce dietary purine intake. Limit intake of seafood/red meat.
2. Acute gout.
   a. Bed rest is important. Early ambulation may precipitate a recurrence.
   b. NSAIDs
      - Treatment of choice in acute gout (indomethacin is traditionally used, but other NSAIDs are effective).
   c. Colchicine
      - An alternative for patients who cannot take NSAIDs or did not respond to NSAIDs.
      - Effective but less favored because 80% of treated patients develop significant nausea/vomiting, abdominal cramps, and severe diarrhea. Compliance tends to be low due to these side effects.
      - It is contraindicated in renal insufficiency and can cause cytopenia.
   d. Corticosteroids
      - Oral prednisone (7- to 10-day course) if patient does not respond to or cannot tolerate NSAIDs and colchicine.
      - Intra-articular corticosteroid injections (if only one joint is involved)—dramatic relief of symptoms.
3. Prophylactic therapy.
   a. Wait until patient has had at least two acute gouty attacks (or perhaps three) before initiating prophylactic therapy. This is because the second attack may take years to occur (if at all), and so the risk-to-benefit ratio for prophylactic medication (allopurinol or uricosuric agents) is not favorable after one gouty attack.
   b. When giving prophylaxis, add either colchicine or an NSAID for 3 to 6 months to prevent an acute attack. The colchicine or NSAID can then be discontinued, and the patient can remain on the uricosuric agent or allopurinol indefinitely.
   c. The choice of whether to use uricosuric drugs or allopurinol depends on how much uric acid is excreted in the urine in a 24-hour period.
      - Uricosuric drugs (probenecid, sulfinpyrazone)—if the 24-hour urine uric acid is <800 mg/day, this indicates undersecretion of urate. These drugs **increase renal excretion** of uric acid; use them only in patients with normal renal function. They are contraindicated if the patient has a history of renal stones.
      - Allopurinol, a xanthine oxidase inhibitor, **decreases uric acid synthesis**—if the 24-hour urine uric acid is **>800 mg/day**, this indicates overproduction. Never give this for acute gout; it makes it worse. Use once-daily dosing. It is well tolerated. Watch for rash or Stevens–Johnson syndrome. Unlike NSAIDS and uricosuric drugs, allopurinol is not contraindicated in kidney dysfunction.

Pseudogout (Calcium Pyrophosphate Deposition Disease)

A. General characteristics

1. Calcium pyrophosphate crystals deposit in joints, leading to inflammation.
2. Risk factors.
   a. Deposition increases with age and with OA of the joints. Therefore, pseudogout is common in **elderly patients with degenerative joint disease.**
   b. Other conditions that may increase crystal deposition include **hemochromatosis, hyperparathyroidism**, hypothyroidism, and Bartter syndrome.

B. Clinical features

1. The most common joints affected are knees and wrists.
2. It is classically monoarticular, but can be polyarticular as well.

C. Diagnosis

1. Joint aspirate is required for definitive diagnosis—**weakly positively birefringent, rod-shaped and rhomboidal crystals** in synovial fluid (calcium pyrophosphate crystals) (Figure 6-8)
2. Radiographs—chondrocalcinosis (cartilage calcification)

D. Treatment

1. Treat the underlying disorder (if identified)
2. Symptomatic management is similar to that for gout
   - First-line therapy includes NSAIDS
   - Colchicine is useful for prophylaxis
   - Intra-articular steroid injections, particularly with triamcinolone
3. Total joint replacement is appropriate if symptoms are debilitating

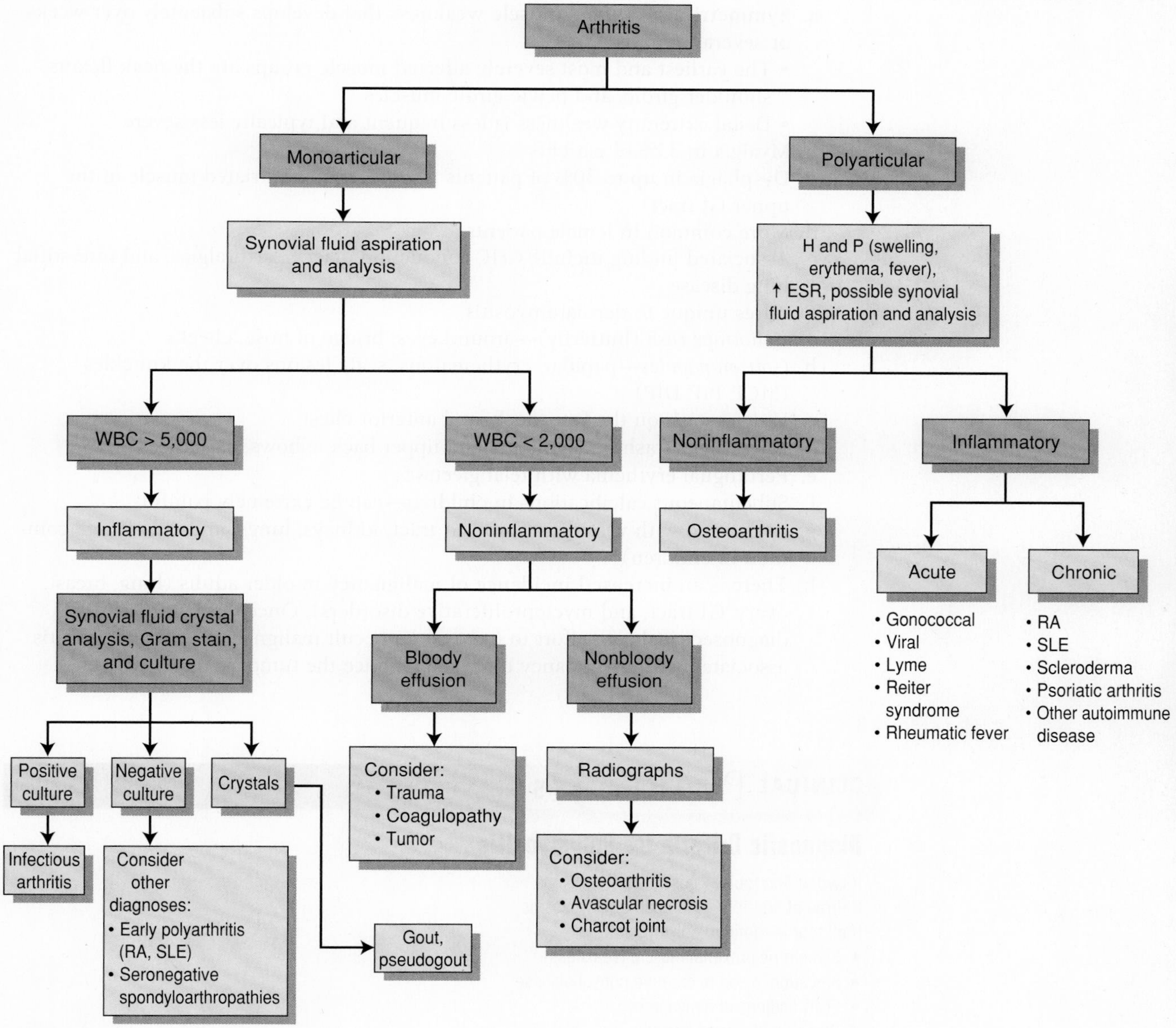

FIGURE 6-8 **Evaluation of joint pain.**

Myopathies and Pain Syndromes

Idiopathic Inflammatory Myopathies

A. General characteristics

1. Classification
   a. **Polymyositis** (does not involve skin)
   b. **Dermatomyositis** (associated with characteristic skin rash)

B. Causes

1. Hypothesis: A genetically susceptible individual plus an environmental trigger leads to immune activation, which results in chronic inflammation.
2. Pathologic changes in muscle
   a. Dermatomyositis—**humoral** immune mechanisms
   b. Polymyositis and inclusion body myositis—**cell-mediated** process

C. Clinical features

1. Features common to both polymyositis and dermatomyositis (see Clinical Pearl 6-5)
   a. **Symmetrical proximal muscle weakness** that develops subacutely over weeks or several months
      - The earliest and most severely affected muscle groups are the neck flexors, shoulder girdle, and pelvic girdle muscles
      - Distal extremity weakness is less frequent and typically less severe
   b. Myalgia in 33% of patients
   c. Dysphagia in up to 30% of patients (involvement of striated muscle in the upper GI tract)
   d. More common in female patients
   e. Associated finding include CHF conduction defects, arthralgias, and interstitial lung disease
2. Features unique to dermatomyositis
   a. *Heliotrope rash* (butterfly)—around eyes, bridge of nose, cheeks
   b. *Gottron papules*—papular, erythematous, scaly lesions over the knuckles (MCP, PIP, DIP)
   c. *V sign*—rash on the face, neck, and anterior chest
   d. *Shawl sign*—rash on shoulders and upper back, elbows, and knees
   e. Periungual erythema with telangiectases
   f. Subcutaneous calcifications in children—can be extremely painful
   g. Associated with vasculitis of the GI tract, kidneys, lungs, and eyes (more common in children)
   h. There is an **increased incidence of malignancy** in older adults (lung, breast, ovary, GI tract, and myeloproliferative disorders). Once dermatomyositis is diagnosed, make an effort to uncover an occult malignancy. Dermatomyositis associated with malignancy often remits once the tumor is removed

CLINICAL PEARL 6-5

Diagnostic Criteria for Polymyositis

If two of first four → possible polymyositis
If three of first four → probable polymyositis
If all four → definite polymyositis

- Symmetric proximal muscle weakness
- Elevation in serum creatine phosphokinase
- EMG findings of a myopathy
- Biopsy evidence of myositis
- Characteristic rash of dermatomyositis

D. Diagnosis

1. Laboratory
   a. CK level is significantly elevated. CK levels correspond to the **degree of muscle necrosis**, so one can monitor the disease severity
   b. LDH, aldolase, AST, ALT elevated
   c. ANA in over 50%
   d. Antisynthetase antibodies (**anti-Jo-1 antibodies**)—abrupt onset of fever, cracked hands, Raynaud phenomenon, interstitial lung disease and fibrosis, arthritis; does not respond well to therapy
   e. Antisignal recognition particle
      - Cardiac manifestations (common)
      - Worst prognosis of all subsets
   f. Anti-Mi-2 antibodies—better prognosis
2. EMG—abnormal in 90% of patients
3. Muscle biopsy
   a. Shows inflammation and muscle fiber fibrosis in *all three*
   b. Dermatomyositis—**perivascular and perimysial**
   c. Polymyositis and inclusion body myositis—**endomysial**

E. Treatment

1. Corticosteroids are the initial treatment
2. Immunosuppressive agents (for patients who do not respond to steroids)—methotrexate, cyclophosphamide, chlorambucil
3. Physical therapy

> **Quick HIT**
> Inclusion body myositis is the "oddball of Inflammatory myopathies" for the following reasons: Affects male patients more than female patients, absence of autoantibodies, distal muscle involvement, and relatively low creatine kinase (CK); prognosis is poor.

Inclusion Body Myositis

A. General characteristics

- More common in men (elderly)
- Insidious onset of slowly progressive proximal **and** distal weakness, often leads to delay in diagnosis
- There is early weakness and atrophy of quadriceps, forearm flexors, and tibialis anterior muscles. Involvement is asymmetrical. Facial weakness occurs in one-third of patients, and dysphagia in one-half of patients
- Patients can also have loss of deep tendon reflexes (nerves are not involved in polymyositis and dermatomyositis)
- Extramuscular manifestations are rare
- Diagnosis—slight elevation of CK levels (relatively low)
- Poor response to therapy
- Not associated with autoantibodies

> **Quick HIT**
> About 10% of people with polymyalgia rheumatica develop **temporal arteritis;** whereas up to 40% to 50% of people with temporal arteritis have coexisting polymyalgia rheumatica.

Polymyalgia Rheumatica

A. General characteristics

1. Usually occurs in **elderly patients** (rare before the age of 50). The mean age of onset is 70, and it is more common in women.
2. The cause is unknown, but an autoimmune process may be responsible. There is a possible genetic link (association with HLA-DR4 allele).
3. Self-limited disease (duration of 1 to 2 years).

B. Clinical features

1. Hip and shoulder muscle pain (bilateral)
   a. Often begins abruptly (but may be gradual)
   b. Stiffness in shoulder and hip regions after a period of inactivity is the most prominent symptom
   c. Pain occurs on movement; muscle strength is normal
   d. Profound morning stiffness is common

2. Constitutional symptoms are usually present: Malaise, fever, depression, weight loss, and fatigue
3. Joint swelling
   a. Up to 20% of patients have synovitis in knees, wrists, or hand joints (can be confused with RA)
   b. Synovitis and tenosynovitis around the shoulder may lead to rotator cuff tendonitis or adhesive capsulitis
4. Signs and symptoms of temporal arteritis (if present)

C. Diagnosis

1. Essentially a clinical diagnosis
2. **ESR is usually elevated** and aids in diagnosis
   a. Almost always >50, frequently >100
   b. Correlates with disease activity

D. Treatment: corticosteroids

1. Response usually occurs within 1 to 7 days. Corticosteroids are not curative, but are effective in suppressing inflammation until the disease resolves itself.
2. After 4 to 6 weeks, begin to taper slowly.
3. Most patients (60% to 70%) can stop corticosteroids within 2 years. A few patients have symptoms for up to 10 years.

••• Fibromyalgia

A. General characteristics

1. Adult women account for 80% to 90% of cases.
2. Chronic nonprogressive course with waxing and waning in severity; many patients improve with time.
3. **Key to diagnosis: multiple trigger points** (points that are tender to palpation)
   a. Symmetrical.
   b. Eighteen characteristic locations have been identified, including occiput, neck, shoulder, ribs, elbows, buttocks, and knees.
4. Etiology is unknown—somatization is not a proven cause.

B. Clinical features

1. **Stiffness**, body aches (musculoskeletal), fatigue.
   a. Pain is constant and aching, and is aggravated by weather changes, stress, sleep deprivation, and cold temperature. It is worse in the morning.
   b. Rest, warmth, and mild exercise improve the pain.
2. Sleep patterns are disrupted, and sleep is unrefreshing.
3. Anxiety and depression are common.

C. Diagnosis

1. Diagnostic criteria
   a. Widespread pain including axial pain for at least 3 months
   b. Pain in at least 11 of the 18 possible tender point sites
2. There are no specific confirmatory tests for fibromyalgia, therefore, it is important to rule out/consider the following conditions: Myofascial syndromes, rheumatoid disease, polymyalgia rheumatica, ankylosing spondylitis, spondyloarthropathy, chronic fatigue syndrome, Lyme disease, hypothyroidism, polymyositis, depression and somatization disorder, and hypertrophic osteoarthropathy.

D. Treatment and management

1. Advise the patient to stay active and engage in low intensity exercise
2. First-line treatment for fibromyalgia is amitriptyline
3. Local anesthetic at trigger points is used acutely
4. Milnacipran (SNRI) and pregabalin are also used
5. Cognitive behavioral therapy; consider psychiatric evaluation

Seronegative Spondyloarthropathies

Ankylosing Spondylitis

A. General characteristics

1. Strong association with **HLA-B27** (90% of patients) (see Table 6-2), however, presence of HLA-B27 should not be considered diagnostic (see Clinical Pearl 6-6).
2. Three times more common in male than in female patients.
3. **Bilateral sacroiliitis** is a prerequisite for making the diagnosis.
4. Onset is in adolescence or young adulthood.
5. It is characterized by "fusion" of the spine in an ascending manner (from lumbar to cervical spine).
6. Course.
   a. There is a slow progression, but the course is highly variable; acute exacerbations are common.
   b. Life expectancy is usually normal.
   c. The first 10 years of the disease can give an indication of long-term severity.

B. Clinical features

1. Low back pain and stiffness (secondary to sacroiliitis)—limited motion in lumbar spine
2. Neck pain and limited motion in cervical spine—occurs later in course of disease
3. **Enthesitis**—inflammation at tendinous insertions into bone (Achilles tendon and supraspinatus tendon)
4. With extensive spinal involvement, the spine becomes brittle and is prone to fractures with minimal trauma. Severe spinal cord injury can occur with such trauma
5. Chest pain and diminished chest expansion—due to thoracic spine involvement
6. Shoulder and hip pain—most commonly the peripheral joints are affected
7. Constitutional symptoms—fatigue, low-grade fever, weight loss
8. Extra-articular manifestations
   a. Eye involvement (most common)—acute **anterior uveitis** or iridocyclitis
   b. Other extra-articular features are rare, but may involve the following systems: Cardiac **(AV heart block and aortic insufficiency)**, renal, pulmonary, and nervous systems
9. Loss of lumbar lordosis can occur as disease advances, leading to inability to stand upright. When severe and symptomatic, this may require spine reconstruction

Quick HIT

In ankylosing spondylitis, low back pain and stiffness are characteristically worse in the morning and better as the day progresses. They **improve with activity** and a hot shower and worsen with rest or inactivity.

CLINICAL PEARL 6-6

Seronegative Spondyloarthropathies

Diseases that belong to seronegative spondyloarthropathies include the following:

- Ankylosing spondylitis
- Reactive arthritis (and Reiter syndrome)
- Psoriatic arthritis
- Arthropathy of IBD
- Undifferentiated spondyloarthropathies

Seronegative spondyloarthropathies have the following **in common:**

- Negative RF
- Strong association with HLA-B27 antigen
- Oligoarthritis (asymmetrical)
- Enthesitis (inflammation at sites of insertion of fascia, ligament, or tendon to bone)
- Inflammatory arthritis (axial and sacroiliac joints)
- Extra-articular features (eyes, skin, genitourinary tract)
- Familial predisposition

Quick HIT

Complications of Ankylosing Spondylitis
- Restrictive lung disease
- Cauda equina syndrome
- Spine fracture with spinal cord injury
- Osteoporosis
- Spondylodiscitis

C. Diagnosis
1. Imaging studies of lumbar spine and pelvis (plain film, MRI, or CT) reveal sacroiliitis—sclerotic changes in the sacroiliac area. Eventually, the vertebral columns fuse, producing "**bamboo spine.**"
2. Elevated ESR in up to 75% of patients (due to inflammation)—nonspecific
3. HLA-B27 is not necessary for diagnosis. Present in 8% of general population

D. Treatment
1. NSAIDs (indomethacin) for symptomatic relief
2. Anti-TNF medications (etanercept, infliximab)
3. Physical therapy (maintaining good posture, extension exercises)
4. Surgery may be necessary in some patients with severe spinal deformity
5. Patients with ankylosing spondylitis who sustain even minor trauma and who complain of neck or back pain should be strictly immobilized to prevent spinal cord injury until thorough imaging studies are obtained

Reactive Arthritis/Reiter Syndrome

Quick HIT

Reactive arthritis is a clinical diagnosis. If any patient has acute asymmetric arthritis that progresses sequentially from one joint to another, reactive arthritis should be in the differential diagnosis.

A. General characteristics
1. Reactive arthritis is asymmetric inflammatory oligoarthritis of lower extremities (upper extremities less common) (see Table 6-7). The arthritis is preceded by an infectious process that is remote from the site of arthritis (1 to 4 weeks prior), usually after enteric or urogenital infections.
2. It occurs mostly in HLA-B27–positive individuals.
3. **Reiter syndrome** is an example of reactive arthritis, but most patients do not have the classic findings of Reiter syndrome (arthritis, uveitis, and urethritis), so the term reactive arthritis is now used.
4. The organisms usually associated with reactive arthritis include *Salmonella, Shigella, Campylobacter, Chlamydia, Yersinia.*

Quick HIT

The term **undifferentiated spondyloarthropathy** is used when a patient has features of reactive arthritis but there is no evidence of previous infection (in the GI or genitourinary tract) and the classic findings of Reiter syndrome are absent.

B. Clinical features
1. Look for evidence of infection (GI or genitourinary) 1 to 4 weeks before the onset of symptoms.
2. Asymmetric arthritis—new joints may be involved sequentially over days. Joints are painful, with effusions and lack of mobility.
3. Fatigue, malaise, weight loss, and fever are common.
4. Joint pain may persist or recur over a long-term period.

C. Diagnosis: Send synovial fluid for analysis (to rule out infection or crystals). There is no test specific to reactive arthritis.

TABLE 6-7 Causes of Joint Pain

Polyarticular Joint Pain	Monoarticular Joint Pain
RA	Osteoarthritis
SLE	Gout
Viral arthritis	Pseudogout
Reiter syndrome	Trauma
Rheumatic fever	Septic arthritis
Lyme disease	Hemarthrosis
Gonococcal arthritis	
Drug-induced arthritis	

D. Treatment

1. NSAIDs are first-line therapy.
2. If there is no response, then try sulfasalazine and immunosuppressive agents such as azathioprine.
3. Antibiotic use is controversial—usually not given.

Psoriatic Arthritis

- Develops in fewer than 10% of patients with psoriasis.
- It is typically gradual in onset. Patients usually have skin disease for months to years before arthritis develops.
- Usually asymmetric and polyarticular. Characteristic "**sausage digits**" and **nail pitting** may also be present.
- Upper extremities most often involved; smaller joints more common than large joints
- Initial treatment is NSAIDs, but persistent arthritis may require methotrexate or anti-TNF agents. Steroids are typically not used.

Vasculitis

Temporal/Giant Cell Arteritis

A. General characteristics

1. Vasculitis of unknown cause; typical patient is >50 years of age; twice as common in women as men (see Clinical Pearl 6-7).
2. The temporal arteries are most frequently affected, but it may involve other arteries, such as the aorta or carotids. Carotid bruits, decreased pulses in the arms, and aortic regurgitation may also be observed.
3. Associated with increased risk of aortic aneurysm and aortic dissection.

B. Clinical features

1. Constitutional symptoms of malaise, fatigue, weight loss, and low-grade fever
2. Headaches—may be severe
3. Visual impairment (in only 25% to 50%)
   a. Caused by involvement of ophthalmic artery
   b. Optic neuritis; amaurosis fugax; may lead to **blindness** in up to 50% if not treated early and aggressively
4. Jaw pain with chewing—intermittent **claudication of jaw/tongue** when chewing
5. Tenderness over temporal artery; absent temporal pulse
6. Palpable nodules
7. **Forty percent of patients also have polymyalgia rheumatica**

C. Diagnosis

1. **ESR elevated** (but normal ESR does not exclude the diagnosis)

CLINICAL PEARL 6-7

Vasculitis

- In all of the vasculitic syndromes, blood vessels are inflamed and vascular necrosis can result. Findings depend on the size of the vessel involved and the location of involvement (target organ ischemia).
- If any patient has a systemic illness that has not been explained by another process (or has ischemia involving one or more systems), entertain the diagnosis of vasculitis.
- Classified according to size of vessel
  - **Large vessel:** Takayasu arteritis, temporal arteritis
  - **Medium vessel:** PAN, Kawasaki disease (a pediatric disease), Wegener granulomatosis, Churg–Strauss syndrome, microscopic polyangiitis
  - **Small vessel:** Henoch–Schönlein purpura, hypersensitivity vasculitis, Behçet syndrome

Quick HIT

Keys to Diagnosing Temporal Arteritis
- Age >50 years
- New headache
- Tender/palpable temporal artery
- High ESR
- Jaw claudication

Quick HIT

If temporal arteritis is suspected, begin prednisone and order a temporal artery biopsy.

Quick HIT

Suspect Takayasu arteritis in a young woman with:
- Decreased/absent peripheral pulses
- Discrepancies of BP (arm vs. leg)
- Arterial bruits

2. Biopsy of the temporal artery has a sensitivity of 90%. A single negative biopsy does not exclude the diagnosis

D. Treatment

1. Use high-dose steroids (prednisone) early to prevent blindness.
   a. Start treatment **immediately**, even if temporal arteritis is only suspected. **Do not wait for biopsy results.** If visual loss is present, admit the patient to the hospital for IV steroids; otherwise, start oral prednisone.
   b. If the diagnosis is confirmed, continue treatment for at least 4 weeks, then taper gradually, but maintain steroid therapy for up to 2 to 3 years. Relapse is likely to occur if steroids are stopped prematurely.
2. Follow up on ESR levels to monitor effectiveness of treatment.
3. Visual loss in one eye may be temporary or permanent. Prompt and aggressive steroid treatment is primarily given to prevent involvement of the other eye, but it may improve the visual outcome in the affected eye as well.
4. Even if untreated, the disease is usually eventually self-limiting in most patients, although vision loss may be permanent.

Takayasu Arteritis

A. General characteristics

1. Most common in young Asian women
2. Granulomatous vasculitis of aortic arch and its major branches—leading to fibrosis and potentially causing to stenosis or narrowing of vessels
3. Diagnosed via arteriogram

B. Clinical features

1. Constitutional symptoms—fever, night sweats, malaise, arthralgias, fatigue
2. Pain and tenderness over involved vessels
3. Absent pulses in carotid, radial, or ulnar arteries; aortic regurgitation may be present
4. Signs and symptoms of ischemia eventually develop in areas supplied by involved vessels
5. Severe complications include limb ischemia, aortic aneurysms, aortic regurgitation, stroke, and secondary HTN due to renal artery stenosis. The main prognostic predictor is the presence or absence of these complications.
6. Causes visual disturbances due to ocular involvement and hemorrhage of retinal arteries.

C. Treatment

1. Steroids such as prednisone may relieve the symptoms.
2. Treat HTN.
3. Surgery or angioplasty may be required to recannulate stenosed vessels. Bypass grafting is sometimes necessary.

Churg–Strauss Syndrome

- Vasculitis involving many organ systems (respiratory, cardiac, GI, skin, renal, neurologic)
- Clinical features include constitutional findings (fever, fatigue, weight loss), prominent respiratory tract findings (**asthma**, dyspnea), skin lesions (subcutaneous nodules, palpable purpura), as well as **eosinophilia**.
- Diagnosis is made by biopsy of lung or skin tissue (prominence of eosinophils). **It is associated with p-ANCA.**
- The prognosis is poor with a 5-year survival of 25% (death is usually due to cardiac or pulmonary complications). With treatment (steroids), the 5-year prognosis improves to 50%.

Wegener Granulomatosis

A. General characteristics: Vasculitis predominantly involving the kidneys and upper and lower respiratory tract (sometimes other organs as well)

B. Clinical features

1. Upper respiratory symptoms (e.g., **sinusitis**); purulent or bloody nasal discharge
2. Oral ulcers (may be painful)
3. Pulmonary symptoms (cough, hemoptysis, dyspnea)
4. Renal involvement (glomerulonephritis—may have rapidly progressive renal failure)
5. Eye disease (conjunctivitis, scleritis)
6. Musculoskeletal (arthralgias, myalgias)
7. Tracheal stenosis
8. Constitutional findings (e.g., fever, weight loss)

C. Diagnosis

1. Chest radiograph is abnormal (nodules or infiltrates).
2. Laboratory findings: Markedly elevated ESR, anemia (normochromic normocytic), hematuria, **positive c-ANCA in 90%** *of patients*—sensitive and specific; thrombocytopenia may be present.
3. Open lung biopsy confirms diagnosis.

D. Prognosis and treatment

1. Prognosis is poor—most patients die within 1 year after the diagnosis.
2. A combination of **cyclophosphamide and corticosteroids** can induce remissions in many patients, but a relapse may occur at any time.
3. Consider renal transplantation if the patient has end-stage renal disease (ESRD).

Quick HIT

Most patients with Wegener granulomatosis also have sinus disease, pulmonary disease, and glomerulonephritis. Renal disease accounts for the majority of deaths.

Polyarteritis Nodosa

A. General characteristics

1. Vasculitis of medium-sized vessels involving the nervous system and GI tract
2. Can be associated with **hepatitis B**, HIV, and drug reactions
3. Pathophysiology: PMN invasion of all layers and fibrinoid necrosis plus resulting intimal proliferation lead to reduced luminal area, which results in ischemia, infarction, and aneurysms
4. Necrosis is segmented leading to "rosary sign" as a result of aneurisms

B. Clinical findings

1. Early symptoms are fever, weakness, weight loss, myalgias and arthralgias, and abdominal pain (bowel angina).
2. Other findings are HTN, mononeuritic multiplex, and livedo reticularis.

C. Diagnosis

1. Diagnosis is made by biopsy of involved tissue or mesenteric angiography.
2. ESR is usually elevated, and p-ANCA may be present.
3. Test for fecal occult blood.

D. Prognosis and treatment: The prognosis is poor, but is improved to a limited extent with treatment. Start with corticosteroids. If polyarteritis nodosa (PAN) is se vere, add cyclophosphamide.

Quick HIT

There is **no pulmonary involvement** in PAN (which distinguishes it from Wegener granulomatosis).

Behçet Syndrome

- An autoimmune, multisystem vasculitic disease; cause is unknown.
- Clinical features: painful, sterile oral and genital ulcerations (**pathergy**), arthritis (knees and ankles most common), **eye involvement** (uveitis, optic neuritis, iritis, conjunctivitis), CNS involvement (meningoencephalitis, intracranial HTN), fever, and weight loss.

- Diagnosis is made by biopsy of involved tissue (laboratory tests are not helpful).
- Treatment is steroids, which are helpful.
- Often presents in Middle Easterners.

Buerger Disease (Thromboangiitis Obliterans)

- Occurs mostly in young men who **smoke cigarettes**
- Acute, **segmental inflammation** of small- and medium-sized arteries and veins, affecting arms and legs
- inflammation in veins leads to superficial nodular phlebitis
- May lead to gangrene and **autoamputation**
- Clinical features include ischemic claudication; cold, cyanotic, painful distal extremities; paresthesias of distal extremities; and ulceration of digits. Raynaud phenomena may also be observed
- Smoking cessation is mandatory to reduce progression

Hypersensitivity Vasculitis

- Small-vessel vasculitis that is a hypersensitivity reaction in response to a drug (penicillin, sulfa drugs), infection, or other stimulus.
- Skin is predominantly involved—palpable purpura, macules, or vesicles (common on lower extremities) can occur. Lesions can be painful.
- Constitutional symptoms (fever, weight loss, fatigue) may be present.
- Diagnosis is made by biopsy of tissue.
- Prognosis is very good—spontaneous remissions are common.
- Withdrawal of the offending agent and steroids are the treatments of choice.

DISEASES OF THE RENAL AND GENITOURINARY SYSTEM

7

Renal Failure

Acute Kidney Injury

A. General characteristics

1. Definition: A rapid decline in renal function, with an increase in serum creatinine level (a relative increase of 50% or an absolute increase of 0.5 to 1.0 mg/dL) (Figure 7-1). The creatinine may be normal despite a markedly reduced glomerular filtration rate (GFR) in the early stages of acute kidney injury (AKI) due to the time it takes for creatinine to accumulate in the body. This condition is also called acute renal failure (ARF).
2. One consensus definition of AKI is called the RIFLE criteria.
   a. **RISK:** 1.5-fold increase in the serum creatinine or GFR decrease by 25% or urine output <0.5 mL/kg/hr for 6 hours.
   b. **INJURY:** Twofold increase in the serum creatinine or GFR decrease by 50% or urine output <0.5 mL/kg/hr for 12 hours.
   c. **FAILURE:** Threefold increase in the serum creatinine or GFR decrease by 75% or urine output of <0.5 mL/kg/hr for 24 hours, or anuria for 12 hours.
   d. **LOSS:** Complete loss of kidney function (i.e., requiring dialysis) for more than 4 weeks.
   e. **ESRD:** Complete loss of kidney function (i.e., requiring dialysis) for more than 3 months.
3. AKI may be oliguric, anuric, or nonoliguric. Severe AKI may occur without a reduction in urine output (nonoliguric AKI).
4. Weight gain and edema are most common findings in patients with AKI. This is due to a positive water and sodium (Na^+) balance.
5. Characterized by **azotemia** (elevated BUN and Cr).
   a. Elevated BUN is also seen with catabolic drugs (e.g., steroids), GI/soft tissue bleeding, and dietary protein intake.
   b. Elevated Cr is also seen with increased muscle breakdown and various drugs. The baseline Cr level varies proportionately with muscle mass.
6. Prognosis
   a. More than 80% of patients in whom AKI develops recover completely. However, prognosis varies widely depending on the severity of renal failure and other comorbidities.
   b. The older the patient and the more severe the insult, the lower is the likelihood of complete recovery.
   c. The most common cause of death is infection (75% of all deaths), followed by cardiorespiratory complications.

Quick HIT

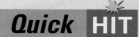

Types of AKI (see Figure 7-1)
- **Prerenal AKI**—decrease in renal blood flow (60% to 70% of cases)
- **Intrinsic AKI**—damage to renal parenchyma (25% to 40% of cases)
- **Postrenal AKI**—urinary tract obstruction (5% to 10% of cases)

B. Categories

1. Prerenal failure (see also Clinical Pearl 7-1)
   a. Most common cause of AKI; potentially reversible

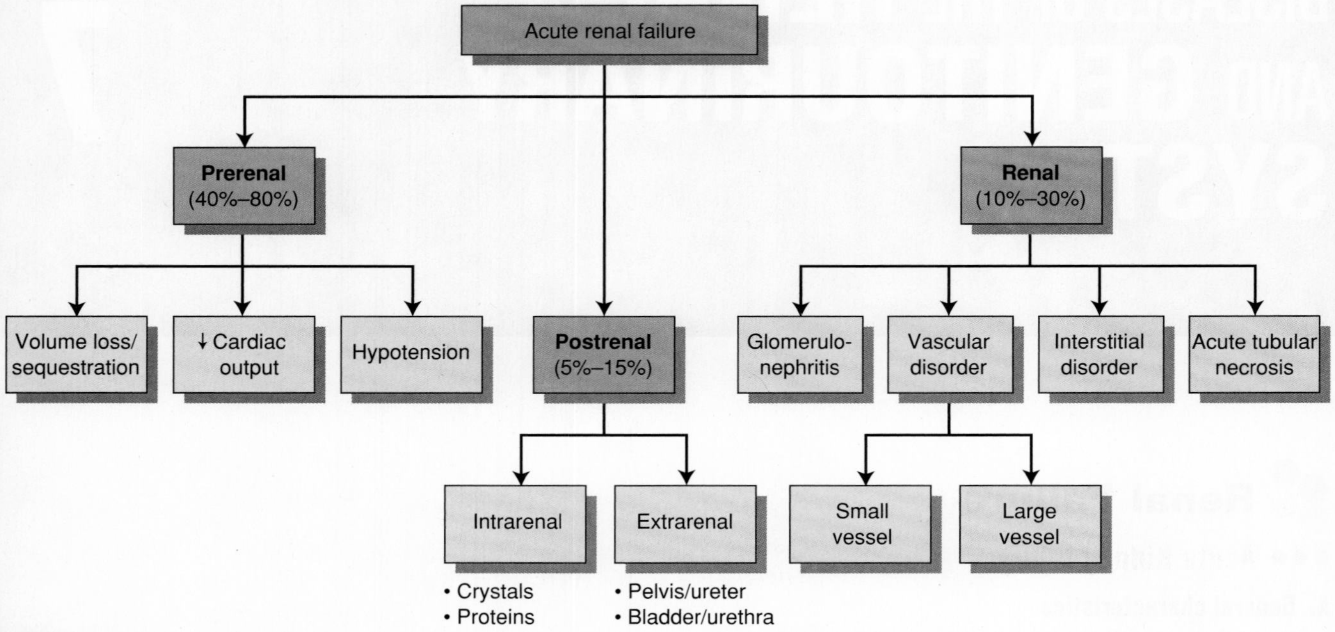

FIGURE 7-1 Causes of AKI.

Quick HIT

Monitoring a Patient with AKI

- Daily weights, intake, and output
- BP
- Serum electrolytes
- Watch Hb and Hct for anemia
- Watch for infection

b. Etiology (decrease in systemic arterial blood volume or renal perfusion)—can complicate any disease that causes hypovolemia, low cardiac output, or systemic vasodilation
  - Hypovolemia—dehydration, excessive diuretic use, poor fluid intake, vomiting, diarrhea, burns, hemorrhage
  - CHF
  - Hypotension (systolic BP below 90 mm Hg), from sepsis, excessive antihypertensive medications, bleeding, dehydration
  - Renal arterial obstruction (kidney is hypoperfused despite elevated blood pressure)
  - Cirrhosis, hepatorenal syndrome
  - In patients with decreased renal perfusion, NSAIDs (constrict afferent arteriole), ACE inhibitors (cause efferent arteriole vasodilation), and cyclosporin can precipitate prerenal failure

CLINICAL PEARL 7-1

Diagnostic Approach in AKI

- History and physical examination.
- The first thing to do is to determine the duration of renal failure. A baseline Cr level provides this information.
- The second task is to determine whether AKI is due to prerenal, intrarenal, or postrenal causes. This is done via a combination of H&P and laboratory findings.
  - Signs of volume depletion and CHF suggest a prerenal etiology.
  - Signs of an allergic reaction (rash) suggest acute interstitial nephritis (an intrinsic renal etiology).
  - A suprapubic mass, BPH, or bladder dysfunction suggests a postrenal etiology.
- Medication review.
- Urinalysis
- Urine chemistry (FENa, osmolality, urine Na^+, urine Cr).
- Renal ultrasound (to rule out obstruction).

TABLE 7-1 Studies to Differentiate Prerenal From Intrinsic AKI

	Prerenal	Intrinsic Renal
Urinalysis	Hyaline casts	Abnormal
BUN/Cr Ratio	>20:1	<20:1
FENa	<1%	>2%–3%
Urine Osmolality	>500 mOsm	250–300 mOsm
Urine Sodium	<20	>40

c. Pathophysiology
- Renal blood flow decreases enough to lower the GFR, which leads to decreased clearance of metabolites (BUN, Cr, uremic toxins)
- Because the renal parenchyma is undamaged, tubular function (and therefore the concentrating ability) is preserved. Therefore, the kidney responds appropriately, conserving as much sodium and water as possible
- This form of AKI is reversible on restoration of blood flow; but if hypoperfusion persists, ischemia results and can lead to acute tubular necrosis (ATN) (see below)

d. Clinical features—signs of volume depletion (dry mucous membranes, hypotension, tachycardia, decreased tissue turgor, oliguria/anuria)

e. Laboratory findings
- **Oliguria—always** found in prerenal failure (this is to preserve volume)
- Increased BUN-to-serum Cr ratio (>**20:1** is the classic ratio)—because kidney can reabsorb urea
- Increased urine osmolality (>500 mOsm/kg H_2O)—because the kidney is able to reabsorb water
- Decreased urine Na^+ (<20 mEq/L with fractional excretion of sodium [FENa] <1%) because Na^+ is avidly reabsorbed
- Increased urine–plasma Cr ratio (>40:1)—because much of the filtrate is reabsorbed (but not the creatinine)
- Bland urine sediment

2. Intrinsic renal failure (see Table 7-1 and Clinical Pearl 7-2)
   a. Kidney tissue is damaged such that glomerular filtration and tubular function are significantly impaired. The kidneys are unable to concentrate urine effectively
   b. Causes
   - Tubular disease (ATN)—can be caused by ischemia (most common cause), nephrotoxins (see Clinical Pearls 7-3 and 7-4)
   - Glomerular disease (acute glomerulonephritis [GN])—for example, Goodpasture syndrome, Wegener granulomatosis, poststreptococcal GN, lupus
   - Vascular disease—for example, renal artery occlusion, TTP, HUS

Quick HIT

Prerenal Failure versus ATN

	Prerenal Failure	ATN
Urine osmolarity	>500	>350
Urine Na^+	<20	>40
FENa	<1%	>1%
Urine sediment	Scant	Full brownish pigment, granular casts with epithelial casts

Quick HIT

Note that prerenal azotemia and ischemic AKI are part of a spectrum of manifestations of renal hypoperfusion. The latter differs in that injury to renal tubular cells occurs.

CLINICAL PEARL 7-2

Rhabdomyolysis

1. Skeletal muscle breakdown caused by trauma, crush injuries, prolonged immobility, seizures, snake bites.
2. Release of muscle fiber contents (myoglobin) into bloodstream. Myoglobin is toxic to kidneys, which can lead to AKI.
3. Presents with markedly elevated creatine phosphokinase (CPK), hyperkalemia, hypocalcemia, hyperuricemia.
4. Treat with IV fluids, mannitol (osmotic diuretic) and bicarbonate (drives K back into cells).

CLINICAL PEARL 7-3

Causes of Acute Tubular Necrosis (ATN)

- **Ischemic AKI**
  - Secondary to **severe decline in renal blood flow,** as in shock, hemorrhage, sepsis, disseminated intravascular coagulation, heart failure.
  - Ischemia results in the death of tubular cells.
- **Nephrotoxic AKI**
  - Injury secondary to substances that directly injure renal parenchyma and result in cell death.
  - Causes include antibiotics (aminoglycosides, vancomycin), radiocontrast agents, NSAIDs (especially in the setting of CHF), poisons, myoglobinuria (from muscle damage, rhabdomyolysis, strenuous exercise), hemoglobinuria (from hemolysis), chemotherapeutic drugs (cisplatin), and kappa and gamma light chains produced in multiple myeloma.

Quick HIT

Three Basic Tests for Postrenal Failure
- Physical examination—palpate the bladder
- Ultrasound—look for obstruction, hydronephrosis
- Catheter—look for large volume of urine

Quick HIT

Diagnosis of AKI is usually made by finding elevated BUN and Cr levels. The patient is usually asymptomatic.

- Interstitial disease—for example, allergic interstitial nephritis, often due to a hypersensitivity reaction to medication (see Tubulointerstitial Diseases section)

c. Clinical features depend on the cause. Edema is usually present. Recovery may be possible but takes longer than in prerenal failure

d. Laboratory findings
- Decreased BUN-to-serum Cr ratio (<20:1, typically closer to 10:1 ratio) in comparison with prerenal failure. Both BUN and Cr levels are still elevated, but less urea is reabsorbed than in prerenal failure
- Increased urine Na^+ (>40 mEq/L with FENa > 2% to 3%)—because Na^+ is poorly reabsorbed
- Decreased urine osmolality (<350 mOsm/kg H_2O)—because renal water reabsorption is impaired
- Decreased urine–plasma Cr ratio (<20:1)—because filtrate cannot be reabsorbed

3. Postrenal failure

a. Least common cause of AKI

b. Obstruction of any segment of the urinary tract (with intact kidney) causes increased tubular pressure (urine produced cannot be excreted), which leads to decreased GFR. Blood supply and renal parenchyma are intact. Note that both kidneys must be obstructed for creatinine to rise.

c. Renal function is restored if obstruction is relieved before the kidneys are damaged.

d. Postrenal obstruction, if untreated, can lead to ATN.

e. Causes
- Urethral obstruction secondary to enlarged prostate (BPH) is the most common cause
- Obstruction of solitary kidney
- Nephrolithiasis
- Obstructing neoplasm (bladder, cervix, prostate, and so on)

CLINICAL PEARL 7-4

Course of ATN

- Onset (insult)
- **Oliguric phase**
  - Azotemia and uremia—average length 10 to 14 days
  - Urine output
- **Diuretic phase**
  - Begins when urine output is >500 mL/day
  - High urine output due to the following: fluid overload (excretion of retained salt, water, other solutes that were retained during oliguric phase); osmotic diuresis due to retained solutes during oliguric phase; tubular cell damage (delayed recovery of epithelial cell function relative to GFR)
- **Recovery phase**—recovery of tubular function

CLINICAL PEARL 7-5

Urine Osmolality

1. Urine osmolality is a measure of urine concentration. The higher the osmolality, the more concentrated the urine.
2. Dehydration in a healthy person leads to increase in urine concentration (osmolality) as follows: Dehydration causes low intravascular volume, which triggers ADH release, which stimulates reabsorption of water from kidney to fill the vasculature. Increased water reabsorption leads to more concentrated urine.
3. In ATN, the tubule cells are damaged and cannot reabsorb water (or sodium); so the urine cannot be concentrated, which leads to low urine osmolality.

- Retroperitoneal fibrosis
- Ureteral obstruction is an uncommon cause because obstruction must be bilateral to cause renal failure

C. Diagnosis

1. Blood tests (see also Clinical Pearl 7-5).
   a. Elevation in BUN and Cr levels.
   b. Electrolytes (K^+, Ca^{2+}, PO_4^{3-}), albumin levels, CBC with differential.
2. Urinalysis (Figure 7-2 and Table 7-2).
   a. A dipstick test positive for protein (3^+, 4^+) suggests intrinsic renal failure due to glomerular insult.

Quick HIT

Obtain the Following in Any Patient with AKI

- Urinalysis
- Urine chemistry
- Serum electrolytes (Na+, K+, BUN, Cr), CBC
- Bladder catheterization to rule out obstruction (diagnostic and therapeutic)
- Renal ultrasound to look for obstruction

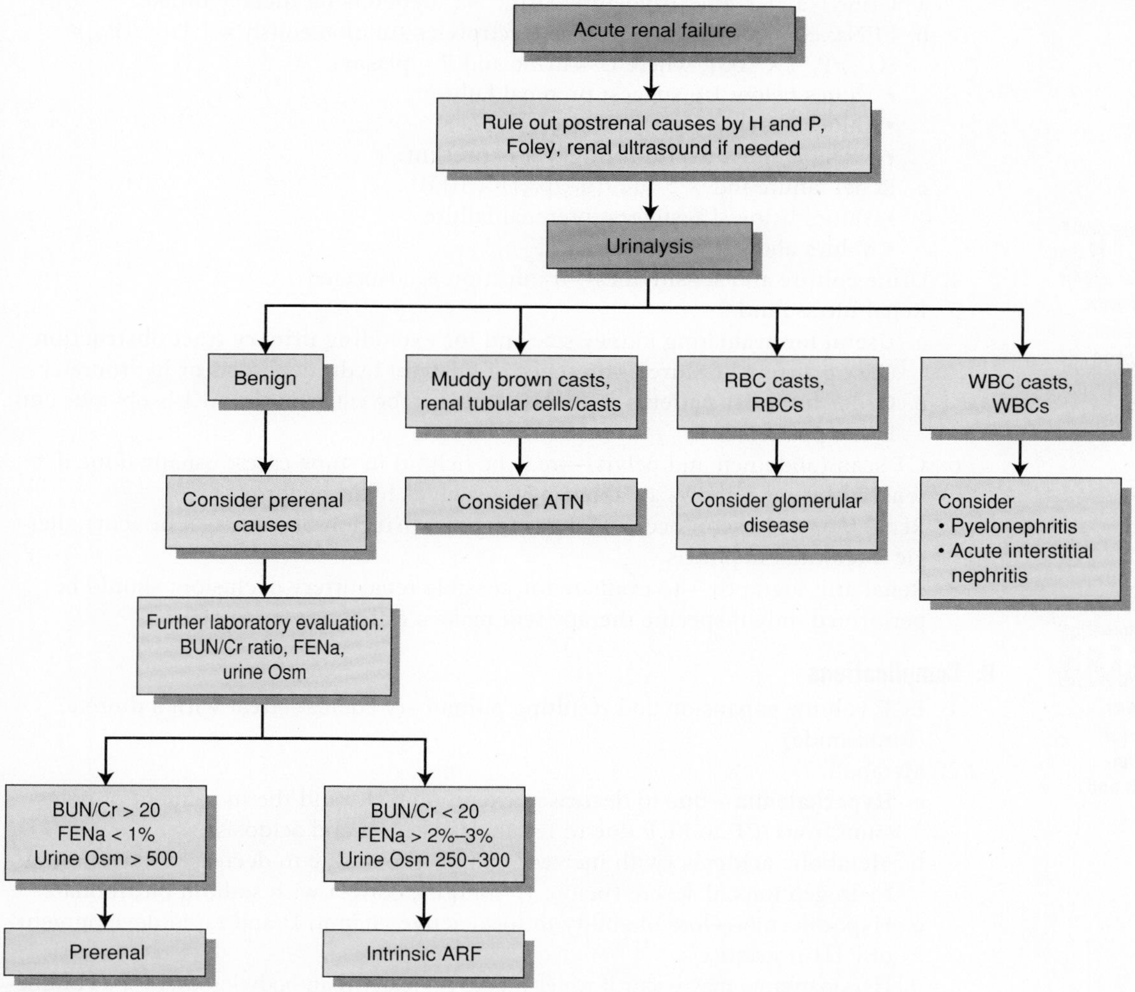

FIGURE 7-2 Evaluation of AKI.

TABLE 7-2 **Urinalysis Findings in Renal Failure**

Cause	Urine Sediment	Protein	Blood
Prerenal	Benign sediment—few hyaline casts	Negative	Negative
Intrarenal			
Acute tubular necrosis	"Muddy brown" casts, renal tubular cells/casts, granular casts	Trace	Negative
Acute glomerulonephritis	Dysmorphic RBCs, RBCs with casts, WBCs with casts, fatty casts	4+	3+
Acute interstitial nephritis	RBCs, WBCs, WBCs with casts, eosinophils	1+	2+
Postrenal	Benign; may or may not see RBCs, WBCs	Negative	Negative

b. Microscopic examination of the urine sediment:
- **Hyaline casts** are devoid of contents (seen in prerenal failure).
- **RBC casts** indicate glomerular disease.
- **WBC casts** indicate renal parenchymal inflammation.
- **Fatty casts** indicate nephrotic syndrome.

3. Urine chemistry—to distinguish between different forms of AKI.
   a. Urine $Na^{+,}$ Cr, and osmolality: Urine Na^+ **depends on dietary intake.**
   b. FENa: collect urine and plasma electrolytes simultaneously = $[(U_{Na})/(P_{Na})/(U_{Cr})/P_{Cr}) \times 100]$, where U = urine and P = plasma.
   - Values below 1% suggest prerenal failure.
   - Values above 2% to 3% suggest ATN.
   - **FENa is most useful if oliguria is present.**

   c. Renal failure index 5 $(u_{Na}/[u_{Cr}/p_{Cr}]) \times 100)$
   - Values below 1% suggest prerenal failure.
   - Values above 1% suggest ATN.
4. Urine culture and sensitivities—if infection is suspected.
5. Renal ultrasound.
   a. Useful for evaluating kidney size and **for excluding urinary tract obstruction (i.e., postrenal failure)**—presence of bilateral hydronephrosis or hydroureter
   b. **Order for most patients with AKI**—unless the cause of the AKI is obvious and is not postrenal
6. CT scan (abdomen and pelvis)—may be helpful in some cases; usually done if renal ultrasound shows an abnormality such as hydronephrosis
7. Renal biopsy—useful occasionally if there is suspicion of acute GN or acute allergic interstitial nephritis
8. Renal arteriography—to evaluate for possible renal artery occlusion; should be performed only if specific therapy will make a difference

Quick HIT

In evaluating a patient with AKI, first exclude prerenal and postrenal causes, and then, if necessary, investigate intrinsic renal causes.

D. Complications

1. ECF volume expansion and resulting pulmonary edema—treat with a diuretic (furosemide)
2. Metabolic
   a. **Hyperkalemia**—due to decreased excretion of K^+ and the movement of potassium from ICF to ECF due to tissue destruction and acidosis
   b. **Metabolic acidosis** (with increased anion gap)—due to decreased excretion of hydrogen ions; if severe (below 16 mEq/L), correct with sodium bicarbonate
   c. Hypocalcemia—loss of ability to form active vitamin D and rapid development of PTH resistance
   d. Hyponatremia may occur if water intake is greater than body losses, or if a volume-depleted patient consumes excessive hypotonic solutions. (Hypernatremia may also be seen in hypovolemic states.)

Quick HIT

In the early phase of AKI, the most common mortal complications are hyperkalemic cardiac arrest and pulmonary edema.

e. Hyperphosphatemia
f. Hyperuricemia
3. Uremia—toxic end products of metabolism accumulate (especially from protein metabolism)
4. Infection
a. A common and serious complication of AKI (occurs in 50% to 60% of cases). The cause is probably multifactorial, but uremia itself is thought to impair immune function
b. Examples include pneumonia, UTI, wound infection, and sepsis

E. Treatment

1. General measures (see also Table 7-3).
a. Avoid medications that decrease renal blood flow (NSAIDs) and/or that are nephrotoxic (e.g., aminoglycosides, radiocontrast agents).
b. Adjust medication dosages for level of renal function.
c. Correct fluid imbalance.
- If volume depleted, give IV fluids. However, many patients with AKI are volume overloaded (especially if they are oliguric or anuric), so diuresis may be necessary.
- The goal is to strike a balance between correcting volume deficits and avoiding volume overload (while maintaining adequate urine output).
- Monitor fluid balance by daily weight measurements (most accurate estimate) and intake–output records.
- Be sure to take into account the patient's cardiac history when considering treatment options for fluid imbalances (i.e., do not give excessive fluid to a patient with CHF).
d. Correct electrolyte disturbances if present.
e. Optimize cardiac output. BP should be approximately 120 to 140/80 to 90.
f. Order dialysis if symptomatic uremia, intractable acidemia, hyperkalemia, or volume overload develop.
2. Prerenal
a. Treat the underlying disorder.
b. Give NS to maintain euvolemia and restore blood pressure—do not give to patients with edema or ascites. May be necessary to stop antihypertensive medications.
c. Eliminate any offending agents (ACE inhibitors, NSAIDs).
d. If patient is unstable, Swan–Ganz monitoring for accurate assessment of intravascular volume.

Quick HIT

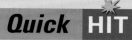

Radiographic contrast media can cause ATN (typically very rapidly) by causing spasm of the afferent arteriole. It can be prevented with saline hydration.

Table 7-3 Prognostic Factors in AKI

Severity of renal failure	Magnitude of increase in Cr Presence of oliguria Fractional excretion of sodium Requirement for dialysis Duration of severe renal failure Marked abnormalities on urinalysis
Underlying health of patient	Age Presence, severity, and reversibility of underlying disease
Clinical circumstances	Cause of renal failure Severity and reversibility of acute process(es) Number and type of other failed organ systems Development of sepsis and other complications

Adapted from Schrier RW, ed. *Diseases of the Kidney and Urinary Tract.* Vol II. 7th ed. Philadelphia, PA: Lippincott Williams & Wilkins, 2001:1128, Table 41-14.

TABLE 7-4 Differentiation of AKI Versus CKD

Favors Chronic	Favors Acute
History of kidney disease, HTN, abnormal urinalysis, edema	—
Small kidney size on renal ultrasound	—
—	Return of renal function to normal with time
Hyperkalemia, acidemia, hyperphosphatemia, anemia	Hyperkalemia, acidemia, hyperphosphatemia, anemia
—	Urine output <500 mL/day without uremic symptoms
Urinalysis with broad casts (i.e., more than two to three WBCs in diameter)	—

Adapted from Schrier RW, ed. *Diseases of the Kidney and Urinary Tract.* Vol II. 7th ed. Philadelphia, PA: Lippincott Williams & Wilkins, 2001:1098, Figure 41-5.

Quick HIT

Whenever a patient has elevated Cr levels, the first thing to do is determine the patient's **baseline** Cr level, if possible. This helps determine whether the patient has AKI, CKD, or chronic renal insufficiency/failure with superimposed AKI. (This condition is known as "acute on chronic" renal failure.)

3. Intrinsic
   a. Once ATN develops, therapy is supportive. Eliminate the cause/offending agent.
   b. If oliguric, a trial of furosemide may help to increase urine flow. This improves fluid balance.
4. Postrenal—a bladder catheter may be inserted to decompress the urinary tract. Consider urology consultation.

Chronic Kidney Disease

A. General characteristics

1. Chronic kidney disease (CKD) is defined as either decreased kidney function (GFR <60 mL/min) or kidney damage (structural or functional abnormalities) for at least 3 months, regardless of cause (see also Table 7-4).
2. Causes
   a. **Diabetes is the most common cause** (30% of cases).
   b. **HTN is responsible for 25% of cases.**
   c. Chronic GN accounts for 15% of cases.
   d. Interstitial nephritis, polycystic kidney disease, obstructive uropathy
   e. Any of the causes of AKI may lead to CKD if prolonged and/or if treatment is delayed.
3. Pathophysiology
   a. Plasma Cr varies inversely with GFR.
   b. Cr clearance is the most common clinical measure of GFR.
   c. An increase in plasma Cr indicates disease progression, whereas a decrease suggests recovery of renal function (assuming muscle mass has not changed). Most laboratories now also report an estimated GFR (eGFR) each time the creatinine is ordered.
4. More common in African-American than in Caucasian patients.

Quick HIT

- **Azotemia** refers to the elevation of BUN.
- **Uremia** refers to the signs and symptoms associated with accumulation of nitrogenous wastes due to impaired renal function. It is difficult to predict when uremic symptoms will appear, but it rarely occurs unless the BUN is >60 mg/dL.

Quick HIT

Diabetes and hypertension are the most common causes of ESRD.

B. Clinical features—any of the following may be present:

1. Cardiovascular
   a. HTN
      - Secondary to salt and water retention—decreased GFR stimulates renin–angiotensin system and aldosterone secretion to increase, which leads to an increase in BP.
      - Renal failure is the most common cause of secondary HTN.
   b. CHF—due to volume overload, HTN, and anemia.
   c. Pericarditis (uremic).

Quick HIT

ESRD is not defined by BUN or creatinine levels. It is a loss of kidney function that leads to laboratory and clinical findings of uremia.

2. GI (usually due to uremia).
   a. Nausea, vomiting.
   b. Loss of appetite (anorexia).
3. Neurologic
   a. Symptoms include lethargy, somnolence, confusion, peripheral neuropathy, and uremic seizures. Physical findings include weakness, asterixis, and hyperreflexia. Patients may show "restless legs"—neuropathic pain in the legs that is only relieved with movement.
   b. Hypocalcemia can cause lethargy, confusion, and tetany.
4. Hematologic
   a. Normocytic normochromic anemia (secondary to deficiency of erythropoietin)—may be severe.
   b. Bleeding secondary to platelet dysfunction (due to uremia). Platelets do not degranulate in uremic environment.
5. Endocrine/metabolic
   a. Calcium–phosphorus disturbances.
      - Decreased renal clearance of phosphate leads to **hyperphosphatemia**, which results in decreased renal production of 1,25-dihydroxy vitamin D. This leads to **hypocalcemia**, which causes secondary hyperparathyroidism.
      - So, **hypo**calcemia and **hyper**phosphatemia are usually seen, but long-standing secondary hyperparathyroidism and calcium-based phosphate binders may sometimes cause **hypercalcemia.**
      - Secondary hyperparathyroidism causes **renal osteodystrophy**, which causes weakening of bones and possibly fractures.
      - Hyperphosphatemia may cause calcium and phosphate to precipitate, which causes vascular calcifications that may result in necrotic skin lesions. This is called **calciphylaxis.**
   b. Sexual/reproductive symptoms due to hypothalamic-pituitary disturbances and gonadal response to sex hormones: in men, decreased testosterone; in women, amenorrhea, infertility, and hyperprolactinemia.
   c. Pruritus (multifactorial etiology)—common and difficult to treat. Dialysis and ultraviolet light.
6. Fluid and electrolyte problems (see Chapter 8).
   a. Volume overload—watch for pulmonary edema.
   b. Hyperkalemia—due to decreased urinary secretion.
   c. Hypermagnesemia—occurs secondary to reduced urinary loss.
   d. Hyperphosphatemia—see above.
   e. Metabolic acidosis—due to loss of renal mass (and thus decreased ammonia production) and the kidney's inability to excrete H^+.
7. Immunologic—uremia inhibits cellular and humoral immunity.

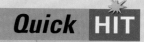

> **Quick HIT**
> When a patient's renal function is irreversibly compromised but not failed, the term chronic renal insufficiency is used. It is generally applied to those with a chronic elevation of serum creatinine to 1.5 to 3.0 mg/dL.

> **Quick HIT**
> Increased susceptibility to infections is a major cause of mortality in patients with CKD.

> **Quick HIT**
> Hypocalcemia leads to secondary hyperparathyroidism, which removes calcium from bones, making them weak and susceptible to fracture.

C. Diagnosis

1. Urinalysis—examine sediment (see AKI).
2. Measure Cr clearance to estimate GFR.
3. CBC (anemia, thrombocytopenia).
4. Serum electrolytes (e.g., K^+, Ca^{2+}, PO_4^{3-}, serum protein)
5. Renal ultrasound—evaluate size of kidneys/rule out obstruction.
   a. Small kidneys are suggestive of chronic renal insufficiency with little chance of recovery.
   b. Presence of normal-sized or large kidneys does not exclude CKD.
   c. Renal biopsy—in select cases to determine specific etiology.

> **Quick HIT**
> In a patient with CKD, symptomatic volume overload and severe hyperkalemia are the most common complications that require urgent intervention.

D. Treatment

1. Diet
   a. Low protein—to 0.7 to 0.8 g/kg body weight per day
   b. Use a low-salt diet if HTN, CHF, or oliguria are present
   c. Restrict potassium, phosphate, and magnesium intake

Quick HIT

Life-threatening Complications in CKD

- Hyperkalemia—obtain an ECG (be aware that potassium levels can be high without ECG changes).
- Pulmonary edema secondary to volume overload—look for recent weight gain.
- Infection (e.g., pneumonia, UTI, sepsis).

2. ACE inhibitors—dilate efferent arteriole of glomerulus
   a. If used early on, they reduce the risk of progression to ESRD because they slow the progression of proteinuria
   b. Use with great caution because they can cause hyperkalemia
3. BP control
   a. Strict control decreases the rate of disease progression
   b. ACE inhibitors are the preferred agents. Multiple drugs, including diuretics, may be required
4. Glycemic control (if the patient is diabetic) prevents worsening of proteinuria
5. Smoking cessation
6. Correction of electrolyte abnormalities
   a. Correct hyperphosphatemia with calcium citrate (a phosphate binder)
   b. Patients with chronic renal disease are generally treated with long-term oral calcium and vitamin D in an effort to prevent secondary hyperparathyroidism and uremic osteodystrophy
   c. Acidosis—treat the underlying cause (renal failure). Patients may require oral bicarbonate replacement
7. Anemia—treat with erythropoietin
8. Pulmonary edema—arrange for dialysis if the condition is unresponsive to diuresis
9. Pruritus—try capsaicin cream or cholestyramine and UV light
10. Dialysis (See indications in the Dialysis section.)
11. Transplantation is the only cure

Quick HIT

Absolute Indications for Dialysis

- **A**cidosis—significant, intractable metabolic acidosis
- **E**lectrolytes—severe, persistent hyperkalemia
- **I**ntoxications—methanol, ethylene glycol, lithium, aspirin
- **O**verload—hypervolemia not managed by other means
- **U**remia (severe)—based on clinical presentation, not laboratory values (e.g., uremic pericarditis is an absolute indication for dialysis)

●●● Dialysis

A. General characteristics

1. Overview
   a. Dialysis is the artificial mechanism by which fluid and toxic solutes are removed from the circulation when the kidneys cannot do so sufficiently.
   b. In all forms of dialysis, the blood interfaces with an artificial solution resembling human plasma (called the dialysate), and diffusion of fluid and solutes occurs across a semipermeable membrane.
   c. **The two major methods of dialyzing a patient are hemodialysis and peritoneal dialysis** (discussed below).
   d. The majority of dialysis patients in the United States receive hemodialysis at hospitals or dialysis centers, but more and more patients are opting for chronic ambulatory peritoneal dialysis (CAPD).
   e. For patients with life-threatening complications of AKI, continuous renal replacement therapy (CRRT) can be used for constant renal support.
2. Settings in which dialysis is considered.
   a. CKD—dialysis serves as a bridge to renal transplantation or as a permanent treatment when the patient is not a transplantation candidate.
   b. AKI—dialysis is often required as a temporary measure until the patient's renal function improves.
   c. Overdose of medications or ingestions of substances cleared by the kidneys—some, but not all medications and toxins can be dialyzed (see Quick Hit).

Quick HIT

Creatinine level is not an absolute indication for dialysis.

B. Specific indications for dialysis

1. Nonemergent indications
   a. Cr and BUN levels are **not** absolute indications for dialysis
   b. Symptoms of uremia
      - Nausea and vomiting
      - Lethargy/deterioration in mental status, encephalopathy, seizures
      - Pericarditis
2. Emergent indications (usually in the setting of renal failure)
   a. Life-threatening manifestations of volume overload
      - Pulmonary edema
      - Hypertensive emergency refractory to antihypertensive agents

b. Severe, refractory electrolyte disturbances, for example, hyperkalemia, hypermagnesemia
c. Severe metabolic acidosis
d. Drug toxicity/ingestions (particularly in patients with renal failure): methanol, ethylene glycol, lithium, aspirin

Quick HIT

Dialyzable Substances
- Salicylic acid
- Lithium
- Ethylene glycol
- Magnesium-containing laxatives

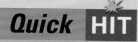

C. Hemodialysis

1. Process
   a. The patient's blood is pumped by an artificial pump outside of the body through the dialyzer, which typically consists of fine capillary networks of semipermeable membranes. The dialysate flows on the outside of these networks, and fluid and solutes diffuse across the membrane.
   b. The patient's blood must be heparinized to prevent clotting in the dialyzer.
2. Frequency: Most hemodialysis patients require 3 to 5 hours of dialysis 3 days per week.
3. Access
   a. Use the central catheter placed using the Seldinger technique most often in the subclavian or jugular vein for temporary access.
   b. Tunneled catheters are placed under the skin which leads to a lower rate of infection. These catheters are often suitable for use up to 6 months.
   c. Arteriovenous fistula.
      - Best form of permanent dialysis access.
      - It requires vascular surgery to connect the radial or brachial artery to veins in the forearm.
      - An audible bruit over the fistula indicates that it is patent.
   d. An alternative to an arteriovenous fistula is an implantable graft—typically made of polytetrafluoroethylene (PTFE).
4. Alternatives to traditional hemodialysis.
   a. Continuous arteriovenous hemodialysis (CAVHD) and continuous venovenous hemodialysis (CVVHD) are often used in hemodynamically unstable patients, such as ICU patients with AKI.
   b. Lower flow rates of blood and dialysate enable dialysis to occur while minimizing rapid shifts in volume and osmolality.
   c. They require highly efficient dialyzers to be effective.
5. Advantages of hemodialysis.
   a. It is more efficient than peritoneal dialysis. High flow rates and efficient dialyzers shorten the period of time required for dialysis.
   b. It can be initiated more quickly than peritoneal dialysis, using temporary vascular access in the emergent setting.
6. Disadvantages of hemodialysis.
   a. It is less similar to the physiology of natural kidney function than is peritoneal dialysis, predisposing the patient to the following:
      - Hypotension due to rapid removal of intravascular volume leading to rapid fluid shifts from the extravascular space into cells.
      - Hypo-osmolality due to solute removal.
   b. Requires vascular access.

D. Peritoneal dialysis

1. Process
   a. The peritoneum serves as the dialysis membrane. Dialysate fluid is infused into the peritoneal cavity, then fluids and solutes from the peritoneal capillaries diffuse into the dialysate fluid, which is drained from the abdomen.
   b. A **hyperosmolar** (high-glucose) solution is used, and water is removed from the blood via osmosis.
2. Frequency: dialysate fluid is drained and replaced every hour in acute peritoneal dialysis, but only once every 4 to 8 hours in CAPD.
3. Access
   a. With CAPD, dialysate is infused into the peritoneal fluid via an implanted catheter.
   b. A temporary catheter is used for acute peritoneal dialysis.

4. Advantages
   a. The patient can learn to perform dialysis on his or her own.
   b. It mimics the physiology of normal kidney function more closely than hemodialysis in that it is more continuous.
5. Disadvantages
   a. High glucose load may lead to hyperglycemia and hypertriglyceridemia.
   b. Peritonitis is a significant potential complication.
   c. The patients must be highly motivated to self-administer it.
   d. Cosmetic—there is increased abdominal girth due to dialysate fluid.

E. Limitations and complications of dialysis

1. Limitations—dialysis does not replicate the kidney's synthetic functions. Therefore, dialysis patients are still prone to erythropoietin and vitamin D deficiency, with their associated complications.
2. Complications associated with hemodialysis.
   a. Hypotension—may result in myocardial ischemia, fatigue, and so on.
   b. The relative hypo-osmolality of the ECF compared with the brain may result in nausea, vomiting, headache, and rarely, seizures or coma.
   c. "First-use syndrome"—chest pain, back pain, and rarely, anaphylaxis may occur immediately after a patient uses a new dialysis machine.
   d. Complications associated with anticoagulation—hemorrhage, hematoma, etc.
   e. Infection of vascular access site—may lead to sepsis.
   f. Hemodialysis-associated amyloidosis of β_2-microglobulin in bones and joints.
3. Complications associated with peritoneal dialysis.
   a. Peritonitis, often accompanied by fever and abdominal pain—usually can be treated with intraperitoneal antibiotics; cloudy peritoneal fluid is key sign.
   b. Abdominal/inguinal hernia—increased risk due to elevated intra-abdominal pressures.
   c. Hyperglycemia—especially with diabetic patients.
   d. Protein malnutrition.

Quick HIT

Asymptomatic Proteinuria
- Asymptomatic transient proteinuria has an excellent prognosis (no further evaluation necessary).
- Asymptomatic **persistent** proteinuria and symptomatic proteinuria require further workup (high chance of renal disease in these patients).

Proteinuria and Hematuria

Proteinuria

A. General characteristics

1. Defined as the urinary excretion of >150 mg protein/24 hours
2. Classification
   a. Glomerular
      - Due to increased glomerular permeability to proteins
      - Can lead to nephrotic syndrome
      - May be seen in all types of GN
      - Protein loss tends to be more severe than in nonglomerular causes
   b. Tubular
      - Small proteins normally filtered at the glomerulus then reabsorbed by the tubules appear in the urine because of abnormal tubules (i.e., due to decreased tubular reabsorption)
      - Proteinuria tends to be less severe
      - Causes include sickle cell disease, urinary tract obstruction, and interstitial nephritis
   c. Overflow proteinuria—increased production of small proteins overwhelms the tubules' ability to reabsorb them (e.g., Bence Jones protein in multiple myeloma)
   d. Other causes of proteinuria (all of the following can affect renal blood flow):
      - UTI
      - Fever, heavy exertion/stress, CHF
      - Pregnancy
      - Orthostatic proteinuria—occurs when the patient is standing but not when recumbent; self-limited and benign

3. Nephrotic syndrome
   a. Key features
      - **Urine protein** excretion rate >3.5 g/24 hours
      - **Hypoalbuminemia**—hepatic albumin synthesis cannot keep up with these urinary protein losses. The result is decreased plasma oncotic pressure, which leads to edema
      - **Edema**—this is often the initial complaint (from pedal edema to periorbital to anasarca, ascites, pleural effusion), and results from hypoalbuminemia. Increased aldosterone secretion exacerbates the problem (increases sodium reabsorption).
      - **Hyperlipidemia** and lipiduria—increased hepatic synthesis of LDL and VLDL because liver is revving up albumin synthesis.
      - Hypercoagulable state (due to loss of certain anticoagulants in the urine)—increased risk of thromboembolic events (deep venous thrombosis, pulmonary embolism, renal vein thrombosis).
      - Increased incidence of infection—results from loss of immunoglobulins in the urine.
   b. Nephrotic syndrome usually indicates significant glomerular disease (either primary or secondary to systemic illness); the underlying cause is abnormal glomerular permeability.
   c. Causes
      - Primary glomerular disease (50% to 75% of cases of nephrotic syndrome)—membranous nephropathy is most common in adults (40% of cases), followed by focal segmental glomerulosclerosis (FSGS) (35%) and membranoproliferative GN (15%). Minimal change disease (MCD) is the most common cause in children (75% of cases).
      - Systemic disease—diabetes, collagen vascular disease, SLE, RA, Henoch–Schönlein purpura, polyarteritis nodosa (PAN), Wegener granulomatosis.
      - Amyloidosis, cryoglobulinemia.
      - Drugs/toxins—captopril, heroin, heavy metals, NSAIDs, penicillamine.
      - Infection—bacterial, viral, protozoal.
      - Multiple myeloma, malignant HTN, transplant rejection.

Quick HIT

Three Key Features of Nephrotic Syndrome
- Proteinuria
- Hypoalbuminemia
- Hyperlipidemia

B. Diagnosis

1. Urine dipstick test (read color changes)
   a. Specific for albumin—detects concentrations of 30 mg/dL or higher
   b. Graded 0, trace, 1+ (15 to 30 mg/dL) through 4+ (>500 mg/dL)
   c. More sensitive to albumin than to immunoglobulins, thus can lead to false-negative results when predominant urinary protein is globulin (e.g., light chains in myeloma)
2. Urinalysis (see Clinical Pearl 7-6)
   a. Initial test once proteinuria is detected by dipstick test
   b. Examination of urine sediment is important
      - RBC casts suggest GN
      - WBC casts suggest pyelonephritis and interstitial nephritis
      - Fatty casts suggest nephrotic syndrome (lipiduria)
   c. If urinalysis confirms the presence of protein, a 24-hour urine collection (for albumin and Cr) is appropriate to establish the presence of significant proteinuria
3. Test for microalbuminuria
   a. Corresponds to albumin excretion of 30 to 300 mg/day
   b. This is below the range of sensitivity of standard dipsticks. Special dipsticks can detect microgram amounts of albumin. If the test result is positive, perform a radioimmunoassay (the most sensitive and specific test for microalbuminuria)
   c. **Microalbuminuria can be an early sign of diabetic nephropathy**
4. Other tests to determine etiology (may or may not be necessary depending on case)
   a. Cr clearance—best test of renal function
   b. Serum BUN and Cr
   c. CBC—to detect anemia due to renal failure

CLINICAL PEARL 7-6

Urinalysis

Collection—a clean-catch, midstream urine sample (after cleaning urethral meatus) is usually adequate for urinalysis and urine culture in adults.

Urinalysis consists of the following three steps:

- Visual inspection of urine—examine color, clarity
- Dipstick reactions
  - pH—this depends on acid-base status. The average is about 6, but can range from 4.5 to 8.0
  - Specific gravity—this is directly proportional to urine osmolality (and therefore solute concentration in urine). Normal is 1.002 to 1.035. It increases with volume depletion and decreases with volume overload. Appropriate changes in specific gravity with volume status of the patient indicate adequate tubular function (i.e., renal concentrating ability)
  - Protein—proteinuria is defined as >150 mg/day; nephrotic syndrome, >3.5 g/day. The following are rough guidelines: Trace = 50 to 150 mg/day; 1+ = 150 to 500 mg/day; 2+ = 0.5 to 1.5 g/day; 3+ = 2 to 5 g/day; 4+ = >5 g/day
  - Glucose—excessive glucose indicates diabetes. Absence of glucosuria does **not** rule out diabetes, however
  - Blood—hematuria—see text
  - Ketones—DKA, starvation
  - Nitrite—suggests presence of bacteria in urine
  - Leukocyte esterase—suggests presence of WBC in urine; if negative, infection is unlikely
- Microscopic examination of urine sediment
  - Look for casts, cells, bacteria, WBCs, RBCs (number, shape), crystals

d. Serum albumin level—varies inversely with degree of proteinuria
e. Renal ultrasound—to detect obstruction, masses, cystic disease
f. Intravenous pyelogram (IVP)—to detect chronic pyelonephritis
g. ANA levels (lupus), antiglomerular basement membrane, hepatitis serology, antistreptococcal antibody titers, complement levels, cryoglobulin studies
h. Serum and urine electrophoresis (myeloma)
i. Renal biopsy—if no cause is identified by less invasive means

C. Treatment

1. Asymptomatic proteinuria.
   a. If it is transient, no further workup or treatment is necessary.
   b. If it is persistent, further testing is indicated. Start by checking BP and examining urine sediment. Treat the underlying condition and associated problems (e.g., hyperlipidemia).
2. Symptomatic proteinuria—further testing is always required.
   a. Treat the underlying disease (diabetes, multiple myeloma, SLE, minimal change disease).
   b. ACE inhibitors (ARB cannot tolerate ACE)—these decrease urinary albumin loss. They are an essential part of treatment for diabetics with HTN and should be started before fixed albuminuria is present.
   c. Diuretics—if edema is present.
   d. Limit dietary protein and sodium.
   e. Treat hypercholesterolemia (using diet or a lipid-lowering agent).
   f. Vaccinate against influenza and pneumococcus—there is an increased risk of infection in these patients.

Quick HIT

Gross hematuria is a common presenting sign in patients with bladder cancer (up to 85% of cases) and patients with renal cell carcinoma (up to 40% of cases).

Hematuria

A. General characteristics

1. Hematuria is defined as >3 erythrocytes/HPF on urinalysis.
2. Microscopic hematuria is more commonly glomerular in origin; gross hematuria is more commonly nonglomerular or urologic in origin.

3. **Consider gross painless hematuria to be a sign of bladder or kidney cancer until proven otherwise.**
4. This may lead to obstruction if large clots form in the lower GU tract. Excessive blood loss can lead to iron deficiency anemia.

B. Causes

1. Kidney stones
2. Infection (UTI, urethritis, pyelonephritis)
3. Bladder or kidney cancer
4. Glomerular disease, immunoglobulin (Ig) A nephropathy
5. Trauma (Foley catheter placement, blunt trauma, invasive procedures)
6. Strenuous exercise (marathon running), fever—hematuria is generally harmless
7. Systemic diseases (SLE, rheumatic fever, Henoch–Schönlein purpura, Wegener granulomatosis, HUS, Goodpasture syndrome, PAN)
8. Bleeding disorders (e.g., hemophilia, thrombocytopenia)
9. Sickle cell disease
10. Medications (cyclophosphamide, anticoagulants, salicylates, sulfonamides)
11. Analgesic nephropathy
12. Polycystic kidney disease, simple cysts
13. BPH—rarely causes isolated hematuria

C. Diagnosis

1. Urine dipstick—sensitivity in identifying hematuria is >90% (Figure 7-3).
2. Urinalysis—crucial in evaluation of hematuria.
   a. Examine urine sediment—this is very important in identifying possible renal disease.
   b. If RBC casts and proteinuria are also present, a glomerular cause is almost always present (usually GN).
   c. If pyuria is present, send for urine culture.
   d. If dipstick is positive for blood, but urinalysis does not reveal microscopic hematuria (no RBCs), hemoglobinuria or myoglobinuria is likely present.
3. Urine specimen—for cytology.
   a. To detect cancers (bladder cancer is the main concern).
   b. **If suspicion for malignancy is high, perform a cystoscopy to evaluate the bladder regardless of cytology results.**
4. Twenty-four–hour urine—test for Cr and protein to assess renal function. Collect if proteinuria is present. (If it is heavy, glomerular disease is likely.)
5. Blood tests—coagulation studies, CBC, BUN/Cr.
6. IVP, CT scan, ultrasound—if no cause is identified by the above tests; look for stones, tumors, cysts, ureteral strictures, or vascular malformations.
7. Renal biopsy—if there is suspicion of glomerular disease.

D. Treatment: Treat the underlying cause; maintain urine volume.

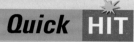

> **Quick HIT**
> Infection (cystitis, urethritis, prostatitis) accounts for 25% and stones for 20% of all cases of atraumatic hematuria.

> **Quick HIT**
> Menstrual blood can contaminate a urine sample and lead to a false-positive dipstick reading for hematuria.

> **Quick HIT**
> If hematuria is microscopic, think of glomerular disease. If gross, think of postrenal causes (trauma, stones, malignancy). Infection can cause either gross or microscopic hematuria.

> **Quick HIT**
> If the patient has no other symptoms associated with hematuria, and thorough workup fails to reveal a cause, the prognosis is excellent. (There is usually mild glomerular/interstitial disease.)

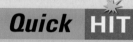

Glomerular Disease (Glomerulonephropathies)

Overview

A. General characteristics

1. Can be primary (intrinsic renal pathology) or secondary (to a systemic disease). Two important categories of glomerular pathology are diseases that present with nephrotic syndrome and those that present with nephritic syndrome. Many conditions have features of both. See Table 7-5.
2. There is a wide range in the rate of disease progression, varying from days to weeks in the acute glomerular diseases, to years in the chronic disorders.

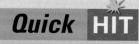

> **Quick HIT**
> Rapid progressive GN is a clinical syndrome that includes any type of GN in which rapid deterioration of renal function occurs over weeks to months, leading to renal failure and ESRD.

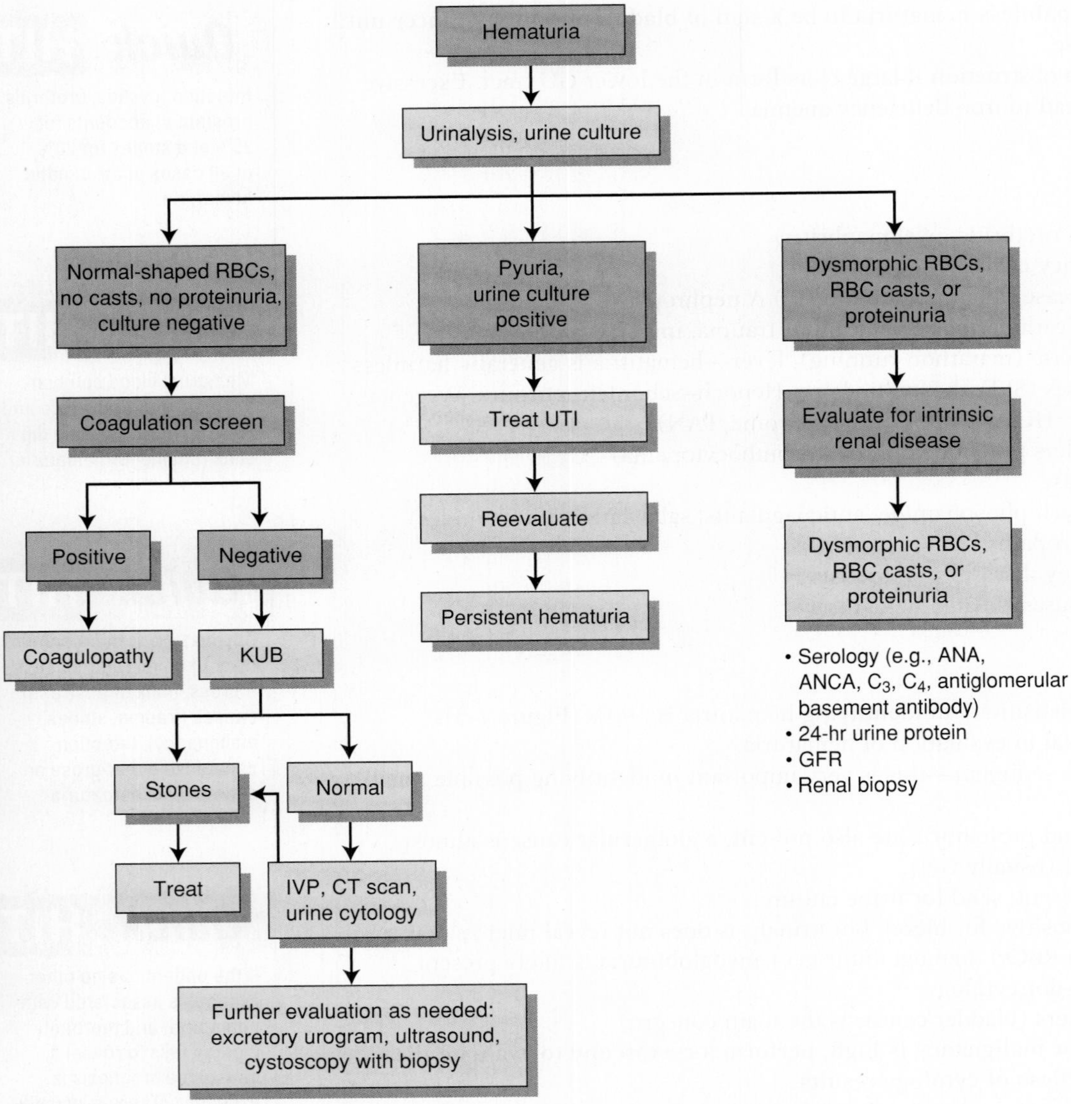

FIGURE 7-3 **Evaluation of hematuria.**

Quick HIT

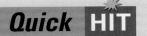

Possible Presentations of Glomerular Disease
- Isolated proteinuria
- Isolated hematuria
- Nephritic syndrome—hematuria, HTN, azotemia
- Nephrotic syndrome—proteinuria, edema, hypoalbuminemia, hyperlipidemia

B. Causes
1. GN is usually caused by immune-mediated mechanisms.
2. Other mechanisms include metabolic and hemodynamic disturbances.

C. Clinical features
1. Glomerular disorders are characterized by impairment in selective filtration of blood, resulting in excretion of larger substances such as plasma proteins and blood cells. As disease advances, GFR decreases proportionately, leading to renal failure and the possible need for dialysis and/or transplantation.
2. The classic features are proteinuria, hematuria, or both. Nephrotic range proteinuria is pathognomonic for glomerular disease.

D. Diagnosis
1. Urinalysis (hematuria, proteinuria, RBC casts)
2. Blood tests (renal function tests)
3. Needle biopsy of the kidney

E. Treatment depends on the disease, but often involves steroids and cytotoxic agents.

TABLE 7-5 Nephritic Versus Nephrotic Syndrome

	Nephritic Syndrome	Nephrotic Syndrome
Pathogenesis	Inflammation of glomeruli due to any of the causes of glomerulonephritis	Abnormal glomerular permeability due to a number of conditions
Causes	Poststreptococcal glomerulonephritis is the most comm on cause, but may be due to any of the causes of glomerulonephritis	Many conditions. Membranous glomerulonephritis is the most common cause in adults. Other causes include diabetes, SLE, drugs, infection, glomerulonephritis (focal segmental and others) Minimal change disease is the most common cause in children
Laboratory Findings	Hematuria AKI—azotemia, oliguria Proteinuria, if present, is mild and not in nephrotic range	Urine protein excretion rate >3.5 g/24 hr Hypoalbuminemia Hyperlipidemia, fatty casts in urine
Clinical Findings	HTN Edema	Edema Hypercoagulable state Increased risk of infection

Primary Glomerular Disorders

A. Minimal change disease

1. Nephrotic syndrome—most common presentation (see also Clinical Pearl 7-7).
2. Most common in children—Hodgkin disease and non-Hodgkin lymphoma have been associated with minimal change disease.
3. No histologic abnormalities on light microscopy; **fusion of foot processes on electron microscopy.**
4. Excellent prognosis; responsive to steroid therapy (4 to 8 weeks), although relapses may occur.
5. Current evidence points to systemic T-cell dysfunction as the most likely root cause of MCD.

B. Focal segmental glomerulosclerosis

1. This accounts for 25% of cases of nephrotic syndrome in adults and is more common in blacks. Hematuria and HTN are often present.
2. It has a fair to poor prognosis. It is generally resistant to steroid therapy—patients develop renal insufficiency within 5 to 10 years of diagnosis. The course is progressive.
3. The treatment regimen is controversial, but remission has been achieved in 50% of patients with the use of cytotoxic agents, steroids, and immunosuppressive agents. ACE/ARBs are also commonly indicated.

CLINICAL PEARL 7-7

Glomerular Disease (GD) Versus Tubular Disease (TD)

1. TD is usually acute, whereas GD is more chronic
2. TD is often caused by toxins (NSAIDs, contrast, myoglobin, drugs); GD is typically not caused by toxins.
3. TD does not cause nephrotic syndrome, GD does.
4. TD does not need biopsy, GD often does.
5. Steroids used for GD, not TD.
6. Immunosuppressive medications used for GD, not TD.

C. Membranous glomerulonephritis

1. Usually presents with nephrotic syndrome; glomerular capillary walls are thickened.
2. Primary disease is idiopathic. The secondary form is due to infection (hepatitis C virus, hepatitis B virus, syphilis, malaria), drugs (gold, captopril, penicillamine), neoplasm, or lupus.
3. Prognosis is fair to good and course is variable; remission is common (in 40% of cases), but renal failure develops in 33% of patients. Steroids do not change survival rate.

D. IgA nephropathy (Berger disease)

1. Asymptomatic recurrent hematuria/mild proteinuria is common. **This is the most common cause of glomerular hematuria.** Gross hematuria after an upper respiratory infection (or exercise) is common.
2. Renal function is usually normal.
3. Mesangial deposition of IgA and C3 are seen on electron microscopy.
4. The prognosis in most patients is good with preservation of renal function (renal insufficiency may develop in 25%).
5. Some advocate steroids for unstable disease, but no therapy has been proven to be effective.

E. Hereditary nephritis (Alport syndrome)

1. X-linked or autosomal dominant inheritance with variable penetrance
2. Features include hematuria, pyuria, proteinuria, high-frequency hearing loss without deafness, progressive renal failure
3. No effective treatment

••• Secondary Glomerular Disorders

A. Diabetic nephropathy—most common cause of ESRD (see Chapter 4)

B. Hypertensive nephropathy—(see Renal Vasculature Disease section)

C. Lupus—(see Chapter 6)

D. Membranoproliferative GN

1. Usually due to hepatitis C infection; other causes include hepatitis B, syphilis, and lupus
2. Common association with cryoglobulinemia
3. The prognosis is poor. Renal failure develops in 50% of patients. Treatment is rarely effective

E. Poststreptococcal GN—most common cause of nephritic syndrome

1. Occurs after infection with group A β-hemolytic streptococcal infection of the upper respiratory tract (or skin—impetigo). The GN develops about 10 to 14 days after infection. Primarily affects children (ages 2 to 6 years).
2. Features include hematuria, edema, HTN, low complement levels, and proteinuria.
3. Antistreptolysin-O may be elevated.
4. It is self-limited (usually resolves in weeks to months) with an excellent prognosis. Some cases develop into rapidly progressive GN (more commonly in adults).
5. Therapy is primarily supportive: antihypertensives, loop diuretics for edema; the use of antibiotics is controversial. Steroids may be helpful in severe cases.

F. Goodpasture syndrome

1. Classic triad of proliferative GN (usually crescentic), pulmonary hemorrhage, and IgG antiglomerular basement membrane antibody.
2. Clinical features: rapidly progressive renal failure, hemoptysis, cough, and dyspnea.
3. Lung disease precedes kidney disease by days to weeks.
4. Renal biopsy shows linear immunofluorescence pattern.

5. Treat with plasmapheresis to remove circulating anti-IgG antibodies. Cyclophosphamide and steroids can decrease the formation of new antibodies.

G. Dysproteinemias—amyloidosis, light chain/heavy chain diseases.

H. Sickle cell nephropathy—(see Renal Vascular Disease section).

I. HIV nephropathy.

1. Characteristics include proteinuria, edema, and hematuria.
2. Histopathology most often resembles a collapsing form of FSGS.
3. Treat with prednisone, ACE inhibitors, and antiretroviral therapy.

J. Wegener granulomatosis—(see Chapter 6).

K. PAN—(see Chapter 6).

Tubulointerstitial Diseases

Acute Interstitial Nephritis

A. General characteristics

1. Inflammation involving interstitium (tissue that surrounds glomeruli and tubules)
2. Accounts for 10% to 15% of cases of AKI
3. Causes
   a. **Acute allergic reaction to medication is the most common cause**—for example, penicillins, cephalosporins, sulfa drugs, diuretics (furosemide, thiazide), anticoagulants, phenytoin, rifampin, allopurinol, proton pump inhibitors.
   b. Infection (especially in children)—due to a variety of agents, including *Streptococcus* spp. and *Legionella pneumophila.*
   c. Collagen vascular diseases—for example, sarcoidosis.
   d. Autoimmune diseases—for example, SLE, Sjögren syndrome.

B. Clinical features

1. Acute interstitial nephritis (AIN) causes AKI and its associated symptoms.
2. Rash, fever, and eosinophilia are the classical findings.
3. Pyuria and hematuria may be present.

C. Diagnosis

1. Renal function tests (increased BUN and Cr levels)
2. Urinalysis
   a. **Eosinophils in the urine suggest the diagnosis, given the proper history and findings**
   b. Mild proteinuria or microscopic hematuria may be present
3. Note that it is often impossible to distinguish AIN from ATN based on clinical grounds alone. Renal biopsy is the only way to distinguish between the two, but is usually not performed given its invasiveness

D. Treatment

1. Removing the offending agent is usually enough to reverse the clinical findings. If creatinine continues to increase after stopping the offending agent, steroids may help.
2. Treat infection if present.

Renal Papillary Necrosis

- Most commonly associated with analgesic nephropathy, diabetic nephropathy, sickle cell disease, urinary tract obstruction, UTI, chronic alcoholism, and renal transplant rejection.
- Diagnosis is typically made by excretory urogram—note change in papilla or medulla.

Quick HIT

Diagnosing AIN
Look for recent infection, start of a new medication, rash, fever, general aches/pains, and signs/symptoms of AKI.

Quick HIT

The diagnosis of AIN can be made if the patient is known to have been exposed to one of the offending agents, and has the following: rash, fever, acute renal insufficiency, and eosinophilia.

Quick HIT

Acute Versus Chronic Interstitial Nephritis
- **Acute** interstitial nephritis causes a rapid deterioration in renal function and is associated with interstitial eosinophils or lymphocytes.
- **Chronic** interstitial nephritis has a more indolent course and is associated with tubulointerstitial fibrosis and atrophy.

Quick HIT

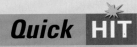

Analgesic Nephropathy Pearls
- Analgesic nephropathy is a form of toxic injury to the kidney due to excessive use of over-the-counter analgesics (those that contain phenacetin, acetaminophen, NSAIDs, or aspirin).
- It can manifest as interstitial nephritis or renal papillary necrosis.
- It may lead to acute or chronic renal failure.

- Variable course: some patients have rapid progression, and others have a more indolent, chronic course.
- Sloughed, necrotic papillae can cause ureteral obstruction.
- Treat the underlying cause, and stop the offending agents (e.g., NSAIDs).

Renal Tubular Acidosis

A. General characteristics

1. Renal tubularacidosis (RTA) is a disorder of the renal tubules that leads to a nonanion gap hyperchloremic metabolic acidosis. Glomerular function is normal (see Table 7-6).
2. It is characterized by a decrease in the H^1 excreted in the urine, leading to acidemia and urine alkalosis.
3. There are three types of RTA (types 1, 2, and 4). (Type 3 RTA is a term that is no longer used.)

B. Type 1 (distal)

1. The defect is an inability to secrete H^+ at the distal tubule (therefore new bicarbonate cannot be generated). This inability to acidify the urine results in metabolic acidosis. Although normally the urine pH can be as low as 4.7, in distal RTA the urine pH cannot be lowered below 6, regardless of the severity of metabolic acidosis.
2. It leads to increased excretion of ions (sodium, calcium, potassium, sulfate, phosphate), with the following effects:
   a. Decrease in ECF volume.
   b. **Hypokalemia.**
   c. **Renal stones/nephrocalcinosis** (due to increased calcium and phosphate excretion into alkaline urine).
   d. Rickets/osteomalacia in children.
3. Leads to hypokalemic, hyperchloremic, nonanion gap metabolic acidosis.
4. Symptoms are secondary to nephrolithiasis and nephrocalcinosis. Up to 70% of patients have kidney stones.
5. Causes: congenital, multiple myeloma, nephrocalcinosis, nephrotoxicity (e.g., amphotericin B toxicity), autoimmune diseases (lupus, Sjögren syndrome), medullary sponge kidney, and analgesic nephropathy
6. Treatment
   a. Correct acidosis with sodium bicarbonate. This can also help prevent kidney stones, which is a major goal of therapy.
   b. Administer phosphate salts (promotes excretion of titratable acid).

TABLE 7-6 Renal Tubular Acidosis (RTA)

Type	Distinguishing Characteristics
1 (distal)	• Inability to secrete H+ • Urine pH >6 • Nephrolithiasis and nephrocalcinosis **do** occur
2 (proximal)	• **Inability to reabsorb HCO_3^-** • **Increased bicarbonate excretion** • Nephrolithiasis and nephrocalcinosis do **not** occur
3 (mixed)	• Rare autosomal recessive disorder: carbonic anhydrase II deficiency • Characteristics of type I and II
4 (hyperaldosteronism)	• Decreased Na^+ absorption and H^+ and K^+ secretion in distal tubule • Results in **hyperkalemia** and **acidic urine** • Nephrolithiasis and nephrocalcinosis are **rare**

C. Type 2 (proximal)

1. The defect is an inability to reabsorb HCO_3^- at the proximal tubule, resulting in **increased excretion of bicarbonate in the urine** and metabolic acidosis. The patient also loses K^+ and Na^+ in the urine
2. Characterized by hypokalemic, hyperchloremic nonanion gap metabolic acidosis (as in type 1 RTA)
3. Causes
   a. Fanconi syndrome (in children)
   b. Cystinosis, Wilson disease, lead toxicity, multiple myeloma, nephrotic syndrome, amyloidosis
   c. The excretion of monoclonal light chains is a common feature, so multiple myeloma should always be ruled out in a patient with proximal RTA
4. Nephrolithiasis and nephrocalcinosis do not occur (as they do in type 1 RTA)
5. Treatment: treat the underlying cause
   a. Do not give bicarbonate to correct the acidosis because it will be excreted in the urine.
   b. Sodium restriction increases sodium reabsorption (and thus bicarbonate reabsorption) in the proximal tubule.

D. Type 4

1. This can result from any condition that is associated with hypoaldosteronism, or increased renal resistance to aldosterone.
2. It is common in patients with interstitial renal disease and diabetic nephropathy.
3. It is characterized by decreased Na^+ absorption and decreased H^+ and K^+ secretion in the distal tubule.
4. Unlike other types of RTA, **type 4 results in hyperkalemia** and acidic urine (although a nonanion gap metabolic acidosis still occurs).
5. Nephrolithiasis and nephrocalcinosis are rare.

Hartnup Syndrome

- Autosomal recessive inheritance of defective amino acid transporter
- Results in decreased intestinal and renal reabsorption of neutral amino acids, such as tryptophan, causing nicotinamide deficiency
- Clinical features are similar to those of pellagra: dermatitis, diarrhea, ataxia, and psychiatric disturbances
- Give supplemental nicotinamide if the patient is symptomatic

Fanconi Syndrome

- Fanconi syndrome is a hereditary or acquired proximal tubule dysfunction that leads to defective transport of some of the following: glucose, amino acids, sodium, potassium, phosphate, uric acid, and bicarbonate.
- It is associated with glucosuria, phosphaturia (leads to skeletal problems: rickets/impaired growth in children; osteomalacia, osteoporosis, and pathologic fractures in adults), proteinuria, polyuria, dehydration, type 2 RTA, hypercalciuria, and hypokalemia.
- Treat with phosphate, potassium, alkali and salt supplementation, as well as adequate hydration.

Renal Cystic Diseases

Autosomal Dominant Polycystic Kidney Disease

A. General characteristics

1. Polycystic kidney disease may be inherited as an autosomal dominant or autosomal recessive trait. Autosomal dominant polycystic kidney disease (ADPKD) is the most common genetic cause of chronic kidney disease (Figure 7-4).

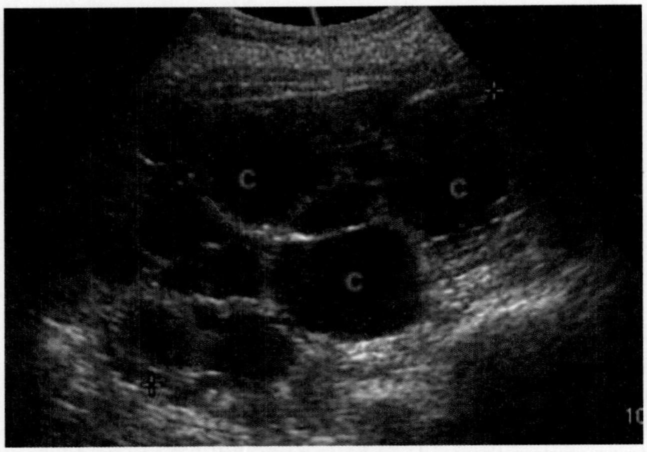

FIGURE 7-4 **Autosomal dominant polycystic kidney disease (ADPKD). Areas in black marked "C" are cysts. *Arrow* marks normal renal parenchyma.**
(Used with permission from Ruden N, Brandon, J, Jeun, B, et al., *University of Virginia Health Sciences Center, Department of Radiology, 2013.*)

2. The course is variable, but ESRD commonly develops in 50% of the patients (by late 50s or 60s); remainder have a normal lifespan. Renal failure occurs from recurrent episodes of pyelonephritis and nephrolithiasis.

B. Clinical features

1. Hematuria
2. Abdominal pain
3. HTN (in >50% of the cases)
4. Palpable kidneys on abdominal examination
5. Complications/associated findings
   a. **Intracerebral berry aneurysm (in 5% to 20% of cases)—most do not rupture**
   b. Infection of renal cysts; bleeding into cysts
   c. Renal failure (late in the disease)
   d. Kidney stones
   e. Heart valve abnormalities (especially mitral valve prolapse)
   f. Cysts in other organs (liver, spleen, pancreas, brain)
   g. Diverticula (colon)
   h. Hernias (abdominal/inguinal)

Quick HIT

ADPKD presents with:
- Pain
- Hematuria
- Infection
- Hypertension
- Kidney stones

C. Diagnosis

1. Ultrasound is confirmatory—multiple cysts appear on the kidney.
2. CT scan and MRI are alternatives.

D. Treatment

1. No curative therapy is available.
2. Drain cysts if symptomatic.
3. Treat infection with antibiotics.
4. Control HTN.

Autosomal Recessive Polycystic Kidney Disease

A. General characteristics

1. Autosomal recessive polycystic kidney disease (ARPKD) was previously called infantile polycystic kidney disease. It is characterized by cysts predominantly in the renal collecting ducts as well as hepatic fibrosis.
2. It is less common compared to the ADPKD, though the true incidence is unknown since many affected newborns die without proper diagnosis.
3. As with ADPKD, there is a wide variability in the level of renal impairment. However, most patients ultimately will experience progressive renal failure.

B. Clinical features

1. Liver involvement is always present, and may be the dominant clinical feature, especially in older individuals.
   a. Hepatic complications include portal HTN and cholangitis.
2. Kidneys are increased in size which may cause severe abdominal distension.
3. HTN
4. Pulmonary insufficiency secondary to pulmonary hypoplasia and enlarged kidneys limiting diaphragmatic movement may be severe. Pulmonary complications are the leading cause of morbidity and mortality in the neonatal period.
5. Newborns with severe ARPKD may present with Potter syndrome, which is the constellation of clinical features associated with decreased amniotic fluid (oligohydramnios). Potter syndrome is characterized by hypoplasia of the lungs, limb abnormalities (e.g., club feet), and characteristic abnormal facies.

C. Diagnosis

1. Some cases are detected prenatally due to the widespread use of ultrasound during pregnancy. Less severe cases may not be detected until much later.
2. Oligohydramnios during pregnancy usually indicates severe disease.
3. Ultrasound will show characteristic renal cysts in the absence of renal cysts in either parent. Ultrasound will also show hepatomegaly and dilated bile ducts.
4. Molecular genetic testing may confirm the disease in cases where the diagnosis is unclear.

D. Treatment

1. No curative therapy is available.
2. Manage respiratory issues in newborns, and treat ESRD with renal replacement therapy.

Medullary Sponge Kidney

- Characterized by cystic dilation of the collecting ducts (Figure 7-5)
- May present with hematuria, UTIs, or nephrolithiasis, or may be asymptomatic
- Thought to be associated with hyperparathyroidism and parathyroid adenoma
- Diagnosed by IVP
- No treatment is necessary other than the prevention of stone formation and the treatment of recurrent UTIs

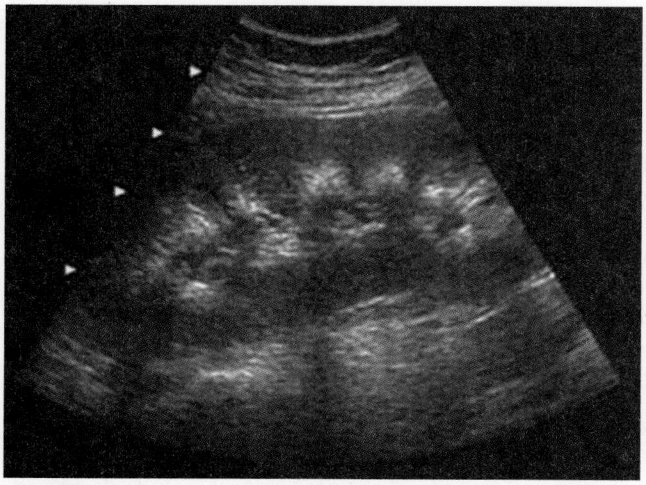

FIGURE 7-5 **Medullary sponge kidney (MSK). Ultrasound usually demonstrates echogenic medullary pyramids.**

(Used with permission from www.kidneyabc.com/medullary-sponge-kidney-diagnosis/559.html)

Simple Renal Cysts

- Very common (50% of the people over age 50); incidence increases with age
- May be single or multiple; usually asymptomatic and discovered incidentally on abdominal ultrasound or other imaging study
- No treatment is necessary in most cases

Renal Vascular Disease

Renal Artery Stenosis (Renovascular Hypertension)

A. General characteristics

1. Renal artery stenosis causes a decrease in blood flow to the juxtaglomerular apparatus. As a result, the renin–angiotensin–aldosterone system becomes activated, leading to HTN.
2. **This is the most common cause of secondary HTN.**

B. Causes

1. Atherosclerosis
   a. Accounts for two-thirds of the cases (most often in elderly men)
   b. Bilateral in up to one-third of the cases
   c. Smoking and high cholesterol levels are predisposing factors
2. Fibromuscular dysplasia
   a. Usually seen in young females
   b. Bilateral in 50% of patients

Quick HIT

ACE inhibitors should be used carefully in patients with renovascular HTN.

C. Clinical features

1. HTN—look for a sudden onset of HTN in a patient without a family history. HTN is often severe (may cause malignant HTN) and refractory to medical therapy.
2. Decreased renal function.
3. Abdominal bruit (RUQ, LUQ, or epigastrium) is present in 50% to 80% of patients; it is especially common in patients with fibromuscular hyperplasia.

Quick HIT

Suspect renovascular HTN in the following situations:
- Malignant HTN
- Sudden onset of HTN
- HTN that suddenly worsens
- HTN that does not respond to standard medical therapy

D. Diagnosis

1. Renal arteriogram is the gold standard, but **contrast dye can be nephrotoxic—do not use it in patients with renal failure.**
2. MRA is a new test that has high sensitivity and specificity. The magnetic dye is not nephrotoxic so it **can** be used in patients with renal failure.
3. Duplex Doppler ultrasonography of the renal arteries and contrast enhanced CT scan may also be helpful in some cases.

E. Treatment

1. Revascularization with percutaneous transluminal renal angioplasty (PRTA) is the initial treatment in most patients; it has a higher success rate and a lower restenosis rate with fibromuscular dysplasia than with the atherosclerotic type.
2. Surgery if PRTA is not successful (bypass).
3. Conservative medical therapy (ACE inhibitors, calcium channel blockers) may be tried alone or in combination with revascularization procedures.

Renal Vein Thrombosis

- May be seen in the following clinical settings: nephrotic syndrome, invasion of renal vein by renal cell carcinoma, trauma, pregnancy/oral contraceptives, extrinsic compression (retroperitoneal fibrosis, aortic aneurysm, lymphadenopathy), or severe dehydration (in infants)
- Clinical features depend on the acuity and severity of the process and include decreased renal perfusion (can lead to renal failure), flank pain, HTN, hematuria, and proteinuria.
- Diagnostic tests include selective renal venography visualizing the occluding thrombus (definitive study) or IVP.
- Anticoagulate to prevent pulmonary embolism.

Atheroembolic Disease of the Renal Arteries

- Refers to showers of cholesterol crystals that dislodge from plaques in large arteries and embolize to the renal vasculature.
- Can occur in other organs as well, such as the retina, brain, or skin
- Refer to cholesterol embolization syndrome in Chapter 1.

Hypertensive Nephrosclerosis

A. Definition: Systemic HTN increases capillary hydrostatic pressure in the glomeruli, leading to benign or malignant sclerosis.

1. Benign nephrosclerosis—thickening of the glomerular afferent arterioles develops in patients with long-standing HTN.
   a. Results in mild to moderate increase in Cr levels, microscopic hematuria, and mild proteinuria.
   b. Advanced disease can lead to ESRD.
2. Malignant nephrosclerosis—this can develop in a patient with long-standing benign HTN or in a previously undiagnosed patient.
   a. Characterized by a rapid decrease in renal function and accelerated HTN due to diffuse intrarenal vascular injury.
   b. African-American men are the most susceptible.
   c. Clinical manifestations include:
      - Markedly elevated BP (papilledema, cardiac decompensation, CNS findings).
      - Renal manifestations: a rapid increase in Cr, proteinuria, hematuria, RBC and WBC casts in urine sediment, and sometimes nephrotic syndrome
      - Microangiopathic hemolytic anemia may also be present.

B. Treatment

1. The most important treatment for both benign and malignant forms is controlling the BP (see Chapter 12). It is not clear which blood pressure agents should be used in the chronic setting, or how effective they are once frank albuminuria is present.
2. In advanced disease, treat as for CKD.

Quick HIT

Nephrosclerosis due to HTN is the second most common cause of ESRD (diabetes is the most common cause).

Scleroderma

In rare cases, this may cause malignant HTN. See Chapter 6.

Sickle Cell Nephropathy

- This refers to a sickling of RBCs in the microvasculature, which leads to infarction. In the kidney this occurs mostly in the renal papilla. Recurrent papillary infarction can lead to papillary necrosis, renal failure, and a high frequency of UTIs.
- Nephrotic syndrome can develop (which can lead to renal failure).
- It progresses to ESRD in approximately 5% of the patients.
- Ischemic injury to the renal tubules can occur, which increases the risk of dehydration (impaired urine concentration), precipitating sickling crises.
- ACE inhibitors may be helpful.

Stones and Obstructions

Nephrolithiasis

A. General characteristics

1. Nephrolithiasis is the development of stones within the urinary tract.
2. Sites of obstruction
   a. Ureterovesicular junction—most common site of impaction
   b. Calyx of the kidney
   c. Ureteropelvic junction
   d. Intersection of the ureter and the iliac vessels (near the pelvic brim)

Quick HIT

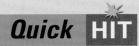

Causes of Hypercalciuria and Hyperoxaluria

Causes of hypercalciuria

- ↑ Intestinal absorption of calcium
- ↓ Renal reabsorption of calcium, leading to ↑ renal excretion of calcium
- ↑ Bone reabsorption of calcium
- Primary hyperparathyroidism
- Sarcoidosis
- Malignancy
- Vitamin D excess

Causes of hyperoxaluria

- Severe steatorrhea of any cause can lead to calcium oxalate stones (due to ↑ absorption of oxalate)
- Small bowel disease, Crohn disease
- Pyridoxine deficiency

3. Risk factors
   a. Low fluid intake—most common and preventable risk factor
   b. Family history
   c. Conditions known to precipitate stone formation (e.g., gout, Crohn disease, hyperparathyroidism, type 1 RTA)
   d. Medications (e.g., loop diuretics, acetazolamide, antacids, chemotherapeutic drugs that cause cell breakdown [uric acid stones])
   e. Male gender (three times more likely to have urolithiasis)
   f. UTIs (especially with urease-producing bacteria)
   g. Dietary factors—low calcium and high oxalate intake
4. Types of stones
   a. Calcium stones (most common form)
      - **Account for 80% to 85% of urinary stones**; composed of calcium oxalate or calcium phosphate (less often) or both
      - Bipyramidal or biconcave ovals
      - Radiodense (i.e., visible on an abdominal radiograph)
      - Secondary to hypercalciuria and hyperoxaluria, which can be due to a variety of causes
   b. Uric acid stones (second most common)
      - Account for 10% of stones
      - A persistently acidic urine pH (<5.5) promotes uric acid stone formation
      - These are associated with hyperuricemia, secondary to gout or to chemotherapeutic treatment of leukemias and lymphomas with high cell destruction. The release of purines from dying cells leads to hyperuricemia
      - Flat square plates
      - **Stones are radiolucent (cannot be seen on an abdominal radiograph)—** require CT, ultrasound, or IVP for detection
   c. Struvite stones (staghorn stones)
      - Account for 5% to 10% of stones
      - Radiodense (visible on an abdominal radiograph); rectangular prisms
      - Occur in patients with recurrent UTIs due to urease-producing organisms (*Proteus, Klebsiella, Serratia, Enterobacter* spp.)
      - They are facilitated by alkaline urine: urea-splitting bacteria convert urea to ammonia, thus producing the alkaline urine.
      - The resultant ammonia combines with magnesium and phosphate to form struvite calculi, which may involve the entire renal collecting system
   d. Cystine stones
      - Account for 1% of urinary stones
      - Genetic predisposition—cystinuria (autosomal recessive)
      - Hexagon-shaped crystals are poorly visualized
5. Clinical course
   a. If a stone is >1 cm, it is unlikely to pass spontaneously. **Stones <0.5 cm usually do pass spontaneously**
   b. Recurrence is common. Up to 50% of the patients have recurrences within 10 years of having the first stone

Quick HIT

Classic Presentation of Nephrolithiasis

- Sudden onset of colicky flank pain that radiates into groin
- Urinalysis showing hematuria

B. Clinical features

1. Renal colic—refers to the pain associated with passing a kidney stone into the ureter, with ureteral obstruction and spasm
   a. Description of pain—begins suddenly and soon may become severe (patient cannot sit still—usually writhes in excruciating pain). Pain may occur in waves or paroxysms
   b. Location of pain—begins in the flank and radiates anteriorly toward the groin (i.e., follows path of the stone)
2. Nausea and vomiting are common.
3. Hematuria (in over 90% of the cases)
4. UTI

C. Diagnosis

1. Laboratory testing
   a. Urinalysis
      - Reveals either microscopic or gross hematuria
      - Reveals an associated UTI if pyuria or bacteriuria are present
      - Examine the urinary sediment for crystals (calcium, cystine, uric acid, or struvite crystals)
      - Determine the urinary pH—alkaline urine might indicate the presence of urease-producing bacteria that cause an infection stone. Acidic urine is suggestive of uric acid stones

   b. Urine culture—obtain if infection is suspected
   c. Twenty-four–hour urine—collect to assess Cr, calcium, uric acid, oxalate, and citrate levels
   d. Serum chemistry—obtain BUN and Cr levels (for evaluation of renal function) and also calcium, uric acid, and phosphate levels
2. Imaging
   a. Plain radiograph of the kidneys, ureter, and bladder (KUB) (Figure 7-6)
      - Initial imaging test for detecting stones
      - Cystine and uric acid stones are not usually visible on plain films

   b. CT scan (spiral CT) without contrast
      - Gold standard for diagnosis. Most sensitive test for detecting stones
      - All stones, even radiolucent ones such as uric acid stones and cystine stones, are visible on the CT scan

   c. IVP
      - Most useful test for defining degree and extent of urinary tract obstruction
      - This is usually not necessary for the diagnosis of renal calculi. IVP may be appropriate for deciding whether a patient needs procedural therapy

   d. Renal ultrasonography
      - Helps in detecting hydronephrosis or hydroureter
      - False-negative results are common in early obstruction. Also, there is a low yield in visualizing the stone

Quick HIT

Hematuria plus pyuria indicates a stone with concomitant infection.

Quick HIT

Having the stone for analysis is very helpful both in treatment and in preventing recurrence. Likewise, reporting a history of stones and their composition (if determined) is very helpful. The patient should attempt to recover the stone that is passed (strain urine).

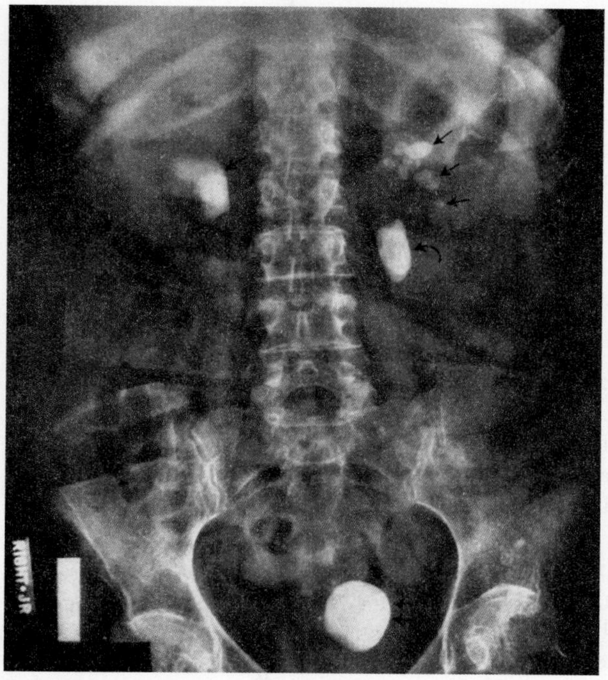

FIGURE 7-6 **Abdominal film (KUB) of renal calculi.**
(From Erkonen WE, Smith, WL. *Radiology 101: The Basics and Fundamentals of Imaging.* Philadelphia, PA: Lippincott Williams & Wilkins, 1998:206, Figure 10-20A.)

- Procedure of choice in patients who cannot receive radiation (i.e., pregnant patients)

D. Treatment

1. General measures (for all types of stones)
   a. Analgesia: IV morphine, parenteral NSAIDs (ketorolac)
   b. Vigorous fluid hydration—beneficial in all forms of nephrolithiasis
   c. Antibiotics—if UTI is present
   d. Outpatient management is appropriate for most patients. Indications for hospital admission include:
      - Pain not controlled with oral medications
      - Anuria (usually in patients with one kidney)
      - Renal colic plus UTI and/or fever
      - Large stone (>1 cm) that is unlikely to pass spontaneously
2. Specific measures (based on severity of pain)
   a. Mild to moderate pain: high fluid intake, oral analgesia while waiting for stone to pass spontaneously (give the patient a urine strainer)
   b. Severe pain (especially with vomiting)
      - Prescribe IV fluids and pain control
      - Obtain a KUB and an IVP to find the site of obstruction
      - If a stone does not pass spontaneously after 3 days, consider urology consult.
   c. Ongoing obstruction and persistent pain not controlled by narcotics—surgery is necessary
      - Extracorporeal shock wave lithotripsy
      - Most common method
      - It breaks the stone apart; once the calculus is fragmented, the stone can pass spontaneously
      - Best for stones that are >5 mm but <2 cm in diameter
      - Percutaneous nephrolithotomy
      - If lithotripsy fails
      - Best for stones >2 cm in diameter
3. Prevention of recurrences
   a. Dietary measures
      - High fluid intake is essential (keep urine volume at 2 L/day)
      - Limit animal protein intake in patients with hyperuricosuria (uric acid stones).
      - Limit calcium intake only if the patient has calcium stones
   b. Pharmacologic measures
      - Thiazide diuretics reduce urinary calcium and have been found to lower recurrence rates, especially in patients with hypercalciuria
      - Allopurinol is effective in preventing recurrence in patients with high uric acid levels in the urine

Urinary Tract Obstruction

A. General characteristics

1. Can lead to renal insufficiency and hydronephrosis (dilation of urinary tract, specifically the pelvis and calyces)
2. More common in men (due to BPH and prostate cancer)
3. Urinary tract obstruction does not usually cause AKI unless the obstruction is bilateral or there is pre-existing renal damage.
4. Classification
   a. Acute versus chronic obstruction
      - Acute obstruction—clinical features are sudden in onset.
      - Chronic obstruction—this causes progressive renal failure/uremia, recurrent infections, and bladder calculi.
   b. Lower versus upper tract obstruction
      - Lower tract obstruction (below ureterovesical junction)—affects urination
      - Upper tract obstruction (above ureterovesical junction)—typically causes renal colic

c. Complete versus partial obstruction
d. Unilateral versus bilateral obstruction (if upper tract)

5. Degree of damage to kidneys and likelihood of return to normal renal function is dependent on the severity and duration of the obstruction
6. Causes
   a. Lower tract obstruction
      - BPH, prostate cancer
      - Urethral stricture, stone
      - Neurogenic bladder (multiple sclerosis, diabetes)
      - Trauma (pelvic fracture or straddle injury)
      - Bladder cancer
   b. Upper tract obstruction
      - Intrinsic causes—kidney stones, blood clots, sloughed papilla, crystal deposition (e.g., uric acid), tumors, strictures, ureteropelvic or ureterovesical junction dysfunction
      - Extrinsic causes—pregnancy, tumors (gynecologic, metastatic), abdominal aortic aneurysm, retroperitoneal fibrosis, endometriosis, prolapse, hematomas, Crohn disease, diverticulitis

Quick HIT

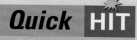

Evaluation of urinary tract obstruction
- Duration of symptoms, UTIs, history of nephrolithiasis, history of surgery
- Suprapubic mass (distended bladder), flank mass (hydronephrosis)
- Features of CKD

B. Clinical features (depend on duration, location, cause, and duration of obstruction)

1. Renal colic and pain—this is more common with acute obstruction (kidney stones, sloughed papilla, blood clot); pain may manifest only during urination. Chronic obstruction may be asymptomatic.
2. Oliguria
3. Recurrent UTIs
4. Hematuria or proteinuria
5. Renal failure

C. Diagnosis

1. **Renal ultrasound is the initial test**—it shows urinary tract dilation. It is very sensitive and specific for identifying hydronephrosis
2. Urinalysis, standard laboratory tests (e.g., CBC, electrolytes, BUN, Cr)
3. KUB—can reveal stones
4. Intravenous urogram—also called IVP
   a. Gold standard for diagnosis of ureteral obstruction
   b. Contraindicated if the patient is pregnant, is allergic to contrast material, or has renal failure
5. Voiding cystourethrography—for lower tract obstruction
6. Cystoscopy—to evaluate urethra and bladder
7. CT scan—to help identify the cause of obstruction

Quick HIT

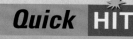

If a patient has an acute obstruction **and** a UTI, emergent diagnostic tests (renal ultrasound or excretory urogram) are indicated. Intervene immediately to relieve the obstruction.

D. Treatment

1. Treatment depends on duration, severity, location, and cause of the obstruction
2. Location of obstruction
   a. Lower urinary tract obstruction
      - Urethral catheter—for acute obstruction
      - Dilatation or internal urethrotomy—if cause is urethral strictures
      - Prostatectomy—if BPH is the cause
   b. Upper urinary tract obstruction
      - Nephrostomy tube drainage—for acute obstruction
      - Ureteral stent (through cystoscope)—if ureteral obstruction
3. Duration and severity of obstruction
   a. Acute complete obstruction—pain or renal failure may be present. This requires immediate therapy
   b. Acute partial obstruction—usually due to stones (see the Treatment section of Nephrolithiasis)
   c. Chronic partial obstruction—this requires immediate therapy only when infection, severe symptoms, renal failure, or urinary retention is present

CLINICAL PEARL 7-8

Prostate-specific Antigen, Digital Rectal Examination, and Transrectal Ultrasonography

- If PSA level >10 ng/mL, TRUS with biopsy is indicated, regardless of DRE findings.
- If DRE is abnormal, TRUS with biopsy is indicated, regardless of PSA level.
- If PSA is <4.0 ng/mL and DRE is negative, annual follow-up is indicated.
- If PSA is 4.1 to 10.0 and DRE is negative, biopsy is usually recommended.

Neoplasms

Prostate Cancer

A. General characteristics: Prostate cancer is the second most common form of cancer in men worldwide (see also Clinical Pearl 7-8). Ninety-five percent are adenocarcinomas.

1. Risk factors
   a. Age (most important risk factor)
   b. African-American race
   c. High-fat diet
   d. Positive family history
   e. Exposure to herbicides and pesticides—certain occupations, such as farming and work in industrial chemical industry, present a higher risk

B. Clinical features

1. Early—it is most commonly asymptomatic. Cancer begins in the periphery of the gland and moves centrally. Thus, obstructive symptoms occur late. In fact, by the time prostate cancer causes urinary obstruction, it often has metastasized to bone or lymph nodes.
2. Later—symptoms due to obstruction of the urethra occur: difficulty in voiding, dysuria, and increased urinary frequency.
3. Late—bone pain from metastases (most commonly vertebral bodies, pelvis, and long bones in legs), weight loss.

Quick HIT

Vertebral metastasis may manifest itself as low back pain in an elderly man with prostate cancer.

C. Diagnosis

1. Digital rectal examination (DRE).
   a. Carcinoma is characteristically hard, nodular, and irregular.
   b. Normal prostate feels like a thenar eminence. Cancer feels like a knuckle. Men with induration, asymmetry, or palpable nodularity of prostate need a biopsy, especially if over age 45.
   c. When palpable, 60% to 70% have spread beyond the prostate.
   d. If DRE is abnormal, transrectal ultrasonography (TRUS) with biopsy is indicated, regardless of the prostate-specific antigen (PSA) level.
2. PSA—not used routinely as a screening test.
   a. PSA is not cancer specific. PSA levels also increase as a result of the following:
      - Prostatic massage (but DRE does not change PSA levels)
      - Needle biopsy
      - Cystoscopy
      - BPH
      - Prostatitis
      - Advanced age
   b. Refinements of the PSA assay—some strategies for improving the diagnostic capability of the PSA test include:
      - Age-adjusted PSA (because PSA normally increases with age).
      - PSA velocity—analysis of the rate of increase in the level with time.

Quick HIT

The combination of DRE and PSA levels can detect up to 60% of prostate cancers while they are still localized.

- Quantifying free and protein-bound forms of serum PSA—PSA produced by prostate cancer tends to be bound by plasma proteins, whereas PSA produced by normal cells is more likely to be free in plasma.
- PSA density—correlation of PSA levels with prostate volume.

3. TRUS with biopsy
   a. May need to repeat biopsies for definitive diagnosis
   b. Indications
      - PSA > 10 ng/dL (or possibly lower). If PSA is >10, chance of finding cancer is over 50%.
      - PSA velocity >0.75 per year
      - Abnormal DRE
4. Other tests in the evaluation include a bone scan, plain radiographs of the pelvis and spine, and a CT scan of the pelvis to evaluate for metastatic disease.

D. Treatment

1. Localized disease (to prostate)—this is usually a curable disease. The definitive therapy is radical prostatectomy. However, watchful waiting is warranted in older men (i.e., those whose remaining natural life expectancy is <10 years) who are asymptomatic. Most common complications of prostatectomy are erectile dysfunction and urinary incontinence.
2. Locally invasive disease—**give radiation therapy plus androgen deprivation** (not curative, but decreases the local spread).
3. Metastatic disease—reduce the amount of testosterone with any of the following:
   a. Orchiectomy (removes testes)—more common in patients who are noncompliant with medical therapy.
   b. Antiandrogens.
   c. Luteinizing hormone–-releasing hormone agonists (leuprolide)
   d. GnRH antagonists—suppress testosterone by binding to receptors in the pituitary without causing a transient surge of LH or FSH (Degarelix).

Quick HIT

Key points about PSA:
1. The higher the PSA, the higher the cancer risk
2. Normal PSA does not rule out prostate cancer
3. Not used as a screening test
4. If patient requests the test, order it

Quick HIT

Stages of Prostate Cancer
- Stage A—nonpalpable, confined to prostate
- Stage B—palpable nodule, but confined to prostate
- Stage C—extends beyond capsule without metastasis
- Stage D—metastatic disease

Renal Cell Carcinoma

A. General characteristics

1. It is twice as common in men as in women.
2. Renal cell carcinoma (RCC) comprises about 85% of primary renal cancers (transitional cell is the second most common).
3. Most cases are sporadic; less than 2% occur as part of autosomal dominant von Hippel–Lindau syndrome.
4. The cause is unknown.
5. Areas of metastasis include the lung, liver, brain, and bone. Tumor thrombus can invade the renal vein or inferior vena cava, resulting in hematogenous dissemination.

B. Risk factors

1. Cigarette smoking
2. Phenacetin analgesics (high use)
3. Adult polycystic kidney disease
4. Chronic dialysis (multicystic disease develops)
5. Exposure to heavy metals (mercury, cadmium)
6. Hypertension

C. Clinical features

1. Hematuria is the most common symptom (gross or microscopic)—occurs in 70% of the patients
2. Abdominal or flank pain—occurs in 50% of the patients
3. Abdominal (flank) mass—occurs in 40% of the patients
4. Weight loss, fever
5. Paraneoplastic syndromes (uncommon)—these tumors can ectopically secrete erythropoietin (causing polycythemia), PTH-like hormone (causing hypercalcemia), renin (causing HTN), cortisol (causing Cushing syndrome), or gonadotropins (causing feminization or masculinization)

Quick HIT

Up to 20% to 30% of cases of renal cell carcinoma are discovered incidentally on a CT scan or ultrasound performed for other reasons.

Quick HIT

The classic triad of hematuria, flank pain, and abdominal mass occurs in less than 10% of patients with renal cell carcinoma.

D. Diagnosis
1. Renal ultrasound—for detection of renal mass
2. Abdominal CT (with and without contrast)—optimal test for diagnosis and staging; perform if ultrasound shows a mass or cysts

E. Treatment—radical nephrectomy (excision of kidney and adrenal gland, including Gerota fascia with excision of nodal tissue along the renal hilum) for stages I to IV

Quick HIT

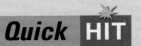

Transitional cell carcinoma accounts for 90% of all bladder cancers. Other types are squamous cell (5%) and adenocarcinoma (2%).

Bladder Cancer

A. General characteristics
1. Bladder carcinoma is the most common type of tumor of the genitourinary tract; 90% of bladder cancers are transitional cell carcinomas. Transitional cell carcinomas can occur anywhere from the kidney to the bladder (e.g., renal pelvis, ureter), but 90% of these carcinomas are in the bladder
2. The most common route of spread is local extension to surrounding tissues
3. **It is likely to recur after removal**
4. Risk factors
   a. Cigarette smoking (major risk factor)
   b. Industrial carcinogens (aniline dye, azo dyes)
   c. Long-term treatment with cyclophosphamide (may cause hemorrhagic cystitis and increase the risk of transitional cell carcinoma)

B. Clinical features
1. Initial presenting sign is **hematuria** in most cases (painless hematuria is the classic presentation).
2. Irritable bladder symptoms, such as dysuria frequency.

C. Diagnosis
1. Urinalysis and urine culture—to rule out infection
2. Urine cytology—to detect malignant cells
3. IVP
4. Cystoscopy and biopsy (definitive test)
5. Chest radiograph and CT scan—for staging

D. Treatment (depends on the stage of the disease)
1. Stage 0 (superficial, limited to mucosa; also known as carcinoma in situ)—intravesical chemotherapy
2. Stage A (involves lamina propria)
   a. Transurethral resection of the bladder tumor
   b. Tends to recur, so frequent cystoscopy and removal of recurrent tumors are indicated
3. Stage B (muscle invasion)—radical cystectomy, lymph node dissection, removal of prostate/uterus/ovaries/anterior vaginal wall, and urinary diversion (e.g., ileal conduit)
4. Stage C (extends to perivesicular fat)—treatment is the same as for stage B
5. Stage D (metastasis to lymph nodes, abdominal organs, or distant sites)—consider cystectomy and systemic chemotherapy

Testicular Cancer

A. General characteristics
1. Most common in men 20 to 35 years of age, but can occur in men of any age
2. Has a relatively high cure rate compared with other cancers
3. Types
   a. Germ cell tumors (account for 95% of all testicular cancers)—most common in men 20 to 40 years of age; curable in >95% of the cases
      - Seminomas (35%)—most common; slow growth and late invasion; most radiosensitive

- Nonseminomatous (65%)—usually contain cells from at least two of the following four types (mixed cell type): embryonal carcinoma (high malignant potential, hemorrhage and necrosis are common; metastases to the abdominal lymphatics and the lungs may occur as an early event); choriocarcinoma (most aggressive type; rare; metastases usually occur by time of diagnosis); teratoma (rarely metastasize); yolk sac carcinoma (rare in men, usually occurs in young boys)

b. Nongerm cell tumors (account for 5% of all testicular cancers)—are usually benign
- Leydig cell tumors are hormonally active—most are benign and are treated with surgery. Prognosis is poor if metastasis occurs. They may secrete a variety of steroid hormones, including estrogen and androgens, and are associated with precocious puberty in children and gynecomastia in adults
- Sertoli cell tumors are usually benign

B. Risk factors

1. Cryptorchidism—surgical correction does not eliminate risk
2. Klinefelter syndrome

C. Clinical features

1. Painless mass/lump/firmness of the testicle—because of lack of pain, may go unnoticed by the patient until advanced.
2. Gynecomastia may be present because some of the nonseminomatous germ cell tumors produce gonadotropins.

D. Diagnosis

1. Physical examination (testicular mass)
2. Testicular ultrasound—initial test for localizing the tumor
3. Tumor markers—helpful in diagnosis, staging, and monitoring response to therapy
   a. β-hCG
   - Always elevated in choriocarcinoma
   - May be elevated in other types of nonseminomatous germ cell tumors as well

   b. AFP
   - Increased in embryonal tumors (in 80% of the cases)
   - Choriocarcinoma and seminoma never have an elevated AFP
4. CT scan and chest radiograph for staging

E. Treatment

1. If testicular cancer is suspected based on physical examination or ultrasound, the testicle should be removed surgically (to confirm diagnosis). An inguinal approach is used because a scrotal incision may lead to tumor seeding of the scrotum.
2. After orchiectomy, perform a CT scan of the chest, abdomen, and pelvis for staging.
3. Perform β-hCG and AFP measurement after orchiectomy for comparison with the preoperative values.
4. Further treatment depends on the histology of the tumor.
   a. Seminoma—inguinal orchiectomy and radiation (very radiosensitive).
   b. Nonseminomatous disease—orchiectomy and retroperitoneal lymph node dissection with or without chemotherapy.

Penile Cancer

- The peak incidence of this tumor is in men in their seventh decade.
- Circumcision may have a protective effect because penile cancer is very rare in those who have been circumcised.
- It is associated with herpes simplex virus and HPV 18 infection.
- It presents as an exophytic mass on the penis.
- Treatment of the primary disease is local excision.

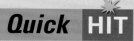

Quick HIT

In a patient with a scrotal mass, perform a careful physical examination to determine its site of origin because testicular cancers are almost always malignant, whereas extratesticular tumors within the scrotum are almost always benign.

Quick HIT

Differential Diagnosis of Testicular Cancer
- Varicocele—dilated, tortuous veins in testicle
- Testicular torsion
- Spermatocele (testicular cyst)
- Hydrocele (fluid in testicle)
- Epididymitis
- Lymphoma

Quick HIT

Staging (Boden–Gibb) of Testicular Cancer
- Stage A—confined to testis/cord
- Stage B—retroperitoneal lymph node spread (below diaphragm)
- Stage C—distant metastasis

Quick HIT

A young man with a firm, painless testicular mass should be presumed to have testicular cancer until proven otherwise.

Quick HIT
Do not confuse testicular cancer with testicular torsion or epididymitis.

Miscellaneous Conditions

Testicular Torsion

- Twisting of the spermatic cord leading to arterial occlusion and venous outflow obstruction; ischemia can lead to testicular infarction.
- Usually seen in adolescents.
- Acute severe testicular pain, swollen and tender scrotum, and an elevated testicle (as twisting occurs, the testicle moves to a higher position in scrotum).
- **This is a surgical emergency:** immediate surgical detorsion and orchiopexy to the scrotum (perform bilaterally to prevent torsion in the contralateral testicle). **If surgery is delayed beyond 6 hours, infarction may occur, and the testicle may not be salvageable.**
- Orchiectomy if a nonviable testicle is found.

Quick HIT
Epididymitis may be difficult to differentiate from testicular torsion.

Epididymitis

- Infection of the epididymis. The common offending organism in children and elderly patients is *Escherichia coli;* in young men, sexually transmitted diseases are more common (gonorrhea, *Chlamydia*).
- A swollen, tender testicle; dysuria; fever/chills; scrotal pain; and a scrotal mass.
- Rule out testicular torsion, and administer antibiotics.

FLUIDS, ELECTROLYTES, AND ACID–BASE DISORDERS

8

Volume Disorders

Approach to Volume Disorders

A. Normal body fluid compartments

1. Men: total-body water (TBW) = 60% of body weight (Figure 8-1).
2. Women: TBW = 50% of body weight.
3. Percentage of TBW decreases with age and increasing obesity (TBW decreases because fat contains very little water).
4. Distribution of water.
   a. Intracellular fluid (ICF) is two-thirds of TBW (or 40% of body weight)—the largest proportion of TBW is in skeletal muscle mass.
   b. Extracellular fluid (ECF) is one-third of TBW (or 20% of body weight).
      - Plasma is one-third of ECF, one-twelfth of TBW, and 5% of body weight.
      - Interstitial fluid is two-thirds of ECF, one-fourth of TBW, and 15% of body weight.
5. Water exchange
   a. Normal intake: 1,500 mL in fluids taken PO per day; 500 mL in solids or product of oxidation.
   b. Normal output.
      - From 800 to 1,500 mL in urine per day is the normal range. Minimum urine output to excrete products of catabolism is about 500 to 600 mL/day, assuming normal renal concentrating ability.
      - Output of 250 mL/day occurs in stool.
      - From 600 to 900 mL/day in insensible losses occurs. This is highly variable but increases with fever, sweating, hyperventilation, and tracheostomies (unhumidified air)—see below.
   c. Remember the Starling equation and forces: fluid shift depends on hydrostatic and oncotic pressures.

Quick HIT

For body fluid compartments, remember the 60-40-20 rule.
- TBW is 60% of body weight (50% for women).
- ICF is 40% of body weight.
- ECF is 20% of body weight (interstitial fluid 15% and plasma 5%).

Quick HIT

Three reasons for oliguria:
- Low blood flow to kidney (assess heart)
- Kidney problem
- Post renal obstruction (place a Foley catheter)

B. Assessing volume status

1. This is not a simple task. For example, a patient with lower extremity edema may be euvolemic, or may be total-body overloaded but intravascularly depleted. Skin turgor and mucous membranes are very difficult to assess and are not always reliable indicators of volume status.
2. Tracking input and output is not an exact science either because there is no accurate way of calculating insensible losses. Monitoring urine output is very important in the assessment of volume status: **Normal urine output in infants is more than 1.0 mL/kg/hr, while normal urine output for an adult is generally regarded as 0.5 to 1.0 mL/kg/hr.** Low urine output could be a sign of volume depletion.
3. Daily weights may give a more accurate assessment of volume trends.

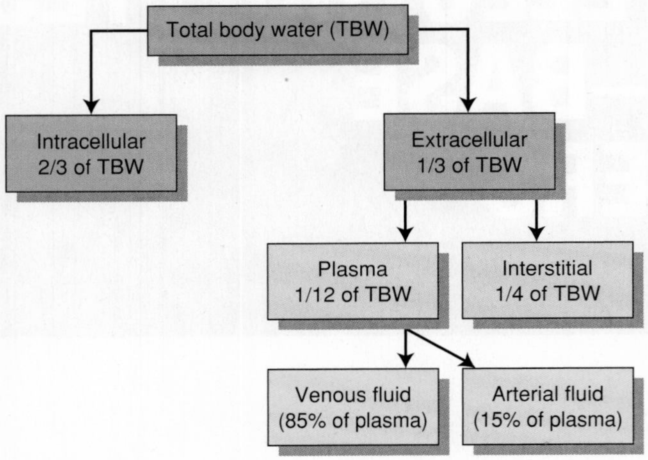

FIGURE 8-1 **Body fluid compartments.**

4. Keep in mind the larger picture of the patient's condition.
   a. In general, patients with sepsis, fever, burns, or open wounds have high insensible losses (and higher metabolic demands).
   b. For each degree of atmospheric temperature over 37°C, the body's water loss increases by approximately 100 mL/day.
   c. Patients with liver failure, nephrotic syndrome, or any condition causing hypoalbuminemia tend to third-space fluid out of the vasculature and may be total-body hypervolemic but intravascularly depleted.
   d. Patients with CHF may have either pulmonary edema or anasarca, depending on which ventricle is involved.
   e. Patients with ESRD are very prone to hypervolemia for obvious reasons.

Quick HIT

If a patient is receiving hypotonic solutions (1/2 NS, 1/4 NS), water is initially transferred from the ECF to intracellular space to equilibrate osmotic pressures in both compartments.

C. Fluid replacement therapy

1. Normal saline (NS)—often used to increase intravascular volume if the patient is dehydrated or has lost blood; usually not the best option in patients with CHF unless the patient needs urgent resuscitation
2. D51/2NS
   a. Often the standard maintenance fluid (often given with 20 mEq of KCl/L of fluid)
   b. Has some glucose, which can spare muscle breakdown, and has water for insensible losses
3. D5W
   a. Used to dilute powdered medicines
   b. May sometimes be indicated in correcting hypernatremia
   c. Only one-twelfth remains intravascular because it diffuses into the TBW compartment, so not effective in maintaining intravascular volume
4. Lactated Ringer solution—This is excellent for replacement of intravascular volume; it is not a maintenance fluid. It is the most common trauma resuscitation fluid. Do not use if hyperkalemia is a concern (contains potassium)

Hypovolemia

A. Causes

1. GI losses due to vomiting, nasogastric suction, diarrhea, fistula drainage, etc.
2. Third-spacing due to ascites, effusions, bowel obstruction, crush injuries, burns
3. Inadequate intake
4. Polyuria—for example, diabetic ketoacidosis (DKA)
5. Sepsis, intra-abdominal and retroperitoneal inflammatory processes
6. Trauma, open wounds, sequestration of fluid into soft tissue injuries

7. Insensible losses—evaporatory losses through the skin (75%) and the respiratory tract (25%)

B. Clinical features

1. CNS findings: mental status changes, sleepiness, apathy, coma
2. Cardiovascular findings (due to decrease in plasma volume): orthostatic hypotension, tachycardia, decreased pulse pressure, decreased central venous pressure (CVP), and pulmonary capillary wedge pressure (PCWP)
3. Skin: poor skin turgor, hypothermia, pale extremities, dry tongue
4. Oliguria
5. Ileus, weakness
6. Acute renal failure due to prerenal azotemia (fractional excretion of sodium <1% and/or BUN/creatinine >20.)

C. Diagnosis

1. Monitor urine output and daily weights. If the patient is critically ill and has cardiac or renal dysfunction, consider placing a Swan–Ganz catheter (to measure CVP and PCWP).
2. Elevated serum sodium, low urine sodium, and a BUN/Cr ratio of >20:1 suggest hypoperfusion to the kidneys, which usually (not always) represents hypovolemia.
3. Increased hematocrit: 3% increase for each liter of deficit.
4. The concentration of formed elements in the blood (RBCs, WBCs, platelets, plasma proteins) increases with an ECF deficit and decreases with an ECF excess.

D. Treatment

1. Correct volume deficit.
   a. Use bolus to achieve euvolemia. Begin with isotonic solution (lactated Ringer or NS).
   b. Again, frequent monitoring of HR, BP, urine output, and weight is essential.
   c. **Maintain urine output at 0.5 to 1 mL/kg/hr.**
   d. Blood loss—replace blood loss with crystalloid at a 3:1 ratio.
2. Maintenance fluid.
   a. D51/2NS solution with 20 mEq KCl/L is the most common adult maintenance fluid. (Dextrose is added to inhibit muscle breakdown.)
   b. There are two methods of calculating the amount of maintenance fluid (see Clinical Pearl 8-1).

Quick HIT

Do **not** combine bolus fluids with dextrose (which can lead to hyperglycemia) or potassium (which can lead to hyperkalemia).

Hypervolemia

A. Causes

1. Iatrogenic (parenteral overhydration)
2. Fluid-retaining states: CHF, nephrotic syndrome, cirrhosis, ESRD

Quick HIT

Most cases of edema result from renal sodium retention.

B. Clinical features

1. Weight gain

Quick HIT

Signs of Volume Overload
- Elevated jugular venous pressure
- Pulmonary rales—due to pulmonary edema
- Peripheral edema

CLINICAL PEARL 8-1

Calculation of Maintenance Fluids

- 100/50/20 rule:
  - 100 mL/kg for first 10 kg, 50 mL/kg for next 10 kg, 20 mL/kg for every 1 kg over 20
  - Divide total by 24 for hourly rate
  - For example, for a 70 kg man: 100 × 10 = 1,000; 50 × 10 = 500, 20 × 50 kg = 1,000. Total = 2,500. Divide by 24 hours: **104 mL/hr**
- 4/2/1 rule:
  - 4 mL/kg for first 10 kg, 2 mL/kg for next 10 kg, 1 mL/kg for every 1 kg over 20
  - For example, for a 70 kg man: 4 × 10 = 40; 2 × 10 = 20; 1 × 50 = 50. Total = **110 mL/hr**

2. Peripheral edema (pedal or sacral), ascites, or pulmonary edema
3. Jugular venous distention
4. Elevated CVP and PCWP
5. Pulmonary rales
6. Low hematocrit and albumin concentration

C. Treatment

1. Fluid restriction
2. Judicious use of diuretics
3. Monitor urine output and daily weights, and consider Swan–Ganz catheter placement depending on the patient's condition

Sodium

Overview of Sodium Homeostasis

A. Salt and water regulation

1. Na^+ regulation is intimately associated with water homeostasis, yet it is regulated by independent mechanisms.
2. Changes in Na^+ **concentration** are a reflection of water homeostasis, whereas changes in Na^+ **content** are a reflection of Na^+ homeostasis.
3. Disturbance of Na^+ balance may lead to hypovolemia or hypervolemia, and disturbance of water balance may lead to hyponatremia or hypernatremia.

B. Sodium homeostasis

1. Sodium is actively pumped out of cells and is therefore restricted to the extracellular space. It is the main osmotically active cation of the ECF.
2. An increase in sodium intake results in an increase in ECF volume, which results in an increase in GFR and sodium excretion. A decline in the extracellular circulating volume results in a decreased GFR and a reduction in sodium excretion.
3. Diuretics inhibit Na^+ reabsorption through various mechanisms in the renal tubular system. Furosemide and other loop diuretics inhibit the Na^+–K^+–Cl^- transporter in the thick ascending limb of the loop of Henle, whereas thiazide diuretics inhibit the Na^+–Cl^- cotransporter at the early distal tubule. However, the majority of Na^+ reabsorption occurs in the proximal tubule.
4. A decrease in renal perfusion pressure results in activation of the renin–angiotensin–aldosterone system. Aldosterone increases sodium reabsorption and potassium secretion from the late distal tubules.

Quick HIT

- Aldosterone increases sodium reabsorption.
- ADH increases water reabsorption.

C. Water homeostasis

1. Osmoreceptors in the hypothalamus are stimulated by plasma hypertonicity (usually >295 mOsm/kg); activation of these stimulators produces thirst.
2. Hypertonic plasma also stimulates the secretion of antidiuretic hormone (ADH) from the posterior pituitary gland. When ADH binds to V_2 receptors in the renal collecting ducts, water channels are synthesized and more water is reabsorbed.
3. ADH is suppressed as plasma tonicity decreases.
4. Ultimately, the amount of water intake and output (including renal, GI, and insensible losses from the skin and the respiratory tract) must be equivalent over time to preserve a steady state.
5. When a steady state is not achieved, hyponatremia or hypernatremia usually occurs.

Quick HIT

- Hyponatremia and hypernatremia are caused by too much or too little **water.**
- Hypovolemia and hypervolemia are caused by too little or too much **sodium.**

Hyponatremia

A. General characteristics

1. This refers to too much water in relation to sodium in the serum.
2. It is typically defined as a plasma Na^+ concentration <135 mmol/L.
3. Symptoms usually begin when the Na^+ level falls to <120 mEq/L. An important exception is increased intracranial pressure (ICP) (e.g., after head injury). As ECF

osmolality decreases, water shifts into brain cells, further increasing ICP. (Therefore, it is critical to keep serum sodium normal or slightly high in such patients.)

B. Causes and classification (based on serum osmolality)

1. **Hypotonic hyponatremia**—"true hyponatremia"—serum osmolality <280 mOsm/kg
   a. Hypovolemic
      - Low urine sodium (<10 mEq/L)—implies increased sodium retention by the kidneys to compensate for **extrarenal losses** (e.g., diarrhea, vomiting, nasogastric suction, diaphoresis, third-spacing, burns, pancreatitis) **of sodium-containing fluid**
      - High urine sodium (>20 mEq/L)—renal salt loss is likely—for example, diuretic excess, decreased aldosterone (ACE inhibitors), ATN
   b. Euvolemic—no evidence of ECF expansion or contraction on clinical grounds
      - SIADH
      - Psychogenic polydipsia
      - Postoperative hyponatremia
      - Hypothyroidism
      - Oxytocin use
      - Administration/intake of a relative excess of free water—if a patient is given D5W (or other hypotonic solution) to replace fluids, or if water alone is consumed after intensive exertion (with profuse sweating)
      - Drugs—haloperidol (Haldol), cyclophosphamide, certain antineoplastic agents
   c. Hypervolemic (low urine sodium)—This is due to water-retaining states. The relative excess of water in relation to sodium results in hyponatremia.
      - CHF
      - Nephrotic syndrome (renal failure)
      - Liver disease
2. Isotonic hyponatremia (pseudohyponatremia)
   a. An increase in plasma solids lowers the plasma sodium **concentration.** But the **amount** of sodium in plasma is normal (hence, **pseudo**hyponatremia)
   b. This can be caused by any condition that leads to elevated protein or lipid levels
3. Hypertonic hyponatremia
   a. Caused by the presence of osmotic substances that cause an **osmotic shift of water out of cells.** These substances cannot cross the cell membrane and therefore create osmotic gradients
   b. These substances include:
      - Glucose—**Hyperglycemia** increases osmotic pressure, and water shifts from cells into ECF leading to a dilutional hyponatremia. For every 100 mg/dL increase in blood glucose level above normal, the serum sodium level decreases about 3 mEq/L. Note that the actual sodium content in the ECF is unchanged.
      - Mannitol, sorbitol, glycerol, maltose
      - Radiocontrast agents

> **Quick HIT**
> Excessive water intake alone rarely leads to hyponatremia because the kidneys have a great capacity to excrete water.

C. Clinical features

1. **Neurologic symptoms predominate**—caused by "water intoxication"—osmotic water shifts, which leads to increased ICF volume, specifically brain cell swelling or cerebral edema
   a. Headache, delirium, irritability
   b. Muscle twitching, weakness
   c. Hyperactive deep tendon reflexes
2. Increased ICP, seizures, coma
3. GI—nausea, vomiting, ileus, watery diarrhea
4. Cardiovascular—hypertension due to increased ICP
5. Increased salivation and lacrimation
6. Oliguria progressing to anuria—**may not be reversible if therapy is delayed**

> **Quick HIT**
> As opposed to acute water intoxication, when hyponatremia develops gradually (over a few days), the clinical features do not appear until a relatively lower sodium level is reached.

D. Diagnosis

1. Plasma osmolality—low in a patient with true hyponatremia (Figure 8-2)

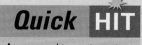

Fluids, Electrolytes, and Acid–base Disorders

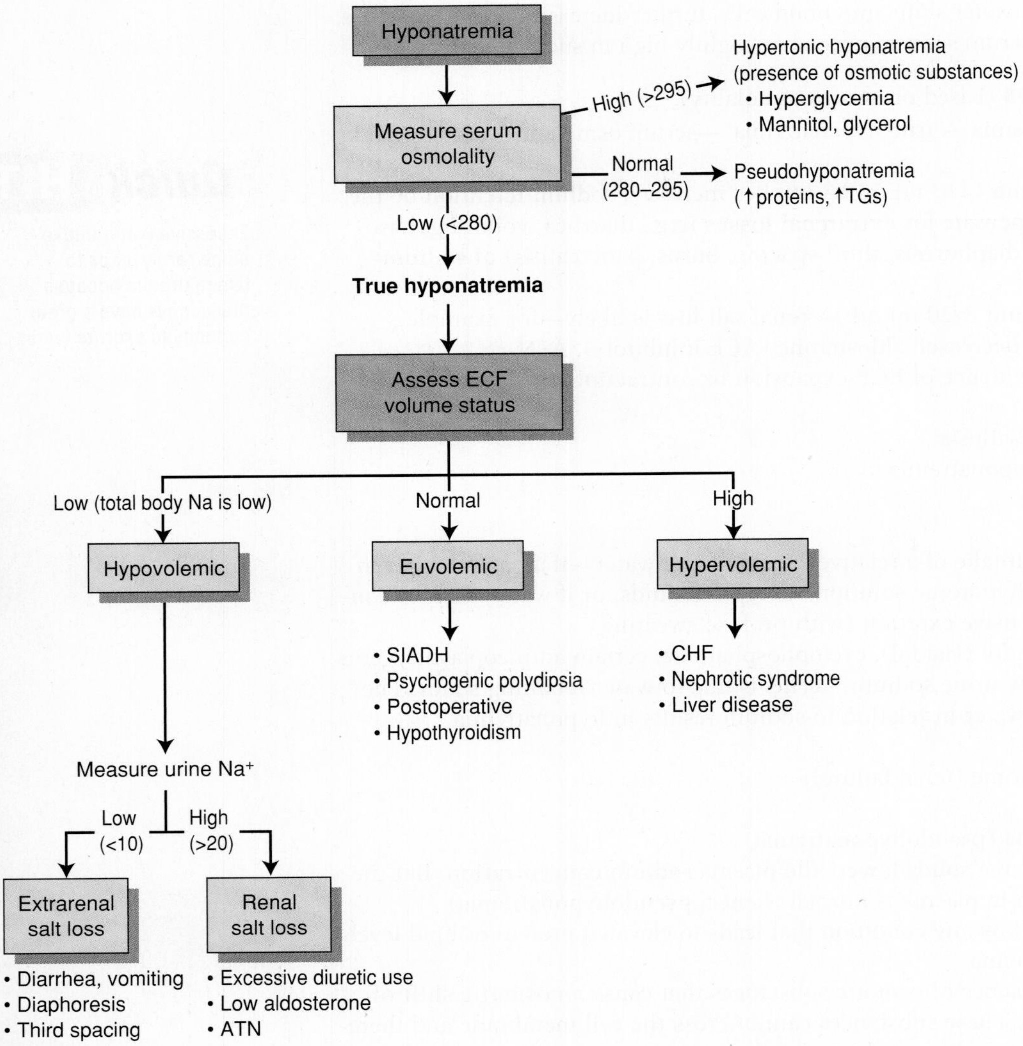

FIGURE 8-2 **Evaluation of hyponatremia.**
(Adapted from Harwood-Nuss A, Wolfson AB. *The Clinical Practice of Emergency Medicine.* 3rd ed. Philadelphia, PA: Lippincott Williams & Wilkins, 2001:849, Figure 173-1.)

2. Urine osmolality
   a. Low if the kidneys are responding appropriately by diluting the urine—for example, primary polydipsia
   b. Elevated if there are increased levels of ADH—for example, SIADH, CHF, and hypothyroidism
3. Urine sodium concentration
   a. Urine Na^+ should be low in the setting of hyponatremia
   b. Urine Na^+ concentration >20 mmol/L is consistent with a salt-wasting nephropathy or hypoaldosteronism. Diuretics may produce this as well
   c. Urine Na^+ concentration <40 mmol/L is consistent with (but does not define) SIADH

Quick HIT

Most cases of hypernatremia are due to the following types of water loss:
- Nonrenal loss: insensible loss, GI tract (diarrhea)
- Renal loss: osmotic diuresis, diabetes insipidus

E. Treatment

1. Isotonic and hypertonic hyponatremias—diagnose and treat the underlying disorder.
2. Hypotonic hyponatremia.
   a. Mild (Na^+ 120 to 130 mmol/L)—withhold free water, and allow the patient to reequilibrate spontaneously.
   b. Moderate (Na^+ 110 to 120 mmol/L)—loop diuretics (given with saline to prevent renal concentration of urine due to high ADH).

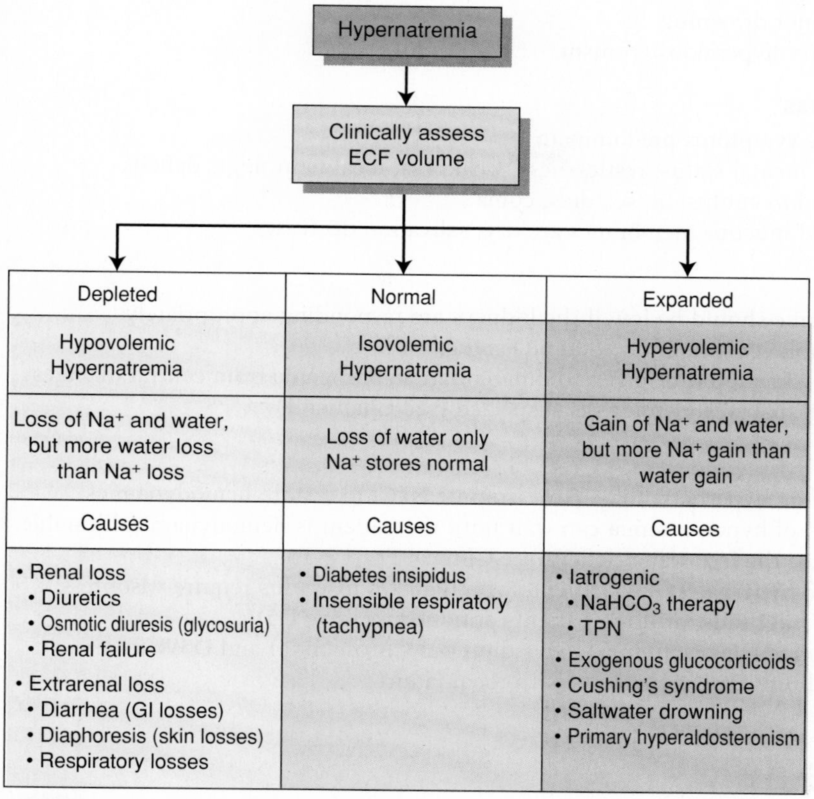

FIGURE **8-3** **Evaluation of hypernatremia.**
(Adapted from Glasscock RJ, Massry SG. *Massry and Glassock's Textbook of Nephrology*. 4th ed. Philadelphia, PA: Lippincott Williams & Wilkins, 2000.)

c. Severe (Na^+ <110 mmol/L or if symptomatic)—give hypertonic saline to increase serum sodium by 1 to 2 mEq/L/hr until symptoms improve.
   - Hypertonic saline rapidly increases the tonicity of ECF.
   - Do not increase sodium more than 8 mmol/L during the first 24 hours. An overly rapid increase in serum sodium concentration may produce **central pontine demyelination.**

Hypernatremia

A. General characteristics

1. Defined as a plasma Na^+ concentration >145 mmol/L
2. Refers to excess sodium in relation to water; can result from water loss or sodium infusion
3. Assess ECF volume clinically, as follows (Figure 8-3):
   a. Hypovolemic hypernatremia (sodium stores are depleted, but more water loss than sodium loss)
      - Renal loss—from diuretics, **osmotic diuresis** (most commonly due to glycosuria in diabetics), renal failure
      - Extrarenal loss—from **diarrhea**, diaphoresis, respiratory losses

   b. Isovolemic hypernatremia (sodium stores normal, water lost)
      - **Diabetes insipidus**
      - Insensible respiratory (tachypnea)

   c. Hypervolemic hypernatremia (sodium excess)—occurs infrequently
      - Iatrogenic—most common cause of hypervolemic hypernatremia (e.g., large amounts of parenteral $NaHCO_3$, TPN)
      - Exogenous glucocorticoids
      - Cushing syndrome

Quick HIT

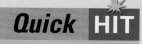

Excessively rapid correction of hypernatremia can lead to **cerebral edema** as water shifts into brain cells. Therefore, the rate of correction should not exceed 12 mEq/L/day (should be <8 mEq/L in the first 24 hours).

- Saltwater drowning
- Primary hyperaldosteronism

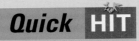

Quick HIT

Clinical features of hypernatremia are secondary to osmotic effects on the brain (water shifts out of brain cells, leaving them dehydrated). Symptoms are more prominent and severe when sodium levels increase rapidly.

B. Clinical features

1. Neurologic symptoms predominate
   a. Altered mental status, restlessness, weakness, focal neurologic deficits
   b. Can lead to confusion, seizures, coma
2. Tissues and mucous membranes are dry; salivation decreases

C. Diagnosis

1. Urine volume should be low if the kidneys are responding appropriately.
2. Urine osmolality should be >800 mOsm/kg.
3. Desmopressin should be given to differentiate nephrogenic from central diabetes insipidus if diabetes insipidus is suspected (see Chapter 4).

D. Treatment

Quick HIT

Calculating free water deficit
Water deficit = TBW (1 − actual Na^+ ÷ desired Na^+)

1. Hypovolemic hypernatremia—Give isotonic NaCl to restore hemodynamics. Correction of hypernatremia can wait until the patient is hemodynamically stable, then replace the free water deficit (see Clinical Pearl 8-1).
2. Isovolemic hypernatremia—Patients with diabetes insipidus require vasopressin. Prescribe oral fluids, or if the patient cannot drink, give D5W.
3. Hypervolemic hypernatremia—Give diuretics (furosemide) and D5W to remove excess sodium. Dialyze patients with renal failure.

Calcium

Calcium Metabolism

A. Normal serum calcium: The normal serum calcium (Ca^{2+}) range is 8.5 to 10.5 mg/dL. Calcium balance is regulated by hormonal control, but the levels are also affected by albumin and pH.

1. Albumin
   a. Calcium in plasma exists in two forms:
      - Protein-bound form: most calcium ions are bound to albumin, so the total calcium concentration fluctuates with the protein (albumin) concentration.
      - Free ionized form: **physiologically active** fraction; under tight hormonal control (PTH), **independent of albumin levels.**
   b. In hypoalbuminemia the total calcium is low, but ionized calcium is normal, and can be estimated by the following formula: total calcium—(serum albumin × 0.8).
2. Changes in pH alter the ratio of calcium binding. An increase in pH increases the binding of calcium to albumin. Therefore, in alkalemic states (especially acute respiratory alkalosis), total calcium is normal, but ionized calcium is low and the patient frequently manifests the signs and symptoms of hypocalcemia.

B. Hormonal control

Quick HIT

Maintenance of calcium balance is a function of PTH, calcitonin, and vitamin D, and their target organs bone, kidney, and gut.

1. PTH—↑ plasma Ca^{2+} and ↓ plasma PO_4^{3-} by acting on:
   a. Bone: ↑ bone resorption
   b. Kidney: ↑ Ca^{2+} reabsorption, ↓ PO_4^{3-} reabsorption
   c. Gut: activation of vitamin D
2. Calcitonin—↓ plasma Ca^{2+} and ↓ plasma PO_4^{3-} by acting on:
   a. Bone: ↓ bone resorption
   b. Kidney: ↓ Ca^{2+} reabsorption, ↑ PO_4^{3-} reabsorption
   c. Gut: ↓ postprandial Ca^{2+} absorption
3. Vitamin D—↑ plasma Ca^{2+} and ↑ plasma PO_4^{3-} by acting on:
   a. Bone: ↑ bone resorption

b. Kidney: ↑ Ca^{2+} reabsorption, ↓PO_4^{3-} reabsorption
c. Gut: ↑ Ca^{2+} absorption, ↑ PO_4^{3-} reabsorption

Hypocalcemia

A. Causes

1. Hypoparathyroidism (most common cause)—usually due to surgery on the thyroid gland (with damage to nearby parathyroids).
2. Acute pancreatitis—deposition of calcium deposits lowers serum Ca^{2+} levels.
3. Renal insufficiency—mainly due to decreased production of 1,25-dihydroxy vitamin D.
4. Hyperphosphatemia—PO_4^{3-} precipitates with Ca^{2+} resulting in calcium phosphate deposition.
5. Pseudohypoparathyroidism—autosomal recessive disease causing congenital end-organ resistance to PTH (so PTH levels are actually high); also characterized by mental retardation and short metacarpal bones.
6. Hypomagnesemia—results in decreased PTH secretion.
7. Vitamin D deficiency
8. Malabsorption—short bowel syndrome.
9. Blood transfusion (with citrated blood)—calcium binds to citrate.
10. Osteoblastic metastases.
11. Hypoalbuminemia—but ionized fraction is normal so hypoalbuminemia is clinically irrelevant.
12. DiGeorge syndrome—caused by a deletion on chromosome 22. Absence of thymic shadow on chest x-ray.

Quick HIT

Ionized calcium may be low with normal serum calcium levels in acute alkalotic states.

B. Clinical features

1. Asymptomatic
2. Rickets and osteomalacia
3. Increased neuromuscular irritability
   a. Numbness/tingling—circumoral in fingers, in toes
   b. Tetany
      - Hyperactive deep tendon reflexes
      - *Chvostek sign*—tapping a facial nerve leads to a contraction (twitching) of facial muscles
      - *Trousseau sign*—Inflate BP cuff to a pressure higher than the patient's systolic BP for 3 minutes (occludes blood flow in forearm). This elicits carpal spasms
   c. Grand mal seizures
4. Basal ganglia calcifications
5. Cardiac manifestations
   a. Arrhythmias
   b. Prolonged QT interval on ECG—hypocalcemia should always be in the differential diagnosis for a prolonged QT interval

Quick HIT

Hospitalized patients frequently have low serum albumin concentrations. Therefore, if you see a low calcium level, look at the albumin level (it is usually low as well). A low serum **ionized calcium** level is much less common.

C. Diagnosis

1. To evaluate for the above-listed etiologies, obtain the following: BUN, Cr, magnesium, albumin, and ionized calcium. Amylase, lipase, and liver function tests may also be warranted.
2. Serum PO_4^{3-}: high in renal insufficiency and in hypoparathyroidism, low in primary vitamin D deficiency
3. PTH
   a. Low in hypoparathyroidism
   b. Elevated in vitamin D deficiency
   c. Very high in pseudohypoparathyroidism

D. Treatment

1. If symptomatic, provide emergency treatment with IV calcium gluconate.
2. For long-term management, use oral calcium supplements (calcium carbonate) and vitamin D.

3. For PTH deficiency.
   a. Replacement therapy with vitamin D (or calcitriol) plus a high oral calcium intake.
   b. Thiazide diuretics—lower urinary calcium and prevent urolithiasis.
4. It is also important to correct hypomagnesemia. It is very difficult to correct the calcium level if the magnesium is not replaced first.

Hypercalcemia

A. Causes

1. Endocrinopathies
   a. Hyperparathyroidism—increased Ca^2+, low PO_4^{3-}
   b. Renal failure—usually results in **hypo**calcemia, but sometimes secondary hyperparathyroidism elevates PTH levels high enough to cause **hyper**calcemia
   c. Paget disease of the bone—due to osteoclastic bone resorption
   d. Hyperparathyroidism, acromegaly, Addison disease
2. Malignancies
   a. Metastatic cancer—bony metastases result in bone destruction due to osteoclastic activity. Most tumors that metastasize to bone cause both osteolytic and osteoblastic activities (prostate cancer, mainly osteoblastic; kidney carcinoma, usually osteolytic)
   b. Multiple myeloma—secondary to two causes
      - Lysis of bone by tumor cells
      - Release of osteoclast-activating factor by myeloma cells
   c. Tumors that release PTH-like hormone (e.g., lung cancer)
3. Pharmacologic
   a. Vitamin D intoxication—increased GI absorption of calcium
   b. Milk-alkali syndrome—hypercalcemia, alkalosis, and renal impairment due to excessive intake of calcium and certain absorbable antacids (calcium carbonate, milk)
   c. Drugs—thiazide diuretics (inhibit renal excretion), lithium (increases PTH levels in some patients, e.g., squamous cell carcinoma)
4. Other
   a. Sarcoidosis—increased GI absorption of calcium
   b. Familial hypocalciuric hypercalcemia—distinguished from primary hyperparathyroidism by a low urine calcium excretion versus a normal or high urine calcium excretion in primary hyperparathyroidism

B. Clinical features

1. "Stones"
   a. Nephrolithiasis
   b. Nephrocalcinosis
2. "Bones"
   a. Bone aches and pains
   b. Osteitis fibrosa cystica ("brown tumors") predisposes to pathologic fractures
3. "Grunts and groans"
   a. Muscle pain and weakness
   b. Pancreatitis
   c. Peptic ulcer disease
   d. Gout
   e. Constipation
4. "Psychiatric overtones"—depression, fatigue, anorexia, sleep disturbances, anxiety, lethargy
5. Other findings
   a. Polydipsia, polyuria
   b. Hypertension
   c. Weight loss
   d. ECG—shortened QT interval
   e. Patients may be asymptomatic

Quick HIT

- In hypercalcemia, ECG shows shortening of the QT interval.
- In hypocalcemia, ECG shows a prolongation of the QT interval.

C. Diagnosis

1. Same laboratory tests as in hypocalcemia
2. Radioimmunoassay of PTH: elevated in primary hyperparathyroidism, low in occult malignancy
3. Radioimmunoassay of PTH-related protein: elevated in malignancy
4. Bone scan or bone survey to identify lytic lesions
5. Urinary cAMP: markedly elevated in primary hyperparathyroidism

D. Treatment

1. Increase urinary excretion
   a. IV fluids (NS)—**first step in management**
   b. Diuretics (furosemide)—further inhibit calcium reabsorption
2. Inhibit bone resorption in patients with osteoclastic disease (e.g., malignancy)
   a. Bisphosphonates (pamidronate)
   b. Calcitonin
3. Give glucocorticoids if vitamin D-related mechanisms (intoxication, granulomatous disorders) and multiple myeloma are the cause of the hypercalcemia. However, glucocorticoids are ineffective in most other forms of hypercalcemia
4. Use hemodialysis for renal failure patients
5. Phosphate is effective but incurs the risk of metastatic calcification

Potassium

Potassium Metabolism

- **Normal K^+ levels:** 3.5 to 5.0 mEq/L.
- **Location in the body**—most of the body's potassium (98%) is intracellular.
- **Hypokalemia**—alkalosis and insulin administration may cause hypokalemia because they cause a shift of potassium into the cells.
- **Hyperkalemia**—acidosis and anything resulting in cell lysis increase serum K^+ (both force K^+ out of cells into the ECF).
- **Potassium secretion**—most of the excretion of potassium occurs through the kidneys (80%); the remainder occurs via the GI tract. Aldosterone plays an important role in renal potassium secretion.

Hypokalemia

A. Causes

1. GI losses
   a. Vomiting and nasogastric drainage (volume depletion and metabolic alkalosis also result)
   b. Diarrhea
   c. Laxatives and enemas
   d. Intestinal fistulas
   e. Decreased potassium absorption in intestinal disorders
2. Renal losses
   a. Diuretics
   b. Renal tubular or parenchymal disease
   c. Primary and secondary hyperaldosteronism
   d. Excessive glucocorticoids
   e. Magnesium deficiency
   f. Bartter syndrome—chronic volume depletion secondary to an autosomal-recessive defect in salt reabsorption in the thick ascending limb of the loop of Henle leads to hyperplasia of juxtaglomerular apparatus, which leads to increased renin levels and secondary aldosterone elevations
3. Other causes
   a. Insufficient dietary intake
   b. Insulin administration

Quick HIT

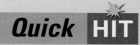

Serum potassium is affected by pH: alkalosis can lead to hypokalemia, whereas acidosis can lead to hyperkalemia.

Quick HIT

Interpretation of urine potassium in hypokalemia
- Low with GI losses (<20 mEq/L)
- High with renal losses (>20 mEq/L)

Quick HIT

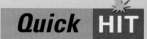

Diarrhea is a common cause of both hypokalemia and non-AG metabolic acidosis.

Quick HIT

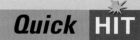

The presence or absence of HTN is useful in differentiating the causes of hypokalemia. If the patient is hypertensive, excessive aldosterone activity is likely. If the patient is normotensive, either GI or renal loss of K^+ is likely.

Quick HIT

Arrhythmias are the most dangerous complications of hypokalemia. ECG changes in hypokalemia appear as follows:
- T wave flattens out; if severe, T wave inverts
- U wave appears

Quick HIT

Always monitor K^+ levels in patients taking digoxin. It is common for these patients to be taking diuretics as well (for CHF), which can cause hypokalemia. **Hypokalemia predisposes the patient to digoxin toxicity.**

c. Certain antibiotics especially Bactrim and amphotericin B
d. Profuse sweating
e. Epinephrine (β_2-agonists)—hypokalemia occurs in 50% to 60% of trauma patients, perhaps due to increased epinephrine levels

B. Clinical features

1. Arrhythmias—prolongs normal cardiac conduction
2. Muscular weakness, fatigue, paralysis, and muscle cramps
3. Decreased deep tendon reflexes
4. Paralytic ileus
5. Polyuria and polydipsia
6. Nausea/vomiting
7. Exacerbates digitalis toxicity
8. Flattening of T waves on EKG. U waves appear if severe

C. Treatment

1. Identify and treat the underlying cause (Figure 8-4).
2. Discontinue any medications that can aggravate hypokalemia.
3. Oral KCl is the preferred (safest) method of replacement and is appropriate in most instances. Always retest the K^+ levels after administration.
   a. Using 10 mEq of KCl increases K^+ levels by 0.1 mEq/L.
   b. It comes in slow-acting and fast-acting forms.

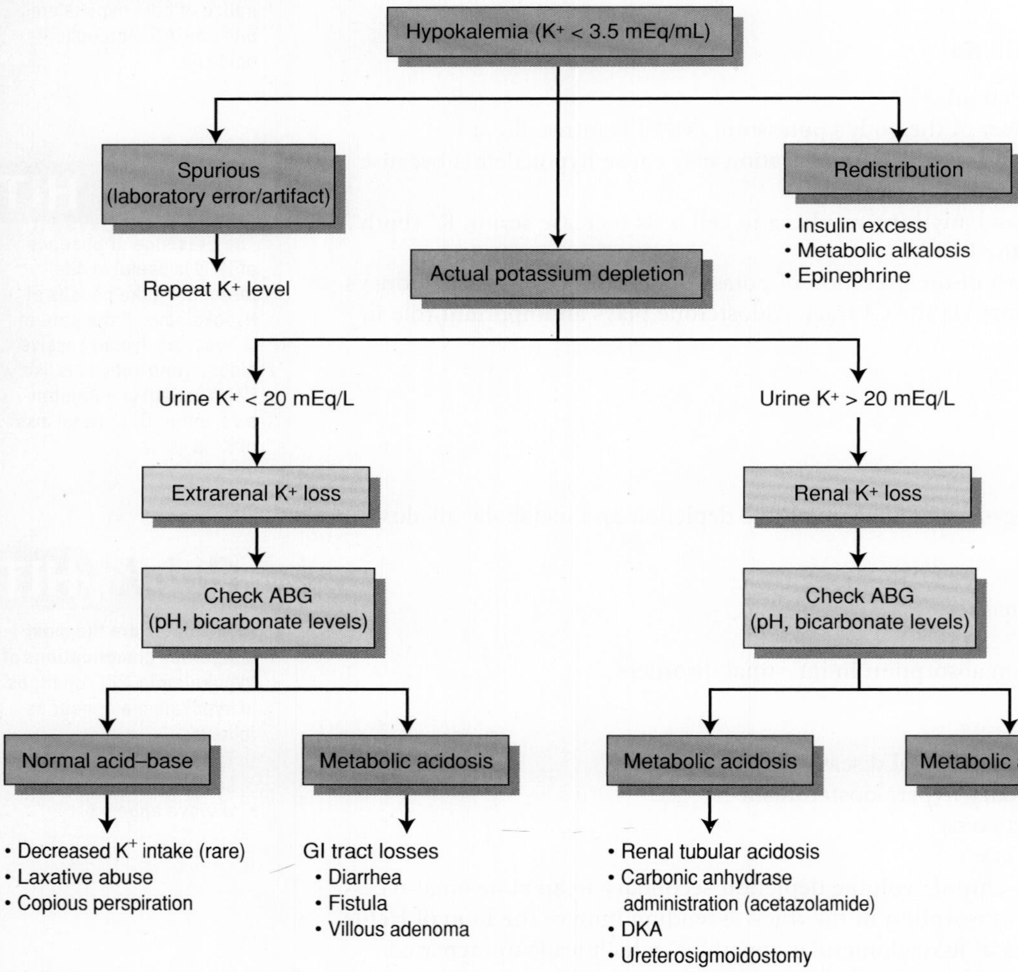

FIGURE 8-4 **Diagnostic evaluation of hypokalemia.**
(Adapted from Humes DH, DuPont HL, Gardner LB, et al. *Kelley's Textbook of Internal Medicine.* 4th ed. Philadelphia, PA: Lippincott Williams & Wilkins, 2000:1165, Figure 146-2.)

4. IV KCl can be given if hypokalemia is severe (<2.5), or if the patient has arrhythmias secondary to hypokalemia.
   a. Give slowly to avoid hyperkalemia.
   b. Monitor K^+ concentration and monitor cardiac rhythm when giving IV potassium.
   c. Infusion pearls.
      - Maximum infusion rate of 10 mEq/hr in peripheral IV line.
      - Maximum infusion rate of 20 mEq/hr in central line.
      - May add 1% lidocaine to bag to decrease pain (potassium burns!)
5. As with calcium, it is difficult to correct the potassium level if any hypomagnesemia is not corrected first.

Hyperkalemia

A. Causes

1. Increased total-body potassium
   a. Renal failure (acute or chronic)
   b. Addison disease
   c. Potassium-sparing diuretics (spironolactone)
   d. Hyporeninemic hypoaldosteronism
   e. ACE inhibitors
   f. Iatrogenic overdose—exercise particular caution when administering potassium to patients with renal failure
   g. Blood transfusion
2. Redistribution—translocation of potassium from intracellular to extracellular space
   a. Acidosis (not organic acidosis)
   b. Tissue/cell breakdown—rhabdomyolysis (muscle breakdown), hemolysis, burns
   c. GI bleeding
   d. Insulin deficiency—Insulin stimulates the Na^+-K^+-ATPase and causes K^+ to shift into cells. Therefore, insulin deficiency and hypertonicity (high glucose) promote K^+ shifts from ICF to ECF
   e. Rapid administration of β-blocker
3. Pseudohyperkalemia (spurious)
   a. This refers to an artificially elevated plasma K^+ concentration due to K^+ movement out of cells immediately before or after venipuncture. Contributing factors include **prolonged use of a tourniquet with or without repeated fist clenching.** This can cause acidosis and subsequent K^+ loss from cells. Nevertheless, plasma (not serum) K^+ should be normal. (Repeat the test to confirm this.)
   b. Additionally, if the sample is not processed quickly, some red blood cells will hemolyze and cause spillage of K^+ leading to a falsely elevated result. The test should be repeated in this case
   c. Other contributing factors include leukocytosis and thrombocytosis

B. Clinical features

1. **Arrhythmias**—The most important effect of hyperkalemia is on the heart (Figure 8-5). Check an ECG immediately in a hyperkalemic patient. With increasing potassium, ECG changes progress through tall, peaked T waves, QRS widening, PR interval prolongation, loss of P waves, and finally a sine-wave pattern.
2. Muscle weakness and (rarely) flaccid paralysis.
3. Decreased deep tendon reflexes.
4. Respiratory failure.
5. Nausea/vomiting, intestinal colic, diarrhea.

C. Treatment

1. If the hyperkalemia is severe, or if ECG changes are present, first give **IV calcium.**
   a. Calcium stabilizes the resting membrane potential of the myocardial membrane—that is, it decreases membrane excitability.
   b. Use caution in giving calcium to patients on digoxin. (Hypercalcemia predisposes the patient to digoxin toxicity.)

Quick HIT

Hyperkalemia inhibits renal ammonia synthesis and reabsorption. Thus, net acid excretion is impaired and results in metabolic acidosis. This further exacerbates hyperkalemia due to K^+ movement out of cells.

Quick HIT

ECG changes in hyperkalemia become prominent when K^+ >6 and include:
- Peaked T waves (by 10 mm)
- A prolonged PR interval
- Widening of QRS and merging of QRS with T wave
- Ventricular fibrillation and cardiac arrest (with increasing levels of K^+)

Quick HIT

Of all electrolyte disturbances, hyperkalemia is the most dangerous and can be the most rapidly fatal.

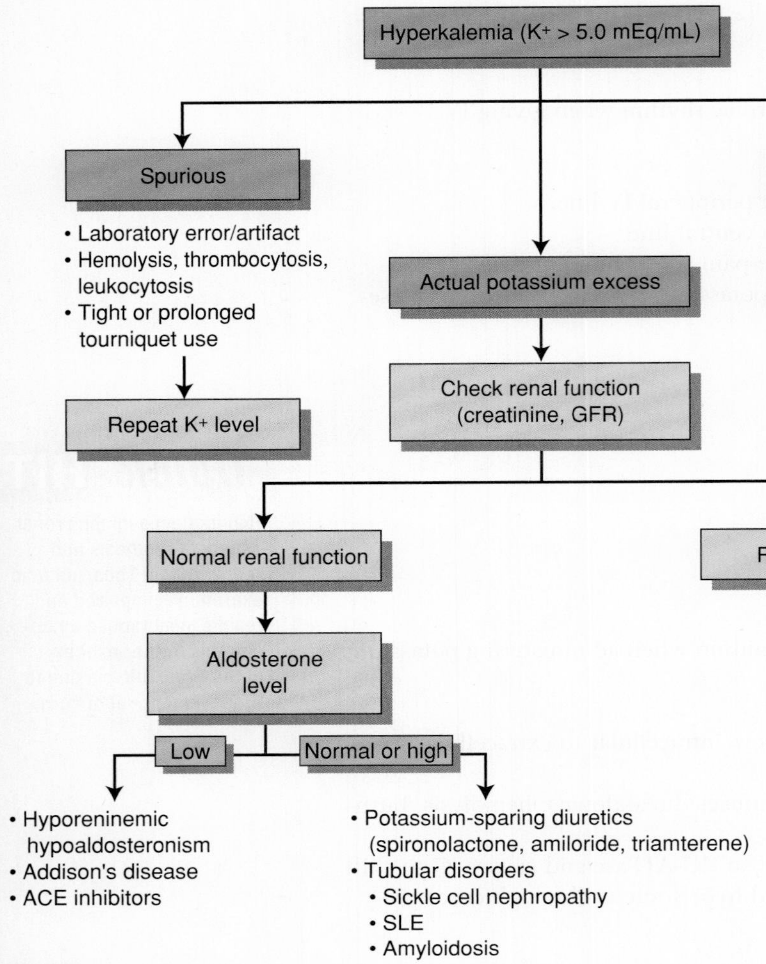

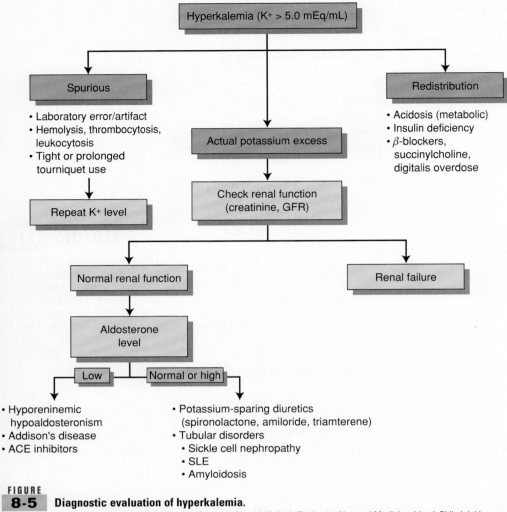

FIGURE 8-5 **Diagnostic evaluation of hyperkalemia.**
(Adapted from Humes DH, DuPont HL, Gardner LB, et al. *Kelley's Textbook of Internal Medicine.* 4th ed. Philadelphia, PA: Lippincott Williams & Wilkins, 2000:1168, Figure 147-1.)

2. Shift potassium into the intracellular compartment.
   a. **Glucose and insulin**—Glucose alone will stimulate insulin from β-cells, but exogenous insulin is more rapid. Give both to prevent hypoglycemia.
   b. Sodium bicarbonate.
      - Increases pH level, which shifts K^+ into cells.
      - An emergency measure in severe hyperkalemia.
3. Remove potassium from the body.
   a. **Kayexalate**—GI potassium exchange resin (Na^+/K^+ exchange in GI tract) absorbs K^+ in the colon, preventing reabsorption (passed in stool).
   b. Hemodialysis.
      - Most rapid and effective way of lowering plasma K^+.
      - Reserved for intractable hyperkalemia and for those with renal failure.
   c. Diuretics (furosemide).

Magnesium

Overview

- **Normal Mg^{2+} levels:** 1.8 to 2.5 mg/dL.
- **Location in the body**—Most of the magnesium in the body (two-thirds) is in bones. The remainder (one-third) is intracellular. Only 1% of magnesium is extracellular.

- **Influences on magnesium excretion**—Many hormones can alter urinary magnesium excretion (e.g., insulin/glucagons, PTH, calcitonin, ADH, and steroids).
- **Magnesium absorption and balance.**
- About 30% to 40% of dietary magnesium is absorbed in the GI tract, but this percentage increases when magnesium levels are low.
- The kidney has a great capacity to reabsorb magnesium and is the major regulator of magnesium balance.

Hypomagnesemia

A. Causes

1. GI causes
   a. Malabsorption, steatorrheic states (most common cause)
   b. Prolonged fasting
   c. Fistulas
   d. Patients receiving TPN without Mg^{2+} supplementation
2. Alcoholism (common cause)
3. Renal causes
   a. SIADH
   b. Diuretics
   c. Bartter syndrome
   d. Drugs: gentamicin, amphotericin B, cisplatin
   e. Renal transplantation
4. Other causes: postparathyroidectomy, DKA, thyrotoxicosis, lactation, burns, pancreatitis, cisplatin

Quick HIT
Hypomagnesemia makes hypokalemia and hypocalcemia more difficult to treat.

B. Clinical features

1. Marked neuromuscular and CNS hyperirritability
   a. Muscle twitching, weakness, tremors
   b. Hyperreflexia, seizures
   c. Mental status changes
2. Effect on calcium levels: **coexisting hypocalcemia is common** because of decreased release of PTH and bone resistance to PTH when Mg^{2+} is low
3. Effect on potassium levels
   a. **Coexisting hypokalemia**—in up to 50% of cases
   b. In muscle and myocardium, when either intracellular Mg^{2+} or K^+ decreases, a corresponding decrease in the other cation takes place
4. ECG changes—prolonged QT interval, T-wave flattening, and ultimately, torsade de pointes

C. Treatment

1. For mild hypomagnesemia—oral Mg^{2+} (e.g., magnesium oxide)
2. For severe hypomagnesemia—parenteral Mg^{2+} (e.g., magnesium sulfate)

Hypermagnesemia

A. Causes

1. Renal failure (most common cause)
2. Early-stage burns, massive trauma or surgical stress, severe ECF volume deficit, severe acidosis
3. Excessive intake of magnesium-containing laxatives or antacids combined with renal insufficiency
4. Adrenal insufficiency
5. Rhabdomyolysis
6. Iatrogenic—in the obstetric setting in women with preeclampsia or eclampsia being treated with magnesium sulfate

B. Clinical features

1. Nausea, weakness

2. Facial paresthesias
3. Progressive loss of deep tendon reflexes (classically the first sign)
4. ECG changes resemble those seen with hyperkalemia (increased P-R interval, widened QRS complex, and elevated T waves)
5. Somnolence leading to coma and muscular paralysis occur late
6. Death is usually caused by respiratory failure or cardiac arrest

C. Treatment

1. Withhold exogenously administered magnesium.
2. Prescribe IV calcium gluconate for emergent symptoms (cardioprotection).
3. Administer saline and furosemide.
4. Order dialysis in renal failure patients.
5. Prepare to intubate if respiratory depression is severe.

Phosphate

Overview

- **Normal phosphate levels:** 3.0 to 4.5 mg/dL.
- **Location in the body**—Most of the phosphorus is in the bones (85%); the remainder is intracellular in soft tissues (15%) and a very small amount (0.1%) in ECF.
- **Influence on phosphate absorption**—Vitamin D controls phosphorus absorption in the GI tract.
- **Phosphate excretion and balance**—PTH controls phosphorus excretion in the kidney—PTH increases renal phosphorus excretion by inhibiting reabsorption. The function of the kidney in maintaining phosphate balance is very important.

> **Quick HIT**
> **Plasma Phosphate Concentration**
> - Normal: 3.0 to 4.5 mg/dL
> - **Hypo**phosphatemia: <2.5 mg/dL
> - **Hyper**phosphatemia: >5 mg/dL

Hypophosphatemia

A. Causes

1. Decreased intestinal absorption due to alcohol abuse, vitamin D deficiency, malabsorption of phosphate, excessive use of phosphate-binding antacids, hyperalimentation (TPN), and/or starvation
2. Increased renal excretion
   a. Excess PTH states (vitamin D deficiency, hyperparathyroidism)
   b. Hyperglycemia (glycosuria), oncogenic osteomalacia, ATN, renal tubular acidosis, and so on
   c. Hypokalemia or hypomagnesemia
3. Other causes: respiratory alkalosis, anabolic steroids, severe hyperthermia DKA, hungry bone syndrome (deposition of bone material after parathyroidectomy)

B. Clinical features

1. None, if the hypophosphatemia is mild.
2. Any of the following, if the hypophosphatemia is severe:
   a. Neurologic: encephalopathy, confusion, seizures, numbness, paresthesias
   b. Musculoskeletal: muscular weakness, myalgias, bone pain, rickets/osteomalacia
   c. Hematologic: hemolysis, RBC dysfunction, WBC dysfunction, platelet dysfunction
   d. Cardiac: cardiomyopathy and myocardial depression secondary to low ATP levels, may lead to cardiac arrest
   e. Rhabdomyolysis
   f. Anorexia
   g. Difficulty in ventilator weaning

> **Quick HIT**
> The most common causes of severe hypophosphatemia are alcohol abuse and DKA.

C. Treatment

1. If mild (>1 mg/dL), oral supplementation: Neutra-Phos capsules, K-Phos tablets, milk (excellent source of phosphate)
2. If severe/symptomatic or if patient is NPO: parenteral supplementation

Hyperphosphatemia

A. Causes

1. Decreased renal excretion of PO_4^{3-} due to renal insufficiency (most common cause), bisphosphonates, hypoparathyroidism, vitamin D intoxication, and/or tumor calcinosis
2. Increased phosphate administration (e.g., PO_4^{3-} repletion or PO_4^{3-} enemas)
3. Rhabdomyolysis, cell lysis, or acidosis (releases PO_4^{3-} into the ECF)

B. Clinical features

1. This results in metastatic calcification and soft tissue calcifications; a calcium–phosphorus product (serum calcium × serum phosphorus) >70 indicates that calcification is likely to occur.
2. The associated hypocalcemia can lead to neurologic changes (tetany, neuromuscular irritability).

C. Treatment

1. Phosphate-binding antacids containing aluminum hydroxide or carbonate (bind phosphate in bowel and prevent its absorption)
2. Hemodialysis (if patient has renal failure)

Acid–base Disorders

Metabolic Acidosis

A. General characteristics

1. Metabolic acidosis is characterized by decreased blood pH and a decreased plasma bicarbonate concentration (see Clinical Pearl 8-2). The goal is to identify the underlying condition that is causing the metabolic acidosis.
2. Anion gap (AG).
   a. AG (mEq/L) = $[Na^+] - ([Cl^-] + [HCO^{3-}])$.
   b. Reflects ions present in serum but unmeasured (i.e., proteins, phosphates, organic acids, sulfates).
   c. Normal values are 5 to 15 mEq/L, but this varies to some extent.
3. Pathophysiology (Figure 8-6).
   a. When fixed acid (lactate) is added, the H^1 from fixed acid is buffered by the bicarbonate system. CO_2 is formed and removed by lungs. $H^+ + HCO_3^- \leftrightarrow H_2CO_3^- \leftrightarrow H_2O + CO_2$. HCO_3^- levels decrease in ECF; therefore, kidneys reabsorb more HCO_3^- (new) to maintain pH.

CLINICAL PEARL 8-2

Effects of Acidosis and Alkalosis

- **Acidosis**
  - Right shift in oxygen–hemoglobin dissociation curve diminishes the affinity of hemoglobin for oxygen (so increases oxygen delivery to tissues)
  - Depresses CNS
  - Decreases pulmonary blood flow
  - Arrhythmias
  - Impairs myocardial function
  - Hyperkalemia
- **Alkalosis**
  - Decreases cerebral blood flow
  - Left shift in oxygen–hemoglobin dissociation curve increases the affinity of hemoglobin for oxygen (so decreases oxygen delivery to tissues)
  - Arrhythmias
  - Tetany, seizures

Fluids, Electrolytes, and Acid–base Disorders

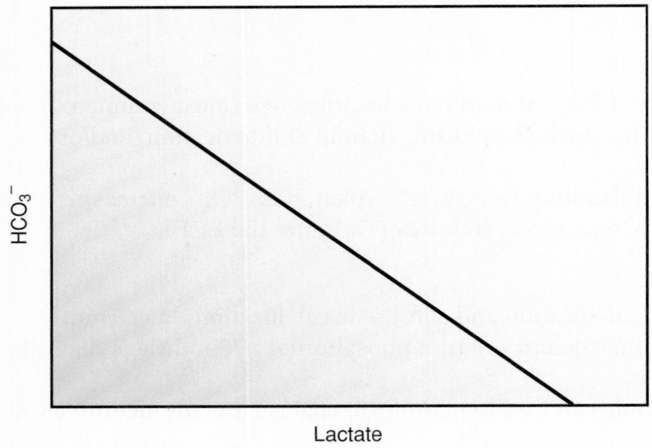

FIGURE 8-6 An increase in lactate results in a decrease in HCO_3^- (due to buffering) in ECF. The kidneys must then reabsorb more HCO_3^- to maintain pH.

Quick HIT

The bicarbonate level obtained in a serum chemistry panel (venous CO_2) is a measured value (more reliable), whereas the level obtained in an arterial blood gas is a calculated value (less reliable).

b. Three situations can arise:
- The change in AG equals the change in HCO_3^- (see Figure 8-7A): simple metabolic acidosis—the addition of acid causes the AG to increase proportionally.
- The change in AG is less than the change in HCO_3^- (see Figure 8-7B): **normal AG acidosis PLUS high AG acidosis**—If after the addition of acid, the HCO_3^- is lower than the calculated prediction, then you started with a lower HCO_3^-.
- The change in AG is greater than the change in HCO_3^- (see Figure 8-7C): **metabolic alkalosis PLUS high AG acidosis**—when you have a high AG, the acid has to be buffered by HCO_3^-, so HCO_3^- decreases. If HCO_3^- does not decrease, it means you started at a higher HCO_3^-.

B. Causes

1. Increased AG acidosis (see also Clinical Pearl 8-3)
   a. Ketoacidosis
   - Diabetes mellitus
   - Prolonged starvation
   - Prolonged alcohol abuse

   b. Lactic acidosis—can occur in many different conditions
   - Low tissue perfusion (decreased oxygen delivery to tissues)
   - Shock states (septic, cardiogenic, hypovolemic)
   - Excessive expenditure of energy (e.g., seizures)

   c. Renal failure—decreased NH_4^+ excretion (thus decreasing net acid)—decreased excretion of organic anions, sulfate, and phosphate increases AG

   d. Intoxication
   - Salicylate (aspirin)
   - Methanol
   - Ethylene glycol

Quick HIT

Salicylate overdose causes both primary respiratory alkalosis **and** primary metabolic acidosis.

CLINICAL PEARL 8-3

Arterial Blood Gas Interpretation

- **CO_2 level**
  - If elevated, think of either respiratory acidosis or compensation for metabolic alkalosis.
  - If low, think of either respiratory alkalosis or compensation for metabolic acidosis.
- **HCO_3^- level**
  - If elevated, think of either metabolic alkalosis or compensation for respiratory acidosis.
  - If low, think of either metabolic acidosis or compensation for respiratory alkalosis.
  - The **base excess/base deficit** values in the arterial blood gas indicate the amount of acid or base that is needed to titrate the plasma pH to 7.40 (with a $PaCO_2$ of 40).

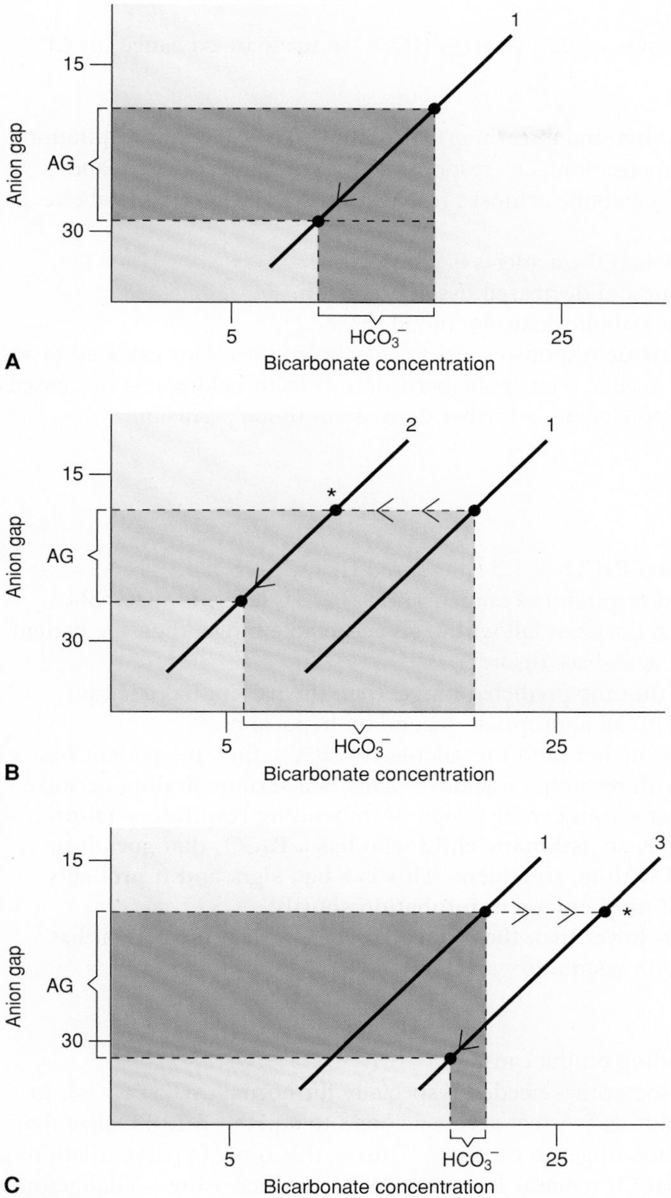

FIGURE 8-7 **A: Simple metabolic acidosis. The change in AG is equal to the change in HCO_3^-. As you add acid, HCO_3^- decreases, and AG increases proportionately. B: Normal anion gap acidosis PLUS high anion gap acidosis. The change in AG is less than the change in HCO_3^-. If after the addition of acid, HCO_3^- is lower than predicted, then you started at a lower HCO_3^- level (*). C: Metabolic alkalosis plus high anion gap acidosis. The change in AG is greater than the change in HCO_3^-. If after the addition of acid, the *decrease* in HCO_3^- is less than expected, then you started at a higher HCO_3^- level (*).**

2. Normal AG acidosis (hyperchloremic metabolic acidosis)—The low HCO_3^- is associated with high Cl^-, so that the AG remains normal
   a. Renal loss of bicarbonate
      - Proximal tubular acidosis—this is characterized by decreased HCO_3^- reabsorption. Causes include multiple myeloma, cystinosis, and Wilson disease
      - Distal tubular acidosis—this is characterized by the inability to make HCO_3^-. Causes include SLE, Sjögren syndrome, and taking amphotericin B.
      - Carbonic anhydrase inhibition (e.g., acetazolamide—a diuretic)
   b. GI loss of HCO_3^-
      - Diarrhea—HCO_3^- loss in diarrhea (**most common cause of non-AG acidosis**)
      - Pancreatic fistulas—pancreatic secretions contain high HCO_3^- levels

- Small bowel fistulas
- Ureterosigmoidostomy—colon secretes HCO_3^- in urine in exchange for Cl^-

C. Clinical features

1. Hyperventilation (deep rhythmic breathing), also known as Kussmaul respiration
   a. This is a typical compensation (i.e., response) for a metabolic acidosis and is a cardinal feature of metabolic acidosis; it is usually seen in severe metabolic acidosis (pH <7.20).
   b. It is less prominent when the acidosis is chronic.
2. Decreased cardiac output and decreased tissue perfusion.
   a. Occurs with severe metabolic acidosis (blood pH <7.2).
   b. Acidosis diminishes tissue responsiveness to catecholamines. This can lead to an undesirable chain of events: poor tissue perfusion → lactic acidosis → decreased cardiac output → hypotension → further decrease in tissue perfusion.

D. Diagnosis

1. History is important.
2. Calculate the AG.
3. Winter formula: **expected $PaCO_2$** = 1.5 (measured HCO_3^-) + 8 ± 2.
   a. Predicts the expected respiratory compensation ($PaCO_2$ level) to metabolic acidosis: If the $PaCO_2$ does not fall within an acceptable range, then the patient has another primary acid–base disorder.
   b. If the $PaCO_2$ falls within the predicted range, then the patient has a simple metabolic acidosis with an appropriate secondary hypocapnia.
   c. If the actual $PaCO_2$ is higher than the calculated $PaCO_2$, then the patient has metabolic acidosis with respiratory acidosis. **This is a serious finding because this failure of compensation can be a sign of impending respiratory failure. The classic example is an asthmatic child who has a $PaCO_2$ that goes from abnormal to normal with no treatment. This is a bad sign, and it probably means the child will need emergent intubation shortly.**
   d. If the actual $PaCO_2$ is lower than the calculated $PaCO_2$, then the patient has metabolic acidosis with respiratory alkalosis.

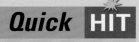

> **Quick HIT**
>
> With metabolic **acidosis,** $PaCO_2$ should decrease. With metabolic **alkalosis,** $PaCO_2$ should increase. This is normal respiratory compensation. **Failure of respiratory compensation indicates an additional primary respiratory acid–base disorder.**

E. Treatment

1. Treatment varies depending on the cause.
2. Sodium bicarbonate is sometimes needed (especially for normal AG acidosis). In correcting metabolic acidosis (correct severe acidosis to a pH of 7.20), realize that this HCO_3^- takes 24 hours to get to the brain. During this time, hyperventilation continues. Therefore, $PaCO_2$ remains low while HCO_3^- is increasing—a dangerous combination ($[H^+] = 24\ [PaCO_2 \div HCO_3^-]$).
3. Mechanical ventilation may be required if the patient is fatigued from prolonged hyperventilation, especially in DKA.

Metabolic Alkalosis

A. General characteristics

1. Metabolic alkalosis is characterized by an increased blood pH and plasma HCO_3^-.
2. Uncomplicated metabolic alkalosis is typically transient, because kidneys can normally excrete the excess HCO_3^-.
3. Consider two events in metabolic alkalosis:
   a. Event that initiates the metabolic alkalosis (loss of H^+ via gastric drainage, vomiting, and so on), or increased HCO_3^- concentration due to ECF volume contraction
   b. Mechanism that **maintains** the metabolic alkalosis due to the kidney's inability to excrete the excess HCO_3^-

> **Quick HIT**
>
> While evaluating a patient with metabolic alkalosis, the first step is to determine whether the ECF volume has contracted or expanded, and why.

B. Causes

1. Saline-sensitive metabolic alkalosis (urine chloride <10 mEq/L)—characterized by **ECF contraction** and hypokalemia.

a. Vomiting or nasogastric suction—When the patient loses HCl, gastric HCO_3^- generation occurs, which causes alkalosis.
b. Diuretics—These decrease the ECF volume. Body HCO_3^- content remains normal, but plasma HCO_3^- increases because of ECF contraction.
c. Villous adenoma of colon, diarrhea with high chloride content.

2. Saline-resistant metabolic alkalosis (urine chloride >20 mEq/L)—characterized by **ECF expansion** and hypertension (due to increased mineralocorticoids).
   a. Most are secondary to adrenal disorders (primary hyperaldosteronism). Increased levels of mineralocorticoid secretion lead to increased tubular reabsorption of Na^+ and HCO_3^-, and an excessive loss of Cl^- in the urine. The result is metabolic alkalosis and expansion of the ECF compartment (because of increased Na^+ reabsorption).
   b. Other causes include Cushing syndrome, severe K^+ deficiency, Bartter syndrome, and diuretic abuse.

Quick HIT

Exogenous bicarbonate loading (administering bicarbonate) can cause metabolic alkalosis, but this usually occurs in ESRD.

Quick HIT

It is useful to distinguish between the following:
- Metabolic alkalosis with volume **contraction** (usually due to fluid loss—e.g., vomiting or diuretics)
- Metabolic alkalosis with volume **expansion** (usually due to pathology of adrenal gland). An easy way to make this distinction is via the chloride concentration in the urine.

C. Clinical features

1. There are no characteristic signs or symptoms.
2. The patient's medical history is most helpful (look for vomiting, gastric drainage, diuretic therapy, and so on).

D. Diagnosis

1. Elevated HCO_3^- level, elevated blood pH.
2. Hypokalemia is common (due to renal loss of K^1).
3. $PaCO_2$ is elevated as a compensatory mechanism (due to hypoventilation). It is rare for a compensatory increase in $PaCO_2$ to exceed 50 to 55 mm Hg (the respiratory rate to achieve this is so low that PaO_2 would be decreased). A higher value implies a superimposed respiratory acidosis.
4. The urine chloride level is very important in distinguishing between saline-sensitive and saline-resistant types.

E. Treatment

1. Treat the underlying disorder that caused the metabolic alkalosis.
2. NS plus potassium will restore the ECF volume if the patient is volume contracted.
3. Address the underlying cause (or prescribe spironolactone) if the patient is volume expanded.

Respiratory Acidosis

A. General characteristics

1. Defined as a reduced blood pH and $PaCO_2$ >40 mm Hg.
2. Renal compensation (increased reabsorption of HCO_3^-) begins within 12 to 24 hours and takes 5 days or so to complete.
   a. Acute respiratory acidosis.
      - There is an immediate compensatory elevation of HCO_3^-.
      - There is an increase of 1 mmol/L for every 10 mm Hg increase in $PaCO_2$.
   b. Chronic respiratory acidosis.
      - Renal adaptation occurs, and HCO_3^- increases by 4 mmol/L for every 10 mm Hg increase in $PaCO_2$.
      - This is generally seen in patients with underlying lung disease, such as chronic obstructive pulmonary disease (COPD).

Quick HIT

Any disorder that reduces CO_2 clearance (i.e., inhibits adequate ventilation) can lead to respiratory acidosis.

B. Causes—alveolar hypoventilation

1. Primary pulmonary diseases—for example, COPD, airway obstruction
2. Neuromuscular diseases—for example, myasthenia gravis
3. CNS malfunction—injury to brainstem
4. Drug-induced hypoventilation (e.g., from morphine, anesthetics, or sedatives)—narcotic overdose in postoperative patients is a possibility (look for pinpoint pupils).
5. Respiratory muscle fatigue

Quick HIT

Increased $PaCO_2$ → increased cerebral blood flow, → increased CSF pressure, which results in generalized CNS depression.

Quick HIT

$PaCO_2$ is primarily determined by respiratory rate and tidal volume.

Quick HIT

Any disorder that increases the respiratory rate inappropriately can lead to respiratory alkalosis.

C. Clinical features

1. Somnolence, confusion, and myoclonus with asterixis.
2. Headaches, confusion, and papilledema are signs of acute CO_2 retention.

D. Treatment

1. Verify patency of the airway.
2. If PaO_2 is low (<60 mm Hg), initiate supplemental oxygen. **Caution:** In patients who are "CO_2 retainers" (e.g., COPD patients), oxygen can exacerbate the respiratory acidosis, so administer oxygen judiciously. (See the discussion under Acute Respiratory Failure in Chapter 2.)
3. Correct reversible causes.
4. Any measure to improve alveolar ventilation.
   a. Aggressive pulmonary toilet.
   b. Correct reversible pulmonary disease (e.g., treat pneumonia).
   c. Remove obstruction.
   d. If there is drug-induced hypoventilation, clear the agent from the body (**naloxone**!).
   e. Administer bronchodilators.
5. Intubation and mechanical ventilation may be necessary to relieve the acidemia and hypoxia that result from hypoventilation. The following situations require intubation:
   a. Severe acidosis.
   b. $PaCO_2$ >60 or inability to increase PaO_2 with supplemental oxygen
   c. If patient is obtunded or shows deterioration in mental status.
   d. Impending respiratory fatigue (ensues with prolonged labored breathing).

Respiratory Alkalosis

A. General characteristics

1. Characterized by an increased blood pH and decreased $PaCO_2$.
2. In order to maintain blood pH within the normal range, HCO_3 must decrease, so renal compensation occurs (i.e., HCO_3^- excretion increases). However, this does not occur acutely, but rather over the course of several hours.
   a. Acutely, for each 10 mm Hg decrease in $PaCO_2$, plasma HCO_3^- decreases by 2 mEq/L and blood pH increases by 0.08 mEq/L.
   b. Chronically, for each 10 mm Hg decrease in $PaCO_2$, plasma HCO_3^- decreases by 5 to 6 mEq/L and blood pH decreases by 0.02 mEq/L.

B. Causes—alveolar hyperventilation

1. Anxiety
2. Pulmonary embolism, pneumonia, asthma
3. Sepsis
4. Hypoxia—leads to increased respiratory rate
5. Mechanical ventilation
6. Pregnancy—increased serum progesterone levels cause hyperventilation
7. Liver disease (cirrhosis)
8. Medication (salicylate toxicity)
9. Hyperventilation syndrome

C. Clinical features

1. Symptoms are mostly related to decreased cerebral blood flow (vasoconstriction): lightheadedness, dizziness, anxiety, paresthesias, and perioral numbness
2. Tetany (indistinguishable from hypocalcemia)
3. Arrhythmias (in severe cases)

D. Treatment

1. Correct the underlying cause.
2. Sometimes this does not need to be treated (e.g., in the case of pregnancy).
3. An inhaled mixture containing CO_2 or breathing into a paper bag may be useful.

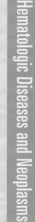

HEMATOLOGIC DISEASES AND NEOPLASMS

9

Anemias

Basics of Anemia

A. General characteristics

1. Anemia is defined as a reduction in Hct or Hb concentration
2. When red cell mass (as measured by Hb or less precisely by Hct) decreases, several compensatory mechanisms maintain oxygen delivery to the tissues. These mechanisms include:
   a. Increased cardiac output (heart rate and stroke volume)
   b. Increased extraction ratio
   c. Rightward shift of the oxyhemoglobin curve (increased 2,3-diphosphoglycerate [2,3-DPG])
   d. Expansion of plasma volume
3. As a general rule, blood transfusion is not recommended unless either of the following is true:
   a. The Hb concentration is <7 g/dL, *OR*
   b. The patient requires increased oxygen-carrying capacity (e.g., patients with coronary artery disease or some other cardiopulmonary disease)
4. If anemia develops rapidly, symptoms are more likely to be present, because there is little time for compensatory mechanisms. When onset is gradual, compensatory mechanisms are able to maintain oxygen delivery, and symptoms may be minimal or absent

B. Clinical features

1. A variety of nonspecific complaints—headache, fatigue, poor concentration, diarrhea, nausea, vague abdominal discomfort
2. Pallor—best noted in the conjunctiva
3. Hypotension and tachycardia
4. Signs of the underlying cause—jaundice if hemolytic anemia, blood in stool if GI bleeding

C. Diagnosis

1. Hb and Hct
   a. Formula for converting Hb to Hct: Hb × 3 = Hct (1 unit of packed RBCs [PRBCs] increases Hb level by 1 point, and Hct by 3 points)
   b. If the patient has good cardiac function and intravascular volume is adequate, low Hb and Hct levels are tolerated—even an Hb of 7 or 8 provides sufficient oxygen-carrying capacity for most patients. However, anemia is not tolerated as well in patients with impaired cardiac function (see Clinical Pearl 9-1)
2. Reticulocyte index
   a. The reticulocyte count is an important initial test in evaluating anemia because it indicates whether effective erythropoiesis is occurring in the bone marrow.

Quick HIT

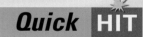

Historical Findings to Consider in Patients with Anemia

- Family history of hemophilia, G6PD deficiency, thalassemia
- Bleeding (melena, recent trauma/surgery, hematemesis)
- Chronic illnesses (e.g., renal failure, autoimmune diseases, malignancies)
- Alcoholism (folate, vitamin B_{12}, iron deficiency)

Quick HIT

Symptoms of anemia are highly variable, depending on how rapidly the hematocrit drops, the underlying condition of the patient, and the hematocrit level the patient typically lives on.

Quick HIT

Pseudoanemia refers to a decrease in hemoglobin and hematocrit secondary to dilution (i.e., secondary to acute volume infusion or overload).

Quick HIT

If H/H reveals anemia, next tests to obtain to determine cause of anemia are reticulocyte count and MCV.

CLINICAL PEARL 9-1

Transfusion Pearls

- PRBCs (contain no platelets or clotting factors).
  - Mix with normal saline to infuse faster (not with lactated Ringer solution because calcium causes coagulation within the IV line).
  - Each unit raises the hematocrit by 3 to 4 points.
  - Each unit may be given to an adult for over 90 to 120 minutes.
  - Always check CBC after the transfusion is completed.
- FFP
  - Contains all of the clotting factors.
  - Contains **no** RBCs/WBCs/platelets.
  - Given for high PT/PTT, coagulopathy, and deficiency of clotting factors—FFP can be given if you cannot wait for Vitamin K to take effect, or if patient has liver failure (in which case Vitamin K will not work).
  - Follow up PT and PTT to assess response.
- Cryoprecipitate
  - Contains factor VIII and fibrinogen.
  - For hemophilia A, decreased fibrinogen (DIC) and vWD.
- Platelet transfusions—1 unit raises platelet count by 10,000.
- Whole blood only for massive blood loss.
- For any patient with massive blood loss, the ideal ratio of platelets: FFP: PRBCs which are transfused should be 1:1:1. Additionally, during massive blood transfusions, blood should be warmed to prevent a decrease in core body temperature.

Effective erythropoiesis is dependent on adequate raw materials (iron, vitamin B_{12}, folate) in the bone marrow, absence of intrinsic bone marrow disease (e.g., aplastic anemia), adequate erythropoietin from the kidney, and survival of reticulocytes (no premature destruction before leaving the bone marrow). See Clinical Pearl 9-2

b. A reticulocyte index >2% implies excessive RBC destruction or blood loss. The bone marrow is responding to increased RBC requirements

c. A reticulocyte index <2% implies inadequate RBC production by the bone marrow

Quick HIT

Note that all causes of anemia are initially normocytic because it takes some time for the abnormal-sized RBCs to outnumber the normal-sized ones.

CLINICAL PEARL 9-2

Hemolytic Transfusion Reactions Are Divided Into Intravascular and Extravascular Hemolysis

- **Intravascular hemolysis** (also called acute hemolytic reactions).
  - Very serious and life-threatening—caused by ABO-mismatched blood transfused into patient. (Usually due to clerical error.) For example, if B blood is given to a type A patient, anti-B IgM antibodies attach to all of the infused B RBCs, they activate a complement pathway, and produce a massive intravascular hemolysis as C9 punches holes through RBC membranes.
  - Symptoms include fever/chills, nausea/vomiting, pain in the flanks/back, chest pain, and dyspnea.
  - Complications include hypovolemic shock (hypotension, tachycardia), DIC, and renal failure with hemoglobinuria.
  - Management involves stopping the transfusion immediately and aggressively replacing the fluid to avoid shock and renal failure, epinephrine for anaphylaxis, dopamine/norepinephrine as needed to maintain blood pressure.
- **Extravascular hemolysis** (also called delayed hemolytic transfusion reaction)
  - Extravascular hemolysis is less severe and in most cases is self-limited; it may occur within 3 to 4 weeks after a transfusion.
  - It is caused by one of the minor RBC antigens. For example, if a patient is Kell antigen-negative and has anti-Kell IgG antibodies from a previous exposure to the antigen, reexposure of her memory B cells to Kell antigen on RBCs will result in synthesis of IgG anti-Kell antibodies. These antibodies coat all of the Kell antigen-positive donor RBCs, which will be removed extravascularly by macrophages in the spleen, liver, and bone marrow.
  - Symptoms are subtle and include fever, jaundice, and anemia.
  - Management: none. The prognosis is good.

3. Blood smear and RBC indices (especially mean corpuscular volume [MCV])—see below

D. Diagnosing the cause of anemia (general approach)

1. If the reticulocyte index <2, examine the smear and RBC indices (Figure 9-1)
   a. If microcytic anemia (MCV<80), the differential diagnosis includes the following:
      - **Iron deficiency anemia—most common cause**
      - Anemia of chronic disease—iron is present in the body but is not available for hemoglobin synthesis (iron trapping in macrophages)
      - Thalassemias—defective synthesis of globin chains
      - Ring sideroblastic anemias (includes lead poisoning, pyridoxine deficiency, toxic effects of alcohol)—this is a defective synthesis of protoporphyrins. Iron accumulates in mitochondria
   b. If macrocytic anemia (MCV >100), the differential diagnosis includes the following:
      - Nuclear defect (MCV increases significantly)—vitamin B_{12} deficiency and folate deficiency

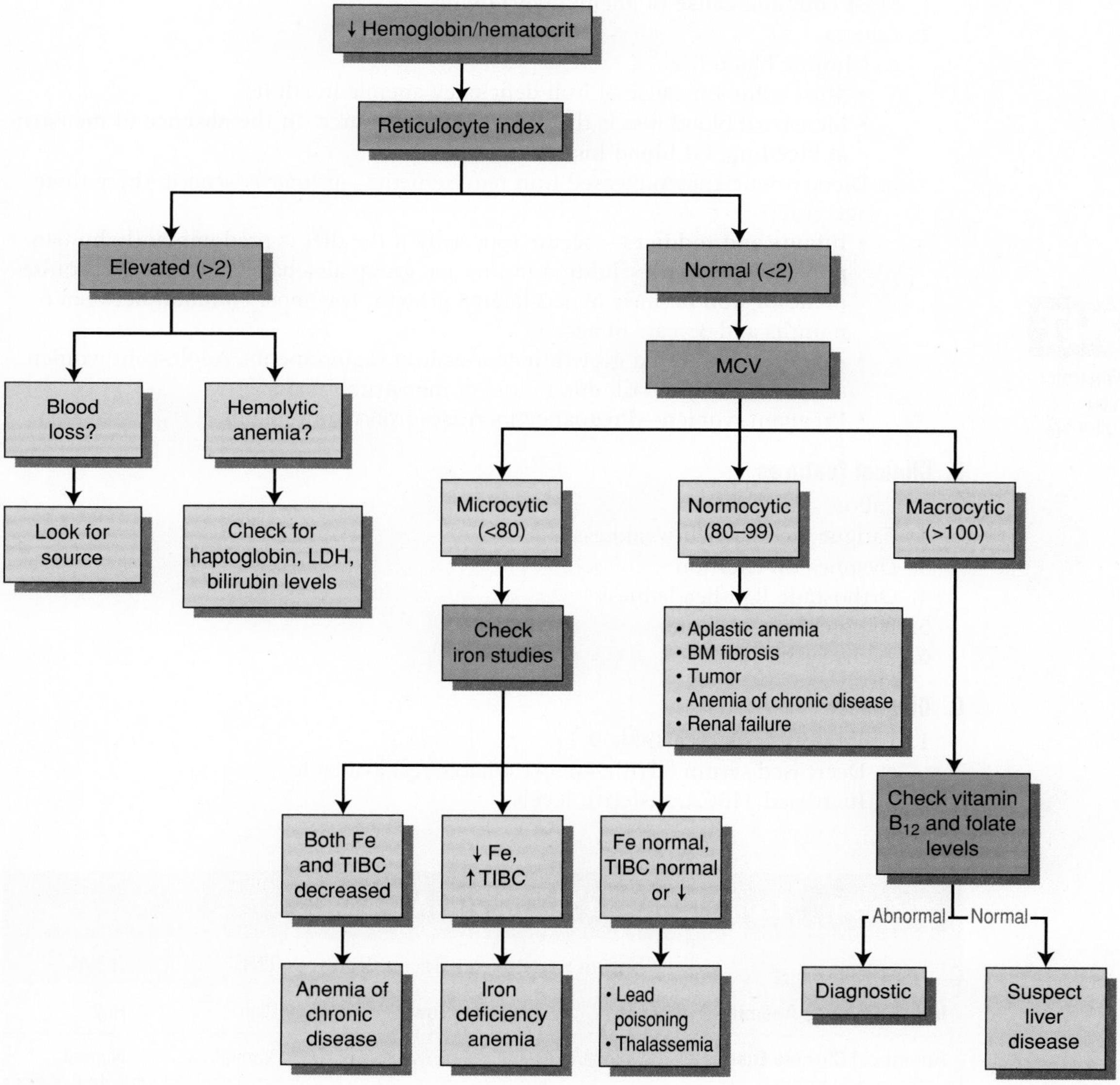

FIGURE 9-1 Evaluation of anemia.

Quick HIT
In an anemic patient, the first step is to assess volume status and hemodynamic stability. If unstable, transfuse PRBCs before attempting to find the cause of the anemia.

- Liver disease (MCV increases up to 115)—due to altered metabolism of plasma lipoproteins into their membranes, altering RBC shape (and increasing volume)
- Stimulated erythropoiesis (MCV increases up to 110)—reticulocytes are larger than mature RBCs, resulting in an increase in polychromatophilic RBCs

c. If normocytic anemia, the differential diagnosis includes the following:
- Aplastic anemia
- Bone marrow fibrosis
- Tumor
- Anemia of chronic disease (chronic inflammation, malignancy)
- Renal failure (decreased erythropoietin production)

2. If the reticulocyte index >2, do the following:
   a. Suspect blood loss—look for the source of the bleeding
   b. Suspect hemolysis (see below)

Microcytic Anemias

Iron Deficiency Anemia

A. Causes

1. **Most common cause of anemia worldwide**
2. Causes
   a. Chronic blood loss
   - Most common cause of iron deficiency anemia in adults
   - Menstrual blood loss is the most common source. **In the absence of menstrual bleeding, GI blood loss is most likely**

   b. Dietary deficiency/increased iron requirements—primarily seen in these three age groups:
   - **Infants and toddlers**—occurs especially if the diet is predominantly human milk (low in iron). Children in this age group also have an increased requirement for iron because of accelerated growth. It is most common between 6 months and 3 years of age
   - **Adolescents**—rapid growth increases iron requirements. Adolescent women are particularly at risk due to loss of menstrual blood
   - **Pregnant women**—Pregnancy increases iron requirements

Quick HIT
In elderly patients with iron deficiency anemia, you must rule out colon cancer.

B. Clinical features

1. Pallor
2. Fatigue, generalized weakness
3. Dyspnea on exertion
4. Orthostatic lightheadedness
5. Hypotension, if acute
6. Tachycardia

C. Diagnosis

1. Laboratory tests (see Table 9-1)
   a. Decreased serum ferritin—most reliable test available
   b. Increased TIBC/transferrin levels

TABLE 9-1 Iron Studies in Microcytic Anemias

	Serum Ferritin	Serum Iron	TIBC	RDW
Iron Deficiency Anemia	Low	Low	High	High
Anemia of Chronic Disease	Normal/high	Low	Normal/low	Normal
Thalassemia	Normal/high	Normal/high	Normal	Normal/high

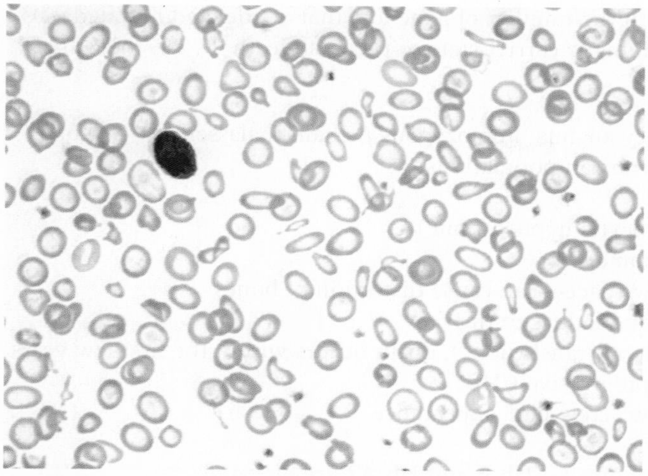

FIGURE 9-2 **Blood smear: iron deficiency anemia.**
(From Pereira I, George T, Arber D. *Atlas of Peripheral Blood.* Philadelphia, PA: Wolters Kluwer Health/Lippincott Williams & Wilkins, 2011.)

c. Low TIBC saturation
d. Decreased serum iron
e. Microcytic, hypochromic RBCs on peripheral smear (Figure 9-2)

2. Bone marrow biopsy—the gold standard, but rarely performed. Indicated if laboratory evidence of iron deficiency anemia is present and no source of blood loss is found
3. If GI bleeding is suspected—guaiac stool test or colonoscopy. Colon cancer is a common cause of GI bleeding in the elderly

D. Treatment

1. Oral iron replacement (ferrous sulfate).
   a. A trial should be given to a menstruating woman. However, in men and postmenopausal women with iron deficiency anemia, attempt to determine the source of blood loss.
   b. Side effects include constipation, nausea, and dyspepsia.
2. Parenteral iron replacement.
   a. Iron dextran can be administered IV or IM.
   b. This is rarely necessary because most patients respond to oral iron therapy. It may be useful in patients with poor absorption, patients who require more iron than oral therapy can provide, or patients who cannot tolerate oral ferrous sulfate.
3. Blood transfusion is **not** recommended unless anemia is severe or the patient has cardiopulmonary disease.

Quick HIT

The MCH and MCHC are of little value clinically. They are neither sensitive nor specific for any diagnosis. However, MCV is very valuable in diagnosing the cause of anemia.

Quick HIT

The RDW measures the variation in RBC size. The RDW is usually abnormal in iron deficiency, but is generally normal in all of the other microcytic anemias.

Thalassemias

A. General characteristics

1. Inherited disorders characterized by inadequate production of either the α- or β-globin chain of hemoglobin
2. They are classified according to the chain that is deficient
3. β-Thalassemias
   a. β-chain production is deficient, but the synthesis of α-chains is unaffected
   b. Excess α-chains bind to and damage the RBC membrane
   c. It is most often found in people of Mediterranean, Middle Eastern, and Indian ancestry
   d. Severity varies with different mutations
4. α-Thalassemias
   a. There is a decrease in α-chains, which are a component of all types of hemoglobins
   b. The β-globin chains form tetramers, which are abnormal hemoglobins

Quick HIT

Iron overload sometimes develops in patients with transfusion-dependent thalassemia, and if untreated this can lead to CHF (symptoms of hemochromatosis). Therefore, these patients are often treated with desferrioxamine (a chelating agent that eliminates excess iron).

c. The severity depends on the number of gene loci that are deleted/mutated—it ranges from an asymptomatic carrier state to prenatal death

B. β-Thalassemias

1. Thalassemia major (Cooley anemia; homozygous β-chain thalassemia)—occurs predominantly in Mediterranean populations
   a. Clinical features
      - Severe anemia (microcytic hypochromic)
      - Massive hepatosplenomegaly
      - Expansion of marrow space—can cause distortion of bones
      - Growth retardation and failure to thrive
      - If untreated (with blood transfusions), death occurs within the first few years of life secondary to progressive CHF
      - Skull x-ray may show "crew-cut" appearance
   b. Diagnosis
      - Hemoglobin electrophoresis—**Hb F and Hb A2 are elevated**
      - Peripheral blood smear—**microcytic hypochromic anemia, target cells may be seen** (Figure 9-3)
   c. Treatment—frequent PRBC transfusions are required to sustain life.
2. Thalassemia minor (heterozygous β-chain thalassemia)
   a. Clinical features: patients are usually asymptomatic. A mild microcytic, hypochromic anemia is the only symptom
   b. Diagnosis: hemoglobin electrophoresis
   c. Treatment: usually not necessary (Patients are not transfusion dependent.)
3. Thalassemia intermedia
   a. Usually involves both β-globin genes
   b. Severity of anemia is intermediate
   c. Patients usually are not transfusion dependent
4. Thalassemia major
   a. Usually diagnosed between 6 and 12 months of age
   b. Characterized by severe anemia with at most a very small amount of β-chain synthesis
   c. Patients are entirely transfusion dependent

Quick HIT

If iron deficiency anemia is suspected, but the anemia does not respond to iron therapy, obtain a hemoglobin electrophoresis to rule out α- and β-thalassemia.

C. α-Thalassemias

1. Silent carriers—mutation/deletion of only one α-locus
   a. Asymptomatic
   b. Normal hemoglobin and hematocrit level
   c. No treatment necessary

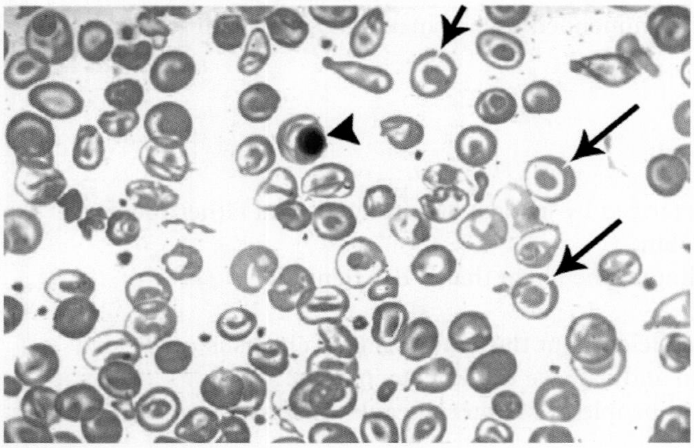

FIGURE 9-3 **Blood smear: thalassemia. Target cells (*arrows*) and circulating nucleated red blood cells (*arrowhead*).**

(From Strayer DS, Rubin, E. *Rubin's Pathology: Clinicopathologic Foundations of Medicine.* Philadelphia, PA: Wolters Kluwer Health/Lippincott Williams & Wilkins, 2014.)

2. α-Thalassemia trait (or minor)—mutation/deletion of two α-loci
   a. Characterized by mild microcytic hypochromic anemia
   b. Common in African-American patients
   c. No treatment necessary
3. Hb H disease—mutation/deletion of three α-loci
   a. Hemolytic anemia, splenomegaly
   b. Significant microcytic, hypochromic anemia
   c. Hemoglobin electrophoresis shows Hb H
   d. Treatment is often the same as for patients with β-thalassemia major. Splenectomy is sometimes helpful
4. Mutation/deletion of all four α-loci—this is either fatal at birth (hydrops fetalis) or shortly after birth

Quick HIT

The most common type of thalassemia is thalassemia minor (β-thalassemia minor is more common than α-thalassemia minor). Both of these conditions can be mistaken for iron deficiency.

Sideroblastic Anemia

- Caused by abnormality in RBC iron metabolism.
- Hereditary or acquired—acquired causes include drugs (chloramphenicol, INH, alcohol), exposure to lead, collagen vascular disease, and neoplastic disease (myelodysplastic syndromes).
- Clinical findings: increased serum iron and ferritin, normal TIBC, TIBC saturation is normal/elevated, which distinguishes it from iron deficiency; **ringed sideroblasts in bone marrow.**
- Treatment: remove offending agents. Consider pyridoxine.

Normocytic Anemias

Anemia of Chronic Disease

- Occurs in the setting of chronic infection (e.g., tuberculosis, lung abscess), cancer (e.g., lung, breast, Hodgkin disease), inflammation (rheumatoid arthritis, systemic lupus erythematosus [SLE]), or trauma. The release of inflammatory cytokines has a suppressive effect on erythropoiesis.
- It may be difficult to differentiate from iron deficiency anemia.
- Laboratory findings: low serum iron, low TIBC, and low serum transferrin levels occur. Serum ferritin levels are increased.
- The anemia is usually normocytic and normochromic, but may be microcytic and hypochromic as well.
- No specific treatment is necessary other than treatment of the underlying process. Do not give iron. The anemia is usually mild and well tolerated.

Aplastic Anemia

A. General characteristics

1. Bone marrow failure leading to **pancytopenia** (anemia, neutropenia, thrombocytopenia)
2. Causes
   a. Idiopathic—majority of cases
   b. Radiation exposure
   c. Medications (e.g., chloramphenicol, sulfonamides, gold, carbamazepine)
   d. Viral infection (e.g., human parvovirus, hepatitis C, hepatitis B, Epstein–Barr virus (EBV), cytomegalovirus, herpes zoster varicella, HIV)
   e. Chemicals (e.g., benzene, insecticides)

B. Clinical features

1. Symptoms of anemia—fatigue, dyspnea
2. Signs and symptoms of thrombocytopenia (e.g., petechiae, easy bruising)
3. Increased incidence of infections (due to neutropenia)
4. Can transform into acute leukemia

Quick HIT

Pernicious anemia is a special case of vitamin B_{12} deficiency. It is an autoimmune disorder resulting in inadequate production of intrinsic factor, which leads to impaired absorption of vitamin B_{12} in the terminal ileum.

C. Diagnosis

1. Normocytic, normochromic anemia.
2. Perform a bone marrow biopsy for definitive diagnosis—this reveals hypocellular marrow and the absence of progenitors of all three hematopoietic cell lines.

D. Treatment

1. Bone marrow transplantation
2. Transfusion of PRBCs and platelets, if necessary (use judiciously)
3. Treat any known underlying causes

Macrocytic Anemias

Vitamin B_{12} Deficiency

A. General characteristics

1. Vitamin B_{12} is involved in two important reactions.
   a. As a cofactor in conversion of homocysteine to methionine.
   b. As a cofactor in conversion of methylmalonyl CoA to succinyl CoA.
2. Vitamin B_{12} stores in the liver are plentiful, and can sustain an individual for 3 or more years.
3. The main dietary sources of vitamin B_{12} are meat and fish.
4. Vitamin B_{12} is bound to intrinsic factor (produced by gastric parietal cells), so it can be absorbed by the terminal ileum.

Quick HIT

In a patient with megaloblastic anemia, always try to determine whether folate or vitamin B_{12} deficiency is the cause, because folate supplements can improve the anemia of vitamin B_{12} deficiency, but not the neurologic impairment. Therefore, **if the vitamin B_{12} deficiency remains untreated, irreversible neurologic disease can result.**

B. Causes (almost all cases are due to impaired absorption)

1. Pernicious anemia (lack of intrinsic factor)—most common cause in the Western hemisphere
2. Gastrectomy
3. Poor diet (e.g., strict vegetarianism); alcoholism
4. Crohn disease, ileal resection (terminal ileum—approximately the last 100 cm)
5. Other organisms competing for vitamin B_{12}
   a. *Diphyllobothrium latum* infestation (fish tapeworm)
   b. Blind loop syndrome (bacterial overgrowth)

Quick HIT

Note that patients with vitamin B_{12} deficiency can have moderate to severe neurologic symptoms with little to no anemia (i.e., blood counts may be normal). Delay in diagnosis and treatment may lead to irreversible neurologic disease.

C. Clinical features

1. Anemia
2. Sore tongue (stomatitis and glossitis)
3. Neuropathy—can distinguish between vitamin B_{12} deficiency and folate deficiency
   a. Demyelination in posterior columns, in lateral corticospinal tracts and spinocerebellar tracts—leads to a loss of position/vibratory sensation in lower extremities, ataxia, and upper motor neuron signs (increased deep tendon reflexes, spasticity, weakness, Babinski sign)
   b. Can lead to urinary and fecal incontinence, impotence
   c. Can lead to dementia—Investigate in the workup for dementia

D. Diagnosis

1. Peripheral blood smear.
   a. Megaloblastic anemia—macrocytic RBCs (MCV >100).
   b. Hypersegmented neutrophils (Figure 9-4).
2. Serum vitamin B_{12} level is low (<100 pg/mL).
3. Serum methylmalonic acid and homocysteine levels—these are elevated in vitamin B_{12} deficiency and are useful if the vitamin B_{12} level is borderline.
4. Antibodies against intrinsic factor can help in the diagnosis of pernicious anemia.
5. Schilling test—historically used to determine if B_{12} deficiency is due to pernicious anemia. Not routinely used now.
   a. Give an IM dose of unlabeled vitamin B_{12} to saturate binding sites.
   b. Give an oral dose of radioactive vitamin B_{12}; measure the amount of vitamin B_{12} in urine and plasma to determine how much vitamin B_{12} was absorbed.

Hematologic Diseases and Neoplasms

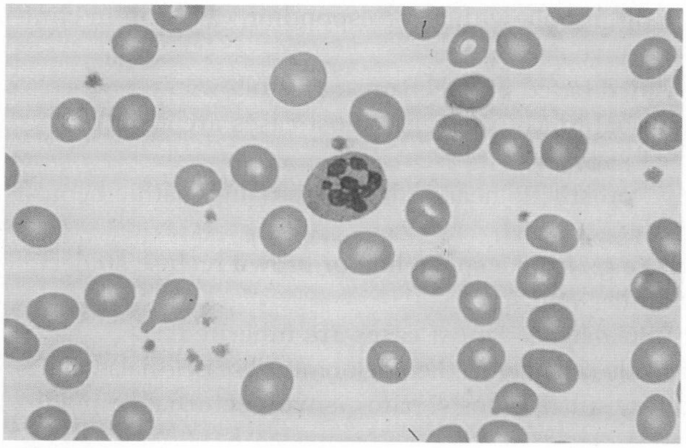

FIGURE **9-4** **Blood smear: hypersegmented neutrophil (vitamin B_{12} deficiency).**
(From Anderson SC. *Anderson's Atlas of Hematology.* Philadelphia, PA: Wolters Kluwer Health/Lippincott Williams & Wilkins, 2003.)

c. Repeat the test (oral radioactive vitamin B_{12}) with the addition of intrinsic factor. If malabsorption is the problem, adding intrinsic factor will not do anything. However, if pernicious anemia is present, adding intrinsic factor will improve serum vitamin B_{12} levels.

E. Treatment: Parenteral therapy is preferred—cyanocobalamin (vitamin B_{12}) IM once per month.

Folate Deficiency

A. General characteristics

1. Folic acid stores are limited. Inadequate intake of folate over a 3-month period can lead to deficiency.
2. Green vegetables are the main source of folate. Overcooking of vegetables can remove folate.

B. Causes

1. Inadequate dietary intake such as "tea and toast" (most common cause)
2. Alcoholism
3. Long-term use of oral antibiotics
4. Increased demand
5. Pregnancy
6. Hemolysis
7. Use of folate antagonists such as methotrexate
8. Anticonvulsant medications (phenytoin)
9. Hemodialysis

C. Clinical features: Similar to those in vitamin B_{12} deficiency without the neurologic symptoms.

D. Treatment: Daily oral folic acid replacement.

Quick HIT

The serum homocysteine level is increased in both folate deficiency and vitamin B_{12} deficiency. However, serum methylmalonic acid levels are only increased with vitamin B_{12} deficiency.

Hemolytic Anemias

Overview

A. General characteristics

1. Premature destruction of RBCs that may be due to a variety of causes.
2. Bone marrow is normal and responds appropriately by increasing erythropoiesis, leading to an elevated reticulocyte count. However, if erythropoiesis cannot keep up with the destruction of RBCs, anemia results.

Quick HIT

The following are relevant in the history of a patient with hemolytic anemia: ethnic background, family history of jaundice/anemia, medications.

Quick HIT

Mechanical heart valves can hemolyze RBCs and lead to hemolytic anemia.

Quick HIT

Laboratory tests in hemolytic anemia:
- Elevated reticulocyte count, LDH
- Decreased haptoglobin and hemoglobin/hematocrit

Quick HIT

Physical injury to RBCs leads to the presence of fragmented RBCs called **schistocytes** and **helmet cells** on the blood smear. This can occur in TTP, DIC, and patients with prosthetic heart valves.

3. Hemolytic anemia can be acute or chronic with a corresponding variation in clinical features.
4. Hemolytic anemias can be classified based on mechanism, as follows:
   a. Hemolysis due to factors external to RBC defects—**most cases are acquired.**
      - Immune hemolysis.
      - Mechanical hemolysis (e.g., prosthetic heart valves, microangiopathic hemolytic anemia).
      - Medications, burns, toxins (e.g., from a snake bite or brown recluse spider); infection (malaria, clostridium), and so on.
   b. Hemolysis due to intrinsic RBC defects—**most cases are inherited.**
      - Hemoglobin abnormality: sickle cell anemia, hemoglobin C disease, thalassemias.
      - Membrane defects: hereditary spherocytosis, paroxysmal nocturnal hemoglobinuria (PNH).
      - Enzyme defects: glucose-6-phosphate dehydrogenase (G6PD) deficiency, pyruvate kinase deficiency.
5. Hemolytic anemias can be classified based on the predominant site of hemolysis, as follows:
   a. Intravascular hemolysis—within the circulation.
   b. Extravascular hemolysis—within the reticuloendothelial system, primarily the spleen.

B. Clinical features

1. Signs and symptoms of anemia
2. Signs and symptoms of underlying disease (e.g., bone crises in sickle cell disease)
3. Jaundice
4. Dark urine color (due to hemoglobinuria, not bilirubin) may be present. This indicates an intravascular process
5. Hepatosplenomegaly, cholelithiasis, lymphadenopathy (in chronic cases)

C. Diagnosis

1. Hb/Hct—level depends on degree of hemolysis and reticulocytosis
2. Elevated reticulocyte count due to increased RBC production
3. Peripheral smear
   a. Schistocytes suggest intravascular hemolysis ("trauma" or mechanical hemolysis) (Figure 9-5)
   b. Spherocytes or helmet cells suggest extravascular hemolysis (depending on the cause)
   c. Sickled RBCs—sickle cell anemia
   d. Heinz bodies in G6PD deficiency
4. Haptoglobin levels—**low** in hemolytic anemias (especially intravascular hemolysis). Haptoglobin binds to hemoglobin, so its absence means that hemoglobin was destroyed

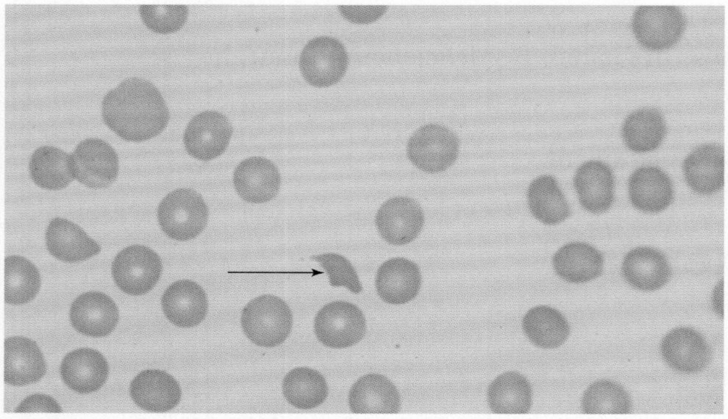

FIGURE 9-5 **Blood smear: schistocytes.**

(From Anderson SC. *Anderson's Atlas of Hematology.* Philadelphia, PA: Wolters Kluwer Health/Lippincott Williams & Wilkins, 2003.)

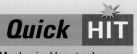

5. LDH level is elevated—LDH is released when RBCs are destroyed
6. Elevated indirect (unconjugated) bilirubin levels due to degradation of heme because RBCs are destroyed
7. Direct Coombs test (detects antibody or complement on RBC membrane)—positive in autoimmune hemolytic anemia (AIHA)
8. Osmotic fragility—see below

D. Treatment

1. Treat underlying cause.
2. Transfusion of PRBCs if severe anemia is present or patient is hemodynamically compromised.
3. Folate supplements (folate is depleted in hemolysis).

Quick HIT

The following may present in patients with hemolytic anemia:

- Jaundice, increased bilirubin
- Decreased haptoglobin
- Increased LDH

Sickle Cell Anemia

A. General characteristics

1. Causes.
   a. **Autosomal recessive** disorder that results when the normal Hb A is replaced by the mutant Hb S. Sickle cell disease is caused by inheritance of two Hb S genes (homozygous).
   b. Hb S may be distinguished from Hb A by electrophoresis because of the substitution of an uncharged valine for a negatively charged glutamic acid at the sixth position of the β-chain.
   c. Under reduced oxygen conditions (e.g., acidosis, hypoxia, changes in temperature, dehydration, and infection) the Hb molecules polymerize, causing the RBCs to sickle. Sickled RBCs obstruct small vessels, leading to ischemia (see Clinical Pearl 9-3).
2. Sickle cell trait.
   a. About 1 in 12 people of African descent carry the sickle cell trait; they are heterozygous. The sickle cell trait also appears in Italians, Greeks, and Saudi Arabians.
   b. Patients with sickle cell trait are not anemic and have a normal life expectancy.
   c. Sickle cell trait is associated with isosthenuria—the inability to concentrate or dilute urine. Patients will have a constant osmolality on urinalysis testing.
3. Screening can identify asymptomatic carriers (sickle cell trait), for whom genetic counseling may be provided.
4. Prognosis.
   a. Survival correlates with the frequency of vaso-occlusive crises—more frequent crises are associated with a shorter lifespan.
   b. If there are more than three crises per year, the median age of death is 35 years. Patients with fewer crises per year live into their 50s.
   c. In general, sickle cell disease reduces life expectancy by 25 to 30 years.

CLINICAL PEARL 9-3

Almost Every Organ Can be Involved in Sickle Cell Disease

- Blood—chronic hemolytic anemia, aplastic crises
- Heart—high-output CHF due to anemia
- CNS—stroke
- GI tract—gallbladder disease (stones), splenic infarctions, abdominal crises
- Bones—painful crises, osteomyelitis, avascular necrosis
- Lungs—infections, acute chest syndrome
- Kidneys—hematuria, papillary necrosis, renal failure
- Eyes—proliferative retinopathy, retinal infarcts
- Genitalia—priapism

Quick HIT

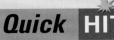

Sickle cell crises vary in severity and frequency among patients. They are typically followed by periods of remission. Some patients have many painful events requiring multiple hospitalizations per year; others have very few crises.

Quick HIT

Vaso-occlusive crises are due to obstruction of microcirculation by sickled RBCs. This leads to ischemia in various organs, producing the characteristic "painful crises."

Quick HIT

Splenic Sequestration Crisis

- Sudden pooling of blood into the spleen results in rapid development of splenomegaly and hypovolemic shock.
- A potentially fatal complication of sickle cell disease (and β-thalassemia) occurring more commonly in children (because they have intact spleens)

B. Clinical features

1. Severe, lifelong **hemolytic anemia.**
   a. Jaundice, pallor.
   b. Gallstone disease (very common)—pigmented gallstones.
   c. The anemia itself is well compensated and is rarely transfusion dependent.
   d. High-output heart failure may occur over time (secondary to anemia)—many adults eventually die of CHF.
   e. Aplastic crises.
      - These are usually provoked by a viral infection such as **human parvovirus B19**, which reduces the ability of the bone marrow to compensate.
      - Treatment is blood transfusion—the patient usually recovers in 7 to 10 days.
2. Findings secondary to vaso-occlusion.
   a. **Painful crises** involving **bone**—bone infarction causes severe pain. This is the most common clinical manifestation.
      - Bone pain usually involves multiple sites (e.g., tibia, humerus, femur). It may or may not be bilateral.
      - The pain is self-limiting and usually lasts 2 to 7 days.
   b. **Hand–foot syndrome** (dactylitis).
      - Painful swelling of dorsa of hands and feet seen in infancy and early childhood (usually 4 to 6 months).
      - Often the first manifestation of sickle cell disease.
      - Caused by avascular necrosis of the metacarpal and metatarsal bones.
   c. **Acute chest syndrome.**
      - Due to repeated episodes of pulmonary infarctions.
      - Clinical presentation is similar to pneumonia.
      - Associated with chest pain, respiratory distress, pulmonary infiltrates, and hypoxia.
   d. Repeated episodes of splenic infarctions—these lead to autosplenectomy as the spleen is reduced to a small, calcified remnant. The spleen is large in childhood but is no longer palpable by 4 years of age.
   e. Avascular necrosis of joints—most common in hip (decreased blood supply to femoral head) and shoulder (decreased blood supply to humeral head)
   f. Priapism.
      - Erection due to vaso-occlusion, usually lasting between 30 minutes and 3 hours.
      - Usually subsides spontaneously, after urine is passed, after light exercise, or after a cold shower.
      - A trial of hydralazine or nifedipine or use of an antiandrogen (e.g., stilbestrol) may prevent further episodes.
      - Sustained priapism (lasting more than 3 hours) is rare (less than 2%), but is a medical emergency.
   g. CVAs (stroke)—the result of cerebral thrombosis; primarily affects children.
   h. Ophthalmologic complications (e.g., retinal infarcts, vitreous hemorrhage, proliferative retinopathy, retinal detachment).
   i. Renal papillary necrosis with hematuria (usually painless).
      - A common complication—up to 20% of patients.
      - Seldom requires hospitalization and may cease spontaneously.
   j. Chronic leg ulcers due to vaso-occlusion (decreased blood flow to superficial vessels)—typically over lateral malleoli.
   k. Abdominal crisis may occur in adulthood—mimics acute abdomen.
3. Infectious complications.
   a. Functional asplenia results in increased susceptibility to infections (particularly encapsulated bacteria such as *Haemophilus influenzae, Streptococcus pneumoniae*).
   b. Predisposition to *Salmonella* osteomyelitis—also due to splenic malfunction.
4. Delayed growth and sexual maturation, especially in boys.

C. Diagnosis: laboratory tests

1. Anemia is the most common finding.
2. Peripheral smear—sickle-shaped RBCs (Figure 9-6).

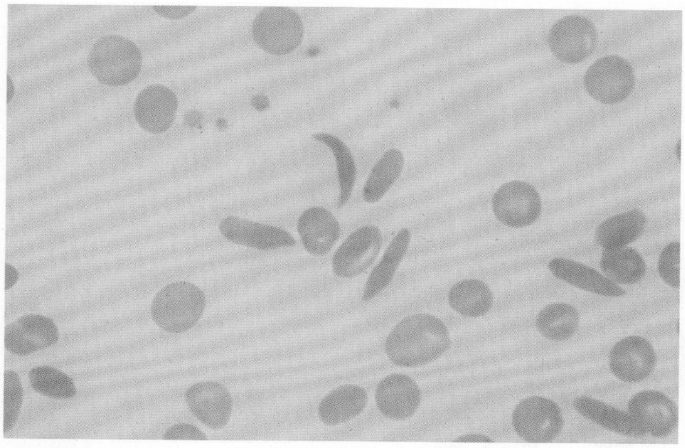

FIGURE 9-6 **Blood smear: sickle cell disease.**
(From Anderson SC. *Anderson's Atlas of Hematology.* Philadelphia, PA: Wolters Kluwer Health/Lippincott Williams & Wilkins, 2003.)

3. Hemoglobin electrophoresis is required for diagnosis. In most cases, diagnosis is made from newborn screening tests.

D. Treatment

1. Advise the patient as follows:
   a. Avoid high altitudes (low oxygen tension can precipitate crisis).
   b. Maintain fluid intake (dehydration can precipitate crisis).
   c. Treat infections promptly (infection/fever can precipitate crisis).
2. Early vaccination for *S. pneumoniae, H. influenzae,* and *Neisseria meningitidis.*
3. Prophylactic penicillin for children until 6 years of age—start at 4 months.
4. Folic acid supplements (due to chronic hemolysis).
5. Management of painful crises.
   a. Hydration—oral hydration if mild episode, otherwise give IV fluids (normal saline).
   b. Morphine for pain control—do not underestimate patient's pain.
   c. Keep the patient warm.
   d. Supplemental oxygen if hypoxia is present.
6. Hydroxyurea.
   a. Enhances Hb F levels, which interferes with the sickling process.
   b. Results in reduced incidence of painful crises.
   c. Accelerates healing of leg ulcers and may reduce recurrence.
7. Blood transfusion.
   a. Not used unless absolutely necessary.
   b. Base the need for transfusion on the patient's clinical condition and not on the Hb levels. Transfusion should be considered in acute chest syndrome, stroke, priapism that does not respond to fluids/analgesia, and cardiac decompensation.
8. Bone marrow transplantation—this has been performed successfully to treat sickle cell anemia, but is not routinely performed due to matched donor availability and risk of complications. It may be more cost-effective in the long run than conservative therapy.
9. Gene therapy offers hope for the future.

Hereditary Spherocytosis

A. General characteristics

1. Hereditary spherocytosis is an autosomal dominant inheritance of a defect in the gene coding for spectrin and other RBC proteins. Spectrin content is decreased but is not totally absent.
2. There is a loss of RBC membrane surface area without a reduction in RBC volume, necessitating a spherical shape. The spherical RBCs become trapped and destroyed in the spleen (by macrophages)—hence the term extravascular hemolysis.

Quick HIT

Causes of Spherocytosis
- Hereditary spherocytosis
- G6PD deficiency
- ABO incompatibility (but not Rh incompatibility)
- Hyperthermia
- AIHA

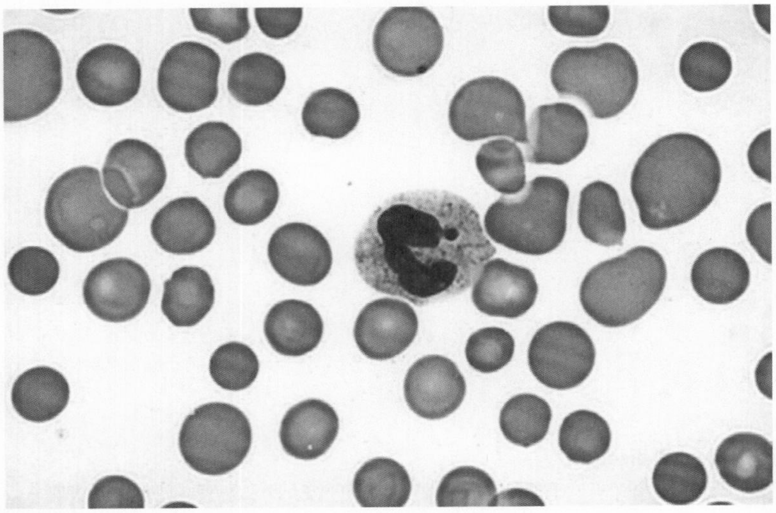

FIGURE 9-7 **Blood smear: spherocytes (hereditary spherocytosis).**
(From Strayer DS, Rubin, E. *Rubin's Pathology: Clinicopathologic Foundations of Medicine.* Philadelphia, PA: Wolters Kluwer Health/Lippincott Williams & Wilkins, 2014.)

Quick HIT

Following splenectomy, patients **must** be immunized against encapsulated organisms—*N. meningitidis, S. pneumoniae, H. influenzae.*

B. Clinical features

1. Hemolytic anemia (can be severe)
2. Jaundice
3. Splenomegaly
4. Gallstones
5. Occasional hemolytic crises

C. Diagnosis

1. RBC **osmotic fragility** to hypotonic saline.
   a. Tests the ability of RBCs to swell in a graded series of hypotonic solutions.
   b. Because of their shape, spherocytes tolerate less swelling before they rupture; thus, they are osmotically fragile. The RBCs undergo lysis at a higher (thus earlier) oncotic pressure.
2. Elevated reticulocyte count, elevated MCHC.
3. Peripheral blood smear would reveal spherocytes (sphere-shaped RBCs) (Figure 9-7).
4. Direct Coombs test result is negative. This is helpful in distinguishing this disease from AIHA, in which spherocytes are also seen.

D. Treatment: Splenectomy is the treatment of choice.

Glucose-6-phosphate Dehydrogenase Deficiency

A. General characteristics

1. An X-linked recessive disorder that primarily affects men.
2. Known precipitants include sulfonamides, nitrofurantoin, primaquine, dimercaprol, fava beans, and infection.
3. Types of G6PD deficiency.
   a. A mild form is present in 10% of African-American men (A-variant)
      - In this form, hemolytic episodes are usually self-limited because they mainly involve only the older RBCs and spare the younger RBCs. (The younger RBCs have sufficient G6PD to prevent RBC destruction.)
      - Hemolytic episodes are usually triggered by infection or by drugs such as antimalarials (primaquine) and sulfur-containing antibiotics (sulfonamide or trimethoprim sulfamethoxazole).
   b. A more severe form is present in people of Mediterranean descent.
      - In this form, young as well as old RBCs are G6PD-deficient.

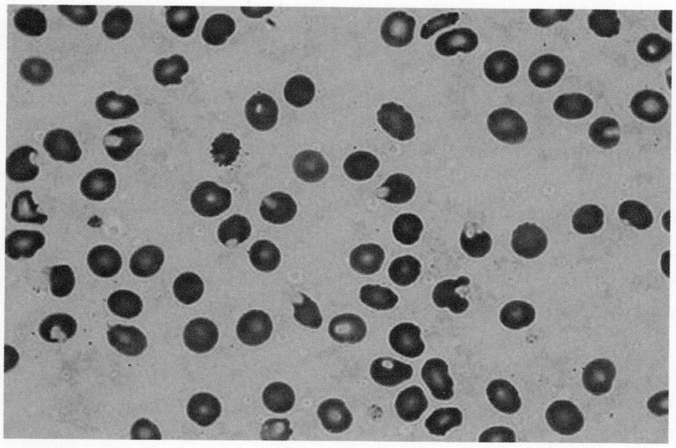

FIGURE 9-8 **Blood smear: bite cells (Glucose-6-phosphate dehydrogenase deficiency).**
(From Farhi D, Chai C, Edelman A, et al. *Pathology of Bone Marrow and Blood Cells.* Philadelphia, PA: Wolters Kluwer Health/Lippincott Williams & Wilkins, 2004.)

- Causes severe hemolytic anemia when exposed to fava beans.
- May require transfusions until the drug is eliminated from the body.

Quick HIT

- Deficiency of G6PD results in an accumulation of unneutralized H2O2, which denatures Hb, precipitating Heinz body formation within RBCs.
- Heinz bodies attach to RBC membranes, reducing their flexibility and making them prone to sequestration by the spleen.

B. Clinical features

1. Episodic hemolytic anemia that is usually drug-induced.
2. Dark urine and jaundice on physical examination.

C. Diagnosis

1. Peripheral blood smear.
   a. Shows "**bite cells**"—RBCs after the removal of the Heinz bodies look as if they have "bites" taken out of them. The "bitten" areas are secondary to phagocytosis of Heinz bodies by splenic macrophages (Figure 9-8).
   b. **Heinz bodies** (abnormal hemoglobin precipitates within RBCs) are visible with special stains.
2. Deficient NADPH formation on G6PD assay.
3. Measurement of G6PD levels is diagnostic; however, G6PD levels may be normal during the hemolytic episode because the RBCs that are most deficient in G6PD have already been destroyed. Repeating the test at a later date facilitates diagnosis.

D. Treatment

1. Avoid drugs that precipitate hemolysis.
2. Maintain hydration.
3. Perform RBC transfusion when necessary.

Autoimmune Hemolytic Anemia

A. General characteristics

1. Production of autoantibodies toward RBC membrane antigen(s) which leads to destruction of these RBCs.
2. The type of antibody produced (immunoglobulin [Ig]G or IgM) determines the prognosis, site of RBC destruction, and response to treatment.
3. The course is variable, but tends to be more fulminant in children than in adults.
4. Warm AIHA (more common than cold AIHA).
   a. Autoantibody is IgG, which binds optimally to RBC membranes at 37°C (hence "warm").
   b. Results in **extravascular hemolysis**—the primary site of RBC sequestration is the spleen. Splenomegaly is a common feature.
   c. Causes.
      - Primary (idiopathic).

- Secondary to lymphomas, leukemias (chronic lymphocytic leukemia [CLL]), other malignancies, collagen vascular diseases (especially SLE), drugs such as α-methyldopa.

5. Cold AIHA.
   a. Autoantibody is IgM, which binds optimally to the RBC membrane at cold temperatures (usually 0°C to 5°C).
   b. Produces complement activation and **intravascular hemolysis**—primary site of RBC sequestration is the liver.
   c. Causes—can be idiopathic (elderly) or due to infection (such as *Mycoplasma pneumoniae* infection or infectious mononucleosis).

B. Clinical features

1. Signs and symptoms of anemia (e.g., fatigue, pallor)
2. Jaundice if significant hemolysis is present
3. Features of the underlying disease

C. Diagnosis

1. Direct Coombs test.
   a. If RBCs are coated with IgG (positive direct Coombs test), then the diagnosis is warm AIHA.
   b. If RBCs are coated with complement alone, then the diagnosis is cold AIHA.
2. If there is a positive cold agglutinin titer, then the diagnosis is cold AIHA.
3. Spherocytes may be present in warm AIHA.

D. Treatment

1. Often, no treatment is necessary in either type of AIHA, because the hemolysis is mild. If it is more severe, the therapeutic approach depends on the type of autoantibody causing the hemolysis.
2. Warm AIHA.
   a. Glucocorticoids are the mainstay of therapy.
   b. Splenectomy—use for patients whose condition does not respond to glucocorticoids.
   c. Immunosuppression (azathioprine or cyclophosphamide) may be beneficial.
   d. RBC transfusions—if absolutely necessary.
   e. Folic acid supplements.
3. Cold AIHA.
   a. Avoiding exposure to cold—prevents bouts of hemolysis and anemia.
   b. RBC transfusions—if absolutely necessary.
   c. Various chemotherapeutic agents.
   d. Steroids are not beneficial.

••• Paroxysmal Nocturnal Hemoglobinuria

A. General characteristics

1. An acquired disorder that affects hematopoietic stem cells and cells of all blood lineages.
2. This is caused by a deficiency of anchor proteins that link complement-inactivating proteins to blood cell membranes. The deficiency of this anchoring mechanism results in an unusual susceptibility to complement-mediated lysis of RBCs, WBCs, and platelets.

B. Clinical features

1. Chronic intravascular hemolysis—results in chronic paroxysmal hemoglobinuria, elevated LDH
2. Normochromic normocytic anemia (unless iron deficiency anemia is present)
3. Pancytopenia
4. Thrombosis of venous systems can occur (e.g., of the hepatic veins [Budd–Chiari syndrome])
5. May evolve into aplastic anemia, myelodysplasia, myelofibrosis, and acute leukemia
6. Abdominal, back, and musculoskeletal pain

C. Diagnosis

1. Ham test: the patient's cells are incubated in acidified serum, triggering the alternative complement pathway, resulting in lysis of PNH cells but not normal cells.
2. Sugar water test: The patient's serum is mixed in sucrose. In PNH, hemolysis ensues.
3. Flow cytometry of anchored cell surface proteins (CD55, CD59)—much more sensitive and specific for PNH.

D. Treatment

1. Glucocorticoids (prednisone) are the usual initial therapy, but many patients do not respond.
2. Bone marrow transplantation.

Platelet Disorders

Thrombocytopenia

A. General characteristics

1. Platelet counts <150,000. Normal is 150,000 to 400,000/mL (Figure 9-9)
2. Causes
   a. Decreased production
      - Bone marrow failure: acquired (aplastic anemia), congenital (Fanconi syndrome), congenital intrauterine rubella
      - Bone marrow invasion: tumors, leukemia, fibrosis
      - Bone marrow injury: drugs (ethanol, gold, cancer chemotherapy agents, chloramphenicol), chemicals (benzene), radiation, infection

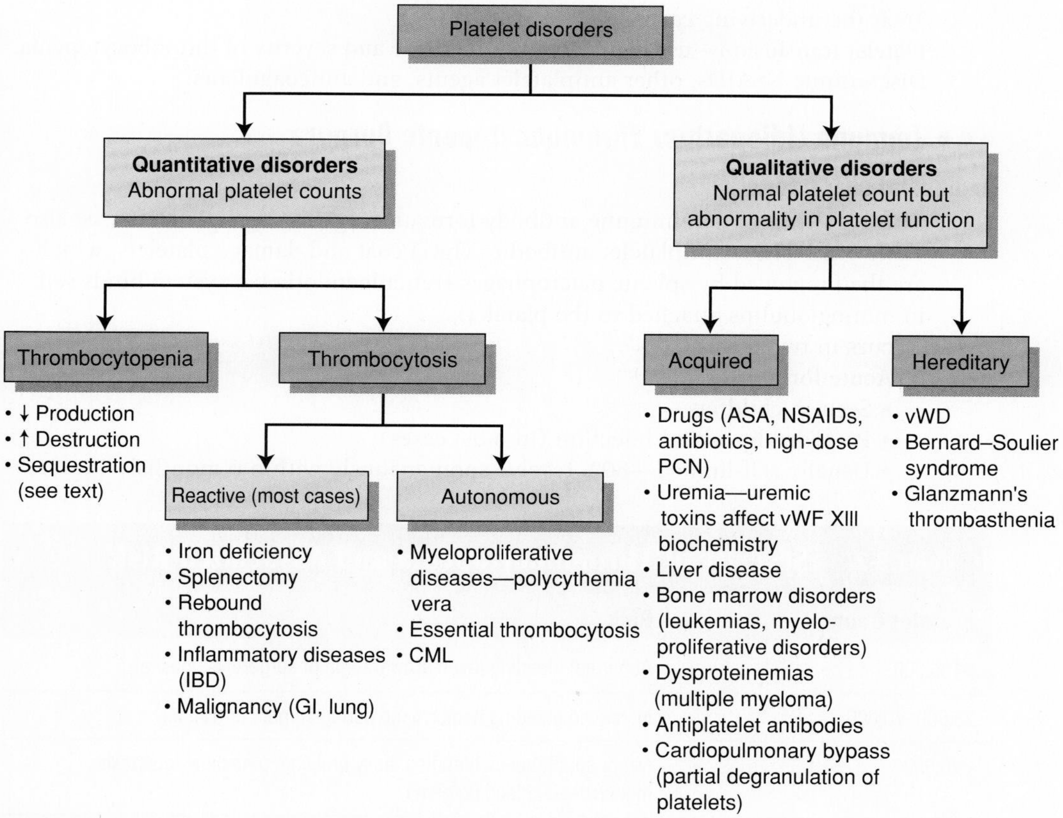

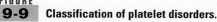

FIGURE 9-9 **Classification of platelet disorders.**

Quick HIT

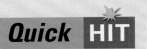

HIT
- HIT type 1: Heparin directly causes platelet aggregation; seen <48 hours after initiating heparin; no treatment is needed.
- HIT type 2: Heparin induces antibody-mediated injury to platelet; seen 3 to 12 days after initiating heparin; heparin should be discontinued immediately.

b. Increased destruction
   - Immune: infection, drug-induced, immune thrombocytopenic purpura (ITP), SLE, heparin-induced thrombocytopenia (HIT) type 2, HIV-associated thrombocytopenia
   - Nonimmune: disseminated intravascular coagulation (DIC), thrombotic thrombocytopenic purpura (TTP), HIT type 1

c. Sequestration from splenomegaly

d. Dilutional—after transfusions or hemorrhage

e. Pregnancy—usually an incidental finding (especially third trimester) but can also occur in setting of preeclampsia or eclampsia (remember HELLP syndrome)

B. Diagnosis
1. CBC—platelet count
2. Bleeding time, prothrombin time (PT), partial thromboplastin time (PTT)
3. To determine the cause of thrombocytopenia, the following may be helpful: examination of peripheral blood smear, bone marrow biopsy

C. Clinical features
1. Cutaneous bleeding: petechiae (most common in dependent areas); confluent petechiae are called purpura, ecchymoses at sites of minor trauma
2. Mucosal bleeding: epistaxis, menorrhagia, hemoptysis, bleeding in GI and genitourinary tracts
3. Excessive bleeding after procedures or surgery
4. Intracranial hemorrhage and heavy GI bleeding can be life-threatening and occur when platelet levels are severely low
5. Unlike coagulation disorders (e.g., hemophilia), heavy bleeding into tissues and joints (hemarthroses, hematomas) is not seen in thrombocytopenia

D. Treatment
1. Treat the underlying cause.
2. Platelet transfusion—use depending on the cause and severity of thrombocytopenia.
3. Discontinue NSAIDs, other antiplatelet agents, and anticoagulants.

Immune (Idiopathic) Thrombocytopenic Purpura

A. General characteristics
1. This results from autoimmune antibody formation against host platelets (see also Table 9-2). These antiplatelet antibodies (IgG) coat and damage platelets, which are then removed by splenic macrophages (reticuloendothelial system binds self-immunoglobulins attached to the platelet)
2. Occurs in two forms
   a. Acute form
      - Seen in children
      - Preceded by a viral infection (in most cases)
      - Usually self-limited—80% resolve spontaneously within 6 months

TABLE 9-2 Severity of Thrombocytopenia and Associated Risk

Platelet Count	Risk
>100,000	Abnormal bleeding (even after trauma or surgery) is unusual
20,000–70,000	Increased bleeding hemorrhage during surgery or trauma
<20,000	Minor spontaneous bleeding: easy bruising, petechiae, epistaxis, menorrhagia, bleeding gums
<5,000	Major spontaneous bleeding: intracranial bleeding, heavy GI bleeding

b. Chronic form
    - Usually seen in adults, most commonly in women between 20 and 40 years of age
    - Spontaneous remissions are rare

B. Clinical features

1. Petechiae and ecchymoses on the skin—many patients will have only very minimal bleeding symptoms despite extremely low platelet counts (<5,000/mL)
2. Bleeding of the mucous membranes
3. No splenomegaly

C. Diagnosis

1. The platelet count is frequently less than 20,000. The remainder of the blood count is normal.
2. Peripheral smear shows decreased platelets.
3. Bone marrow aspiration shows increased megakaryocytes.
4. There is an increased amount of platelet-associated IgG.

D. Treatment

1. Adrenal corticosteroids
2. IV immune globulin—saturates the reticuloendothelial system binding sites for platelet-bound self-immunoglobulin, so there is less platelet uptake and destruction by the spleen
3. Splenectomy—induces remission in 70% to 80% of the cases of chronic ITP
4. Platelet transfusions—for life-threatening and serious hemorrhagic episodes
5. Two new drugs, romiplostim and eltrombopag, have been approved for splenectomy-resistant patients. Both these drugs work as thrombopoietin receptor agonists to increase platelet production

Thrombotic Thrombocytopenic Purpura

A. General characteristics

1. TTP is a rare disorder of platelet consumption. **Patients with TTP lack functional ADAMTS13**, a protease that cleaves von Willebrand factor (vWF). Ultralarge vWF multimers build-up in the blood as a result of this deficiency.
2. Microthrombi (mostly platelet thrombi) occlude small vessels leading to microangiopathic hemolytic anemia—any organ may be involved. They cause mechanical damage to RBCs (schistocytes on peripheral smear)
3. This is a life-threatening emergency that is responsive to therapy (see below). If untreated, death occurs within a few months.

> **Quick HIT**
>
> **TTP**
> - There is no consumption of clotting factors in TTP, so PT and PTT are normal.
> - TTP = HUS + fever + altered mental status
> - HUS = microangiopathic hemolytic anemia + thrombocytopenia + renal failure

B. Clinical features

1. Hemolytic anemia (microangiopathic)
2. Thrombocytopenia
3. Acute renal failure (mild)
4. Fever
5. Fluctuating, transient neurologic signs—can range from mental status change to hemiplegia

C. Treatment

1. Plasmapheresis (large volume).
    a. Begin as soon as diagnosis is established (delay in treatment is life-threatening).
    b. Response is usually good (monitor platelet count, which should increase).
2. Corticosteroids and splenectomy—may be of benefit in some cases.
3. Platelet transfusions are contraindicated.

Heparin-induced Thrombocytopenia

- Occurs when antibodies are formed against the heparin-platelet factor 4 complex.
- Can occur with use of any amount of heparin. Mostly occurs with unfractionated heparin. Low-molecular-weight heparin (LMWH) has a much lower risk of HIT.

- Drop in platelets a few days after heparin administration. Platelets aggregate ("clump") leading to venous thrombosis (deep vein thrombosis [DVT], pulmonary embolism [PE])
- Decrease in platelet count by 50% suggests HIT.
- Diagnostic tests: antiplatelet factor IV antibody or serotonin release assay.
- Treatment: stop heparin. If anticoagulation is indicated (venous thrombosis), give a thrombin inhibitor such as lepirudin, argatroban, and dabigatran.
- Avoid heparin in the future in any patient who has developed an episode of HIT.

Quick HIT
Main complication of HIT is venous thrombosis—DVT or PE.

Bernard–Soulier Syndrome

- Autosomal recessive disease.
- Disorder of platelet adhesion (to subendothelium) due to deficiency of platelet glycoprotein GPIb-IX.
- On peripheral blood smear, platelets are abnormally large.
- Platelet count is mildly low.

Glanzmann Thrombasthenia

- Autosomal recessive disease.
- Disorder of platelet aggregation due to deficiency in platelet glycoprotein GPIIb-IIIa.
- Bleeding time is prolonged.
- Platelet count is normal.

Quick HIT
The **ristocetin assay** can be used to test for vWD.

Disorders of Coagulation

von Willebrand Disease

A. General characteristics

1. Autosomal dominant disorder characterized by deficiency or defect of factor VIII-related antigen (vWF) (see also Table 9-3).
2. vWF enhances platelet aggregation and adhesion (the first steps in clot formation). It also acts as a carrier of factor VIII in blood.
3. **The most common inherited bleeding disorder (affects 1% to 3% of population).**
4. There are three major subtypes with varying severity.
   a. Type 1 (most common form)—decreased levels of vWF.
   b. Type 2 (less common)—exhibits qualitative abnormalities of vWF.
   c. Type 3 (least common form)—absent vWF (very severe disease).

Quick HIT
Factor VIII has two portions: the coagulant portion (factor VIII coagulant protein) and an antigenic portion (factor VIII antigenic protein). The latter is synonymous with vWF.

Quick HIT
Other causes of impaired platelet function include uremia as well as the use of NSAIDs and aspirin.

TABLE 9-3 vWF Versus Factor VIII Coagulant Protein

	vWF (Also Known as Factor VIII-Related Antigenic Protein)	Factor VIII Coagulant Protein
Site of Synthesis	Endothelial cells and megakaryocytes	Liver
Functions	• Platelet adhesion—mediates the adhesion of platelets to the injured vessel walls (i.e., it reacts with platelet GPIb/IX and subendothelium) • Binds the factor VIII coagulant protein and protects it from degradation	Fibrin clot formation
Inheritance Pattern	Autosomal dominant	X-linked recessive
vWD	Low	Reduced
Hemophilia	Normal	Very low

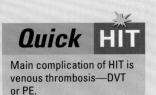

B. Clinical features

1. Cutaneous and mucosal bleeding—epistaxis, easy bruising, excessive bleeding from scratches and cuts, gingival bleeding.
2. Menorrhagia (affects more than 50% of women with von Willebrand Disease [vWD]).
3. GI bleeding is possible.

C. Diagnosis

1. Diagnosis is derived from clinical findings and laboratory information, which can be variable.
2. **Prolonged bleeding time** (but normal platelet count)—PTT may be prolonged (a normal PTT does not exclude this diagnosis).
3. Decreased plasma vWF, decreased factor VIII activity.
4. Reduced ristocetin-induced platelet aggregation.

D. Treatment

1. DDAVP (desmopressin)—induces endothelial cells to secrete vWF.
   a. Treatment of choice for type 1 vWD (the most common type).
   b. Some patients with type 2 vWD may respond to DDAVP, but it is not effective in type 3 vWD.
2. Factor VIII concentrates (containing high-molecular-weight vWF).
   a. Give to all patients with vWD (any type) after major trauma or during surgery.
   b. Recommended for type 3 vWD (and type 2 patients not responsive to DDAVP).
3. Cryoprecipitate is not recommended as treatment for vWD because it carries the risk of viral transmission.
4. Avoid aspirin/NSAIDs as well as intramuscular injections (exacerbate bleeding tendency).

Hemophilia A

A. General characteristics

1. X-linked recessive disorder—affects male patients primarily (approximately 1 in 10,000 male patients).
2. Caused by deficiency or defect of factor VIII coagulant protein.
3. Bleeding tendency is related to factor VIII activity (see Table 9-4).

B. Clinical features

1. Hemarthrosis
   a. Knees are the most common site, but any joint can be involved.
   b. Progressive joint destruction can occur secondary to recurrent hemarthroses.
      - Maintaining normal factor VIII levels (by prophylactic administration of factor VIII concentrate) can minimize joint destruction

Quick HIT

- In many patients, vWD is mild, and is not diagnosed until surgery or trauma.
- In general, bleeding in vWD is much milder than in hemophilia. Spontaneous hemarthroses do not occur.

Quick HIT

First line treatment for vWD is desmopressin. If no response, give Factor VIII concentrate.

Quick HIT

Suspect hemophilia if unsuspected hemorrhage occurs in a male patient with a positive family history.

TABLE 9-4 Classification of Severity of Hemophilia

Classification	Amount (or Activity) of Factor VIII	Clinical Feature
Subclinical	10% of normal factor VIII	Usually asymptomatic
Mild factor VIII deficiency	5%–10% of normal factor VIII	Bleeding after injuries/surgery
Moderate factor VIII deficiency	1%–5% of normal factor VIII	Rare spontaneous bleeding; severe bleeding after trauma or surgery
Severe factor VIII deficiency—accounts for about 60% of all cases—diagnosed in infancy or early childhood	<1% of normal factor VIII	Spontaneous bleeding in joints (hemarthrosis) and soft tissues; severe hemorrhage after surgery and trauma

Quick HIT

More than 75% of patients with hemophilia A and about 50% of patients with hemophilia B are HIV-positive. However, these statistics should be decreasing with time, thanks to modern screening of donor blood.

Quick HIT

Detection of Factor VIII Inhibitor
- If normal plasma is mixed with plasma from a hemophiliac patient, PTT becomes normal.
- If PTT fails to normalize, this is diagnostic of the presence of a factor VIII inhibitor.

Quick HIT

- PT: reflects extrinsic pathway (prolonged by warfarin)
- PTT: reflects intrinsic pathway (prolonged by heparin)
- Thrombin time: measure of fibrinogen concentration
- Bleeding time: reflects platelet function

Quick HIT

- Normal PT = 11 to 15 seconds
- Normal PTT = 25 to 40 seconds
- Normal bleeding time = 2 to 7 minutes

- Synovectomy (arthroscopic) or radiosynovectomy may be needed if severe recurrent hemarthrosis occur despite optimal medical management

2. Intracranial bleeding
   a. Second most common cause of death (AIDS due to past history of transfusion [before screening was initiated] is most common)
   b. Any head trauma is potentially life-threatening and requires urgent evaluation
3. Intramuscular hematomas
4. Retroperitoneal hematomas
5. Hematuria or hemospermia

C. Diagnosis

1. Prolonged PTT (see also Table 9-4)
2. Low factor VIII coagulant level and normal levels of vWF

D. Treatment

1. Acute hemarthrosis
   a. Analgesia (codeine with or without acetaminophen)—avoid aspirin and NSAIDs
   b. Immobilization of the joint, ice packs, nonweight bearing
2. Clotting factor replacement
   a. Factor VIII concentrate is the mainstay of therapy (both plasma-derived and recombinant factor VIII are available)—for acute bleeding episodes and before surgery or dental work
   b. Cryoprecipitate and fresh frozen plasma (FFP) are not recommended because of the risk of viral transmission
3. DDAVP—this may be helpful in patients with mild disease. It can increase the levels of factor VIII up to fourfold
4. Gene therapy offers hope for the future

Hemophilia B

- Caused by deficiency of factor IX
- X-linked recessive disorder
- Much less common than hemophilia A
- Clinical features are identical to those of hemophilia A
- Treatment involves administration of factor IX concentrates. DDAVP does not play a role in treatment

Disseminated Intravascular Coagulation

A. General characteristics

1. DIC is characterized by abnormal activation of the coagulation sequence, leading to formation of microthrombi throughout the microcirculation. This causes consumption of platelets, fibrin, and coagulation factors. Fibrinolytic mechanisms are activated, leading to hemorrhage. Therefore, bleeding and thrombosis occur simultaneously
2. Most common in critically ill patients (in ICU), but can occur in healthy patients as well
3. Can be acute (and fatal), or more gradual
4. Causes
   a. Infection—most common cause, especially gram-negative sepsis, but any infection can cause DIC
   b. Obstetric complications (placenta and uterus have increased tissue factor)—amniotic fluid emboli (often acute and fatal); retained dead fetus (often chronic); abruptio placentae
   c. Major tissue injury—trauma, major surgery, burns, fractures
   d. Malignancy—lungs, pancreas, prostate, GI tract, acute promyelocytic leukemia (APL)
   e. Shock, circulatory collapse
   f. Snake venom (rattlesnakes)

TABLE 9-5 Laboratory Findings for Bleeding Disorders

Condition	Platelet Count	Bleeding Time	PT	PTT
Hemophilia	NL[a]	NL	NL	Increased
vWD	NL	Increased	NL	Increased
ITP	Decreased	Increased	NL	NL
TTP	Decreased	Increased	NL	NL
DIC	Decreased	Increased	Increased	Increased
Heparin	NL or decreased	NL	NL	Increased
Warfarin	NL	NL	Increased	NL
Liver disease	NL	NL	Increased	Increased

[a]NL = normal.

B. Clinical features

1. Bleeding tendency (more common in acute cases)
   a. Superficial hemorrhage (ecchymoses, petechiae, purpura)
   b. Bleeding from GI tract, urinary tract, gingival or oral mucosa
   c. Oozing from sites of procedures, incisions, and so on
2. Thrombosis—occurs most often in chronic cases. End-organ infarction may develop; all tissues are at risk, especially the CNS and kidney

C. Diagnosis

1. The following are all increased: (see Table 9-5)
   a. PT, PTT, bleeding time, TT
   b. Fibrin split products (due to activation of fibrinolytic system)
   c. D-dimer
2. The following are decreased:
   a. **Fibrinogen level (a normal/elevated fibrinogen essentially rules out the diagnosis)**
   b. Platelet count (thrombocytopenia)
3. Peripheral smear reveals schistocytes from damage of RBCs as they go through the microcirculation (with microthrombi)

D. Treatment

1. Management of the condition that precipitated DIC.
2. Supportive measures may be indicated if severe hemorrhage is present (these are only temporizing measures).
   a. Cryoprecipitate replaces clotting factors and fibrinogen.
   b. FFP replaces all the clotting factors.
   c. Platelet transfusions are not recommended in DIC unless counts drop below ~30,000.
   d. Low doses of heparin (IV or SC) inhibit clotting and can prevent consumption of clotting factors. The use of heparin is controversial; give only in rare cases in which thrombosis dominates the clinical picture.
   e. Other supportive measures include oxygen and IV fluids. Maintain BP and renal perfusion.

Vitamin K Deficiency

A. General characteristics

1. Several clotting factors depend on vitamin K as a cofactor in their synthesis by the liver (factors II, VII, IX, and X; proteins C and S). The process is posttranslational modification (γ-carboxylation)

Quick HIT

Whenever a coagulopathy is present, consider vitamin K deficiency and liver disease in the differential diagnosis (in addition to DIC).
- Liver disease: PT and PTT are elevated, but TT, fibrinogen, and platelets are usually normal.
- Vitamin K deficiency: PT is prolonged, but PTT, TT, platelet count, and fibrinogen level S are normal.

Quick HIT

Complications of DIC
- Hemorrhage—Intracranial bleeding is a common cause of death.
- Thromboembolism—stroke, PE, bowel infarction, acute renal failure, arterial occlusion.

Quick HIT

All critically ill patients are at risk for DIC.

Quick HIT

The fat-soluble vitamins include vitamin A, D, E, and K.

Quick HIT

Vitamin K deficiency is most commonly seen in critically ill patients (who are NPO and on antibiotics).

Quick HIT

Factor VII has the shortest half-life (3 to 5 hours) of all clotting factors, so prolonged PT is the first laboratory finding.

Quick HIT

Prolonged PT is a poor prognostic indicator in cirrhosis because synthesis of clotting factors is not **significantly** impaired until liver disease is advanced.

Quick HIT

Patients with AT III deficiency do not respond to heparin. (Heparin requires the presence of AT III.)

Quick HIT

Patients with antiphospholipid antibody syndrome usually have a prolonged PTT during laboratory testing. This is because the antibody interferes with the test, and is a *false* prolongation.

2. Sources of vitamin K include diet (e.g., leafy green vegetables) and synthesis by intestinal bacterial flora
3. Causes
   a. Broad-spectrum antibiotics (suppression of gut flora) in patients who are NPO (inadequate dietary intake)
   b. Patients on TPN (unless vitamin K is added)
   c. Malabsorption of fat-soluble vitamins (small bowel disease, inflammatory bowel disease, obstructive jaundice)
   d. Warfarin—a vitamin K antagonist (causes production of inactive clotting factors)

B. Clinical features

1. Hemorrhage—serious bleeding can develop.
2. PT is initially prolonged (factor VII has the shortest half-life). PTT prolongation follows (as other factors diminish).

C. Treatment

1. Vitamin K replacement (oral or subcutaneous)—it may take a few days for PT to return to normal.
2. If bleeding is severe and emergency treatment is necessary, FFP should be transfused.

Coagulopathy of Liver Disease

A. General characteristics

1. All clotting factors are produced by the liver (except vWF).
2. Liver disease must be severe for coagulopathy to develop. Therefore, if the coagulopathy is due to liver failure, the overall prognosis for the patient is very poor.
3. The following are the reasons coagulopathy develops in liver failure:
   a. There is a decreased synthesis of clotting factors.
   b. Cholestasis leads to decreased vitamin K absorption, which leads to vitamin K deficiency.
   c. Hypersplenism (splenomegaly due to portal hypertension) causes thrombocytopenia.

B. Clinical features

1. Abnormal bleeding—GI bleeding is the most common, primarily due to varices secondary to portal hypertension, but exacerbated by the coagulopathy.
2. Prolonged PT and PTT (especially PT).

C. Treatment

1. FFP (contains all clotting factors)—if PT or PTT is prolonged or if bleeding is present
2. Vitamin K in certain cases (cholestasis)
3. Platelet transfusion—if thrombocytopenia is present
4. Cryoprecipitate—if there is a deficiency of fibrinogen

Inherited Hypercoagulable States

A. Causes

1. Antithrombin (AT) III deficiency
   a. Autosomal dominant inheritance
   b. AT III is an inhibitor of thrombin, so a deficiency leads to increased thrombosis
2. Antiphospholipid antibody syndrome
   a. Acquired hypercoagulability state
   b. Can present with arterial or venous thrombosis, recurrent fetal loss, or thrombocytopenia
   c. The antibody may be against lupus anticoagulants, anticardiolipin, and β_2-microglobulin, among others
3. Protein C deficiency
   a. Autosomal dominant inheritance

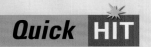

CLINICAL PEARL 9-4

Secondary Hypercoagulable States or Risk Factors

- Malignancy (especially pancreas, GI, lung, and ovaries)
- Antiphospholipid antibody syndrome—the lupus anticoagulant
- Pregnancy—up to 2 months postpartum
- Immobilization, causing stasis of blood
- Myeloproliferative disorders
- Oral contraceptives
- Postoperative state (especially after orthopedic procedures)
- Trauma
- Nephrotic syndrome
- HIT or DIC
- PNH
- Heart failure—causes stasis of blood

b. Protein C is an inhibitor of factors V and VIII, so a deficiency leads to unregulated fibrin synthesis

4. Protein S deficiency—protein S is a cofactor of protein C, so a deficiency leads to decreased protein C activity
5. Factor V Leiden (activated protein C resistance)
   a. A mutation in factor V gene
   b. Most common hereditary hypercoagulability disorder among Caucasians
   c. Protein C can no longer inactivate factor V, leading to unregulated prothrombin activation, and thus an increase in thrombotic events
6. Prothrombin gene mutation
7. Hyperhomocysteinemia

Quick HIT

In many cases, inherited hypercoagulable diseases cause thrombotic events when other risk factors (e.g., immobilization, pregnancy) are also present.

B. Clinical features

1. Venous thromboembolisms (DVT and PE) are the most common sequelae. Such hypercoagulable disorders are usually not diagnosed until the patient has had several episodes of DVT or PE (see Clinical Pearl 9-4).
2. Suspect an inherited hypercoagulable state if one or more of the following are present:
   a. The patient has a family history of DVT, PE, or thrombotic events.
   b. The patient has recurrent episodes of DVT, PE, or thrombotic events.
   c. The patient's first thrombotic event was before age 40.
   d. The patient experiences thrombosis in unusual sites (e.g., in mesenteric veins, inferior vena cava, renal veins, or cerebral veins).

Quick HIT

- Check for any secondary hypercoagulable states or risk factors (see Clinical Pearl 9-4) in any patient with a DVT, PE, or any thrombotic event, especially if recurrent. Once these are ruled out, search for an inherited hypercoagulable state.
- It is very important to identify the patient with an inherited hypercoagulable state because prophylactic anticoagulation should be started and genetic counseling may be appropriate.

C. Diagnosis: Functional assays are available for AT, antiphospholipid antibodies, protein C, protein S, factor V Leiden, prothrombin gene mutation, and hyperhomocysteinemia.

D. Treatment

1. Standard treatment for DVT or PE as in patients without primary hypercoagulable states.
2. Patients with any of these disorders who have had two or more thromboembolic events should be permanently anticoagulated with warfarin.

Anticoagulation

Heparin

A. Mechanism of action

1. Potentiates the action of AT to primarily inhibit clotting factors IIa and Xa
2. Prolongs PTT

> **Quick HIT**
> **Options for DVT prophylaxis**
> - LMWH
> - Low-dose unfractionated heparin
> - Pneumatic compression boots

3. Half-life of standard heparin is 1 hour. It is longer for LMWHs (longer than 3 hours and up to 24 hours, depending on the product)

B. Indications for use

1. Venous thromboembolism: DVT, PE
2. Acute coronary syndromes: unstable angina, myocardial infarction
3. Low-dose standard heparin or LMWH for DVT prophylaxis
4. Atrial fibrillation in acute setting
5. After vascular bypass grafting

C. Administration

1. Standard heparin
   a. A therapeutic dose is usually given intravenously, initiated with a bolus of 70 to 80 U/kg and followed by continuous IV infusion (15 to 18 U/kg/hr infusion). Therapeutic PTT is usually 60 to 90 seconds, but this varies depending on the clinical situation
   b. Therapeutic heparin is now often monitored using antifactor Xa levels
   c. A prophylactic dose is given subcutaneously—low-dose heparin (5,000 U SC subcutaneously every 12 hours). PTT monitoring is not necessary with SC dosing
2. LMWH
   a. Therapeutic dose—given as a weight-adjusted dose
   b. Prophylactic dose—varies depending on type of product

D. Adverse effects

1. Bleeding
2. HIT—lower incidence with LMWHs
3. Possible osteoporosis—lower incidence with LMWHs
4. Transient alopecia
5. Rebound hypercoagulability after removal due to depression of AT III

E. Contraindications to heparin

1. Previous HIT
2. Active bleeding, GI bleeding, intracranial bleeding
3. Hemophilia, thrombocytopenia
4. Severe HTN
5. Recent surgery on eyes, spine, brain

F. Reversing the effects of heparin and LMWHs

1. The half-life of standard heparin is short, so it will cease to have an effect within 4 hours of its cessation.
2. One can give protamine sulfate to reverse the effects of heparin if necessary (effectiveness is not proven, but it is the only potential antidote that exists in the case of severe bleeding).
3. LMWH has a longer half-life than standard heparin, so it takes longer for the effects to fade.

> **Quick HIT**
> Administer FFP if severe bleeding occurs (for patients on either warfarin or heparin).

Low-molecular-weight Heparin

A. Mechanism of action

1. LMWHs mostly inhibit factor Xa (equivalent inhibition of factor Xa as standard heparin), but have less inhibition of factor IIa (thrombin) and platelet aggregation.
2. They cannot be monitored by PT or PTT because they do not affect either.
3. Examples include enoxaparin, dalteparin, and tinzaparin.

B. Indications for use

1. LMWHs are being used more now because of their greater convenience compared with standard heparin, as well as a decreased risk of side effects (HIT, osteoporosis).
   a. They are given subcutaneously (no IV administration).
   b. PTT monitoring is not necessary.

c. They are easier to use as an outpatient—the patient may be discharged if stable, and the patient can continue LMWH until the level of long-term anticoagulation (warfarin) is therapeutic.
2. Excreted via kidneys—use cautiously in patients with renal dysfunction.
3. It is much more expensive than standard heparin, but often more cost-effective in the long run due to reduced testing, nursing time, and length of hospital stay.

Warfarin

A. Mechanism of action

1. A vitamin K antagonist—leads to a decrease in vitamin K-dependent clotting factors (II, VII, IX, X) and proteins C and S
2. Causes prolongation of PT (and increase in INR)
3. It takes 4 to 5 days for the anticoagulant effect to begin. Therefore, start heparin as well if the goal is acute anticoagulation because heparin has an immediate effect. Once warfarin is therapeutic (check by INR), then stop the heparin and continue warfarin for as long as necessary

B. Indications for use: Same as heparin but used for long-term anticoagulation.

C. Administration

1. Given orally.
2. Heparin is initiated first—as soon as PTT is therapeutic, initiate warfarin. Continue heparin for at least 4 days after starting warfarin. Once INR is therapeutic on warfarin, stop the heparin.
3. The level of anticoagulation is monitored by the INR. In most cases, an INR of 2 to 3 is therapeutic. However, patients with mechanical heart valves need coagulation with goal INR of 2.5 to 3.5.

D. Adverse effects

1. Hemorrhage.
2. Skin necrosis is a rare but serious complication. It is caused by rapid decrease in protein C (a vitamin K-dependent inhibitor of factors Va and VIIIa).
3. **Teratogenic—avoid during pregnancy**!
4. Should not be given to alcoholics or to any patient who is prone to frequent falls because an intracranial bleed in a patient on warfarin can be catastrophic.

E. Reversing the effects of warfarin

1. Discontinue warfarin and administer vitamin K.
2. The half-life of warfarin is much longer than that of heparin—it takes 5 days to correct the effects of warfarin on stopping the medication. Vitamin K infusion corrects an abnormal PT within 4 to 10 hours if the patient has normal liver function.
3. Giving vitamin K makes it difficult to return the patient to therapeutic INR levels if anticoagulation is to be continued.

Quick HIT

If rapid reversal of acute bleeding from warfarin is indicated, give FFP.

Clopidogrel

A. Mechanism of action

1. Blocks the binding of ADP to a specific platelet ADP receptor $P2Y_{12}$, which reduces platelet activation and aggregation
2. Increases the bleeding time

B. Indications for use

1. Acute coronary syndromes: unstable angina, myocardial infarction, NSTEMI
2. Pretreatment for patients undergoing PCI
3. After PCI—patients should typically receive at least 1 year of clopidogrel (and aspirin) after stent placement
4. Peripheral artery disease

C. Administration

1. Given orally
2. For patients with STEMI who will undergo treatment with primary PCI, a loading dose of clopidogrel is associated with better outcomes than pretreatment with placebo. There is some debate about the appropriate dose, but 600 mg seems to provide the best ratio of benefit to associated bleeding risk
3. Patients should receive daily clopidogrel after receiving a stent for any indication. The dose is typically 75 mg/day for at least 12 months, with the first 6 months being the most important

D. Adverse effects

1. Bleeding
2. Bruising/purpura
3. Some animal models suggest that proton pump inhibitors (PPIs) interfere with the conversion of clopidogrel to its active metabolite, decreasing the effectiveness of clopidogrel. For this reason, many people suggest not using clopidogrel with PPIs

Next Generation Anticoagulants

A. Direct factor Xa inhibitors—rivaroxaban, apixaban, edoxaban

1. Inhibit factor Xa directly (as opposed to stimulating AT like heparin)
2. Currently approved for DVT prophylaxis in surgical patients and stroke prophylaxis in patients

B. Direct thrombin (factor II) inhibitors—lepirudin, argatroban, dabigatran

1. Inhibitor thrombin directly
2. Lepirudin, argatroban, and dabigatran are used currently for treatment of HIT

Oncology

- A detailed description of many cancers can be found in the appropriate anatomical chapter of this book (i.e., lung cancers in pulmonary chapter, colon cancer in GI).

Epidemiology

- In order of occurrence, the most common cancers in males are prostate, lung, and colon. The cancers with the highest mortality in males are lung, followed by prostate and colon.
- In order of occurrence, the most common cancers in females are breast, lung, and colon. The cancers with the highest mortality in females are lung, followed by breast and colon.
- The number one avoidable risk factor for most cancers is smoking. All patients should be encouraged to stop smoking.
- Other etiologic agents in cancer include viruses (Hepatitis B/C for hepatocellular carcinoma, HPV in cervical cancer), chemicals (asbestos, ethanol, aflatoxin, cadmium, silica), and UV light.

Cancer Prevention and Screening

- Breast cancer—annual mammogram beginning at age 40 years for females.
- Cervical cancer—Quadrivalent HPV vaccine (Gardasil) protects against high-risk HPV, approved in females ages 9 to 26 years old. Begin annual pap smears at age 21 even if not sexually active.
- Colorectal cancer (CRC)—begin colonoscopy screening (q10 years) for average risk people. If first-degree CRC, begin screening at age 40 or 10 years before the age of diagnosis of relative (whichever earlier).
- Prostate cancer—despite ongoing trials, currently there is no consensus that screening with measuring prostate-specific antigen (PSA) levels decreases mortality.
- Lung cancer—screen any previous or current smoker (with minumum 30 pack years history) for lung cancer using low-dose CT between ages 55 to 80, annually (NLST trial showed 20% reduction in mortality in CT cohort vs. chest x-ray cohort).

Principles of Cancer Staging and Therapy

- Cancer is usually treated by three disciplines—surgery, chemotherapy, and radiation.
- Clinical staging is usually performed by clinical examination and imaging techniques (PET, CT, MRI scans). TNM staging is most commonly employed. T (T1-T4) describes the size of the primary tumor and whether it has invaded any nearby tissue, N (N1-N3) describes extent of tumor spread to regional lymph nodes, and M (M0 or M1) indicates presence or absence of any distant metastatic disease.
- Pathologic staging is defined after surgical resection and can give more precise information with regards to local or distant spread of the tumor.

A. Surgical oncology

1. Goal is to resect primary tumor with negative margins
2. Many times these surgeries involve excision or sampling of locoregional lymph nodes
3. Closely work with medical and radiation oncologists to determine optimal treatment plan based on accurate clinical staging and evidence-based medicine

B. Radiation oncology

Basics of Radiation Therapy

1. Therapy using ionizing radiation that is generated by either megavoltage linear accelerators, heavy ions (protons, neutrons, carbon ions), or radioisotopes (i.e., iodine-131 for thyroid cancer).
2. Can either be given via an external beam (EBRT or stereotactic radiosurgery), sealed source that is implanted in or near a tumor (brachytherapy), or as a radiation source conjugated to antibodies (radioimmunotherapy).

Mechanism of Action

1. Photons interact with biologic matter and deposit energy into DNA either directly or indirectly (through generation of reactive oxygen species) that leads to DNA damage.
2. DNA double-strand breaks are the critical determinant of cellular response to radiation and eventual cell death.

Clinical Radiation Oncology

1. Radiation is primarily used in conjunction with surgery as adjuvant therapy to prevent local tumor recurrence. However, with the advent of new technologies that allow for dose escalation while sparing normal tissues, radiation is also used as definitive therapy (stereotactic radiosurgery for inoperable brain tumors and early stage lung cancers), or as neoadjuvant therapy to shrink tumors prior to surgery.

C. Medical oncology

Chemotherapy

1. Primary use is when cancer has spread systemically with distant metastatic disease.
2. Also used in the adjuvant setting to prevent tumor recurrence and neoadjuvant setting to decrease size of tumor to make it resectable. Chemotherapy is definitive therapy for most leukemias to consolidate disease and to induce a remission.

Mechanisms of Action

1. The list of chemotherapeutic agents is too vast to be covered in this section but key categories are DNA alkylating agents (melphalan, cyclophosphamide, cisplatin, carboplatin), antimetabolites (methotrexate, cytarabine, gemcitabine, fluorouracil), antimicrotubule agents (vincristine, paclitaxel, docetaxel), topoisomerase inhibitors (irinotecan, topotecan), and anthracyclines (doxorubicin, daunorubicin, bleomycin).
2. Next generation chemotherapeutic agents are attempting to target specific mutations that give rise to cancer and drive oncogenesis. Examples of these include imatinib (targets the tyrosine kinase that is aberrantly upregulated in the majority of chronic myelogenous leukemias), trastuzumab (blocks Her2/neu receptor

Quick HIT

Oncologic emergencies which necessitate immediate treatment include hypercalcemia (IV fluids, diuretics, bisphosphonates), spinal cord compression (steroids, get MRI, surgical consult), pericardial tamponade (pericardiocentesis), and tumor lysis syndrome (IV fluids, treat individual electrolyte abnormalities).

Quick HIT

A conservative approach to all breast masses in women over the age of 30 is a biopsy. Most test questions will make it obvious if they want you to do anything other than biopsy the mass.

in breast cancers with amplification of this oncogene), and cetuximab (epidermal growth factor receptor inhibitor).

Breast Cancer

A. Risk factors—prior history of breast cancer, age, family history of breast cancer, female gender, prior thoracic radiation, smoking, alcohol consumption, and anything which increases the number of menstrual cycles (early menarche, late menopause, nulliparity).

B. Breast cancer is rare in women under 35. Instead, think of fibroadenoma if a young woman presents with a round, movable mass which changes in size over the course of the menstrual cycle. Other breast masses which may occur at any age include cysts (benign if not bloody after aspiration and does not recur) and fibrocystic changes (bilateral breast pain caused by cyclic hormonal stimulation).

C. The premalignant in situ breast cancers are ductal carcinoma in situ (DCIS) and lobular carcinoma in situ (LCIS). These entities are usually distinguished histologically.

1. DCIS represents a broad spectrum of diseases which arises from the ductal elements of the breast. It is often found on screening mammogram, and a mass may or may not be present. As this is a marker for the possible development of invasive ductal carcinoma (typically in the same breast), treat with lumpectomy or mastectomy if negative margins cannot be achieved. Radiation and systemic chemotherapy are used less often depending on the specific lesion in question.
2. LCIS arises from the lobular elements of the breast. The lesion is typically found incidentally during biopsy of another breast lesion, and a mass is rarely palpable. It leads to an increased risk of breast cancer in either breast. Unfortunately, removal of the lesion does not reduce the risk of progression to invasive cancer. Treatment is variable, but may include close observation, selective estrogen receptor modulators, and prophylactic bilateral mastectomy.

D. The two most common types of breast cancer are invasive ductal carcinoma, accounting for over 70% of invasive cancers, and invasive lobular carcinoma.

1. Patients may present with a palpable mass, palpable lymph nodes, skin dimpling, nipple retraction, or no symptoms at all (found on mammogram).
2. The diagnosis of both should be confirmed with tissue biopsy. The biopsy should also include testing for the estrogen/progesterone receptor, and Her-2/neu amplification status.
3. Treatment typically starts with surgery, with adjuvant radiotherapy if the tumor has not spread to sentinel lymph nodes to decrease tumor recurrence.
4. For all small lesions (typically <1 cm) without lymph node involvement there is no need for postsurgical chemotherapy. However, for large lesions in premenopausal women, systemic chemotherapy is recommended after surgery. For postmenopausal women with large lesions or lymph node involvement, either chemotherapy or Tamoxifen/Herceptin is recommended, depending on the status of the estrogen receptor.

Plasma Cell Disorders

Monoclonal Gammopathy of Undetermined Significance

- Common in the elderly (up to 10% in patients >75 years of age).
- Asymptomatic premalignant clonal plasma cell proliferation.
- Diagnosis: IgG spike <3.0 g; less than 10% plasma cells in bone marrow; Bence Jones proteinuria <1 g/24 hours. There should also be NO end-organ damage (lytic bone lesions, anemia, hypercalcemia, etc.)
- Fewer than 20% develop multiple myeloma in 10 to 15 years. However, several studies have shown that almost all patients with multiple myeloma had a preceding monoclonal gammopathy of undetermined significance (MGUS).
- No specific treatment is necessary, just close observation.

Multiple Myeloma

A. General characteristics

1. Multiple myeloma is neoplastic proliferation of a single plasma cell line that produces monoclonal immunoglobulin. This leads to enormous copies of one specific immunoglobulin (usually of the IgG or IgA type).
2. Incidence is increased after age 50; it is twice as common in African-American patients as in Caucasian patients.
3. The etiology is unclear.
4. As the disease process advances, bone marrow elements are replaced by malignant plasma cells. Therefore, anemia, leukopenia, and thrombocytopenia may be present in advanced disease.

B. Clinical features

1. Skeletal manifestations
   a. Bone pain due to osteolytic lesions, fractures, and vertebral collapse—occurs especially in the low back or chest (ribs) and jaw (mandible)
   b. Pathologic fractures
   c. Loss of height secondary to collapse of vertebrae
2. Anemia (normocytic normochromic)—present in most patients due to bone marrow infiltration and renal failure
3. Renal failure—mainly due to the following conditions:
   a. Myeloma nephrosis—immunoglobulin precipitation in renal tubules leads to tubular casts of **Bence Jones** protein
   b. Hypercalcemia also plays a role in renal decompensation
4. Recurrent infections
   a. Secondary to deprivation of normal immunoglobulins; therefore, humoral immunity is affected
   b. **Most common cause of death**—up to 70% of patients die of infection (lung or urinary tract most common)
5. Cord compression may occur secondary to a plasmacytoma or fractured bone fragment. Though rare, this constitutes a medical emergency. Get MRI of entire spine and start steroids immediately

C. Diagnosis

1. Serum and urine protein electrophoresis
   a. Monoclonal spike due to a malignant clone of plasma cells synthesizing a single Ig (usually IgG) called a monoclonal protein (M-protein)
   b. Serum monoclonal protein is present in 85% of patients, and 75% have a urine monoclonal protein
2. Plain radiographs detect lytic bone lesions
3. Bone marrow biopsy is essential for diagnosis and reveals at least 10% abnormal plasma cells
4. Other laboratory findings
   a. Hypercalcemia (due to bone destruction)
   b. Increased total protein in serum due to paraproteins in blood (hyperglobulinemia)
   c. Peripheral smear—RBCs are in **rouleaux formation**, which resembles a stack of poker chips. The hyperglobulinemia causes the RBCs to stick together (Figure 9-10)
   d. Substantially elevated ESR
   e. Urine—large amounts of free light chains called Bence Jones protein
   f. Leukopenia, thrombocytopenia, and anemia may be present, especially in advanced disease
   g. Elevated creatinine

D. Treatment

1. In contrast to the premalignant conditions MGUS and smoldering multiple myeloma, patients with full-blown MM require treatment.

Quick HIT

The signs of multiple myeloma can be remembered using the mnemonic CRAB for **C**alcium (hypercalcemia), **R**enal failure, **A**nemia, and **B**one lesions (lytic)

Quick HIT

Low hemoglobin, high calcium, high serum protein, and poor renal function suggest multiple myeloma.

Quick HIT

Diagnostic criteria for multiple myeloma: at least 10% abnormal plasma cells in bone marrow **plus** one of the following:
- M-protein in the serum
- M-protein in the urine
- Lytic bone lesions (well-defined radiolucencies on radiographs)—predominantly found in the skull and axial skeleton

Quick HIT

Almost all patients with multiple myeloma have an M-protein in either the serum or urine.

Quick HIT

- Radiographs show punched-out lytic lesions, osteoporosis, or fractures in 75% of patients with multiple myeloma.
- Osteolytic lesions are secondary to the release of osteoclast-activating factor by the neoplastic plasma cells.

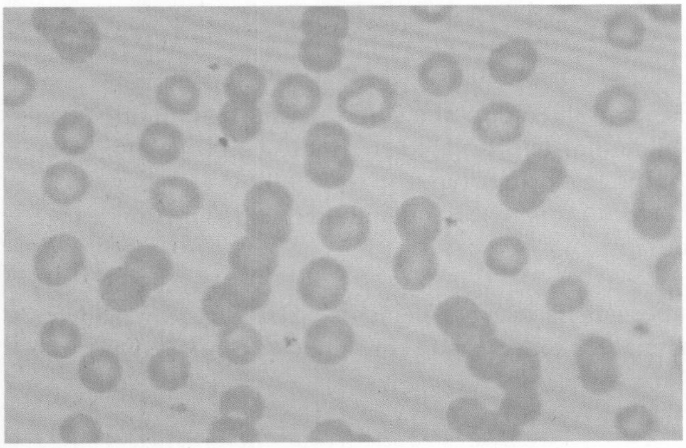

FIGURE **9-10** **Rouleaux formation (multiple myeloma).**
(From Anderson SC. *Anderson's Atlas of Hematology.* Philadelphia, PA: Wolters Kluwer Health/Lippincott Williams & Wilkins, 2003.)

2. The preferred treatment for multiple myeloma is autologous hematopoietic cell transplantation (HCT), as this has been shown to have better survival rates when compared to chemotherapy. However, this treatment is usually reserved for younger and relatively asymptomatic patients. If you are considering HCT, you SHOULD NOT start chemotherapy, as this would preclude a patient from having HCT later on.
3. Systemic chemotherapy—preferred initial treatment (alkylating agents) for patients who are not transplant candidates.
4. Radiation therapy—if no response to chemotherapy and if disabling pain is present.

Waldenström Macroglobulinemia

- Malignant proliferation of plasmacytoid lymphocytes. These cells produce IgM paraprotein, which is very large and causes hyperviscosity of the blood.
- Diagnosis: IgM >5 g/dL; Bence Jones proteinuria in 10% of cases; **absence of bone lesions.**
- Clinical features: fatigue, weight loss, neurologic symptoms, lymphadenopathy, splenomegaly, anemia, abnormal bleeding, and hyperviscosity syndrome (due to elevated IgM).
- There is no definitive cure. Use chemotherapy and plasmapheresis for hyperviscosity syndromes.

Lymphomas

Hodgkin Lymphoma

A. General characteristics

1. Bimodal age distribution: X_1 = 15 to 30 years of age; X_2 = >50 years of age
2. Lymph node histology divides the disease into four subtypes
   a. Lymphocyte predominance (5%)—few Reed–Sternberg cells and many B cells
   b. Nodular sclerosis (70%)—occurs more frequently in women; bands of collagen envelope pools of Reed–Sternberg cells
   c. Mixed cellularity (25%)—large numbers of Reed–Sternberg cells in a pleomorphic background
   d. Lymphocyte depletion (<1%)—lacking in mix of reactive cells; associated with the worst prognosis
3. Staging is based on physical examination, CT scan (chest, abdomen, pelvis), and bone marrow biopsy. **Ann Arbor staging system:**
   a. Stages
      - Stage I: confined to single lymph node
      - Stage II: involvement of two or more lymph nodes but confined to same side of diaphragm

Quick HIT
Multiple myeloma has a poor prognosis with a median survival of only 2 to 4 years with treatment, and only a few months without treatment. The 5-year survival rate is about 10%.

Quick HIT
Hyperviscosity syndrome can lead to retinal vessel dilation with resulting hemorrhage and possible blindness.

Quick HIT
- Lymphomas are cancers of the lymphatic system. There are two types: Hodgkin disease and NHL.
- Lymphadenopathy is usually the first finding in lymphomas.

Quick HIT
The histologic type does not greatly influence the prognosis of Hodgkin disease (with the exception of the lymphocyte-depleted type, which has the worst prognosis). Treatment is effective in most patients with the other histologic types of Hodgkin disease.

Quick HIT
Chemotherapy and radiation therapy in combination achieve cure rates of over 70% in Hodgkin disease.

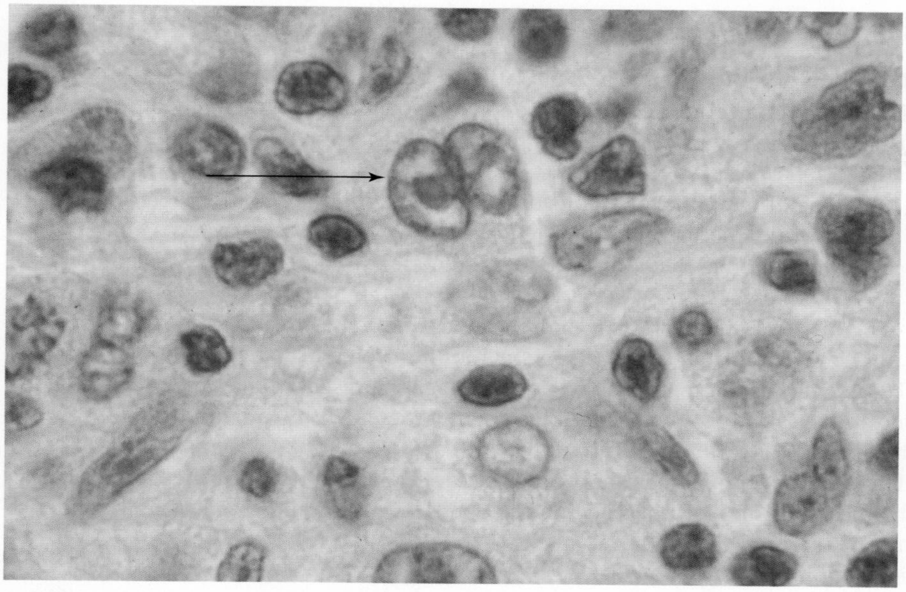

FIGURE 9-11 **Reed–Sternberg cells (Hodgkin lymphoma).**
(From Anderson SC. *Anderson's Atlas of Hematology.* Philadelphia, PA: Wolters Kluwer Health/Lippincott Williams & Wilkins, 2003.)

- Stage III: both sides of diaphragm involved
- Stage IV: dissemination of disease to extralymphatic sites

b. Suffixes
- A: No symptoms
- B: Fever, weight loss, night sweats (presence of these constitutional symptoms worsens the prognosis)

B. Clinical features

1. Most common symptom is a painless lymphadenopathy
2. Supraclavicular, cervical, axillary, mediastinal lymph nodes
3. Spreads by continuity from one lymph node to adjacent lymph nodes
4. Other presentations may or may not be present, including B symptoms (fever, night sweats, weight loss), pruritus, and cough (secondary to mediastinal lymph node involvement)

C. Diagnosis

1. Lymph node biopsy—the presence of **Reed–Sternberg cells** is required to make the diagnosis (Figure 9-11)
   a. Neoplastic, large cell with two or more nuclei; look like owl's eyes
   b. Usually B-cell phenotype
   c. Reed–Sternberg cells may be found in other neoplasms
   d. May be rare in the nodular sclerosis variant
2. Presence of inflammatory cell infiltrates—This distinguishes Hodgkin lymphoma from non-Hodgkin lymphoma (NHL). The inflammatory cells present are reactive to the Reed–Sternberg cells. These include plasma cells, eosinophils, fibroblasts, and T and B lymphocytes.
3. CXR and CT scan (chest, abdomen)—to detect lymph node involvement
4. Bone marrow biopsy—to evaluate bone marrow involvement
5. Laboratory findings—leukocytosis, eosinophilia; level of ESR elevation sometimes corresponds with disease activity

D. Treatment consists mainly of chemotherapy and radiation therapy to the involved field.

1. Stages I, II, and IIIA can be treated with radiotherapy alone. However, some physicians advocate the use of chemotherapy in these patients as well.
2. Stages IIIB and IV require chemotherapy.

Quick HIT

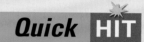

Key Epidemiologic Associations with NHL
- Burkitt lymphoma in regions of Africa
- Patients with HIV and HIV-associated lymphomas
- Adult T-cell lymphoma in Japan and the Caribbean

Quick HIT

It is beyond the scope of this chapter to give a detailed account of each specific type of NHL. Focus on the general clinical presentations as well as certain commonly tested pathologic features—see highlighted points in Table 9-6.

Quick HIT

Rituximab, **a monoclonal antibody against CD20** antigen, is often used in combination with CHOP therapy to treat NHL and other cancers with better outcomes than CHOP alone.

Quick HIT

Staging NHL—Stages I–IV depend on the extent of disease.
- Stage I—single lymph node involved (or one extralymphatic site)
- Stage II—two or more lymph nodes on the same side of the diaphragm (or localized involvement of one lymph node region and a contiguous extralymphatic site)
- Stage III—lymph node involvement on both sides of the diaphragm
- Stage IV—disseminated involvement of one or more extralymphatic organs with or without lymph node involvement

Non-Hodgkin Lymphoma

A. General characteristics

1. NHL is a diverse group of solid tumors which occurs with the malignant transformation and growth of B or T lymphocytes or their precursors in the lymphatic system.
   a. The type of lymphocyte involved and its level of differentiation determine the course of the disease and its prognosis.
   b. B-cell lymphomas account for 85% of all cases; T-cell lymphomas account for 15% of all cases.
   c. The disease usually starts in lymph nodes and may spread to blood and bone marrow. The primary tumor may be found in the GI tract.
2. NHL is twice as common as Hodgkin disease. At presentation, patients with NHL tend to have a more advanced disease than patients with Hodgkin disease.
3. The etiology of NHL is still unknown.
4. NHL is the sixth most common cause of cancer-related death in the United States. The mean age of onset varies with subtype. There is an increased overall incidence with increasing age.
5. Risk factors for NHL.
   a. HIV/AIDS.
   b. Immunosuppression (e.g., organ transplant recipients).
   c. History of certain viral infections (e.g., EBV, HTLV-1).
   d. History of *Helicobacter pylori* gastritis (risk of primary associated gastric lymphoma).
   e. Autoimmune disease—for example, Hashimoto thyroiditis or Sjögren syndrome (risk of mucosa-associated lymphoid tissue [MALT]).
6. Classification.
   a. There are more than 20 different subtypes of NHL, and they are often arranged into unique classification systems. One such classification system stratifies them according to histologic grade: **low grade** (or indolent), **intermediate grade**, and **high grade** (see Table 9-6).

B. Clinical features

1. Lymphadenopathy—sometimes the only manifestation of disease.
   a. Lymph nodes are usually painless, firm, and mobile.
   b. Enlargement of lymph nodes is often rapid.
   c. Supraclavicular, cervical, and axillary nodes are involved most often.
2. B symptoms—less common than in Hodgkin lymphoma.
3. Hepatosplenomegaly, abdominal pain, or fullness.
4. Recurrent infections, symptoms of anemia, or thrombocytopenia—due to bone marrow involvement.
5. Various other findings are possible (e.g., superior vena cava obstruction, respiratory involvement, bone pain, skin lesions).

C. Diagnosis

1. Lymph node biopsy—for definitive diagnosis. **Any lymph node >1 cm present for more than 4 weeks that cannot be attributed to infection should be biopsied.**
2. Other tests that may help in diagnosis:
   a. CXR—may reveal hilar or mediastinal adenopathy.
   b. CT scan (chest, abdomen, pelvis)—to determine extent of disease spread and patient's response to treatment.
   c. Serum LDH and β_2-microglobulin are indirect indicators of tumor burden.
   d. If alkaline phosphatase is elevated, bone or liver involvement is likely.
   e. If liver function tests or bilirubin is elevated, liver involvement is likely.
   f. CBC.
   g. Serum electrolytes, renal function tests.
   h. Bone marrow biopsy.

Quick HIT

- Low-grade lymphomas—Cure is rare. Median survival is 5 to 7 years.
- Intermediate-grade lymphomas—Fifty percent of patients can be cured with aggressive therapy. Median survival is about 2 years.
- High-grade lymphomas—Up to 70% can be cured with aggressive therapy. Median survival without treatment is a few months.

TABLE 9-6 **Non-Hodgkin Lymphomas**

Grade[a]	Type[a]	Key Features	Prognosis
Indolent or Low Grade	Small lymphocytic lymphoma	• **Closely related to CLL;** more common in elderly patients • **Indolent course**	• Eventually results in widespread lymph node involvement with dissemination to liver, spleen, and bone marrow • Most patients with localized disease can be cured with radiotherapy, but only 15% of patients do have localized disease • Median survival is approximately 10 yrs
	Follicular, predominantly small, cleaved-cell lymphoma	• **Most common form of NHL** • Mean age of onset is 55 • May transform into diffuse, large cell; associated with translocation: t(14;18) • Indolent course • **Presents with painless, peripheral lymphadenopathy**	
Intermediate	Diffuse, large-cell lymphoma	• Predominantly B-cell origin • Middle-aged and elderly patients • **Locally invasive; presents as large extranodal mass**	• 85% cure rate with CHOP therapy
High Grade	Lymphoblastic lymphoma	• **T-cell lymphoma;** more common in children • **May progress to T-ALL** • 50% of patients have B symptoms	• **Aggressive with rapid dissemination,** but may respond to combination chemotherapy
	Burkitt (small noncleaved-cell) lymphoma	• **B-cell lymphoma;** more common in children • Two types: African and American; the African variety involves facial bone and jaw, whereas the American variety often involves abdominal organs (hepatomegaly, abdominal masses, lymphadenopathy) • **African variety linked with EBV infection** • **Associated with specific translocation: t(8;14)**	• Grave prognosis unless treated very aggressively with chemotherapy • Treatment may cure 50%–60% of patients
Miscellaneous Lymphomas	Mycosis fungoides	• T-cell lymphoma of the skin • Presents with **eczematoid skin lesions** that progress to generalized erythroderma • **Cribriform shape of lymphocytes** • Disseminate to lymph nodes, blood, and other organs	• Depends on degree of dissemination (<2 yrs if dissemination has occurred) • Potentially curable (with radiation, topical chemotherapy) if limited to skin
	Sézary syndrome	Involves skin as well as blood stream	
	HIV-associated lymphomas	Not a discrete entity: usually Burkitt or diffuse, large-cell lymphoma	• Very poor prognosis

[a]Not all types for each grade are included in this table.

D. Treatment

1. This varies depending on the stage and subtype of NHL. There is not always a standard treatment for a given type of NHL.
2. Indolent forms of NHL are not curable, but have a 5-year survival rate of 75%. These patients are treated in a variety of ways, depending on the patient's age, comorbidities, stage of disease, and wishes, as follows:
   a. Observation.
   b. Chemotherapy (single-agent or combination).
   c. Radiation therapy.
3. Intermediate and high-grade NHLs may be curable with aggressive treatments, but if complete remission is not achieved, survival is usually less than 2 years. In general, aggressive forms are treated with multiple regimens of combination chemotherapy (e.g., CHOP) and radiation therapy.
4. Very high-dose chemotherapy with bone marrow transplantation is a last resort.

Quick HIT

CHOP therapy consists of:
- **C**yclophosphamide
- **H**ydroxydaunomycin (doxorubicin)
- **O**ncovin (vincristine)
- **P**rednisone

Quick HIT

Acute leukemias account for 60% of all leukemias, 25% are CLL and 15% are CML.

Quick HIT

General Evaluation in Patients with Leukemias (acute or chronic)
Evaluate the patient for:
- Evidence of infection
- Evidence of bleeding or easy bruising
- Lymphadenopathy, hepatosplenomegaly
- Signs of anemia
- Fatigue, weight loss

Quick HIT

For testing purposes, the age of a patient can be a simple yet important aid to confirming the correct leukemia diagnosis. Patients less than 15 most likely have ALL, while those greater than 65 typically have CLL. AML and CML both typically present from age 40 to 60.

Leukemias

Acute Leukemias

A. General characteristics

1. Two types
   a. Acute myelogenous leukemia (AML)
      - Neoplasm of myelogenous progenitor cells
      - AML occurs mostly in adults (accounts for 80% of adult acute leukemias)
      - Risk factors include exposure to radiation, myeloproliferative syndromes, Down syndrome, and chemotherapy (e.g., alkylating agents)
      - Response to therapy is not as favorable as in acute lymphoblastic leukemia (ALL)
      - One important variant of AML is APL. This condition is characterized by t(15;17) and often presents with pancytopenia. Patients may be very sick, so treatment should be started with all-trans retinoic acid (ATRA) without delay along with concurrent chemotherapy once the diagnosis is confirmed (see Clinical Pearl 9-5)

   b. ALL
      - ALL is a neoplasm of early lymphocytic precursors. Histology reveals a predominance of lymphoblasts
      - **ALL is the most common malignancy in children under age 15 in the United States**
      - It is the leukemia most responsive to therapy
      - Poor prognostic indicators are as follows: age <2 or >9; WBC $>10^5/\text{mm}^3$; and/or CNS involvement
      - Presence of any of the following is associated with an increased risk for CNS involvement: B-cell phenotype, increased LDH, rapid leukemic cell proliferation
2. Many patients with acute leukemias can be cured if they are treated aggressively. However, the most aggressive acute leukemias can be fatal within months

B. Clinical features

1. Anemia and associated symptoms
2. Increased risk of bacterial infections (due to neutropenia)
   a. Pneumonia, urinary tract infection, cellulitis, pharyngitis, esophagitis
   b. Associated with high morbidity and mortality; potentially life-threatening
3. Abnormal mucosal or cutaneous bleeding (due to thrombocytopenia)—for example, epistaxis, bleeding at puncture sites, petechiae, ecchymosis
4. Splenomegaly, hepatomegaly, lymphadenopathy
5. Bone and joint pain (invasion of periosteum)
6. CNS involvement—diffuse or focal neurologic dysfunction (e.g., meningitis, seizures)

CLINICAL PEARL 9-5

Leukemias

- Leukemias are characterized by neoplastic proliferation of abnormal WBCs. As these abnormal WBCs accumulate, they interfere with the production of normal WBCs, as well as the production of erythrocytes and platelets, resulting in anemia and thrombocytopenia.
- Leukemias are classified in two ways.
  - The type of WBC affected.
    - If granulocytes or monocytes are affected, myelogenous leukemia is present.
    - If lymphocytes are affected, lymphocytic leukemia is present.
  - The maturity of cells affected and the rapidity of disease progression.
    - Acute leukemias are characterized by rapid progression and affect immature cells (i.e., immature cells proliferate before maturation).
    - Chronic leukemias progress slowly and affect mature cells.

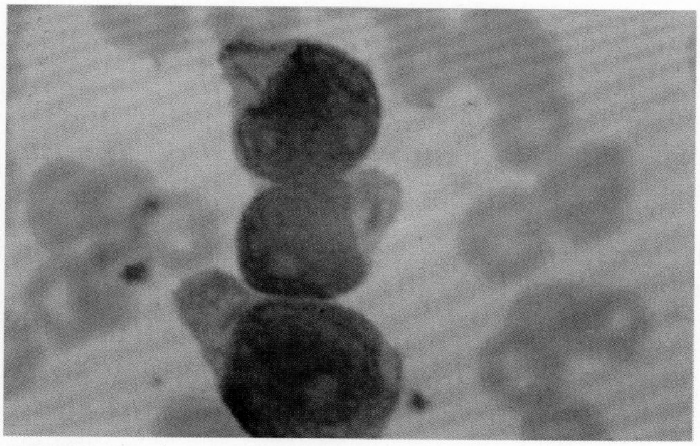

FIGURE 9-12 **Auer rods (acute myelogenous leukemia).**
(From Handin RI, Lux SE, Stossel TP. *Blood: Principles and Practice of Hematology.* Philadelphia: Lippincott Williams & Wilkins, 2003.)

7. Testicular involvement (ALL)
8. Anterior mediastinal mass (T-cell ALL)
9. Skin nodules (AML)

C. Diagnosis

1. Laboratory findings
   a. The WBC count is variable (from 1,000/mm^3 to 100,000/mm^3). There are significant numbers of blast cells (immature cells) in peripheral blood
   b. Anemia
   c. Thrombocytopenia—monitor platelet counts regularly
   d. Granulocytopenia—puts the patient at high risk for infection
   e. Electrolyte disturbances (hyperuricemia, hyperkalemia, hyperphosphatemia)
2. Bone marrow biopsy is required for diagnosis
   a. In ALL, you will see proliferation of lymphoblasts in the bone marrow (20% or greater)
   b. In AML, you will see Auer rods, especially if it is the APL phenotype (Figure 9-12)

D. Treatment

1. Treatment of emergencies.
   a. Blood cultures, antibiotics for infections.
   b. Blood transfusion for anemia and platelet transfusion for bleeding, if necessary
2. Aggressive, combination chemotherapy in high doses for several weeks is appropriate to obtain remission (i.e., absent leukemic cells in bone marrow). Once remission occurs, maintenance therapy is used for months or years to prevent recurrence.
   a. ALL: More than 75% of children with ALL achieve complete remission (compared with 30% to 40% of adults). Relapses, when they occur, usually respond to treatment. With aggressive therapy, survival rates in children can be up to 15 years or longer. Up to 50% of patients are cured.
   b. AML: This is more difficult to treat and does not respond as well to chemotherapy. Survival rates are considerably lower despite intensive treatment. Bone marrow transplantation gives the best chance of remission or cure.
3. Bone marrow transplantation.

Chronic Lymphocytic Leukemia

A. General characteristics

1. CLL is the most common leukemia that occurs after age 50. Most patients with CLL are >60 years of age. It is the most common leukemia in the Western world.
2. The cause is unknown.

Quick HIT

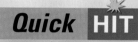

Auer rods (granules and eosinophilic rods inside malignant cells) are present in AML but not ALL.

Quick HIT

Tumor Lysis Syndrome
- This is a potential complication of chemotherapy seen in acute leukemia and high-grade NHL.
- Rapid cell death with release of intracellular contents causes hyperkalemia, hyperphosphatemia, and hyperuricemia.
- Treat as a medical emergency.

3. Monoclonal proliferation of lymphocytes that are morphologically mature but functionally defective (i.e., they do not differentiate into antibody-manufacturing plasma cells).
4. In general, this is the least aggressive type of leukemia, and CLL patients survive longer than those with acute leukemias or chronic myeloid leukemia (CML). The course is variable, but may follow a prolonged indolent course. Many patients die of other causes.
5. The most recent WHO classification released in 2008 describes CLL as identical to the indolent NHL B-cell neoplasm small lymphocytic leukemia. That is, they are considered the same disease at different stages.

B. Clinical features

1. Usually asymptomatic at time of diagnosis; CLL may be discovered on a routine CBC (lymphocytosis).
2. Generalized painless lymphadenopathy (lymph nodes are nontender), splenomegaly.
3. Frequent respiratory or skin infections due to immune deficiency.
4. In more advanced disease: fatigue, weight loss, pallor, skin rashes, easy bruising, bone tenderness, and/or abdominal pain.

> **Quick HIT**
> AIHAs can be seen in patients with CML.

C. Diagnosis

1. Laboratory findings
   a. CBC—WBC: 50,000 to 200,000
   b. Anemia, thrombocytopenia, and neutropenia are common
   c. Peripheral blood smear is often diagnostic
      - Absolute lymphocytosis—almost all of the WBCs are mature, small lymphocytes
      - Presence of **smudge cells**—"fragile" leukemic cells that are broken when placed on a glass slide
   d. Flow cytometry of the peripheral blood will show clonal population of B cells
2. Bone marrow biopsy—presence of infiltrating leukemic cells in bone marrow

> **Quick HIT**
> Remember that the cells of the myeloid line are erythrocytes, granulocytes, and platelets.

D. Treatment

1. Chemotherapy has little effect on overall survival, but is given for symptomatic relief and reduction of infection. Patients are often observed until symptoms develop.
2. Prognosis is variable depending on the number of lymph node sites involved and the presence or absence of anemia/thrombocytopenia.

> **Quick HIT**
> Differentiating benign leukemoid reaction from CML leukemoid reaction
> - Usually no splenomegaly
> - Increased leukocyte alkaline phosphatase
> - History of a precipitating event (e.g., infection)
> - CML—opposite to the above findings

Chronic Myeloid Leukemia

A. General characteristics

1. Neoplastic, clonal proliferation of myeloid stem cells.
2. Patients are usually older than 40 years of age.
3. CML follows an indolent (chronic) course for many years before it transforms to acute leukemia. The end point of the disease course is usually an acute phase (or **blast crisis**), which is an accelerated phase of blast and promyelocyte production.
4. It is associated with translocation t(9,22). The fusion of the BCR gene on chromosome 22 with the ABL1 gene on chromosome 9 results in the Philadelphia chromosome—present in more than 90% of patients. The abnormal chromosome results in a constitutively active tyrosine kinase protein, which is targeted by imatinib. Note that patients without the Philadelphia chromosome have shorter survival times and respond more poorly to treatment.

> **Quick HIT**
> Treat CML with TKIs, either imatinib, dasatinib, or nilotinib.

B. Clinical features

1. Most patients present in the chronic phase (85%). These patients may be asymptomatic at the time of diagnosis—disease discovered on routine blood work.
2. Constitutional symptoms are also common presenting symptoms—fevers, night sweats, anorexia, weight loss.
3. Recurrent infections, easy bruising/bleeding, symptoms of anemia.

4. Splenomegaly, hepatomegaly, lymphadenopathy.
5. Patients may also present in more advanced stages, either the accelerated phase or blast crisis.

C. Diagnosis

1. Laboratory findings
   a. Marked leukocytosis—WBCs from 50,000 to 200,000 with a left shift toward granulocytes
   b. Small numbers of blasts and promyelocytes
   c. Eosinophilia
   d. Peripheral smear—leukemic cells in the peripheral blood: myelocytes, metamyelocytes, bands, and segmented form
   e. **Decreased leukocyte alkaline phosphatase activity**
   f. Thrombocytosis
   g. Bone marrow biopsy: leukemic cells

D. Treatment

1. Treatment for CML is one of the great stories of modern medicine. After the mechanism was elucidated, the oral tyrosine kinase inhibitor (TKI) imatinib was developed. This drug targets the dysfunctional chimeric protein bcr-abl formed by the t(9,22) Philadelphia chromosome. Second-generation TKIs are now available, and early results have shown them to be even better.
2. Unfortunately, patients who present in a blast crisis still have very poor outcomes. The TKIs can still be attempted in these patients. Stem cell transplantation is also an option.

Quick HIT

Imatinib is current standard of care for CML.

Myeloproliferative Disorders

Polycythemia Vera

A. General characteristics

1. Malignant clonal proliferation of hematopoietic stem cells leading to excessive erythrocyte production.
2. The increase in RBC mass occurs independent of erythropoietin.
3. The median survival with treatment is about 9 to 14 years.
4. Mutations in the JAK2 tyrosine kinase are found in >90% of polycythemia vera cases.

B. Clinical features

1. Symptoms due to hyperviscosity: headache, dizziness, weakness, **pruritus**, visual impairment, dyspnea
2. **Thrombotic phenomena**—DVT, CVA, myocardial infarction, portal vein thrombosis
3. **Bleeding**—GI or genitourinary bleeding, ecchymoses, epistaxis
4. Splenomegaly, hepatomegaly
5. HTN

C. Diagnosis

1. Rule out causes of secondary polycythemia (e.g., hypoxemia, carbon monoxide exposure)
2. CBC
   a. **Elevated RBC count, hemoglobin, hematocrit (usually >50)**
   b. Thrombocytosis, leukocytosis may be present
3. Serum erythropoietin levels are reduced
4. Elevated vitamin B_{12} level
5. Hyperuricemia is common
6. Bone marrow biopsy confirms the diagnosis

D. Treatment

1. Repeated phlebotomy to lower hematocrit

Quick HIT

An often-tested presentation for PV is a patient who complains of severe pruritus after a hot bath or shower.

Quick HIT

Diagnostic Criteria for Polycythemia Vera
Must have all three major criteria or any two major criteria plus any two minor criteria:

Major Criteria
- Elevated RBC mass (men >36 L/kg; women >32 L/kg)
- Arterial oxygen saturation >92%
- Splenomegaly

Minor Criteria
- Thrombocytosis (platelet count >400 × 109/L)
- Leukocytosis >12 × 109/L
- Leukocyte alkaline phosphatase >100 (no fever or infection)
- Serum vitamin B_{12} >900 pg/mL

Myelodysplastic Syndromes

A. General characteristics

1. Myelodysplastic syndromes are a class of acquired clonal blood disorders. They are characterized by ineffective hematopoiesis, with apoptosis of myeloid precursors. The result is pancytopenia, despite a normal or hypercellular bone marrow
2. They occur more commonly in elderly patients, and are slightly more common in men
3. Causes
   a. Usually idiopathic
   b. Exposure to radiation, immunosuppressive agents, and certain toxins are known risk factors for development of myelodysplastic syndromes
4. They are classified into subtypes according to findings on bone marrow biopsy and peripheral smear
5. The prognosis, although variable, is generally poor and the end result is often progression to acute leukemia

Quick HIT

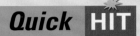

Hyperviscosity and elevated total blood volume in polycythemia vera account for most of the clinical findings.

B. Clinical features

1. They are often asymptomatic in the early stages. Pancytopenia may be an incidental finding on a routine blood test.
2. They may present with manifestations of anemia, thrombocytopenia, or neutropenia.

Quick HIT

Thrombotic and hemorrhagic complications in polycythemia vera can be life-threatening.

C. Diagnosis

1. Bone marrow biopsy typically shows dysplastic marrow cells with blasts or ringed sideroblasts.
2. CBC with peripheral smear shows the following:
   a. Normal or mildly elevated MCV.
   b. Low reticulocyte count.
   c. Other abnormalities may include **Howell–Jolly bodies**, basophilic stippling, nucleated RBCs, hypolobulated neutrophilic nuclei, and large, agranular platelets.
3. Cytogenic studies often reveal chromosomal abnormalities or mutated oncogenes.

Quick HIT

Clinical features in myelodysplastic syndromes are due to bone marrow failure and mimic those of aplastic anemia.

D. Treatment

1. Treatment is mainly supportive.
   a. RBC and platelet transfusions are the mainstays of treatment.
   b. Erythropoietin may help to reduce the number of blood transfusions necessary.
   c. Granulocyte colony-stimulating factor can be an effective adjunctive treatment for neutropenic patients.
   d. Vitamin supplementation, particularly with vitamins B_6, B_{12}, and folate, is important given the large turnover of marrow cells.
2. Pharmacologic therapies have variable results.
   a. Immunosuppressive agents.
   b. Chemotherapy.
   c. Androgenic steroids.
3. Bone marrow transplantation is the only potential cure.

Essential Thrombocythemia

- Defined as platelet count >600,000/mm^3.
- A diagnosis of exclusion. Reactive thrombocytosis (due to infection, inflammation, bleeding, and so on) and other myeloproliferative disorders must be excluded.
- It is primarily manifested by thrombosis (e.g., CVA), or paradoxically and less frequently, bleeding (due to defective platelet function). It is a disease with high morbidity but low mortality.
- Other findings may include splenomegaly, pseudohyperkalemia, and elevated bleeding time. Erythromelalgia is burning pain and erythema of the extremities due to microvascular occlusions.
- Peripheral smear shows hypogranular, abnormally shaped platelets.
- Bone marrow biopsy shows an increased number of megakaryocytes.
- JAK2 tyrosine kinase mutation seen in 40% to 50% of cases.
- Treatment usually involves antiplatelet agents such as anagrelide and low-dose aspirin. Hydroxyurea is sometimes used for severe thrombocytosis.

INFECTIOUS DISEASES

10

Infections of the Upper and Lower Respiratory Tracts

Pneumonia

A. General characteristics

1. There are two types of pneumonia: community-acquired and nosocomial
   a. Community-acquired pneumonia (CAP)
      - Occurs in the community or within first 72 hours of hospitalization
      - Can be typical or atypical
      - **Most common bacterial pathogen is *Streptococcus pneumoniae***
   b. Nosocomial pneumonia
      - Occurs during hospitalization after first 72 hours
      - **Most common bacterial pathogens are gram-negative rods (*Escherichia* coli, *Pseudomonas*) and *Staphylococcus aureus***
2. There are two recommended methods of prevention
   a. Influenza vaccine—give yearly to people at increased risk for complications and to healthcare workers
   b. Pneumococcal vaccine—for patients >65 years and for younger people at high risk (e.g., those with heart disease, cochlear implants, sickle cell disease, pulmonary disease, diabetes, alcoholic cirrhosis, or asplenic individuals)

B. Typical CAP

1. Common agents
   a. *S. pneumoniae* (60%)
   b. *Haemophilus influenzae* (15%)
   c. Aerobic gram-negative rods (6% to 10%)—*Klebsiella* (and other Enterobacteriaceae)
   d. *S. aureus* (2% to 10%)
2. Clinical features
   a. Symptoms
      - Acute onset of fever and shaking chills
      - Cough productive of thick, purulent sputum
      - Pleuritic chest pain (suggests pleural effusion)
      - Dyspnea
   b. Signs
      - Tachycardia, tachypnea
      - Late inspiratory crackles, bronchial breath sounds, increased tactile and vocal fremitus, dullness on percussion
      - Pleural friction rub (associated with pleural effusion)
3. Chest radiograph (CXR)
   a. Lobar consolidation
   b. Multilobar consolidation indicates very serious illness

Quick HIT

- "Classic" CAP presents with a sudden chill followed by fever, pleuritic pain, and productive cough.
- The "atypical pneumonia" syndrome, associated with *Mycoplasma* or *Chlamydia* infection, often begins with a sore throat and headache followed by a nonproductive cough and dyspnea.

Quick HIT

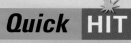

Most cases of CAP result from aspiration of oropharyngeal secretions because the majority of organisms that cause CAP are **normal inhabitants of the pharynx.**

Quick HIT

S. pneumoniae accounts for up to 66% of all cases of bacteremic pneumonia, followed by *H. influenzae,* influenza virus, and *Legionella* spp.

Quick HIT

Studies have shown that if vital signs are entirely normal, the probability of pneumonia in outpatients is less than 1%.

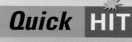

Quick HIT

"Atypical" pneumonia refers to organisms not visible on Gram stain and not culturable on standard blood agar.

Quick HIT

Sputum Culture CAP

- The value of routine sputum collection for Gram stain and culture is controversial. The Infectious Disease Society of America has recently advocated performing sputum Gram stain and culture in all patients hospitalized with CAP.
- A good sputum specimen has >25 PMNs and <10 epithelial cells per low-power field.

C. Atypical CAP

1. Common agents
   a. *Mycoplasma pneumoniae* (most common)
   b. *Chlamydia pneumoniae*
   c. *Chlamydia psittaci*
   d. *Coxiella burnetii* (Q fever)
   e. *Legionella* spp.
   f. Viruses: influenza virus (A and B), adenoviruses, parainfluenza virus, RSV
2. Clinical features
   a. Symptoms
      - Insidious onset—headache, sore throat, fatigue, myalgias
      - Dry cough (no sputum production)
      - Fevers (chills are uncommon)
   b. Signs
      - Pulse-temperature dissociation—normal pulse in the setting of high fever is suggestive of atypical CAP
      - Wheezing, rhonchi, crackles
   c. CXR
      - Diffuse reticulonodular infiltrates
      - Absent or minimal consolidation

D. Diagnosis

1. PA and lateral CXR required to confirm the diagnosis (Figure 10-1) (see also Clinical Pearls 10-1 and 10-2).
   a. Considered sensitive—if CXR findings are not suggestive of pneumonia, do not treat the patient with antibiotics.

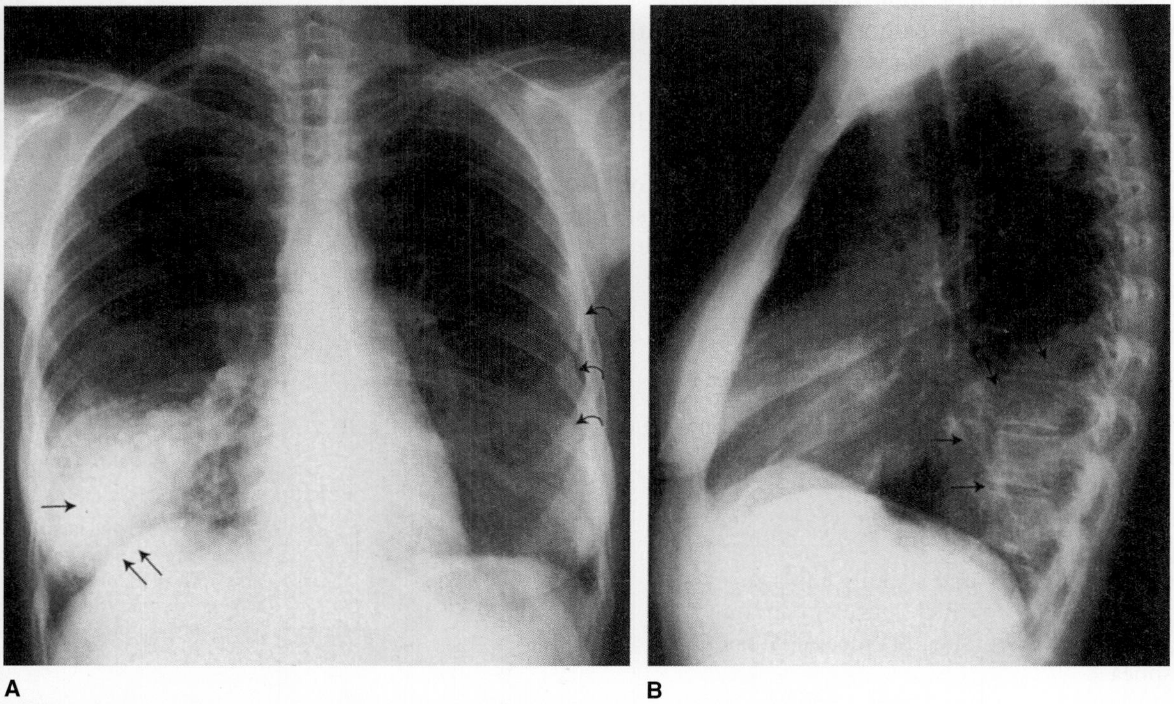

FIGURE 10-1 **Chest PA (A) and lateral (B) radiographs: Right lower lobe pneumonia (*straight arrows*). On the PA radiograph, the right cardiac border is clearly visible, and the right hemidiaphragm is partially silhouetted (*double straight arrows*). These findings indicate that the infiltrate is posterior or in the right lower lobe as confirmed on the lateral radiograph (*straight arrows*).**

(From Erkonen WE, Smith WL. *Radiology 101: The Basics and Fundamentals of Imaging.* Philadelphia, PA: Lippincott Williams & Wilkins, 1998:110, Figure 6-54A and B.)

CLINICAL PEARL 10-1

General Approach to Diagnosis of CAP

The first task is to **differentiate lower respiratory tract infection from the other causes of cough and from upper respiratory infection.**

- If nasal discharge, sore throat, or ear pain predominates, upper respiratory infection is likely.
- Once lower tract infection is suspected, the next task is to differentiate between pneumonia and acute bronchitis. Unfortunately, clinical features (cough, sputum, fever, dyspnea) are not reliable in differentiating between the two.
- CXR is the only reasonable method of differentiating between pneumonia and acute bronchitis.

b. After treatment, changes evident on CXR usually lag behind the clinical response (up to 6 weeks).
c. Changes include interstitial infiltrates, lobar consolidation, and/or cavitation.
d. False-negative chest radiographs occur with neutropenia, dehydration, infection with PCP (*Pneumocystis carinii* pneumonia), and early disease (<24 hours).

2. Pretreatment expectorated sputum for Gram stain and culture—low sensitivity and specificity, but still worthwhile tests because antimicrobial resistance is an increasing problem.
   a. Sputum Gram stain—try to obtain in all patients.
      - Commonly contaminated with oral secretions.
      - A good specimen has a sensitivity of 60% and specificity of 85% for identifying gram-positive cocci in chains (*S. pneumoniae*).
   b. Sputum culture—try to obtain in all patients requiring hospitalization.
      - Specificity is improved if the predominant organism growing on the culture media correlates with the Gram stain.
3. Special stains of the sputum in selected cases.
   a. Acid-fast stain (*Mycobacterium* spp.) if tuberculosis (TB) is suspected.
   b. Silver stain (fungi, *P. carinii*) for HIV/immunocompromised patients.
4. Urinary antigen assay for *Legionella* in selected patients.
   a. This test is very sensitive.
   b. The antigen persists in the urine for weeks (even after treatment has been started).
5. Consider two pretreatment blood cultures from different sites. Blood cultures positive in 5% to 15% of cases.

E. Treatment of CAP

1. Decision to hospitalize.
   a. **The decision to hospitalize or treat as an outpatient is probably the most important decision to be made and is based on severity of disease** (see Table 10-1).
   b. Patients are stratified into five classes based on severity (see Table 10-1). The pneumonia severity index can serve as a general guideline, but clinical judgment is critical in making this decision. The decision to admit the patient is not based on a specific organism (one does not have this information when making this decision).

CLINICAL PEARL 10-2

Pneumonia Pearls

- In alcoholics, think of Klebsiella pneumonia; in immigrants, think of TB.
- In nursing home residents, consider a nosocomial pathogen and predilection for the upper lobes (e.g., *Pseudomonas*).
- HIV-positive patients are at risk for *P. carinii* and *M. tuberculosis*, but are still more likely to have a typical infectious agent.
- *Legionella* pneumonia is common in organ transplant recipients, patients with renal failure, patients with chronic lung disease, and smokers and presents with GI symptoms and hyponatremia. *Legionella* pneumonia is rare in healthy children and young adults.

Quick HIT

Patients admitted to the hospital with suspected pneumonia should get:
- CXR (PA and lateral)
- Laboratory tests—CBC and differential, BUN, creatinine, glucose, electrolytes
- O2 saturation
- Two pretreatment blood cultures
- Gram stain and culture of sputum
- Antibiotic therapy

Quick HIT

Radiographic changes and clinical findings do not help in identifying the causative pathogen in CAP.

Quick HIT

Test for microbial diagnosis for outpatients is not required. Empiric treatment is often successful if CAP is suspected.

Quick HIT

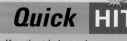

If patient is hypoxic or hypotensive, admit to hospital.

Quick HIT

Uncomplicated CAP in patients without significant comorbidities, treat with azithromycin or clarithromycin. If patient has comorbidities, give a fluoroquinolone.

TABLE 10-1 Pneumonia Severity Index

Patient Characteristic	Points
Demographics	
Male	Female
Nursing home resident	1 Age (yr)
1 Age (yr)	–10
	110
Comorbid illness	
Neoplastic disease	130
Liver disease	120
Congestive heart failure	110
Cerebrovascular disease	110
Renal failure	110
Physical examination	
Altered mental status	120
Respiratory rate >30	120
Systolic BP <90	120
Temp <95°F or >104°F	115
Heart rate >125	110
Laboratory and radiographic findings	
Arterial pH <7.35	130
BUN >64	120
Sodium <130	120
Glucose >250	110
Hematocrit <30%	110
Partial pressure of arterial oxygen <60 or oxygen saturation <90%	110
Pleural effusion	110

ADD TOTAL POINTS FOR RISK ASSESSMENT:

Total Points	Risk	Risk Class	% Mortality	Treat as
No predictors	Low	I	0.1	Outpatient
<70	Low	II	0.6	Outpatient
71–90	Low	III	2.8	Inpatient (briefly)
91–130	Moderate	IV	8.2	Inpatient
>130	High	V	29.2	Inpatient

Adapted from Fine MJ, Auble TE, Yealy DM, et al. A prediction rule to identify low-risk patients with community-acquired pneumonia. *N Engl J Med.* 1997;336:243–250.

2. Antimicrobial therapy.
   a. Because the specific cause is usually not determined on initial evaluation, empiric therapy is often required.
   b. For outpatients.
      - In people younger than 60 years of age, the most common organisms are *S. pneumoniae, Mycoplasma, Chlamydia,* and *Legionella.* Macrolides (azithromycin or clarithromycin) or doxycycline cover all of these organisms and are the first-line treatment. Fluoroquinolones are alternative agents. Penicillins or cephalosporins do not cover the atypical organisms in this age group.

- In older adults and patients with comorbidities (more likely to have typical CAP) or those treated with antibiotics in the last 3 months, a fluoroquinolone is the first-line agent (levofloxacin, moxifloxacin). A second- or third-generation cephalosporin is the first-line treatment.
- For outpatients, treatment is continued for 5 days. Do not stop treatment until patient has been afebrile for 48 hours.

c. For hospitalized patients, a fluoroquinolone alone or a third-generation cephalosporin plus a macrolide (i.e., ceftriaxone plus azithromycin) is appropriate.

F. Treatment of hospital-acquired pneumonia

1. **Treatment is tailored toward gram-negative rods (any of the following three are appropriate):**
   a. **Cephalosporins with pseudomonal coverage: ceftazidime or cefepime**
   b. **Carbapenems: imipenem**
   c. **Piperacillin/tazobactam**
2. **Macrolides are not used (as they are in CAP)**

G. Complications

1. Pleural effusion ("parapneumonic effusions")—See Chapter 2.
   a. Can be seen in more than 50% of patients with CAP on routine CXR. Empyema is infrequent in these patients.
   b. Most of these effusions have an uncomplicated course and resolve with treatment of the pneumonia with antibiotics.
   c. Thoracentesis should be performed if the effusion is significant (>1 cm on lateral decubitus film). Send fluid for Gram stain, culture, pH, cell count, determination of glucose, protein, and LDH levels.
2. Pleural empyema occurs in 1% to 2% of all cases of CAP (up to 7% of hospitalized patients with CAP). See Chapter 2.
3. Acute respiratory failure may occur if the pneumonia is severe.

••• Ventilator Associated Pneumonia

A. Patients on mechanical ventilation are at risk of developing pneumonia because the normal mucociliary clearance of the respiratory tract is impaired (cannot cough). Also, positive pressure impairs the ability to clear colonization.

B. Findings to help with diagnosis: new infiltrate on chest x-ray, purulent secretions from endotracheal tube, fever, rising WBC count.

C. Bronchoalveolar lavage (BAL)—bronchoscope passed into lungs to get cultures.

D. Treatment is with a combination of the following three different drugs:

1. Cephalosporin (ceftazidime or cefepime) OR penicillin (piperacillin/tazobactam) OR carbapenem (imipenem).
2. Aminoglycoside OR fluoroquinolone.
3. Vancomycin OR linezolid.

••• Lung Abscess

A. General characteristics

1. Abscess in the lung parenchyma results when infected lung tissue becomes necrotic and forms suppurative cavitary lesions. The typical case is aspiration of a large volume of oropharyngeal contents or food, with resulting pneumonia and necrosis when adequate treatment is not administered. Most patients who have aspiration pneumonia are treated promptly, thereby avoiding abscess formation.
2. By definition, a lung abscess is formed by one or more cavities, each >2 cm in diameter.
3. Lung abscesses can be complications of the following:
   a. Aspiration of organisms.

Quick HIT

For outpatients, treatment is continued for 5 days. Do not stop treatment until patient has been afebrile for 48 hours.

Quick HIT

Pleural effusion is common in patients with pneumonia. Progression to empyema (infected, loculated pleural fluid) requires chest tube drainage.

Quick HIT

Lung Abscess Pearls

- The dependent zones of the lungs are most likely to be infected by aspirated contents—the posterior segments of the upper lobes and superior segments of the lower lobes.
- Aspirated material is more likely to affect the right lung due to the angle of the right main stem bronchus from the trachea.

b. Acute necrotizing pneumonia (gram-negative rods).
c. Hematogenous spread of infection from distant site.
d. Direct inoculation with contiguous spread.
4. Microbiologic causes are mainly bacteria that colonize the oropharynx.
a. Oral anaerobes: *Prevotella, Peptostreptococcus, Fusobacterium, Bacteroides* spp.
b. Other bacteria: *S. aureus, S. pneumoniae,* and aerobic gram-negative bacilli
5. Epidemiology/risk factors.
a. The main risk factor is predisposition to aspiration. This may be seen in patients with alcoholism, drug addition, CVA, seizure disorders, general anesthesia, or a nasogastric or endotracheal tube.
b. Poor dental hygiene increases the content of oral anaerobes.
c. Edentulous patients are **less** likely to aspirate oropharyngeal secretions.

B. Clinical features

1. The majority of cases have an indolent onset; some present more acutely.
2. Common symptoms and signs.
   a. Cough—Foul-smelling sputum is consistent with anaerobic infection. It is sometimes blood tinged.
   b. Shortness of breath.
   c. Fever, chills.
   d. Constitutional symptoms: fatigue, malaise, weight loss.

C. Diagnosis

1. CXR
   a. This reveals thick-walled cavitation with air–fluid levels.
   b. Look for abscess in dependent, poorly ventilated lobes.
2. CT scan may be necessary to differentiate between abscess and empyema.
3. Sputum Gram stain and culture has low sensitivity and specificity.
4. Consider obtaining cultures via bronchoscopy or transtracheal aspiration rather than simple expectoration to avoid contamination with oral flora.

D. Treatment

1. Hospitalization is often required if lung abscess is found. Postural drainage should be performed.
2. Antimicrobial therapy.
   a. Antibiotic regimens include coverage for the following:
      - Gram-positive cocci—ampicillin or amoxicillin/clavulanic acid, ampicillin/sulbactam, or vancomycin for *S. aureus.*
      - Anaerobes—clindamycin or metronidazole.
      - If gram-negative organisms are suspected, add a fluoroquinolone or ceftazidime.
   b. Continue antibiotics until the cavity is gone or until CXR findings have improved considerably—this may take months!

Tuberculosis

A. General characteristics

1. Microbiology
   a. Most commonly caused by *Mycobacterium tuberculosis*
   b. Mycobacteria are acid-fast bacilli (AFB)—considered slow growing but hardy organisms
   c. Inhibited by the cellular arm of the immune system
2. Transmission
   a. Transmission occurs via inhalation of aerosolized droplets containing the active organism
   b. Only those people with active TB are contagious (e.g., by coughing, sneezing)
   c. People with primary TB are not contagious

Quick HIT

TB is the most common cause of death due to infection worldwide.

3. Pathophysiology
   a. Primary TB
      - Bacilli are inhaled and deposited into the lung, then ingested by alveolar macrophages
      - Surviving organisms multiply and disseminate via lymphatics and the bloodstream. Granulomas form and "wall off" the mycobacteria. The granulomas in oxygen-rich areas, such as the lungs, allow these organisms to remain viable (they are aerobes). After the resolution of the primary infection, the organism remains dormant within the granuloma
      - An insult to the immune system may activate the TB at any time
      - Only 5% to 10% of individuals with primary TB will develop active disease in their lifetime
   b. Secondary TB (reactivation)
      - Occurs when the host's immunity is weakened (e.g., HIV infection, malignancy, immunosuppressants, substance abuse, poor nutrition)
      - Usually manifests in the most oxygenated portions of the lungs—the apical/posterior segments
      - Produces clinical manifestations of TB
      - Can be complicated by hematogenous or lymphatic spread, resulting in miliary TB
   c. Extrapulmonary TB
      - Individuals with impaired immunity may not be able to contain the bacteria at either the primary or the secondary stage of the infection
      - This may result in active disease throughout the body
      - It is common in patients with HIV because their cellular immunity is impaired
4. Risk factors (almost all patients with TB have one or more of the following):
   a. HIV-positive patients
   b. Recent immigrants (within the past 5 years)
   c. Prisoners
   d. Healthcare workers
   e. Close contacts of someone with TB
   f. Alcoholics
   g. Diabetics
   h. Glucocorticoid use
   i. Hematologic malignancy
   j. Injection drug users

B. Clinical features

1. Primary TB
   a. **Usually asymptomatic**
   b. Pleural effusion may develop
   c. If the immune response is incomplete, the pulmonary and constitutional symptoms of TB may develop. This is known as progressive primary TB
2. Secondary (active) TB
   a. Constitutional symptoms—fever, night sweats, weight loss, and malaise are common
   b. Cough progresses from dry cough to purulent sputum. Hemoptysis suggests advanced TB
   c. Apical rales may be present on examination
3. Extrapulmonary TB
   a. May involve any organ. The lymph nodes, pleura, genitourinary tract, spine, intestine, and meninges are some of the common sites of infection
   b. Miliary TB refers to hematogenous dissemination of the tubercle bacilli
      - May be due to a reactivation of dormant, disseminated foci or a new infection
      - Also common in patients with HIV
      - May present with organomegaly, reticulonodular infiltrates on CXR, and choroidal tubercles in the eye

Quick HIT

Radiographic Findings in Primary TB
- Ghon complex—calcified primary focus with an associated lymph node
- Ranke complex—when Ghon complex undergoes fibrosis and calcification

Quick HIT

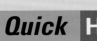

Diagnosis of TB is challenging in HIV patients because:
- PPD skin test result is negative.
- Patients have "atypical" CXR findings.
- Sputum smears are more likely to be negative.
- Granuloma formation may not be present in the late stages.

C. Diagnosis

1. Must have a high index of suspicion, depending on patient's risk factors and presentation
2. CXR
   a. Classic findings are **upper lobe infiltrates with cavitations**
   b. Other possible findings
      - Pleural effusion(s)
      - *Ghon complex* and *Ranke complex:* evidence of healed primary TB
      - Atypical findings common in immunocompromised patients
3. Sputum studies (sputum acid-fast testing)
   a. Definitive diagnosis is made by sputum culture—growth of *M. tuberculosis*
   b. Obtain three morning sputum specimens—culture takes 4 to 8 weeks
   c. PCR can detect specific mycobacterial DNA more rapidly
   d. Diagnosis is sometimes made by finding AFB on microscopic examination, but this is not definitive because other mycobacteria may colonize airways
4. Tuberculin skin test (PPD test)
   a. Tuberculin skin test is a screening test to detect those who may have been exposed to TB. It is not for diagnosis of active TB, but rather of latent (primary) TB (if positive, a chest x-ray is used to diagnose active TB). PPD is not a screening test for everyone, only patients with one or more of the risk factors mentioned above should have this test. If patient is symptomatic or has abnormal chest x-ray, order a sputum acid-fast test, not a PPD
   b. Inject PPD into the volar aspect of forearm. Measure the amount of induration 48 to 72 hours later. Positive result is interpreted as follows:
      - The result is positive if induration ≥15 mm in patients with no risk factors
      - In certain high-risk populations (e.g., those who live in high-prevalence areas, immigrants in the last 5 years, the homeless, prisoners, healthcare workers, nursing home residents, close contact of someone with TB, alcoholics, diabetics), 10 mm of induration is considered positive
      - For patients with HIV, steroid users, organ transplant recipients, close contacts of those with ACTIVE TB, or those with radiographic evidence of primary TB, induration of 5 mm is positive
   c. If a patient has never had a PPD test before, repeat the test in 1 to 2 weeks if the first test is negative (first test may be false negative). The results of the second test (whether positive or negative) are used for management
   d. If PPD test is positive, a chest x-ray is needed to rule out active disease. Once active disease is excluded, 9 months of isoniazid treatment is initiated. A patient with a positive PPD test has a 10% lifetime risk of TB, and this risk is reduced to 1% after 9 months of isoniazid treatment
   e. Many persons born outside of United States have been Bacille Calmette–Guerin (BCG)-vaccinated, which may cause a positive PPD skin test. However, this does not affect treatment decisions. If a patient has a positive PPD test, isoniazid for 9 months is indicated even if the patient had prior BCG vaccine

Quick HIT

Patients previously vaccinated with BCG will have a positive PPD test but this does not affect treatment decisions.

Quick HIT

INH should always be started with Vitamin B6 (pyridoxine) to prevent symptoms of deficiency, which include stomatitis, glossitis, cheilosis, convulsions, hyperirritability, peripheral neuropathy, and sideroblastic anemia.

Infectious Diseases

D. Treatment

1. Patients with active TB must be isolated until sputum is negative for AFB.
   a. First-line therapy is a four-drug regimen: isoniazid (INH), rifampin, pyrazinamide, and ethambutol or streptomycin.
   b. The initial treatment regimen consists of 2 months of treatment with the four-drug regimen. After this initial 2-month phase, a phase of 4 months is recommended using INH and rifampin.
2. Prophylactic treatment for latent (primary) TB (i.e., positive PPD skin test): consists of 9 months of INH **after** active TB has been excluded (negative CXR, sputum, or both).

Quick HIT

- For a positive TB exposure and a positive PPD test (but no active disease), treatment is INH only.
- If the patient has active TB, multiagent therapy is indicated.

••• Influenza

- Orthomyxovirus is transmitted via respiratory droplets, typically occurring in winter months.

- Antigenic types A and B are responsible for the clinical syndrome known as the "flu."
- Annual epidemics are due to minor genetic reassortment and usually are not life-threatening except in the very young, the very old, the immunocompromised, and hosts with significant medical comorbidities.
- Rarely occurring pandemics are due to major genetic recombination and are often fatal, even in young, otherwise healthy hosts.
- Clinical findings are a rapid onset of fever, chills, malaise, headache, nonproductive cough, and sore throat. Nausea may also be present.
- Treatment is largely supportive. Antiviral agents are available but these antiviral agents are only indicated in patients with severe disease (requiring hospitalization) or at high risk of complications and must be given within the first 48 hours of illness. Give antibiotics only for secondary bacterial infections. (See Chapter 12 for vaccination recommendations.)
- A neuraminidase inhibitor (zanamivir or oseltamivir) is the recommended antiviral agent.

Quick HIT

All TB medications can cause hepatotoxicity. Discontinue treatment only if liver transaminases rise to 3 to 5 times the upper limit of normal.

Infections of the Central Nervous System

Meningitis

A. General characteristics

1. This refers to inflammation of the meningeal membranes that envelop the brain and spinal cord. It is usually associated with infectious causes, but noninfectious causes (such as medications, SLE, sarcoidosis, and carcinomatosis) also exist.
2. Pathophysiology
   a. Infectious agents frequently colonize the nasopharynx and respiratory tract.
   b. These pathogens typically enter the CNS via one of the following:
      - Invasion of the bloodstream, which leads to hematogenous seeding of CNS.
      - Retrograde transport along cranial (e.g., olfactory) or peripheral nerves.
      - Contiguous spread from sinusitis, otitis media, surgery, or trauma.
3. Can be classified as acute or chronic, depending on onset of symptoms.
   a. Acute meningitis—onset within hours to days.
   b. Chronic meningitis—onset within weeks to months; commonly caused by mycobacteria, fungi, Lyme disease, or parasites.
4. Another important distinction is bacterial versus aseptic (described below).
5. Acute bacterial meningitis.
   a. Causes
      - Neonates—Group B streptococci, *E. coli*, *Listeria monocytogenes*.
      - Children >3 months—*Neisseria meningitidis*, *S. pneumoniae*, *H. influenzae*.
      - Adults (ages 18 to 50)—*S. pneumoniae*, *N. meningitidis*, *H. influenzae*.
      - Elderly (>50)—*S. pneumoniae*, *N. meningitidis*, *L. monocytogenes*.
      - Immunocompromised—*L. monocytogenes*, gram-negative bacilli, *S. pneumonia*.
   b. Complications
      - Seizures, coma, brain abscess, subdural empyema, DIC, respiratory arrest.
      - Permanent sequelae—deafness, brain damage, hydrocephalus.
6. Aseptic meningitis
   a. Aseptic meningitis is caused by a variety of nonbacterial pathogens, frequently viruses such as enterovirus and herpes simplex virus (HSV). It can also be caused by certain bacteria, parasites, and fungi.
   b. **It may be difficult to distinguish it clinically from acute bacterial meningitis.** If there is uncertainty in diagnosis, treat for acute bacterial meningitis.
   c. It is associated with a better prognosis than acute bacterial meningitis.

Quick HIT

Acute bacterial meningitis is a medical emergency requiring prompt recognition and antibiotic therapy. It is frequently fatal, even with appropriate treatment.

Quick HIT

Acute Bacterial Meningitis (clinical features)
Characteristic triad includes:
- Fever
- Nuchal rigidity
- Change in mental status

B. Clinical features

1. Symptoms (any of the following may be present)
   a. Headache (may be more severe when lying down)
   b. Fevers

c. Nausea and vomiting
d. Stiff, painful neck
e. Malaise
f. Photophobia
g. Alteration in mental status (confusion, lethargy, even coma)

2. Signs (any of the following may be present)
a. Nuchal rigidity: stiff neck, with resistance to flexion of spine (may be absent)
b. Rashes
• Maculopapular rash with petechiae—purpura is classic for *N. meningitidis*
• Vesicular lesions in varicella or HSV
c. Increased ICP and its manifestations—for example, papilledema, seizures
d. Cranial nerve palsies
e. *Kernig sign*—inability to fully extend knees when patient is supine with hips flexed (90 degrees)
• Caused by irritation of the meninges
• Only present in approximately half of patients with bacterial meningitis
f. *Brudzinski sign*—flexion of legs and thighs that is brought on by passive flexion of neck for same reason as above; also present in only half of patients with bacterial meningitis

C. Diagnosis

1. CSF examination (LP)—Perform this if meningitis is a possible diagnosis unless there is evidence of a space-occupying lesion (see Table 10-2). Also note the opening pressure.
a. Examine the CSF. Cloudy CSF is consistent with a pyogenic leukocytosis.
b. CSF should be sent for the following: cell count, chemistry (e.g., protein, glucose), Gram stain, culture (including AFB), and cryptococcal antigen, or India ink.
c. Bacterial meningitis—pyogenic inflammatory response in CSF.
• Elevated WBC count—PMNs predominate.
• Low glucose.
• High protein.
• Gram stain—positive in 75% to 80% of patients with bacterial meningitis.
d. Aseptic meningitis—nonpyogenic inflammatory response in CSF.
• There is an increase in mononuclear cells. Typically a lymphocytic pleocytosis is present.
• Protein is normal or slightly elevated.
• Glucose is usually normal.
• CSF may be completely normal.
2. CT scan of the head is recommended before performing an LP if there are focal neurologic signs or if there is evidence of a space-occupying lesion with elevations in ICP.
3. Obtain blood cultures before antibiotics are given.

Infectious Diseases

TABLE 10-2 CSF Findings in Bacterial Versus Aseptic Meningitis

	Normal	Bacterial Meningitis	Aseptic Meningitis
WBC count (cells/mm^3)	<5	>1,000 (1,000-20,000)	<1,000
WBC differential	All lymphocytes or monocytes; no PMNs	Mostly PMNs	Mostly lymphocytes and monocytes
Glucose (mg/dL)	50–75	Low	Normal
Protein (mg/dL)	<60	High	Moderate elevation

TABLE 10-3 Empiric Treatment for Acute Bacterial Meningitis

Age or Risk Factor	Likely Etiology	Empiric Treatment
Infants (<3 mo)	Group B streptococci, *E. coli, Klebsiella* spp., *L. monocytogenes*	Cefotaxime + ampicillin + vancomycin (aminoglycoside if <4 weeks)
3 mo to 50 yrs	*N. meningitidis, S. pneumoniae, H. influenzae*	Ceftriaxone or cefotaxime + vancomycin
>50 yrs	*S. pneumoniae, N. meningitidis, L. monocytogenes*	Ceftriaxone or cefotaxime + vancomycin + ampicillin
Impaired cellular immunity (e.g., HIV)	*S. pneumoniae, N. meningitidis, L. monocytogenes*, aerobic gram-negative bacilli (including *P. aeruginosa*)	Ceftazidime + ampicillin + vancomycin

D. Treatment

1. Bacterial meningitis.
   a. Empiric antibiotic therapy—Start immediately after LP is performed. If a CT scan must be performed or if there are anticipated delays in LP, give antibiotics first. Pathogen can often still be identified from CSF several hours after administration of antibiotics.
   b. Intravenous (IV) antibiotics.
      - Initiate immediately if the CSF is cloudy or if bacterial infection is suspected.
      - Begin empiric therapy according to the patient's age (see Table 10-3).
      - Modify treatment as appropriate based on Gram stain, culture, and sensitivity findings.
   c. Steroids—if cerebral edema is present.
   d. Vaccination
      - Vaccinate all adults >65 years for *S. pneumoniae*.
      - Vaccinate asplenic patients for *S. pneumoniae, N. meningitidis*, and *H. influenzae* (organisms with capsules).
      - Vaccinate immunocompromised patients for meningococcus.
   e. Prophylaxis (e.g., rifampin or ceftriaxone)—For all close contacts of patients with meningococcus, give 1 dose of IM ceftriaxone.
2. Aseptic meningitis.
   a. No specific therapy other than supportive care is required. The disease is self-limited.
   b. Analgesics and fever reduction may be appropriate.

Encephalitis

A. General characteristics

1. Encephalitis is a diffuse inflammation of the brain parenchyma and is often seen simultaneously with meningitis
2. It is usually viral in origin. Nonviral causes, however, must also be considered
   a. Viral causes
      - Herpes (HSV-1)
      - Arbovirus—for example, Eastern equine encephalitis, West Nile virus
      - Enterovirus—for example, polio
      - Less common causes—for example, measles, mumps, EBV, CMV, VZV, rabies, and prion diseases such as Creutzfeldt–Jakob disease
   b. Nonviral infectious causes
      - Toxoplasmosis
      - Cerebral aspergillosis
   c. Noninfectious causes
      - Metabolic encephalopathies
      - T-cell lymphoma

Quick HIT

Differential diagnosis in patients with fever and altered mental status: infection
- Sepsis, UTI/urosepsis, pneumonia, bacterial meningitis, intracranial abscess, subdural empyema, medication/drugs
- Neuroleptic malignant syndrome (haloperidol, phenothiazines)
- Delirium tremens, metabolic
- Thyroid storm

3. Risk factors
   a. AIDS—patients with AIDS are especially at risk for toxoplasmosis when the CD4 count is <200
   b. Other forms of immunosuppression
   c. Travel in underdeveloped countries
   d. Exposure to insect (e.g., mosquito) vector in endemic areas
   e. Exposure to certain wild animals (e.g., bats) in an endemic area for rabies
4. The overall mortality associated with viral encephalitis is approximately 10%.

B. Clinical features

1. Patients often have a prodrome of headache, malaise, and myalgias.
2. Within hours to days, patients become more acutely ill.
3. Patients frequently have signs and symptoms of meningitis (e.g., headache, fever, photophobia, nuchal rigidity).
4. In addition, patients have altered sensorium, possibly including confusion, delirium, disorientation, and behavior abnormalities.
5. Focal neurologic findings (e.g., hemiparesis, aphasia, cranial nerve lesions) and seizures may also be present.

C. Diagnosis

1. Routine laboratory tests (to rule out nonviral causes) include CXR, urine and blood cultures, urine toxicology screen, and serum chemistries.
2. Perform an LP to examine CSF, unless the patient has signs of significantly increased ICP.
   a. Lymphocytosis (>5 WBC/mL) with normal glucose is consistent with viral encephalitis (similar CSF as in viral meningitis). CSF cultures are usually negative.
   b. **CSF PCR** is the most specific and sensitive test for diagnosing many various viral encephalitides, including HSV-1, CMV, EBV, and VZV.
3. MRI of the brain is the imaging study of choice.
   a. Can rule out focal neurologic causes, such as an abscess.
   b. Increased areas of T2 signal in the frontotemporal localization are consistent with HSV encephalitis.
4. EEG can be helpful in diagnosing HSV-1 encephalitis—it would show unilateral or bilateral temporal lobe discharges.
5. Brain biopsy is indicated in an acutely ill patient with a focal, enhancing lesion on MRI without a clear diagnosis.

Quick HIT

Not all brain abscesses are bacterial—especially in immunocompromised hosts!
- *Toxoplasma gondii* and fungi in patients with AIDS
- *Candida* spp., *Aspergillus* spp., or zygomycosis in neutropenic patients

D. Treatment

1. Supportive care, mechanical ventilation if necessary
2. Antiviral therapy
   a. There is no specific antiviral therapy for most causes of viral encephalitis
   b. HSV encephalitis—acyclovir for 2 to 3 weeks
   c. CMV encephalitis—ganciclovir or foscarnet
3. Management of possible complications
   a. Seizures—require anticonvulsant therapy
   b. Cerebral edema—treatment may include hyperventilation, osmotic diuresis, and steroids

Infections of the Gastrointestinal Tract (see also Chapter 3)

Viral Hepatitis

A. General characteristics

1. Hepatitis simply means inflammation of the liver. There are many noninfectious types of hepatitis, such as alcoholic hepatitis, drug-induced hepatitis, and autoimmune hepatitis, and numerous hereditary diseases that can cause hepatitis.

2. Causes of viral hepatitis.
   a. There are five well-understood, main categories of viral hepatitis: hepatitis A, B, C, D, and E. Hepatitis viruses are often abbreviated by their type (i.e., HAV is hepatitis A virus, HBV is hepatitis B virus, and so forth.)
   b. Other viruses that can cause one form or another of hepatitis are EBV, CMV, and HSV. These are not commonly associated with hepatitis in immunocompetent patients.
3. Transmission varies depending on the specific virus.
   a. Hepatitis A and E are transmitted via the fecal–oral route and are more prevalent in developing countries.
   b. Hepatitis E is particularly prevalent in India, Pakistan, southeast Asia, and parts of Africa.
   c. **Hepatitis B is transmitted parenterally or sexually.** Perinatal transmission is also possible and is a significant health issue in parts of Africa and Asia.
   d. Hepatitis D requires the outer envelope of the hepatitis B surface antigen (HB_SAG) for replication and therefore can be transmitted only as a coinfection with HBV, or as a superinfection in a chronic HBV carrier.
   e. **The main route of transmission for hepatitis C is parenteral**, and it is therefore more prevalent in IV drug users. Sexual or perinatal transmission is not common.
   f. **Hepatitis B, C, and D are the types that can progress to chronic disease.**

Quick HIT

- **Hepatitis B** is associated with PAN.
- **Hepatitis C** is associated with cryoglobulinemia.

B. Clinical features

1. Classified as acute (<6 months of liver inflammation) or chronic (>6 months of persistent liver inflammation) (Figure 10-2)
2. Acute hepatitis has a wide spectrum of clinical presentations, ranging from virtually asymptomatic to fulminant liver failure
   a. General clinical features
      - Jaundice—look first in the sclera, because this may be the first place jaundice can be detected, especially in black patients
      - Dark-colored urine may be present (due to conjugated hyperbilirubinemia)
      - RUQ pain

Quick HIT

Generally, HAV and HEV cause a more mild form of hepatitis and do not become chronic.

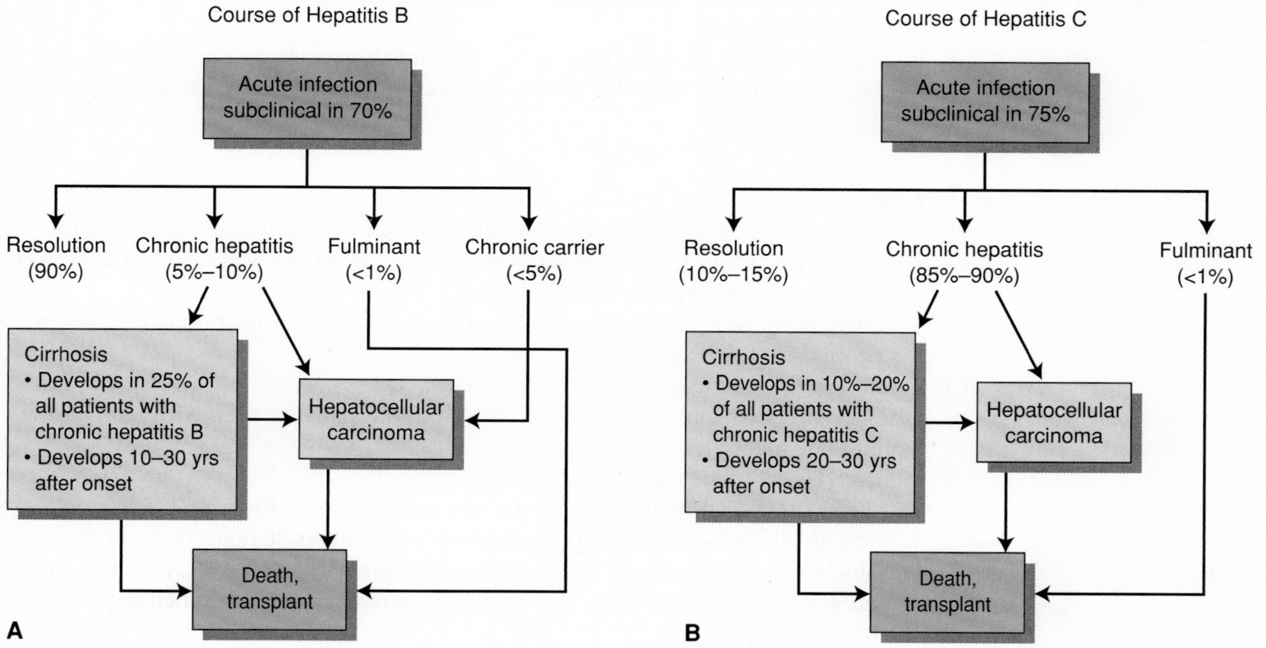

FIGURE 10-2 A: Course of hepatitis B. B: Course of hepatitis C.

Quick HIT

If transaminases are markedly elevated (>500), think of acute viral hepatitis, shock liver, or drug-induced hepatitis.

- Nausea and vomiting
- Fever and malaise
- Hepatomegaly may also be present

b. In severe cases, acute hepatitis may result in liver failure and its complications. This is known as fulminant hepatitis (uncommon) and may be life-threatening. It occurs more commonly in hepatitis B, D, and E than in other types. Complications include:
  - Hepatic encephalopathy—Look for **asterixis** and **palmar erythema**
  - Hepatorenal syndrome
  - Bleeding diathesis—this occurs only when liver function is very compromised

c. Sometimes acute hepatitis may only present with transient flu-like symptoms such as fever, myalgias, and malaise

d. Acute HBV may also present with a serum sickness-like illness

e. Hepatitis C typically does not cause significant **acute** illness

3. Chronic hepatitis also has a wide variety of presentations. Some patients are asymptomatic ("chronic carriers") and may only present with late complications of hepatitis, such as cirrhosis or hepatic cell carcinoma (HCC)
   a. Chronic hepatitis occurs after acute hepatitis in 1% to 10% of patients with HBV and >80% patients with HCV
   b. It is categorized based on the grade of inflammation, the stage of fibrosis, and the etiology of disease
   c. The risk of developing cirrhosis or HCC is 25% to 40% in patients with chronic HBV and 10% to 25% in patients with chronic HCV

Quick HIT

Look for positive HB_sAg and positive IgM anti-HBc to check for hepatitis B infection.

C. Diagnosis

1. Serum serology—the presence of serum antigens and immunoglobulins is the most important factor for diagnosing viral hepatitis. These are helpful for determining the acuity or chronicity of illness as well as adequate immunity (see Clinical Pearl 10-3).
2. PCR is used to detect viral RNA to diagnose HCV.
3. LFTs—Elevation of serum transaminases is not diagnostic, but LFTs are helpful.
   a. ALT (SGPT) is typically elevated more than AST (SGOT) for all forms of viral hepatitis (the opposite of alcoholic hepatitis).
   b. In acute hepatitis, ALT is usually >1,000. It is generally not as high as in drug-induced hepatitis.
   c. In chronic HBV, ALT can also be >1,000, but this varies. In chronic HCV, ALT is generally lower than this due to destruction of hepatocytes from longevity of disease.

D. Treatment

1. Active (vaccine) and passive (immunoglobulin) immunization are available for both hepatitis A and B. It is the standard of care for infants and healthcare workers to be vaccinated for HBV (see Chapter 12).
2. Travelers often receive vaccinations for HAV. Passive immunization can be given for people who are exposed to the virus.
3. Treatment for hepatitis A and E is supportive.
4. Chronic HBV—treat with interferon (IFN)-α. Alternatively, treat with lamivudine (nucleoside analog).
5. Chronic HCV—treat with IFN-α and ribavirin.
   a. Newer direct-acting antiviral agents can possibly cure chronic HCV. They include telaprevir, boceprevir, simeprevir, paritaprevir, ledipasvir, ombitasvir, sofosbuvir, and dasabuvir but they are very expensive. Get a HCV viral load and genotype if considering this option because treatment regimen depends on HCV genotype.
6. Consider liver transplantation in advanced disease, although recurrence can occur after transplantation. Hepatitis C is the most frequent indication for liver transplantation in the United States.

CLINICAL PEARL 10-3

Hepatitis Serology

Hepatitis A

- Hepatitis A antibody (anti-HAV)
  - Anti-HAV is detectable during acute infection and persists for life, so its presence does not distinguish between active disease and immunity. IgM-specific antibody denotes acute infection.

Hepatitis B

- HB_sAg
  - Present in acute or chronic infection
  - Detectable as early as 1 to 2 weeks after infection
  - It persists in chronic hepatitis regardless of whether symptoms are present. If virus is cleared, then HB_sAg is undetectable
- Hepatitis B e antigen (HB_eAg)
  - Reflects active viral replication, and presence indicates infectivity
  - Appears shortly after HB_sAg
- Anti-HB_sAg antibody (anti-HBs)
  - Present after vaccination or after clearance of HB_sAg—usually detectable 1 to 3 months after infection
  - In most cases, presence of anti-HBs indicates immunity to HBV
- Hepatitis B core antibody (anti-HBc)
  - Assay of IgM and IgG combined
  - Useful because it may be the only serologic marker of HBV infection during the "window period" in which HB_sAg is disappearing, but anti-HB_sAg is not yet detectable
  - Does not distinguish between acute and chronic infection, and presence does not indicate immunity
- Viral load
  - HBV DNA measured by PCR; if it persists for more than 6 weeks, patient is likely to develop chronic disease

Hepatitis C

- Hepatitis C antibody
  - Key marker of HCV infection
  - Sometimes not detectable until months after infection, so its absence does not rule out infection
- Viral load: HCV RNA measured by PCR
  - Detectable 1 to 2 weeks after infection—more sensitive than HCV antibody

Hepatitis D

- Hepatitis D antibody (anti-HDV)
  - Presence indicates HDV superinfection
  - The antibody may not be present in acute illness, so repeat testing may be necessary

Botulism

A. General characteristics

1. Results from ingestion of **preformed toxins** produced by spores of *Clostridium botulinum*. Improperly stored food (e.g., home-canned foods) can be contaminated with these spores. Toxins can be inactivated by cooking food at high temperatures (e.g., 100°C [212°F] for 10 minutes).
2. Wound contamination is another source.
3. Inhalation botulism has been reported in laboratory workers but is not a common occurrence. Could be a possible threat as a bioterrorist weapon.

B. Clinical features

1. The severity of illness ranges widely, from mild, self-limiting symptoms, to rapidly fatal disease.
2. Abdominal cramps, nausea, vomiting, and diarrhea are common.
3. **The hallmark clinical manifestation is symmetric, descending flaccid paralysis.** It starts with dry mouth, diplopia, and/or dysarthria. Paralysis of limb musculature occurs later.

Quick HIT

Differential diagnosis of food-borne botulism includes:
- Guillain–Barré syndrome—characteristically ascending paralysis, but one variety (Fischer) can be descending
- Eaton–Lambert syndrome
- Myasthenia gravis—EMG studies differentiate
- Diphtheria
- Tick paralysis

C. Diagnosis

1. The definitive diagnosis is identification of toxin in serum, stool, or gastric contents (bioassay).
2. Identifying *C. botulinum* alone in food is **not** a reliable diagnostic indicator.

D. Treatment

1. Admit the patient and observe respiratory status closely. Gastric lavage is helpful only within several hours after ingestion of suspected food.
2. If suspicion of botulism is high, administer antitoxin (toxoid) as soon as laboratory specimens are obtained (do not wait for the results).
3. For contaminated wounds—(in addition to the above) wound cleansing and penicillin.

Intra-abdominal Abscess

- Causes include spontaneous bacterial peritonitis, pelvic infection (e.g., tubo-ovarian abscess), pancreatitis, perforation of the GI tract, and osteomyelitis of the vertebral bodies with extension into the retroperitoneal cavity.
- Usually polymicrobial in origin.
- Diagnose using CT scan or ultrasound.
- Treatment typically involves drainage of the abscess.
- The antibiotic regimen should include broad coverage against gram-negative rods, enterococci, and anaerobes.

Infections of the Genitourinary Tract

Lower Urinary Tract Infections

Quick HIT

More than 90% of uncomplicated UTIs are caused by *E. coli, S. saprophyticus,* and *Enterococcus* spp. A small percentage is caused by *Proteus, Klebsiella, Enterobacter,* and *Pseudomonas.*

Quick HIT

Noninfectious causes of cystitis or cystitis-like symptoms:
- Cytotoxic agents (e.g., cyclophosphamide)
- Radiation to the pelvis
- Dysfunctional voiding
- Interstitial cystitis

A. General characteristics

1. Urinary tract infections (UTIs) are much more common in women than in men. Up to 33% of all women experience a UTI in their lifetime. The most common UTI is uncomplicated acute cystitis.
2. The majority of UTIs are caused by ascending infection from the urethra. Colonization of the vaginal area by pathogens from the fecal flora leads to ascension via the urethra into the bladder.
3. Common organisms.
   a. *E. coli* (most common)—causes 80% of cases.
   b. Other organisms—*Staphylococcus saprophyticus, Enterococcus, Klebsiella, Proteus* spp., *Pseudomonas, Enterobacter,* and yeast (such as *Candida* spp.)

B. Risk factors

1. Female gender—greater risk due to the shorter female urethra and vaginal colonization of bacteria
2. Sexual intercourse
   a. Often the trigger of a UTI in women, thus the term "honeymoon cystitis"
   b. Use of diaphragms and spermicides increases risk further (alters vaginal colonization)
3. Pregnancy
4. Indwelling urinary catheters—risk factor for hospitalized patients
5. Personal history of recurrent UTIs
6. Host-dependent factors—increase risk for recurrent or complicated UTIs
   a. Diabetes—diabetic patients are at risk for upper UTI
   b. Patients with spinal cord injury
   c. Immunocompromised state
   d. Any structural or functional abnormality that impedes urinary flow (e.g., incomplete voiding, neurogenic bladder, BPH, vesicoureteral reflux, calculi)
7. Male risk factors
   a. Uncircumcised males are at higher risk due to bacterial colonization of the foreskin

b. Anal intercourse
c. Vaginal intercourse with a female colonized with uropathogens

C. Clinical features

1. Dysuria—commonly expressed as burning on urination
2. Frequency
3. Urgency
4. Suprapubic tenderness
5. Gross hematuria is sometimes present
6. **In lower UTIs, fever is characteristically absent**

D. Diagnosis

1. Dipstick urinalysis
   a. Positive urine leukocyte esterase test—presence of leukocyte esterase reflects pyuria
   b. Positive nitrite test for presence of bacteria (gram-negative)—nitrite test is sensitive and specific for detecting Enterobacteriaceae. But it lacks sensitivity for other organisms, so a negative test should be interpreted with caution
   c. Combining the above two tests yields a sensitivity of 85% and specificity of 75%
2. Urinalysis (clean-catch midstream specimen)
   a. Adequacy of collection
      - The presence of epithelial (squamous) cells indicates vulvar or urethral contamination
      - If contamination is suspected, perform a straight catheterization of the bladder
   b. Criteria for UTI
      - Bacteriuria: >1 organism per oil-immersion field. Bacteriuria without WBCs may reflect contamination and is not a reliable indicator of infection
      - Pyuria is the most valuable finding for diagnosis: Greater than or equal to 10 leukocytes/μL is abnormal
   c. Other findings—hematuria and mild proteinuria may be present. Hematuria in and of itself does not require extended therapy
3. Urine Gram stain
   a. A count of $>10^5$ organisms/mL represents significant bacteriuria
   b. It is 90% sensitive and 88% specific
4. Urine culture
   a. Confirms the diagnosis (high specificity). Obtaining a urine culture is warranted if symptoms are not characteristic of UTI, if a complicated infection is suspected, or if symptoms persist despite prior antibiotic treatment
   b. Traditional criteria: $\geq 10^5$ CFU/mL of urine from a clean-catch sample; misses up to one-third of UTIs
   c. Colony counts as low as 10^2 to 10^4 CFU/mL are adequate for diagnosis if clinical symptoms are present
5. Blood cultures—only indicated if patient is ill and urosepsis is suspected
6. IVP, cystoscopy, and excretory urography are not recommended unless structural abnormalities or obstruction is suspected

E. Complications

1. Complicated UTI
   a. Any UTI that spreads beyond the bladder (e.g., pyelonephritis, prostatitis, urosepsis)—risk factors for upper UTI: pregnancy, diabetes, and vesicoureteral reflux
   b. Any UTI caused by structural abnormalities, metabolic disorder, or neurologic dysfunction
2. UTI during pregnancy—increased risk of preterm labor, low birth weight, and other complications, especially in advanced pregnancy
3. Recurrent infections
   a. Usually due to infection with new organism, but sometimes is a relapse due to unsuccessful treatment of the original organism

Quick HIT

Urine culture and sensitivity may modify antibiotic therapy, but most UTIs are treated based on urinalysis and Gram stain results. Obtain cultures under the following conditions: patient age ≥65 years, diabetes, recurrent UTIs, presence of symptoms for 7 days or more, use of a diaphragm.

Quick HIT

Asymptomatic Bacteriuria
- To diagnose asymptomatic bacteriuria, two successive positive cultures ($\geq 10^5$ CFU/mL) must be present.
- Treat asymptomatic bacteriuria only in pregnancy or before urologic surgery.

Quick HIT

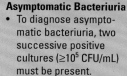

On UA, most important finding is white blood cells.

Quick HIT

Complicated UTI is caused by functional or structural abnormalities of the urinary tract or underlying disease. The following groups of patients are considered to have complicated UTI:
- Men
- Diabetics, renal failure
- Pregnancy
- History of pyelonephritis in last year
- Urinary tract obstruction, indwelling catheter, stent, nephrostomy tube
- Antibiotic-resistant organism
- Immunocompromised patients (e.g., HIV patients, transplant recipients)

b. Risk factors include impaired host defenses, pregnancy, vesicoureteral reflux, and sexual intercourse in women
c. Generally the consequences are not significant unless the patient is at risk for upper UTI

Quick HIT
For uncomplicated UTI, empiric treatment is appropriate—do not wait for culture results.

Quick HIT
If complicated UTI, extend antibiotic treatment to 7 days.

F. Treatment

1. Acute uncomplicated cystitis—that is, nonpregnant women. Several options exist:
   a. Oral TMP/SMX (Bactrim) for 3 days.
   b. Nitrofurantoin (5 to 7 days)—do not give if early pyelonephritis is suspected.
   c. Fosfomycin (single dose)—do not give if early pyelonephritis is suspected.
   d. Amoxicillin is a less popular alternative due to increasing antimicrobial resistance.
   e. Fluoroquinolones (ciprofloxacin in 3-day regimen) is a reasonable alternative to the above-mentioned agents.
   f. Treat presumptively for pyelonephritis if the condition fails to respond to a short course of antibiotics.
   g. Phenazopyridine (Pyridium) is a urinary analgesic; it can be given for 1 to 3 days for dysuria.
2. Pregnant women with UTI.
   a. Treat with ampicillin, amoxicillin, or oral cephalosporins for 7 to 10 days.
   b. Avoid fluoroquinolones (can cause fetal arthropathy).
3. UTIs in men.
   a. Treat as with uncomplicated cystitis in women, but for 7 days.
   b. Urologic workup is required in all men presenting with UTI unless there is an obvious underlying risk factor (catheterization, etc.).
4. Recurrent infections.
   a. If relapse occurs within 2 weeks of cessation of treatment, continue treatment for 2 more weeks and obtain a urine culture.
   b. Otherwise treat as for uncomplicated cystitis. If the patient has more than two UTIs per year, give chemoprophylaxis.
      - Single dose of TMP/SMX after intercourse or at first signs of symptoms.
      - Alternative low-dose prophylactic antibiotics (e.g., low-dose TMP/SMX) for 6 months.

Pyelonephritis

A. General characteristics

1. Pyelonephritis is an infection of the upper urinary tract.
   a. It is usually caused by ascending spread from the bladder to the kidney.
   b. Uncomplicated pyelonephritis is limited to the renal pyelocalyceal-medullary region.
   c. Vesicoureteral reflux facilitates this ascending spread. See above for other risk factors.
2. Organisms
   a. *E. coli* (most frequent cause).
   b. Other gram-negative bacteria include *Proteus, Klebsiella, Enterobacter,* and *Pseudomonas* spp.
   c. Gram-positive bacteria (less common) include *Enterococcus faecalis* and *S. aureus.*
3. Complications (unusual).
   a. Sepsis occurs in 10% to 25% of patients with pyelonephritis. May lead to shock.
   b. Emphysematous pyelonephritis—caused by gas-producing bacteria in diabetic patients.
   c. Chronic pyelonephritis and scarring of the kidneys—rare unless underlying renal disease exists.

B. Clinical features

1. Symptoms
   a. Fever, chills
   b. Flank pain

c. Symptoms of cystitis (may or may not be present)
d. Nausea, vomiting, and diarrhea (sometimes present)

2. Signs
a. Fever with tachycardia
b. Patients generally appear more ill than patients with cystitis
c. Costovertebral angle tenderness—unilateral or bilateral
d. Abdominal tenderness may be present on examination

C. Diagnosis

1. Urinalysis
a. Look for pyuria, bacteriuria, and **leukocyte casts**
b. As in cystitis, hematuria and mild proteinuria may be present
2. Urine cultures—obtain in all patients with suspected pyelonephritis
3. Blood cultures—obtain in ill-appearing patients and all hospitalized patients
4. CBC—leukocytosis with left shift
5. Renal function—this is usually preserved. Impairment is usually reversible, especially with IV fluids
6. Imaging studies—perform these if treatment fails or in any patient with complicated pyelonephritis. Consider renal ultrasound, CT, IVP, or retrograde ureterogram

D. Treatment

1. For uncomplicated pyelonephritis.
a. Use outpatient treatment if the patient can take oral antibiotics. Treat based on Gram stain:
- TMP/SMX or a fluoroquinolone for 10 to 14 days is effective for most gram-negative rods.
- Amoxicillin is appropriate for gram-positive cocci (enterococci, *S. saprophyticus*).
- A single dose of ceftriaxone or gentamicin is often given initially before starting oral treatment.

b. Repeat urine culture 2 to 4 days after cessation of therapy.
c. If symptoms fail to resolve within 48 hours, adjust treatment based on urine culture.
d. Failure to respond to appropriate antimicrobial therapy suggests a functional or structural abnormality; perform a urologic investigation.

2. If the patient is very ill, elderly, pregnant, unable to tolerate oral medication, or has significant comorbidities, or if urosepsis is suspected
a. Hospitalize the patient and give IV fluids.
b. Treat with antibiotics.
- Start with parenteral antibiotics (broad-spectrum)—ampicillin plus gentamicin or ciprofloxacin are common initial choices.
- If blood cultures are negative, treat with IV antibiotics until the patient is afebrile for 24 hours, then give oral antibiotics to complete a 14- to 21-day course.
- If blood cultures are positive (urosepsis), treat with IV antibiotics for 2 to 3 weeks.

3. For recurrent pyelonephritis.
a. If relapse is due to the same organism despite appropriate treatment, treat for 6 weeks.
b. If relapse is due to a new organism, treat with appropriate therapy for 2 weeks.

Prostatitis

A. General characteristics

1. Acute bacterial prostatitis
a. Less common than chronic bacterial prostatitis
b. Occurs more commonly in younger men
c. Pathophysiology
- Ascending infection from the urethra and reflux of infected urine
- May occur after urinary catheterization
- Other causes—direct or lymphatic spread from the rectum
- Hematogenous spread (rare)

Quick HIT

Acute Versus Chronic Prostatitis

- Acute prostatitis is a more serious condition than chronic prostatitis, and urgent treatment is necessary.
- Acute prostatitis is much more obvious clinically (fever, exquisitely tender prostate), whereas chronic prostatitis is difficult to diagnose because the prostate may not be tender and findings are variable.

Quick HIT

Avoid prostatic massage in patients with acute bacterial prostatitis because it may cause bacteremia. In fact, rectal examination may be skipped if the diagnosis is straightforward, given the risk of inducing bacteremia.

Quick HIT

Recurrent exacerbations are common in chronic prostatitis if not treated adequately. Recurrent UTI is very common in these patients.

Quick HIT

Eighty percent of cases of reactive arthritis (formerly Reiter syndrome) are associated with chlamydial infection.

d. Gram-negative organisms predominate (e.g., *E. coli, Klebsiella, Proteus, Pseudomonas, Enterobacter,* and *Serratia* spp.)

2. Chronic bacterial prostatitis
   a. More common than acute bacterial prostatitis; true prevalence is difficult to determine because many cases are asymptomatic and are diagnosed incidentally
   b. It most commonly affects men 40 to 70 years of age
   c. It has the same routes of infection as acute bacterial prostatitis. It may develop from acute bacterial prostatitis
   d. Organisms are similar to those in acute prostatitis

B. Clinical features

1. Acute prostatitis
   a. Fever, chills—patients may appear toxic.
   b. Irritative voiding symptoms—dysuria, frequency, and urgency are common.
   c. Perineal pain, low back pain, and urinary retention may be present as well.
2. Chronic prostatitis
   a. Patients may be asymptomatic. Patients do not appear ill. Fever is uncommon.
   b. Patients frequently have recurrent UTIs with irritative voiding and/or obstructive urinary symptoms.
   c. There is dull, poorly localized pain in the lower back, perineal, scrotal, or suprapubic region.

C. Diagnosis

1. DRE—there is a boggy, exquisitely tender prostate in acute disease. In chronic disease, prostate is enlarged and usually nontender.
2. Urinalysis—numerous (sheets of) WBCs are present in acute bacterial prostatitis.
3. Urine cultures—almost always positive in acute prostatitis.
4. Chronic prostatitis—the presence of WBCs in expressed prostatic secretions suggests diagnosis. Urine cultures may be positive (chronic bacterial prostatitis) or negative (nonbacterial prostatitis).
5. Obtain CBC and blood cultures if patient appears toxic or if sepsis is suspected.

D. Treatment

1. Acute prostatitis.
   a. If it is severe and the patient appears toxic, hospitalize the patient and initiate IV antibiotics.
   b. If it is mild, treat on an outpatient basis with antibiotics—TMP/SMX or a fluoroquinolone and doxycycline. Treat for 4 to 6 weeks.
   c. The patient usually responds to therapy.
2. Chronic prostatitis.
   a. Treat with a fluoroquinolone. For chronic bacterial prostatitis, a prolonged course is recommended but does not guarantee complete eradication.
   b. It is very difficult to treat. Recurrences are common.

Sexually Transmitted Diseases

Genital Warts

- These are caused by HPV.
- **They are the most common** sexually transmitted disease (**STD**).
- **See Chapter 11**, Common Dermatologic Problems, Inflammatory, Allergic, and Autoimmune Skin Conditions, Warts.

Chlamydia

A. General characteristics

1. **Chlamydia is the most common bacterial STD.** The organism is an intracellular pathogen.

2. Many patients are coinfected with gonorrhea (up to 40% of women and 20% of men).
3. The incubation period is 1 to 3 weeks.

B. Clinical features

1. Many cases are asymptomatic (80% of women, 50% of men).
2. Men who are symptomatic may have any of the following: dysuria, purulent urethral discharge, scrotal pain and swelling, and fever.
3. Women who are symptomatic may have purulent urethral discharge, intermenstrual or postcoital bleeding, and dysuria.

C. Diagnosis

1. Diagnostic tests include culture, enzyme immunoassay, and molecular tests such as PCR. Serologic tests are not used for *Chlamydia.*
2. Molecular diagnostic tests are replacing culture as the screening test of choice due to higher sensitivity.
3. Sexually active adolescents (particularly females) should be screened for chlamydial infection even if they are asymptomatic.

D. Treatment

1. Azithromycin (oral one dose) or doxycycline (oral for 7 days).
2. Treat all sexual partners.

Quick HIT

Chlamydia infection is a risk factor for cervical cancer, especially when there is a history of multiple infections.

Quick HIT

Complications of Chlamydia

- Complications in men include epididymitis and proctitis.
- Complications in women include pelvic inflammatory disease, salpingitis, tubo-ovarian abscess, ectopic pregnancy, and Fitz-Hugh–Curtis syndrome. **Chlamydia is a leading cause of infertility in women due to tubal scarring.**

Gonorrhea

A. General characteristics

1. The responsible organism is *Neisseria gonorrhoeae* (a gram-negative, intracellular diplococcal organism).
2. Gonorrhea is usually asymptomatic in women but symptomatic in men. Therefore, complications occur more often in women due to undetected disease.
3. It is almost always transmitted sexually (except with neonatal transmission).
4. Coinfection with *Chlamydia trachomatis* occurs in 30% of patients (more common in women).

B. Clinical features

1. Men
   a. Gonorrhea is asymptomatic in up to 10% of carriers. These asymptomatic carriers can still transmit the disease
   b. Most men have symptoms involving the urethra—for example, purulent discharge, dysuria, erythema and edema of urethral meatus, and frequency of urination
2. Women
   a. **Most women are asymptomatic or have few symptoms**
   b. Women may have symptoms of cervicitis or urethritis—for example, purulent discharge, dysuria, intermenstrual bleeding, and dyspareunia
3. Disseminated gonococcal infection (occurs in 1% to 2% of cases; more common in women)—possible findings:
   a. Fever, arthralgias, tenosynovitis (of hands and feet)
   b. Migratory polyarthritis/septic arthritis, endocarditis, or even meningitis
   c. Skin rash (usually on distal extremities)

C. Diagnosis

1. Gram stain of urethral discharge showing organisms within leukocytes is highly specific for gonorrhea.
2. Obtain cultures in all cases—in men from the urethra; in women from the endocervix. May treat empirically because culture results take 1 to 2 days to return.
3. Consider testing for syphilis and HIV.
4. Obtain blood cultures if disease has disseminated.

Quick HIT

In gonorrhea, infection of the pharynx, conjunctiva, and rectum can occur.

Quick HIT

Gonorrheal Complications

- Pelvic inflammatory disease, with possible infertility and chronic pelvic pain
- Epididymitis, prostatitis (uncommon)
- Salpingitis, tubo-ovarian abscess
- Fitz-Hugh–Curtis syndrome (perihepatitis)—RUQ pain; elevated LFTs
- Disseminated gonococcal infection

D. Treatment

1. Ceftriaxone (IM, one dose) is preferred because it is also effective against syphilis. Other options are oral cefixime, ciprofloxacin, or ofloxacin.
2. Also give azithromycin (one dose) or doxycycline (for 7 days) to cover coexistent chlamydial infection.
3. If disseminated, hospitalize the patient and initiate ceftriaxone (IV or IM for 7 days).

HIV and AIDS

A. General characteristics

1. Pathophysiology
   a. The most common virus associated with HIV is the HIV type 1 human retrovirus
   b. The virus attaches to the surface of CD4+ T lymphocytes (targets of HIV-1); it enters the cell and uncoats, and its RNA is transcribed to DNA by reverse transcriptase
   c. Billions of viral particles are produced each day by activated CD4 cells. When the virus enters the lytic stage of infection, CD4 cells are destroyed. It is the depletion of the body's arsenal of CD4 cells that weakens the **cellular immunity** of the host
2. Transmission is usually sexual or parenteral. Other than semen and blood, fluids that transmit the disease are breast milk and vaginal fluid
   a. Risk of Transmission:
      - Needlestick injury—1 in 300
      - Vaginal (male to female)—1 in 1,000
      - Vaginal (female to male)—1 in 3,000
      - Anal receptive—1 in 100
      - Mother to child—1 in 3 without medications. With medications, risk is under 2 in 100
   b. Caesarian delivery is indicated if viral load is over 1,000 copies. If CD4 count is high (over 500) and viral load is low (under 1,000), C-section is not necessary
3. Mortality is usually secondary to opportunistic infection, wasting, or cancer
4. High-risk individuals: homosexual or bisexual men, IV drug abusers, blood transfusion recipients before 1985 (before widespread screening of donor blood), heterosexual contacts of HIV-positive individuals, unborn and newborn babies of mothers who are HIV positive

Quick HIT

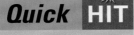

It is important (but often difficult) to identify patients with primary HIV infection because of the benefits of early antiretroviral therapy. A high index of suspicion is necessary.

B. Clinical features

1. Primary infection (see also Clinical Pearl 10-4).
   a. A mononucleosis-like syndrome about 2 to 4 weeks after exposure to HIV. Duration of the illness is brief (3 days to 2 weeks).
   b. Symptoms include fever, sweats, malaise, lethargy, headaches, arthralgias/myalgias, diarrhea, sore throat, lymphadenopathy, and a truncal maculopapular rash.
2. Asymptomatic infection (seropositive, but no clinical evidence of HIV infection).
   a. CD4 counts are normal (>500/mm^3).
   b. Longest phase (lasts 4 to 7 years, but varies widely, especially with treatment).
3. Symptomatic HIV infection (pre-AIDS).
   a. First evidence of immune system dysfunction.
   b. Without treatment, this phase lasts about 1 to 3 years.
   c. The following frequently appear:
      - Persistent generalized lymphadenopathy.
      - Localized fungal infections (e.g., on fingernails, toes, mouth).
      - Recalcitrant vaginal yeast and trichomonal infections in women.
      - Oral hairy leukoplakia on the tongue.
      - Skin manifestations that include seborrheic dermatitis, psoriasis exacerbations, molluscum, and warts.
      - Constitutional symptoms (night sweats, weight loss, and diarrhea).

Quick HIT

The course of HIV varies considerably from patient to patient. However, the typical course can be divided into the following four phases: primary infection, asymptomatic infection, symptomatic infection, and full-blown AIDS.

Quick HIT

The combination of ELISA and Western blot yields an overall sensitivity and specificity of >99%.

CLINICAL PEARL 10-4

HIV Serology

CD4 Cell Count

- It is the best indicator of the status of the immune system and of the risk for opportunistic infections and disease progression.
- It is used to determine when to initiate antiretroviral therapy and PCP prophylaxis. It is also useful in assessing the response to antiretroviral therapy.
- If untreated (no retroviral therapy), the CD4 cell count decreases at an average rate of about 50 per year.
- If >500, the immune system is essentially normal. HIV-related infection or illness is unlikely.
- If 200 to 500, there is an increased risk of HIV-related problems, such as herpes zoster, TB, lymphoma, bacterial pneumonias, and Kaposi sarcoma. However, many patients are asymptomatic at these CD4 levels.
- Most opportunistic infections occur when the CD4 count falls below 200.

Viral Load (HIV-1 RNA Levels)

- Used to assess response to and adequacy of antiretroviral therapy; provides complementary prognostic information to the CD4+ count.
- If the viral load is still >50 after about 4 months of treatment, modification in the regimen may be needed.
- Do not stop antiretroviral therapy even if viral loads are undetectable for years. Latently infected cells can lead to reappearance of viral RNA once therapy is stopped.
- Measure the plasma HIV RNA levels and the CD4 cell count at the time of diagnosis and every 3 to 4 months thereafter.

4. AIDS
   a. Marked immune suppression leads to disseminated opportunistic infections and malignancies.
   b. CD4 count is <200 cells/mm^3.
   c. Pulmonary, GI, neurologic, cutaneous, and systemic symptoms are common (see Table 10-4).

C. Diagnosis

1. PCR RNA viral load test—patients with acute HIV infection have very high levels of viremia. This test is repeated to assess effectiveness of therapy.
2. p24 antigen assay—less costly but less sensitive alternative to viral load testing.

TABLE 10-4 Clinical Manifestation of AIDS

System	Condition	Comments
Pulmonary	Community-acquired bacterial pneumonia PCP	Recurrent bacterial pneumonia (two or more episodes per year) is 20 times more common in HIV-1 patients with low CD4 cell counts (<200/mm^3) than in those with normal counts • Seventy percent of patients acquire PCP at some point; often the initial opportunistic infection establishes the diagnosis of AIDS • **Leading cause of death in patients with AIDS** • **Occurs when CD4 count is ≤200** • Clinical findings: fever, nonproductive cough, shortness of breath (with exertion at first, then occurring at rest) • CXR: diffuse interstitial infiltrates; negative radiographs in 10%–15% of patients with PCP • Treatment: TMP-SMX (PO or IV) for 3 weeks; steroid therapy if patient is hypoxic or has elevated A–a gradient • Prophylaxis: Oral TMP-SMX, 1 dose daily, is recommended
	Tuberculosis (other infections)	Negative PPD test results are frequent among AIDS patients due to immunosuppression • CMV or MAC: **increased risk when the CD4 count <50** • *C. neoformans*, *Histoplasma capsulatum*, neoplasms (Kaposi sarcoma)

(*continued*)

TABLE 10-4 Clinical Manifestation of AIDS (*Continued*)

System	Condition	Comments
Nervous system	AIDS dementia	• Progressive process in 33% of patients • Early stages: subtle impairment of recent memory and other cognitive deficits • Later stages: changes in mental status, aphasia, motor abnormalities
	Toxoplasmosis	• Usually a reactivation of latent infection of *Toxoplasma gondii* • Symptoms both of a mass lesion (discrete deficits, headache) and of encephalitis (fever, altered mental status) • CT scan or MRI shows characteristic findings: multiple (more than three) **contrast-enhanced mass lesions in the basal ganglia and subcortical white matter**
	Cryptococcal meningitis	• Diagnosed by identifying organisms in CSF by cryptococcal antigen, culture, or **staining with India ink** • Treat with amphotericin B for 10–14 days. Follow this with 8–10 weeks of oral fluconazole. Lifelong maintenance therapy with fluconazole is indicated
	Other CNS infections	Bacterial meningitis, histoplasmosis, CMV, progressive multifocal leukoencephalopathy (PML), HSV, neurosyphilis, TB
	Noninfectious CNS diseases	CNS lymphoma, CVA, metabolic encephalopathies
Gastrointestinal	Diarrhea	Most common GI complaint; caused by a variety of pathogens (*E. coli, Shigella, Salmonella, Campylobacter,* CMV, *Giardia, Cryptosporidium, Isospora belli, Mycobacterium avium-intracellulare*). Antibiotic therapy is also a common cause
	Oral lesions	Oral thrush (candidiasis), HSV or CMV (ulcers), oral hairy leukoplakia (EBV infection), Kaposi sarcoma
	Esophageal involvement	Candidiasis is most common cause of dysphagia; also CMV and HSV—**seen with CD4 counts <100**
	Anorectal disease	Proctitis—*N. gonorrhoeae, C. trachomatis,* syphilis, HSV
Dermatologic	Kaposi sarcoma	• More common in homosexual men than in other groups • Painless, raised brown-black or purple papules (common sites: face, chest, genitals, oral cavity) • Widespread dissemination can occur
	Infections	HSV infections, molluscum contagiosum, secondary syphilis, warts, shingles, and many other skin conditions/infections occur with higher frequency
Miscellaneous	CMV infection	• Common cause of serious opportunistic viral disease • Disseminated disease is common and usually involves the GI or pulmonary systems • Most important manifestation is retinitis—unilateral visual loss that can become bilateral if untreated (seen in 5%–10% of AIDS patients) • Colitis and esophagitis are other findings • Treat with ganciclovir or foscarnet
	Mycobacterium avium complex (MAC)	• Most common opportunistic bacterial infection in AIDS patients. Wasting syndrome (weight loss, fever), lymphadenopathy, anemia • MAC causes disseminated disease in 50% of AIDS patients. MAC occurs in patients with advanced AIDS and fewer than 50 CD4 cells • Diarrhea and weight loss are constitutional symptoms
	HIV-1 wasting syndrome	Profound involuntary loss of more than 10% of body weight in conjunction with **either** of the following: • Chronic diarrhea (two or more stools per day for more than 1 mo) • Fever and persistent weakness for a similar period in the absence of another cause
	Malignancies	• Kaposi sarcoma • Non-Hodgkin lymphoma—rapidly growing mass lesion in CNS • Primary CNS lymphoma

3. Seroconversion occurs 3 to 7 weeks after infection and confirms the diagnosis.
   a. Enzyme-linked immunosorbent assay (ELISA) method.
      - Screening test for detecting antibody to HIV; becomes positive 1 to 12 weeks after infection.
      - A negative ELISA essentially excludes HIV (99% sensitive) as long as the patient has not had a subsequent exposure before testing (before seroconversion).
      - If positive, Western blot test should be performed for confirmation.

Infectious Diseases

TABLE 10-5 AIDS Indicator Diseases

Candidiasis, invasive
Cervical cancer, invasive
Coccidioidomycosis, extrapulmonary
Cryptococcosis, extrapulmonary
Cryptosporidiosis of >1-mo duration
Cytomegalovirus disease outside lymphoreticular system
Encephalopathy, HIV-related
Herpes simplex infection of >1-mo duration or visceral herpes simplex
Salmonella bacteremia, recurrent
Histoplasmosis, extrapulmonary
Isosporiasis of >1-mo duration
Kaposi sarcoma
Lymphoma: primary central nervous system, immunoblastic, or Burkitt
Mycobacterial disease, disseminated or extrapulmonary
M. tuberculosis infection
PCP
Pneumonia, recurrent (more than one episode in 1 yr)
Progressive multifocal leukoencephalopathy
Toxoplasmosis, cerebral
Wasting syndrome due to HIV

Modified from Stoller JK, Ahmad M, Longworth DL. The Cleveland Clinic Intensive Review of Internal Medicine. 3rd ed. Philadelphia, PA: Lippincott Williams & Wilkins, 2002:188, Table 15.6.

b. Western blot test is a specific test used to confirm a positive result on an ELISA test.

4. Diagnosis of AIDS.
   a. Depends principally on the identification of an indicator condition or on finding in an HIV-1-seropositive patient a CD4 cell count lower than 200.
   b. There are many indicator conditions **(AIDS-defining illnesses).** (See Table 10-5.)

D. Treatment

1. Antiretroviral therapy (Table 10-6)
   a. Indications
      - Symptomatic patients regardless of CD4 count
      - Asymptomatic patients with CD4 count <500
   b. Triple-drug regimens known as highly active antiretroviral therapy (HAART): To target and prevent HIV replication at three different points along the replication process, use two nucleoside reverse transcriptase inhibitors and either of the following:
      - A nonnucleoside reverse transcriptase inhibitor
      - A protease inhibitor
   c. Monitor the response to treatment using plasma HIV RNA load—the goal is to reduce the viral load to undetectable levels

Quick HIT

Antiretroviral Therapy in HIV

- The importance of strict (i.e., 100%) adherence to the triple-drug regimen cannot be overemphasized, because even minor deviations may result in drug resistance. This has been improved in recent years by combining the medications into a single pill for patients.
- Do not initiate triple-drug therapy in a patient who is not willing or able to fully comply with the prescribed regimen.

TABLE 10-6 **Antiretroviral Therapy**

Drug	Mechanism	Toxicity
Nucleoside Reverse Transcriptase Inhibitors (NRTIs)		
Abacavir (ABC) Didanosine (ddI) Emtricitabine (FTC) Lamivudine (3TC) Stavudine (d4T) Tenofovir (TDF) (only nucleotide) Zalcitabine (ddC) Zidovudine (ZDV, formerly AZT)	Competitively inhibit reverse transcriptase by lacking 3′ OH group. All are nucleosides and require phosphorylation to be active except tenofovir. ZDV used in pregnancy.	Bone marrow suppression, peripheral neuropathy, megaloblastic anemia (ZDV), pancreatitis (ddI)
Nonnucleoside Reverse Transcriptase Inhibitors (NNRTIs)		
Efavirenz (contraindicated in pregnancy) Nevirapine Delavirdine (contraindicated in pregnancy)	Noncompetitively inhibit reverse transcriptase. Do not require phosphorylation.	Rash and hepatotoxicity. CNS symptoms with efavirenz.
Protease Inhibitors		
Atazanavir Darunavir Fosamprenavir Indinavir (crystal-induced nephropathy) Ritonavir ("boost" by inhibiting P450) Saquinavir ("boost" by inhibiting P450)	Inhibited protease (*pol* gene), which cleaves polypeptide products. All end in -navir.	Hyperglycemia, hyperlipidemia, GI intolerance, lipodystrophy
Integrase Inhibitors		
Raltegravir	Inhibit integration into host cell.	Hypercholesteremia
Fusion Inhibitors		
Enfuvirtide Maraviroc	Binds gp41, inhibits entry. Binds CCR-5, inhibits interaction with gp120.	Eosinophilia causing skin reaction at injection site.

   d. It is generally recommended that HAART therapy be continued in pregnant patients with HIV
2. Opportunistic infection prophylaxis
   a. Pneumocystic pneumonia (PCP), formerly *P. carinii*, now named *Pneumocystis jiroveci*
      - Occurs in patients with AIDS when CD4 cell count is <200 and patient is not on prophylaxis
      - Dyspnea, dry cough, fever
      - Tests: chest x-ray (bilateral interstitial infiltrates), LDL level (always elevated), ABG (hypoxia or increased A–a gradient), sputum stain for pneumocystis (very specific but not sensitive), bronchoscopy with BAL (most accurate test)
      - TMP/SMX is the preferred agent
   b. TB
      - Screen all patients with a yearly PPD test
      - Prescribe isoniazid plus pyridoxine if the patient has positive PPD
   c. Atypical mycobacteria—*Mycobacterium avium* complex (MAC)
      - Start prophylaxis when CD4 cell count is <100
      - Clarithromycin and azithromycin are prophylactic agents
   d. Toxoplasmosis
      - Give this to patients with CD4 count <100
      - TMP/SMX is the preferred agent
3. Vaccination **(no live-virus vaccines!)**
   a. Pneumococcal polysaccharide vaccine (Pneumovax)—every 5 to 6 years
   b. Influenza vaccine—yearly
   c. Hepatitis B vaccine (if not already antibody-positive) (See Chapter 12.)

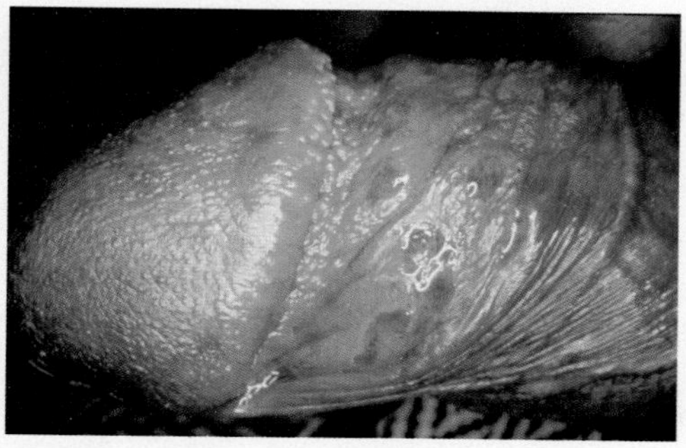

FIGURE **10-3** **Herpes simplex virus.**
(From Goodheart HP. *Goodheart's Photoguide of Common Skin Disorders.* 2nd ed. Philadelphia, PA: Lippincott Williams & Wilkins, 2003, Figure 19.13).

Herpes Simplex

A. General characteristics

1. There are two types of HSV: HSV-1 and HSV-2. Both are very prevalent in the general population (Figure 10-3).
   a. HSV-1 is typically associated with lesions of the oropharynx.
   b. HSV-2 is associated with lesions of the genitalia (see Table 10-7).
   c. Both viruses, however, can cause either genital or oral lesions.

TABLE 10-7 **Clinical Manifestations of Genital Ulcers With Regional Lymphadenopathy**

Genital Lesions	Incubation (Days)	Type	Pain	Number	Duration
Primary syphilis	3–90	Clean ulcer, raised	No	Usually single	3–6 wks
Primary herpes simplex virus	1–26	Grouped papules, vesicles, pustules, ulcers	Yes	Often multiple	1–3 wks
Chancroid	1–21	Purulent ulcer, shaggy border	Yes	Single in men, multiple in women	Progressive
Lymphogranuloma venereum	3–21	Papule, vesicle, ulcer	No	Usually single	Few days
Granuloma inguinale	8–80	Nodules, coalescing granulomatous ulcers	No	Single or multiple	Progressive
Inguinal Adenopathy	**Onset**	**Pain**	**Type**	**Frequency**	**Constitutional Symptoms**
Primary syphilis	Same time	No	Firm	80%, 70% bilateral	Absent
Primary herpes simplex virus	Same time	Yes	Firm	80%, usually bilateral	Common
Chancroid	Same time	Yes	Fluctuant, may fistulize	50%–65%, usually unilateral	Uncommon
Lymphogranuloma venereum	2–6 wks later	Yes	Indurated, fluctuant, may fistulize	Unilateral, one-third bilateral	Common
Granuloma inguinale	Variable	—	Suppurating pseudobubo	10%	1%–5%

From Stoller JK, Ahmad M, Longworth DL. *The Cleveland Clinic Intensive Review of Internal Medicine.* 3rd ed. Philadelphia, PA: Lippincott Williams & Wilkins, 2002:168, Table 14.3.

Infectious Diseases

2. Pathophysiology: After inoculation, the HSV replicates in the dermis and epidermis, then travels via sensory nerves up to the dorsal root ganglia. It resides as a latent infection in the dorsal root ganglia, where it can be reactivated at any time and reach the skin through peripheral nerves.
3. Transmission
   a. HSV is transmitted by contact with people who have active ulcerations or shedding of virus from mucous membranes. HSV-1 is typically associated with transmission through nonsexual personal contact (e.g., kissing), and HSV-2 through sexual contact.
   b. Most people acquire HSV-1 in childhood, and more than 80% of adults have been infected with HSV-1.
   c. The incidence of HSV-2 has increased in recent years.
   d. Episodes of genital herpes frequently may be asymptomatic or may produce symptoms that often go unrecognized. Virus is still shed, and the infected person is contagious.
   e. Contracting one form of herpes confers some degree of cross-immunity, rendering primary infection with the other form of herpes less severe.
   f. Infection with genital herpes is associated with an increased risk of contracting HIV.

Quick HIT

Recurrences of HSV
- Recurrences are associated with the following: stress, fever, infection, and sun exposure.
- Recurrent episodes tend to become shorter in duration and less frequent over time.

B. Clinical features

1. HSV-1
   a. Primary infection is usually asymptomatic and often goes unnoticed.
   b. When symptomatic, primary infection is associated with systemic manifestations (e.g., fevers, malaise) as well as oral lesions (described below).
   c. Oral lesions involve groups of vesicles on patches of erythematous skin. Herpes labialis (cold sores) are most common on the lips (usually painful, heal in 2 to 6 weeks).
   d. HSV-1 is associated with Bell palsy as well.
2. HSV-2
   a. Primary infection results in more severe and prolonged symptoms, lasting up to 3 weeks in duration.
   b. Recurrent episodes are milder and of shorter duration, usually resolving within 10 days. There is also a decrease in the frequency of episodes over time.
   c. Constitutional symptoms (e.g., fever, headache, malaise) often present in primary infection.
   d. HSV-2 presents with painful genital vesicles or pustules (see Figure 10-3). Other findings are tender inguinal lymphadenopathy and vaginal and/or urethral discharge.
3. Disseminated HSV
   a. Usually limited to immunocompromised patients.
   b. May result in encephalitis, meningitis, keratitis, chorioretinitis, pneumonitis, and esophagitis.
   c. Rarely, pregnant women may develop disseminated HSV, which can be fatal to the mother and fetus.
4. Neonatal HSV (vertical transmission at time of delivery) is associated with congenital malformations, intrauterine growth retardation (IUGR), chorioamnionitis, and even neonatal death.
5. Ocular disease—either form of herpes simplex can cause keratitis, blepharitis, and keratoconjunctivitis.

Quick HIT

Herpetic Whitlow
- HSV infection of the finger caused by inoculation into open skin surface. Common in healthcare workers.
- Painful vesicular lesions erupt at the fingertip.
- It may cause fever and axillary lymphadenopathy.
- Treat with acyclovir. Do not mistake for paronychia. Incision and drainage should NOT be done for herpetic whitlow.

C. Diagnosis

1. The diagnosis can be made clinically when characteristic lesions are recognized.
2. If there is uncertainty, perform the following tests to confirm the diagnosis.
   a. Tzanck smear—quickest test.
      - Perform by swabbing the base of the ulcer and staining with Wright stain.
      - This shows multinucleated giant cells. It does not differentiate between HSV and VZV.

b. **Culture of HSV is the gold standard of diagnosis.**
   - Perform by swabbing the base of the ulcer.
   - Results are available within 2 to 3 days.

c. Direct fluorescent assay and ELISA.
   - 80% sensitive.
   - Results available within minutes to hours.

D. Treatment

1. There is no cure available for either type of herpes simplex. Antiviral treatment provides symptomatic relief and reduces the duration of symptoms (see below).
2. Mucocutaneous disease
   a. Treat with oral and/or topical acyclovir for 7 to 10 days.
   b. Valacyclovir and famciclovir have better bioavailability.
   c. Oral acyclovir may be given as prophylaxis for patients with frequent recurrences.
   d. Foscarnet may be given for resistant disease in immunocompromised patients.
3. Disseminated HSV warrants hospital admission. Treat with parenteral acyclovir.

Syphilis

A. General characteristics

1. It is caused by *Treponema pallidum* spirochetes and transmitted by **direct sexual contact** with infectious lesions.
2. It is a systemic illness with four stages (see below). The late stages can be prevented by early treatment.

Quick HIT

Primary syphilis is characterized by a hard chancre (indurated, painless ulcer with clean base).

B. Clinical features

1. Primary stage
   a. **Chancre**—a **painless**, crater-like lesion that appears on the genitalia 3 to 4 weeks after exposure (Figure 10-4)
   b. Heals in 14 weeks, even without therapy
   c. Highly infectious—anyone who touches the lesion can transmit the infection
2. Secondary stage
   a. This may develop 4 to 8 weeks after the chancre has healed. **A maculopapular rash is the most characteristic finding in this stage**
   b. Other possible manifestations: flu-like illness, aseptic meningitis, hepatitis
   c. Patients are contagious during this stage
   d. About one-third of untreated patients with secondary syphilis develop latent syphilis
3. Latent stage
   a. Latent stage is defined as the presence of positive serologic test results in the absence of clinical signs or symptoms. Two-thirds of these patients remain asymptomatic; one-third develop tertiary syphilis

Quick HIT

Most common presentations for syphilis include:
- Genital lesion (chancre)
- Inguinal lymphadenopathy
- Maculopapular rash of secondary syphilis

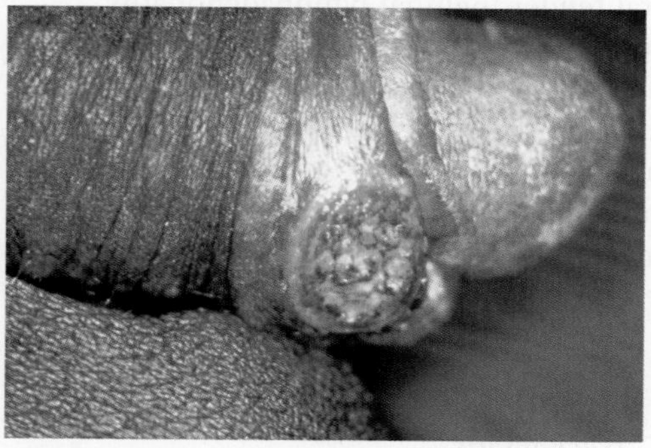

FIGURE 10-4 Chancre of primary syphilis.
(From Goodheart HP. *Goodheart's Photoguide of Common Skin Disorders*. 2nd ed. Philadelphia, PA: Lippincott Williams & Wilkins, 2003, Figure 19.15).

b. It is called early latent syphilis if serology has been positive for <1 year. During this time, the patient may relapse back to the secondary phase.
c. It is called late latent syphilis if serology has been positive for >1 year. Patients are not contagious during this time and do not have any symptoms of the disease.

4. Tertiary stage
   a. One-third of untreated syphilis patients in the latent phase enter this stage
   b. It occurs years after the development of the primary infection (up to 40 years later)
   c. Major manifestations include cardiovascular syphilis, neurosyphilis, and gummas (subcutaneous granulomas)
   d. Neurosyphilis is characterized by dementia, personality changes, and **tabes dorsalis** (posterior column degeneration)
   e. It is very rare nowadays due to treatment with penicillin

Quick HIT

Diagnosis of syphilis: first obtain VDRL and RPR. If positive, confirm with FTA-ABS.

Quick HIT

RPR or VDRL may be falsely positive in patients with SLE.

C. Diagnosis

1. Dark-field microscopy (definitive diagnostic test)—examines a sample of the chancre with visualization of spirochetes. May be required in patients presenting with chancre because serology might not be positive yet.
2. Serologic tests (most commonly used tests).
   a. Nontreponemal tests—RPR, VDRL (most commonly used).
      - High sensitivity—ideal for screening.
      - Specificity is only around 70%. If positive, confirmation is necessary with the specific treponemal tests.
   b. Treponemal tests—FTA-ABS, MHA-TP.
      - More specific than nontreponemal tests
      - Not for screening, just for confirmation of a positive nontreponemal test.
3. All patients should be tested for HIV infection.

D. Treatment

1. Antibiotics are effective in early syphilis but less so in late syphilis.
2. Benzathine penicillin g (one dose IM) is the preferred agent. If the patient is allergic to penicillin, give oral antibiotics (doxycycline, tetracycline) for 2 weeks.
3. If the patient has late latent syphilis or tertiary syphilis, give penicillin in three doses IM once per week.
4. Repeat nontreponemal tests every 3 months to ensure adequate response to treatment. Titers should decrease fourfold within 6 months. If they do not, that may signal treatment failure or reinfection.

Chancroid

Quick HIT

Diagnosis of Chancroid
- Painful genital ulcer(s)
- Tender lymphadenopathy
- Syphilis ruled out (negative, dark-field examination for *T. pallidum* and negative serologic tests)
- HSV ruled out based on clinical presentation or negative culture for HSV

- Caused by *Haemophilus ducreyi*, a gram-negative rod.
- Transmission through sexual contact.
- Incubation period of 2 to 10 days
- There are no systemic findings. Disseminated infection does not occur.
- Clinical features: **painful genital ulcer(s)** that can be deep with ragged borders and with a purulent base (Figure 10-5); unilateral tender inguinal lymphadenopathy ("buboes") that appears 1 to 2 weeks after ulcer.
- Diagnosis is made clinically. Rule out syphilis and HSV and consider testing for HIV. No serologic tests are available, and culture of the organism is not practical because it requires special media that are not widely available.
- Treatment options include azithromycin (oral, one dose), ceftriaxone (IM, one dose), or an oral course of azithromycin, erythromycin, or ciprofloxacin.
- With treatment, most ulcers resolve in 1 or 2 weeks.

Lymphogranuloma Venereum

- A sexually transmitted disease **caused by *C. trachomatis*.**
- Clinical features—painless ulcer at the site of inoculation that may go unnoticed. A few weeks later, tender inguinal lymphadenopathy (usually unilateral) and constitutional symptoms develop.

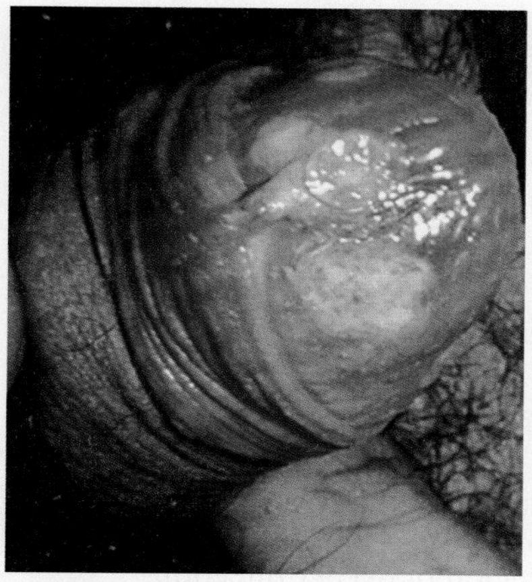

FIGURE 10-5 **Chancroid.**
(From Goodheart HP. *Goodheart's Photoguide of Common Skin Disorders.* 2nd ed. Philadelphia, PA: Lippincott Williams & Wilkins, 2003, Figure 19.14).

- If untreated, proctocolitis may develop with perianal fissures and rectal stricture; obstruction of lymphatics may lead to elephantiasis of genitals.
- Diagnosis is made by serologic tests (complement fixation, immunofluorescence).
- The treatment is doxycycline (oral for 21 days).

Pediculosis Pubis (Pubic Lice)

- Pediculosis pubis (pubic lice or "crabs") is a common STD caused by *Phthirus pubis* (the pubic or crab louse).
- It can be transmitted through sexual contact, clothing, or towels.
- **Severe pruritus** in the genital region is characteristic. Other hairy areas of the body can be involved.
- Diagnosis is made by examination of hair under microscope (or possibly with the naked eye)—identification of adult lice or nits.
- Treat with permethrin 1% shampoo (Elimite)—apply to all hairy regions from neck down and wash off after several hours. Sexual partner(s) should also be treated. Combs, clothes, and bed linens should be washed thoroughly.

Quick HIT
There are three forms of pediculosis: pediculosis capitis (head lice), pediculosis corpora (body lice), and pediculosis pubis (pubic lice or "crabs").

Wound and Soft Tissue Infections

Cellulitis

A. General characteristics

1. Cellulitis is an inflammatory condition of **skin and subcutaneous tissue.**
2. It is caused by a wide variety of bacteria, the most common being group A streptococci or *S. aureus.*
3. **Likely bacterial pathogens are based on patient histories.** Bacteria gain entry through breaks in the skin: IV catheters, incisions, immersion in water, and bites or wounds. Venous stasis diseases, lymphedema, and diabetic ulcers also are associated with cellulitis (see Table 10-8).
4. If untreated, cellulitis may lead to potentially life-threatening bacteremia.

Quick HIT
Patients with cellulitis are predisposed to recurrences in the same area because of damage that occurs to the local lymphatic vessels.

B. Clinical features

1. Classic findings of inflammation: erythema, warmth, pain, swelling
2. Fever (may or may not be present)

C. Diagnosis

1. The diagnosis is essentially clinical.
2. Obtain blood cultures if the patient has a fever.

Quick HIT
Spread to the face is a worrisome complication of cellulitis, and any evidence of orbital involvement is a medical emergency requiring urgent evaluation by an ophthalmologist.

TABLE 10-8 Common Pathogens in Cellulitis

Means of Bacterial Invasion	Likely Pathogen
Local trauma, breaks in skin	Group A Streptococcus *(S. pyogenes)*
Wounds, abscesses	*S. aureus*
Immersion in water	*P. aeruginosa, Aeromonas hydrophila, Vibrio vulnificus*
Acute sinusitis	*H. influenzae*

3. Obtain tissue cultures if there is a wound, ulcer, or site of infection.
4. Obtain imaging (plain film, MRI) if there is suspicion of deeper infection.

D. Treatment

1. Base treatment on suspected pathogens from the patient history. Most patients require parenteral antibiotic therapy.
2. Treat with a staphylococcal penicillin (e.g., oxacillin, nafcillin) or a cephalosporin (e.g., cefazolin).
3. Continue IV antibiotics until signs of infection improve. Follow up with oral antibiotics for 2 weeks.

Erysipelas

- Erysipelas is a cellulitis that is usually confined to the dermis and lymphatics (see also Clinical Pearl 10-5).
- It is usually caused by group A streptococci (other forms of streptococci less commonly).
- The classic presentation is a well-demarcated, fiery red, painful lesion, most commonly on the lower extremities and the face. High fever and chills may be present.
- Predisposing factors include lymphatic obstruction (e.g., after radical mastectomy), local trauma or abscess, fungal infections, diabetes mellitus, and alcoholism.
- Complications include sepsis, local spread to subcutaneous tissues, and necrotizing fasciitis.
- Treatment for uncomplicated cases is IM or oral penicillin or erythromycin; otherwise treat as for cellulitis. Has a high rate of recurrence.

Necrotizing Fasciitis

- Necrotizing fasciitis is a life-threatening infection of deep soft tissues that rapidly tracks along fascial planes.
- Common bacterial causes include *Streptococcus pyogenes* and *Clostridium perfringens*.
- Risk factors include recent surgery, diabetes, trauma, and IV drug use.
- Clinical features may include fever and pain out of proportion to appearance of skin in early stages, so a high index of suspicion is important. Extension of infection leads to thrombosis of microcirculation, resulting in tissue necrosis, discoloration, crepitus, and cutaneous anesthesia.
- It may rapidly progress to sepsis, toxic shock syndrome (TSS), and multiorgan failure.

CLINICAL PEARL 10-5

Differentiating Deep Vein Thrombosis (DVT) From Cellulitis

- Like cellulitis, acute DVT also presents with erythema, warmth, and tenderness in the affected extremity.
- Inflammation in DVT is usually restricted to the posterior calf.
- Because Homans sign and the palpation of venous cords are not sensitive in detecting DVT, venous Doppler must sometimes be performed to differentiate between cellulitis and acute DVT.

- Antibacterial treatment alone is not sufficient. **Rapid surgical exploration and excision of devitalized tissue is an absolute necessity!**
- Broad-spectrum parenteral antimicrobial therapy is warranted.

Lymphadenitis

- This is inflammation of a lymph node (single or multiple) usually caused by local skin or soft tissue bacterial infection (often hemolytic streptococci and staphylococci).
- It presents with fever, tender lymphadenopathy of regional lymph nodes, and red streaking of skin from the wound or area of cellulitis.
- Complications include thrombosis of adjacent veins, sepsis, and even death if untreated.
- Helpful diagnostic studies include blood and wound cultures.
- It usually responds well to treatment. Treat with appropriate antibiotics (penicillin G, antistaphylococcal penicillin, or cephalosporin) and warm compresses. Wound drainage may ultimately be necessary.

Tetanus

A. General characteristics

1. Causes
   a. It is caused by neurotoxins produced by spores of *Clostridium tetani*, a gram-positive anaerobic bacillus.
   b. *C. tetani* proliferates and produces its **exotoxin** in contaminated wounds. The exotoxin blocks inhibitory transmitters at the neuromuscular junction.
2. Patients at risk are those who have incomplete or no tetanus immunization (see Chapter 12).

B. Clinical features

1. The classic and earliest symptom is hypertonicity and contractions of the masseter muscles, resulting in *trismus*, or "lockjaw."
2. Progresses to severe, generalized muscle contractions including:
   a. *Risus sardonicus*—grin due to contraction of facial muscles.
   b. *Opisthotonos*—arched back due to contraction of back muscles.
3. Sympathetic hyperactivity.

C. Diagnosis

1. The diagnosis is mainly clinical.
2. Obtain wound cultures, but they are not a reliable means of diagnosis.

D. Treatment

1. Admit the patient to the ICU and provide respiratory support if necessary (see also Table 10-9). Give diazepam for tetany.
2. Neutralize unbound toxin with passive immunization—give a single IM dose of tetanus immune globulin (TIG).
3. Provide active immunization with tetanus/diphtheria toxoid (Td).

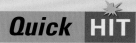

Quick HIT

The following types of wounds are most likely to result in tetanus:
- Wounds contaminated with dirt, feces, or saliva
- Wounds with necrotic tissue
- Deep puncture wounds

Quick HIT

The incubation period for tetanus ranges from about 2 days to 2 weeks. The onset of symptoms is characteristically gradual (1 to 7 days).

TABLE 10-9 Guide to Tetanus Immunization in Wound Management

History of Immunization (Td Doses)	Clean, Minor Wounds		Other Wounds	
	Td	TIG	Td	TIG
≥3 known Td doses	No	No	No	No
<3 doses, unknown status, or >10 yrs since last booster	Yes	No	Yes	Yes

Td, tetanus/diphtheria toxoid; TIG, tetanus immune globulin.

4. Thoroughly clean and debride any wounds with tissue necrosis.
5. Give antibiotics (metronidazole or penicillin G), although efficacy is somewhat controversial.

Quick HIT

Common Bugs in Osteomyelitis
- Catheter septicemia: *S. aureus*
- Prosthetic joint: coagulase-negative staphylococci
- Diabetic foot ulcer: polymicrobial organisms
- Nosocomial infections: *Pseudomonas* spp.
- IV drug abuse, neutropenia: fungal species, *Pseudomonas* spp.
- Sickle cell disease: *Salmonella* spp.

Quick HIT

Up to 10% of patients with open fractures eventually develop osteomyelitis. Use of orthopedic hardware increases this risk (foreign body is the site of bacterial colonization).

Quick HIT

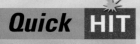

Osteomyelitis of the vertebral body due to *M. tuberculosis* is called **Pott disease.**

Infections of the Bones and Joints

Osteomyelitis

A. General characteristics

1. Osteomyelitis refers to inflammatory destruction of bone due to infection.
2. There are two main categories of osteomyelitis.
   a. Hematogenous osteomyelitis (most common in children)—occurs secondary to sepsis.
   b. Direct spread of bacteria from any of the following:
      - An adjacent infection (e.g., infected diabetic foot ulcer, decubitus ulcer).
      - Trauma (e.g., **open fractures**).
      - Vascular insufficiency (e.g., peripheral vascular disease).
3. The most common microorganisms causing osteomyelitis are *S. aureus* and coagulase-negative staphylococci.
4. Osteomyelitis can involve any bone. Common locations include long bones (tibia, humerus, femur), foot and ankle, and vertebral bodies.

B. Risk factors (for complications or chronic osteomyelitis)

1. Open fractures
2. Diabetes mellitus (causes predisposition to infection and peripheral vascular disease)
3. Use of illicit IV drugs
4. Sepsis

C. Clinical features

1. Pain over the involved area of bone is the most common finding.
2. Localized erythema, warmth, or swelling may be present.
3. Systemic symptoms (e.g., fever, headache, fatigue) may be present, but are inconsistent findings.
4. A draining sinus tract through the skin may form in chronic disease.

D. Diagnosis

1. WBC count—may or may not be elevated and is not useful for diagnosis
2. ESR and CRP
   a. These are fairly nonspecific, but if these markers of inflammation are elevated in the appropriate clinical setting, seriously consider a diagnosis of osteomyelitis. However, a normal ESR and CRP do not exclude the diagnosis
   b. **Both ESR and CRP are very useful in monitoring the response to therapy**
3. **Needle aspiration** of infected bone or bone biopsy (obtained in operating room)—**most direct and accurate means of diagnosis.** Culture results can determine the specific antibiotic therapy
4. Plain radiography
   a. The earliest radiographic changes (periosteal thickening or elevation) are not evident for at least 10 days
   b. Lytic lesions are only apparent in advanced disease
5. Radionucleotide bone scans—usually positive within 2 to 3 days of infection, but are relatively nonspecific (can be positive in metastatic bone disease, trauma, or overlying soft tissue inflammation)
6. **MRI is generally the most effective imaging study for diagnosing osteomyelitis and assessing the extent of disease process**

E. Treatment: Give IV antibiotics for extended periods (4 to 6 weeks). Initiate antibiotic therapy only after the microbial etiology is narrowed based on data from cultures. General guidelines:

1. Empiric therapy requires antibiotics with high bone penetration including cephalosporins (cefazolin, ceftriaxone, cefuroxime), fluroquinolones (levofloxacin, ciprofloxacin, moxifloxacin), vancomycin, linezolid, daptomycin, and clindamycin. Rifampin can also be added as adjunct to help with biofilm penetration.
2. Add an aminoglycoside and possibly a β-lactam antibiotic if there is a possibility of infection with a gram-negative organism.
3. Surgical debridement of infected necrotic bone is an important aspect of treatment.

Quick HIT

Chronic osteomyelitis refers to bone necrosis and soft tissue compromise or to a relapse of previously treated osteomyelitis. It is very challenging to treat and almost impossible to completely eradicate.

Acute Infectious Arthritis

A. General characteristics

1. Acute infectious arthritis occurs when microorganisms (usually bacteria) invade the joint space (not the bone itself), where they release endotoxins and trigger cytokine release and neutrophil infiltration. These inflammatory reactions ultimately lead to erosion and destruction of the joint.
2. Pathogenesis—microorganisms penetrate the joint via the following mechanisms:
   a. Hematogenous spread—most common route.
   b. Contiguous spread from another locus of infection (e.g., osteomyelitis, abscess, or cellulitis).
   c. Traumatic injury to joint.
   d. Iatrogenic (e.g., from arthrocentesis, arthroscopy).
3. Microbiology
   a. The most common offender is bacteria.
   b. Acute bacterial arthritis can be caused by any of the following:
      - ***S. aureus* is the most common agent overall in adults and children.** Various streptococcal species are also frequently involved.
      - An important gram-negative agent is *N. gonorrhoeae*. **Gonococcal arthritis is the most common cause of acute infectious arthritis in young, sexually active adults (see also Clinical Pearl 10-6).**
      - Consider gram-negative organisms such as *Pseudomonas aeruginosa* or *Salmonella* spp. if there is a history of sickle cell disease, immunodeficiency, or IV drug abuse.
4. Other risk factors for acute infectious arthritis.
   a. Prior joint damage (e.g., rheumatoid arthritis).
   b. Joint prosthesis
   c. Diabetes mellitus

Quick HIT

If patient has a painless range of motion of involved joint, septic arthritis is very unlikely, even in the presence of erythema. Micromotion of joint causes severe pain in septic arthritis.

B. Clinical features

1. The joint is swollen, warm, and painful.
   a. **The range of motion (active or passive) is very limited.**
   b. An effusion can be palpated.
2. Constitutional symptoms such as fever, chills, and malaise are common.

Quick HIT

Septic Arthritis

- **The most common joint affected is the knee.** The hip, wrist, shoulder, and ankle may also be involved.
- Patients with immunosuppression or connective tissue diseases may have polyarticular arthritis (and a worse prognosis).

Infectious Diseases

CLINICAL PEARL 10-6

Gonococcal Arthritis

- This presents with acute monoarthritis or oligoarthritis, and often progresses within days in a migratory or additive pattern.
- Knees, wrists, hands, and ankles are the most commonly involved.
- Tenosynovitis is often present in the hands and feet.
- Fever, chills, and rash (macules, papules, and/or pustules) are signs of disseminated gonococcal infection. If the patient has disseminated gonococcal infection, admit to the hospital.
- After the joint is initially aspirated, repeated aspiration is unnecessary (unlike in other causes of septic arthritis), and antibiotics alone usually lead to improvement. Treat presumptively for chlamydial infection (e.g., with doxycycline).
- Consider testing for HIV and syphilis. Educate the patient about the risks of sexual practices.

C. Diagnosis

1. **Perform a joint aspiration ("tap") and analysis of synovial fluid in all patients suspected of having a septic joint.** Order the following studies on aspirated synovial fluid.
   a. WBC count with differential—usually >50,000 WBCs/mm^3 with >80% PMNs—the most helpful test.
   b. Gram stain of fluid—positive in approximately 75% of gram-positive cases, but only 30% to 50% of gram-negative cases.
   c. Culture—aerobic and anaerobic.
   d. Crystal analysis—keep in mind that acute gout may present like septic arthritis.
   e. PCR of synovial fluid—this may be useful if gonococcal arthritis is suspected but Gram stain and cultures are negative.
2. Blood cultures are positive in >50% of all cases (frequently negative in gonococcal arthritis).
3. Other laboratory abnormalities.
   a. Leukocytosis—present in about half of patients with a septic joint.
   b. Elevated ESR—elevated in up to 90% of patients with septic joint.
   c. Elevated CRP—useful in monitoring clinical improvement.
4. Imaging studies.
   a. Plain radiographs—generally not useful unless joint damage is severe.
   b. CT or MRI—helpful if the sacroiliac or facet joints are involved.
5. Obtain cultures from appropriate mucosal surfaces (e.g., genitourinary tract) if gonococcal arthritis is suspected.

D. Treatment

1. Prompt antibiotic treatment.
   a. Do not delay in initiating antimicrobial therapy when acute infectious arthritis is suspected.
   b. If the Gram stain result is negative but acute bacterial arthritis is still suspected, treat empirically based on the clinical scenario (see Table 10-10) until culture and sensitivity results are available.
2. Drainage
   a. Daily aspiration of affected joint as long as effusion persists is one treatment option. However, surgical drainage is recommended to prevent further damage to the articular cartilage that occurs with persistent infectious process. Certain joints are amenable to arthroscopic drainage (shoulder, knee) whereas others are not (hip, wrist, elbow, ankle) and should be opened.

Quick HIT

Complications of Septic Arthritis
- Destruction of joint and surrounding structures (e.g., ligaments, tendons), leading to stiffness, pain, and loss of function
- Avascular necrosis (if hip is involved)
- Sepsis

TABLE 10-10 Medical Treatment of Acute Bacterial Arthritis

Adult (Relatively Healthy): Treat for *S. aureus*	Patient Is Immunocompromised or Has Significant Risk Factors for Gram-negative Arthritis	Young Adult With History and Presentation Consistent with Gonococcal Arthritis
Parenteral, β-lactamase–resistant penicillin (e.g., oxacillin) or first-generation cephalosporin × 4 wks	Parenteral, broad-spectrum antibiotics (with gram-negative coverage) (e.g., a third-generation cephalosporin or aminoglycoside) for 3–4 wks	Parenteral, third-generation cephalosporin (e.g., ceftriaxone) until there is improvement
Treat with vancomycin if MRSA is suspected	For pseudomonal infection, use aminoglycoside + extended-spectrum penicillin	Switch to an oral agent with gram-negative coverage (e.g., ciprofloxacin 3–10 days) once there is clinical improvement

Zoonoses and Arthropod-borne Diseases

Lyme Disease

A. General characteristics

1. Three major endemic areas in the United States
   a. Northeastern seaboard (from Maine to Maryland)
   b. Midwest (north central states—e.g., Minnesota, Wisconsin)
   c. West coast (Northern California)
2. Incubation period is 3 to 32 days
3. Transmission cycle
   a. Caused by spirochete *Borrelia burgdorferi*
   b. Transmitted by ticks—commonly the deer tick *Ixodidae scapularis*
   c. The tick is hosted by white-footed mice (immature ticks), white-tailed deer (mature ticks), and brief and unfortunate encounters with humans

B. Clinical features

1. Stage 1—early, localized infection.
   a. **Erythema migrans** is the hallmark skin lesion at site of the tick bite. Characteristically it is a large, painless, well-demarcated target-shaped lesion, commonly seen on the thigh, groin, or axilla (Figure 10-6).
   b. Multiple lesions signify that hematogenous spread has occurred (see below).
2. Stage 2—early, disseminated infection.
   a. Infection spreads via lymphatics and the bloodstream within days to weeks after the onset of erythema migrans.
   b. Clinical features: intermittent flu-like symptoms, headaches, neck stiffness, fever/chills, fatigue, malaise, musculoskeletal pain.
   c. After several weeks, about 15% of patients develop one or several of the following (usually resolve within several months):
      - Meningitis (Brudzinski and Kernig signs negative).
      - Encephalitis.
      - Cranial neuritis (often bilateral facial nerve palsy).
      - Peripheral radiculoneuropathy (motor or sensory).
   d. Within weeks to months of onset of symptoms, about 8% will have cardiac manifestations (e.g., AV block, pericarditis, carditis). These usually only last for several weeks, but recurrence is not uncommon.
3. Stage 3—late, persistent infection (months to years after initial infection).
   a. Arthritis—This occurs in 60% of untreated patients; it typically affects the large joints (especially knees). Chronic arthritis will develop in some patients.

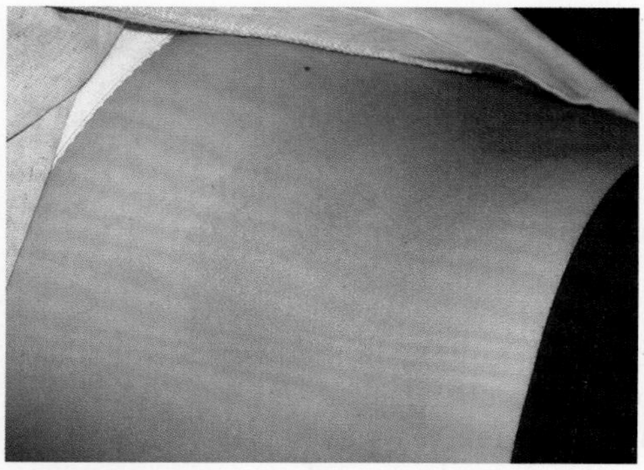

FIGURE 10-6 **Erythema migrans (Lyme disease).**
(From Goodheart HP. *Goodheart's Photoguide of Common Skin Disorders*. 2nd ed. Philadelphia, PA: Lippincott Williams & Wilkins, 2003, Figure 7.19).

Quick HIT

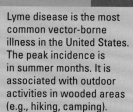

Lyme disease is the most common vector-borne illness in the United States. The peak incidence is in summer months. It is associated with outdoor activities in wooded areas (e.g., hiking, camping).

Quick HIT

- Patients with tick bites should be followed up closely for the appearance of erythema migrans, but the majority of tick bites do not result in infection.
- A vaccine against B. *burgdorferi* has been developed but was taken off the market due to lack of use in the medical community.

CLINICAL PEARL 10-7

Lyme Serology

- IgM antibodies peak 3 to 6 weeks after the onset of symptoms. If a few months have passed since the onset of disease, IgM levels are basically worthless.
- IgG antibodies slowly increase and remain elevated in patients with disseminated illness. If a patient has had Lyme disease in the past and now has symptoms consistent with new illness, IgG levels will not indicate whether the infection is acute or chronic.
- Patients with a history of distant Lyme disease may have elevated IgG levels despite adequate antibiotic treatment.
- IgG antibodies cross-react with *T. pallidum,* but patients with Lyme disease will not have a positive VDRL.

b. Chronic CNS disease—subacute, mild encephalitis, transverse myelitis, or axonal polyneuropathy.
c. Acrodermatitis chronica atrophicans (a rare skin lesion)—reddish-purple plaques and nodules on the extensor surfaces of the legs.

Quick HIT

Early treatment with antibiotics is extremely important because later sequelae of disease can usually be prevented. Treatment in later stages is usually effective, but recovery may be delayed.

C. Diagnosis

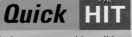

1. Clinical diagnosis—In early, localized disease, documented erythema migrans in a patient with a history of tick exposure in an endemic area obviates the need for laboratory confirmation. Treat empirically.
2. **Serologic studies—most important tests to confirm a clinical suspicion of Lyme disease (see also Clinical Pearl 10-7)**
   a. ELISA is used to detect serum IgM and IgG antibodies during the first month of illness.
   b. Western blot is used to confirm positive or equivocal results.

D. Treatment

1. Early localized disease.
   a. If it is confined to the skin, 10 days of antibiotic therapy is adequate.
   b. If there is any evidence of spread beyond the skin, extend treatment to 20 to 30 days.
   c. For early Lyme disease.
      - Oral doxycycline (for 21 days)—contraindicated in pregnant women and in children <8 years of age.
      - Amoxicillin and cefuroxime are alternative agents.
      - Erythromycin may be given to pregnant patients with penicillin allergies.
2. Treatment of complications such as facial nerve palsy, arthritis, or cardiac disease is prolonged antibiotic therapy (30 to 60 days). For meningitis or other CNS complications, treat with IV antibiotics for 4 weeks.

Rocky Mountain Spotted Fever

A. General characteristics

1. Caused by the intracellular bacteria *Rickettsia rickettsii.*
2. Ticks feeding on various mammals serve as vectors for disease transmission.
3. The major endemic areas include the southeastern, midwestern, and western United States. Peak incidence is in the spring and summer months due to increased outdoor activity.
4. Pathophysiology of disease.
   a. Organisms enter the host cells via tick bites, multiply in the vascular endothelium, and spread to different layers of the vasculature.
   b. Damage to the vascular endothelium results in increased vascular permeability, activation of complement, microhemorrhages, and microinfarcts.

B. Clinical features

1. The onset of symptoms is typically 1 week after the tick bite.

2. It classically presents with a sudden onset of fever, chills, malaise, nausea, vomiting, myalgias, photophobia, and headache.
3. Papular rash usually appears after 4 to 5 days of fever. **Rash starts peripherally (wrists, forearms, palms, ankles, and soles) but then spreads centrally** (to the rest of the limbs, trunk, and face). It becomes maculopapular, and eventually petechial.
4. It may lead to interstitial pneumonitis.

C. Diagnosis

1. Diagnosis is primarily clinical. Laboratory abnormalities may include elevated liver enzymes and thrombocytopenia.
2. Acute and convalescent serology and immunofluorescent staining of skin biopsy are confirmatory tests.

D. Treatment

1. Doxycycline—usually given for 7 days; given intravenously if the patient is vomiting.
2. CNS manifestations or pregnant patients—give chloramphenicol.

Malaria

A. General characteristics

1. A protozoal infection caused by one of four organisms
   a. *Plasmodium falciparum*
   b. *Plasmodium ovale*
   c. *Plasmodium vivax*
   d. *Plasmodium malariae*
2. Prevalent in tropical climates, parts of Africa and the Middle East
3. Transmitted via mosquito bite in endemic areas

B. Clinical features

1. Symptoms may include fever and chills, myalgias, headache, nausea, vomiting, and diarrhea.
2. Fever pattern varies depending on cause
   a. *P. falciparum*—fever is usually constant
   b. *P. ovale* and *P. vivax*—fever usually spikes every 48 hours
   c. *P. malariae*—fever usually spikes every 72 hours

C. Diagnosis

1. Identify organism on peripheral blood smear
2. Blood smear must have **Giemsa stain**

D. Treatment

1. Use chloroquine phosphate unless resistance is suspected. In many countries, chloroquine resistance is so prevalent that it should be assumed.
2. If chloroquine resistance is suspected, give quinine sulfate and tetracycline. Alternative agents are atovaquone–proguanil and mefloquine.
3. *P. falciparum* infection may require IV quinidine and doxycycline.
4. Relapses can occur in *P. vivax* and *P. ovale* infection as a result of dormant hypnozoites in the liver. Add a 2-week regimen of primaquine phosphate for these types of malarial infection.
5. Prophylaxis is important for travelers to endemic regions. Mefloquine is the agent of choice in chloroquine-resistant areas. Chloroquine can be used in areas where chloroquine resistance has not been reported.

Rabies

A. General characteristics

1. A devastating, deadly viral encephalitis
2. Contracted from a bite or scratch by an infected animal; infection from a corneal transplant has been documented as well

Quick HIT

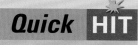

The onset of illness in malaria usually occurs weeks to months after infection, but it is dependent on the specific cause.

Quick HIT

P. falciparum infection is by far the most serious and life-threatening cause of malaria.

Quick HIT

Side effects of medications can be a factor in choosing appropriate malaria prophylaxis:
- Atovaquone–proguanil is contraindicated in patients with renal disease and pregnancy.
- Mefloquine is contraindicated in patients with seizures and psychiatric conditions.
- Chloroquine is well tolerated and can be used in pregnancy.

Primaquine is contraindicated in patients with G6PD deficiency due to precipitation of hemolytic anemia.

3. More prevalent in developing countries where rabies vaccination of animals is not widespread

B. Clinical features

1. The incubation period typically ranges from 30 to 90 days, but varies considerably.
2. Once symptoms are present, rabies is almost invariably fatal.
3. Symptoms (in progressive order).
   a. Pain at site of bite.
   b. Prodromal symptoms of sore throat, fatigue, headache, nausea, and/or vomiting.
   c. Encephalitis—confusion, combativeness, hyperactivity, fever, and seizures may be present.
   d. Hydrophobia—inability to drink, laryngeal spasm with drinking, hypersalivation ("foaming at mouth"), usually progresses to coma and death.
   e. Some patients may present with ascending paralysis.

> **Quick HIT**
> **Pre-exposure prophylaxis**—Rabies vaccine is available for at-risk individuals (e.g., those with potential occupational exposure, such as veterinarians, wildlife officials, and laboratory workers).

C. Diagnosis

1. Virus or viral antigen can be identified in infected tissue. Virus can be isolated in saliva as well.
2. Fourfold increase in serum antibody titers.
3. Identification of **Negri bodies** histologically.
4. PCR detection of virus RNA.

D. Treatment (postexposure management)

1. Clean the wound thoroughly with soap.
2. For wild animal bites (e.g., bat or raccoon), the animal should be captured if possible, destroyed, and sent to a laboratory for immunofluorescence of brain tissue.
3. If a patient was bitten by a healthy dog or cat in an endemic area, the animal should be captured and observed for 10 days. If there is no change in the animal's condition, then it most likely does not have rabies.
4. For known rabies exposure, both of the following should be performed.
   a. Passive immunization—administer the human rabies immunoglobulin to patients, into the wound as well in the gluteal region.
   b. Active immunization—administer the antirabies vaccine in three IM doses into the deltoid or thigh over a 28-day period.

Other Zoonoses

- Table 10-11 covers leptospirosis, ehrlichiosis, tularemia, Q fever, and cat scratch fever.

Common Fungal Infections

Candidiasis

A. General characteristics

1. *Candida* species are oval, budding yeasts known for their formation of hyphae and long pseudohyphae. They normally colonize humans, and it is the overgrowth of these organisms that results in the clinical pathology of candidiasis
2. *Candida albicans* is the most common cause of candidiasis
3. Risk factors for candidiasis
   a. Antibiotic therapy
   b. Diabetes mellitus
   c. Immunosuppressive therapy
   d. Immunocompromised hosts (increased risk for both mucocutaneous and systemic candidiasis)

B. Clinical features

1. Typical presentation is the mucocutaneous growth. The most common affected areas are:

TABLE 10-11 **Other Zoonoses and Arthropod-borne Diseases**

Disease	Organism	Transmission	Reservoir	Clinical Findings	Diagnosis	Treatment
Leptospirosis	*Leptospira* spp. (spirochetes)	Contaminated water	Rodents, farm animals	**Anicteric:** rash, LAN,[a] ↑ LFTs	Isolation of organism in blood or urine CTX[a] **Icteric:** renal and/or liver failure, vasculitis, vascular collapse	Oral antibiotics: tetracycline or doxycycline; if severe, IV penicillin G
Ehrlichiosis	*Ehrlichia* spp. (intracellular, gram-negative bacteria)	Tick bite	Deer	Fever, chills, malaise ± rash **Complications:** renal failure, GI bleeding	Clinical; confirm by serology	Oral tetracycline or doxycycline × 1 week
Tularemia	*Francisella tularensis* (small gram-negative bacillus)	Tick bite, animal bites, handling carcass	Rabbits, other rodents	Fever, headache, nausea; ulcer at site of tick bite; painful LAN	Isolation of organism in blood or wound CTX	IM streptomycin or gentamicin
Q fever	*C. burnetii* (gram-negative organism)	Blood, ingestion of infected milk, inhalation	Farm animals	**Acute:** constitutional symptoms, nausea, vomiting **Chronic:** endocarditis	Serology; CXR—multiple opacities in acute illness	**Acute:** doxycycline or fluoroquinolone **Chronic:** rifampin
Cat scratch disease	*Bartonella henselae* (gram-negative bacillus)	Scratch from a flea-infested cat	Cats, fleas	LAN or lymphadenitis; systemic symptoms rare	Serology, clinical	Usually self-limited; if severe, oral doxycycline or ciprofloxacin

[a]LAN, lymphadenopathy; CTX, culture.

a. Vagina—"yeast infection"
   - This results in a thick, white, "cottage cheese-like" vaginal discharge
   - The discharge characteristically is painless but does cause pruritus
b. Mouth, oropharynx—"thrush"
   - This causes thick, white plaques that adhere to the oral mucosa
   - Usually painless
   - Unexplained oral thrush should raise suspicion of HIV infection
c. Cutaneous candidiasis
   - This causes erythematous, eroded patches with "satellite lesions" (Figure 10-7)
   - It is more common in obese diabetic patients; it appears in skin folds, underneath breasts, and in macerated skin areas
d. GI tract (e.g., esophagus)
   - Candida esophagitis may cause significant odynophagia
   - It may also be asymptomatic

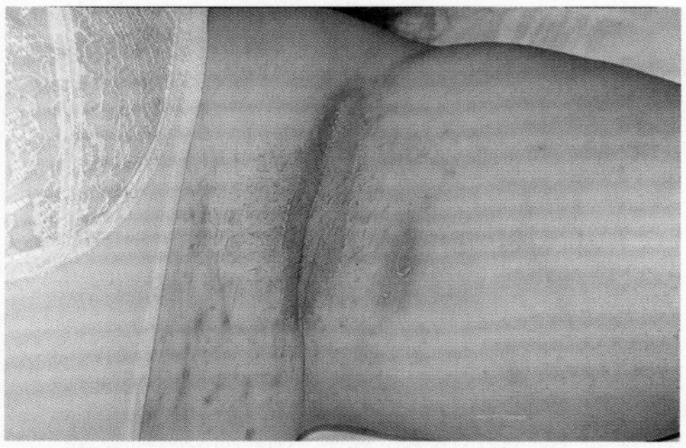

FIGURE 10-7 **Cutaneous candidiasis (axilla).**
(From Goodheart HP. *Goodheart's Photoguide of Common Skin Disorders.* 2nd ed. Philadelphia, PA: Lippincott Williams & Wilkins, 2003, Figure 3.25).

2. Disseminated or invasive disease may occur in immunocompromised hosts. Manifestations include sepsis/septic shock, meningitis, and multiple abscesses in various organs.

C. Diagnosis

1. Mucocutaneous candidiasis diagnosis is primarily clinical; KOH preparation demonstrates yeast.
2. Invasive candidiasis is diagnosed by blood or tissue culture.

D. Treatment

1. Remove indwelling catheters or central lines.
2. Acceptable treatments for oropharyngeal candidiasis.
   a. Clotrimazole troches (dissolve in the mouth) five times per day.
   b. Nystatin mouthwash ("swish and swallow") three to five times per day; only for oral candidiasis.
   c. Oral ketoconazole or fluconazole for esophagitis.
3. Vaginal candidiasis—miconazole or clotrimazole cream.
4. Cutaneous candidiasis—oral nystatin powder, keeping skin dry.
5. For systemic candidiasis, use amphotericin B or fluconazole. New, alternative antifungal agents include voriconazole and caspofungin.

Aspergillus

A. General characteristics

1. *Aspergillus* spp. spores are found everywhere in the environment. Typically, disease occurs when spores are inhaled into the lung.
2. There are three main types of clinical syndromes associated with *Aspergillus* (see clinical features below).
3. Invasive aspergillosis is usually limited to severely immunocompromised patients. It should be considered in any immunocompromised patient with fever and respiratory distress despite use of broad-spectrum antibiotics.

B. Clinical features

1. Allergic bronchopulmonary aspergillosis.
   a. A type I hypersensitivity reaction to *Aspergillus*.
   b. It presents with **asthma and eosinophilia.** Recurrent exacerbations are common.
2. Pulmonary aspergilloma.
   a. Pulmonary aspergilloma is caused by inhalation of spores into the lung. Patients with a history of sarcoidosis, histoplasmosis, TB, and bronchiectasis are at risk.
   b. It presents with chronic cough; hemoptysis may be present as well.
   c. It may resolve spontaneously or invade locally.
3. Invasive aspergillosis.
   a. This occurs when hyphae invade the lung vasculature, resulting in thrombosis and infarction.
   b. Hosts are typically at-risk patients with acute leukemia, transplant recipients, and patients with advanced AIDS.
   c. It usually presents with acute onset of fever, cough, respiratory distress, and diffuse, bilateral pulmonary infiltrates.
   d. It is transmitted via hematogenous dissemination, and may invade the sinuses, orbits, and brain.

C. Diagnosis

1. CXR reveals a dense pulmonary consolidation and sometimes a **fungus ball.**
2. Definitive diagnosis of invasive aspergillosis is by tissue biopsy, but diagnosis is presumed when *Aspergillus* is isolated from the sputum of a severely immunocompromised/neutropenic patient with clinical symptoms.
3. Blood cultures are usually not helpful because they are rarely positive.

D. Treatment

1. For allergic bronchopulmonary aspergillosis, patients should avoid exposure to *Aspergillus;* corticosteroids may be beneficial.
2. For pulmonary aspergilloma, patients with massive hemoptysis may require a lung lobectomy.
3. For invasive aspergillosis, treat with IV amphotericin B, voriconazole, or caspofungin.
4. Suspicion of head or brain involvement warrants prompt evaluation (imaging studies). Surgery may be required.

Cryptococcosis

A. General characteristics

1. Caused by *Cryptococcus neoformans,* a budding, round yeast with a thick polysaccharide capsule
2. Associated with pigeon droppings
3. Most commonly seen in patients with advanced AIDS
4. Infection is due to inhalation of fungus into lungs. Hematogenous spread may involve the brain and meninges

B. Clinical features

1. CNS disease—meningitis or meningoencephalitis; brain abscess is also possible
   a. CNS disease is a life-threatening condition that requires aggressive treatment (see below). It should always be on the differential diagnosis of an HIV-positive patient with a fever and headache. If untreated, it is almost invariably fatal.
   b. Symptoms include fever, headache, irritability, dizziness, confusion, and possibly seizures. The onset may be insidious.
2. Isolated pulmonary infection may also occur.

C. Diagnosis

1. LP is absolutely essential if meningitis is suspected.
   a. Latex agglutination detects cryptococcal antigen in the CSF.
   b. India ink smear shows encapsulated yeasts.
2. Tissue biopsy is characterized by **lack of inflammatory response.**
3. The organism may also be present in urine and blood.

D. Treatment

1. Use amphotericin B with flucytosine for approximately 2 weeks, followed by oral fluconazole.
2. The duration of therapy varies depending on follow-up CSF cultures.

Other Fungal Infections

- Table 10-12 covers blastomycosis, histoplasmosis, coccidioidomycosis, and sporotrichosis.

Common Parasitic Infections

- Table 10-13 covers cryptosporidiosis, amebiasis, giardiasis, ascariasis, hookworm, pinworm (enterobiasis), tapeworm, and schistosomiasis.

Fever and Sepsis

Fever of Unknown Origin

A. General characteristics

1. Defining fever of unknown origin (FUO)
   a. Classically defined as having the following necessary criteria:
      - Fever >38.3°C (101°F)

TABLE 10-12 Other Important Fungal Infections

Infection	Organism	Transmission	Findings	Diagnosis	Treatment
Blastomycosis	*Blastomyces dermatitidis* (dimorphic fungus)	Inhalation of spores from the environment	Disseminated infection → chronic, indolent disease: constitutional symptoms, LAN, pneumonia	CTX from urine, sputum, body fluids	PO itraconazole × 6–12 mo Amphotericin B for meningitis
Histoplasmosis	*H. capsulatum* (dimorphic fungus with septate hyphae)	Exposure to bird/bat droppings (endemic in Ohio and Mississippi River valleys)	Flu-like symptoms, erythema nodosum, hepatosplenomegaly	Demonstration of yeast in body fluids or skin	PO itraconazole; amphotericin B for severe infection or ↓ immunocompromised host
Coccidioidomycosis	*Coccidioides immitis* (dimorphic fungus)	Inhalation of spores	Asymptomatic or nonspecific respiratory symptoms	Visualization of fungus in fluids or skin	PO fluconazole or itraconazole × 6 mo IV amphotericin B for severe infection or ↓ immunocompromised host
			Dissemination → focal CNS findings	Visualization of fungus in fluids or skin	
Sporotrichosis	*Sporothrix schenckii* (dimorphic, cigar-shaped yeast)	Invasion of skin by thorn or other plant material Keyword: gardening	Lymphocutaneous form: hard, subcutaneous nodules → ulcerate and drain Disseminated form: pneumonia, meningitis	Visualization of yeast in tissue or body fluids or serology	Potassium iodide × 1–2 mo or itraconazole × 3–6 mo Disseminated: amphotericin B

LAN, lymphadenopathy; CTX, culture.

Quick HIT

Persistence of fever in the ICU, despite antimicrobial therapy, should raise the index of suspicion for:
- Fungal infection
- Antimicrobial resistance
- Infections requiring surgical intervention (e.g., occult abscess, wound necrosis)
- Drug fever

- Continuing "on several occasions" for at least 3 weeks
- No diagnosis over this time period despite 1 week of inpatient workup

b. Because of changes in medical practice, this definition has been altered: Three outpatient visits now substitute for 1 week in the hospital

2. Causes
   a. Infection—most common cause
      - TB and other mycobacterial infection
      - Occult abscesses (e.g., hepatic, retroperitoneal)
      - UTI/complicated UTI
      - Endocarditis
      - Sinusitis
      - HIV
      - Infectious mononucleosis and other viruses
      - Malaria and other parasitic infections
   b. Occult neoplasms are the second most common cause, particularly:
      - Lymphoma (especially Hodgkin lymphoma)
      - Leukemia
   c. Collagen vascular disease
      - SLE
      - Still disease
      - Polyarteritis nodosa (PAN)
      - Temporal arteritis
      - Polymyalgia rheumatica
   d. Other causes (in no particular order)
      - Granulomatous disease (e.g., sarcoidosis, Crohn disease)
      - Drug fevers (e.g., sulfonamides, penicillin, quinidine, barbiturates, "diet pills" [with phenolphthalein])

TABLE 10-13 Important Parasitic Infections

Infection	Organism	Transmission/ Life Cycle	Findings	Diagnosis	Treatment
Cryptosporidiosis	*Cryptosporidium* spp. (spore-forming protozoa)	Fecal–oral route	Watery diarrhea ↓ Severe diarrhea in an immunocompromised host	Stool sample: see oocytes	Supportive care
Amebiasis	*Entamoeba histolytica* (protozoan)	Fecal–oral route Contaminated water/ food, anal–oral sexual contact	Bloody diarrhea, tenesmus, abdominal pain ± liver abscess	Stool sample: see trophozoites	Iodoquinol or paromomycin Metronidazole for liver abscess
Giardiasis	*Giardia lamblia* (protozoan)	Fecal–oral route (as in amebiasis) Hints: daycare, camping	Watery diarrhea Chronic infection; weight loss	Stool sample: see cysts or trophozoites	Metronidazole
Ascariasis	*Ascaris lumbricoides* (roundworms = nematodes)	Ingestion of food or water contaminated by human feces	Varies: no symptoms, postprandial abdominal pain, or vomiting Heavy worm burden: bowel, pancreatic duct or common bile duct obstruction	Stool sample: see eggs or adult worms	Albendazole, mebendazole, or pyrantel pamoate
Hookworm	*Ancylostoma duodenale* or *Necator americanus* (roundworm)	Larvae invade skin → travel to lung → coughed and swallowed → reside in intestine	Usually no symptoms Cough, anemia, malabsorption, weight loss, eosinophilia	Stool sample: see adult worms	Mebendazole or pyrantel pamoate
Enterobiasis (pinworm)	*Enterobius vermicularis* (roundworm)	Fecal–oral route (self-infection with anus–hand–mouth contact) Common in children	Perianal pruritus, worse at night	"Tape test": see eggs on tape after it is placed near the anus	Mebendazole or pyrantel pamoate
Tapeworm (cestodes)	*Taenia saginata* (beef), *Taenia solium* (pork), *Diphyllobothrium latum* (fish)	Eating raw or undercooked meat	Usually asymptomatic Possible nausea, abdominal pain, weight loss Fish tapeworm: vitamin B_{12} deficiency	Tape test for *D. latum*, stool sample (see eggs)	Praziquantel; vitamin B_{12} if deficient
Schistosomiasis (trematodes)	*Schistosoma mansoni, Schistosoma haematobium, Schistosoma japonicum*	Penetration of human skin (in contaminated fresh water) → migrate to lungs → to portal vein → to venules of mesentery, bladder, or ureters	*S. mansoni* and *S. japonicum:* fever, diarrhea (acute) → liver fibrosis, portal HTN (chronic) *S. haematobium:* urinary tract granulomas → bladder polyps and fibrosis, dysuria	Demonstration of eggs in urine or feces	Praziquantel

- Pulmonary embolism
- Hemolytic anemia
- Familial Mediterranean fever
- Gout
- Subacute thyroiditis
- Factitious illnesses

Quick HIT

FUO is obviously a term of exclusion, and is not itself a diagnosis. In patients with persistent unexplained fevers, continue diagnostic testing until the cause is found.

B. Clinical features

1. Manifestations that **may** accompany fever but are not specific to any specific entity
   a. Chills—ironic sensation of cold, often with shivering
   b. Rigors—severe form of chills with pronounced shivering and chattering of teeth
   c. Night sweats
   d. Change in mental status—especially at extremes of age
2. Look for systemic manifestations of some of the more common causes of FUO (e.g., skin changes, constitutional symptoms, anemia, weight loss).

C. Diagnosis

1. Careful history and physical examination—with attention to medications, travel, immune system competency, and review of systems
2. Laboratory tests
   a. CBC with differential
   b. Urinalysis
   c. Cultures of blood, sputum, CSF, urine, and stool when indicated by clinical presentation
   d. Analysis and culture of abnormal fluid collections (e.g., joint, pleural)
   e. Complement assay
   f. PPD when TB is on the differential
   g. Other laboratory values: LFTs, ESR, ANA, rheumatoid factor, TSH
3. Imaging studies
   a. CXR, CT scan of the chest and abdomen—to detect tumors and abscesses
   b. Tagged WBC scan—sometimes helpful
   c. MRI, ultrasound, and echocardiogram may be appropriate, depending on the clinical situation
4. Invasive diagnostic procedures—biopsy of lymph node, bone marrow, or other tissue when there is a high suspicion of tumor or abscess
5. Observation is sometimes necessary to make a diagnosis

D. Treatment

1. Antibiotics and corticosteroids may mask the patterns of fever response (see also Clinical Pearl 10-8). Base empiric treatment with antibiotics on the severity of illness.

CLINICAL PEARL 10-8

Approach to Fever

- There is no uniformly accepted definition, but most sources define fever as body temperature >37.5°C (99.5°F) measured by a modern oral thermometer.
- Measurement—Readings obtained using rectal thermometers are slightly higher than oral or axillary thermometer readings.
- Hyperthermia versus fever.
  - Hyperthermia is an elevation in body temperature not caused by "raising the thermostat" (i.e., no change in the hypothalamic set-point).
  - Hyperthermia is usually caused by the inability of the body to dissipate heat.
  - Causes of hyperthermia include neuroleptic malignant syndrome, malignant hyperthermia, and heat stroke.
  - Hyperthermia does not respond to antipyretics, but rather to external cooling measures (e.g., ice, fans) and medications specific to the cause (e.g., dantrolene for malignant hyperthermia).
  - Fever occurs when there is an elevation in the hypothalamic set-point. It is a natural response to an inflammatory process.
  - Fever usually responds to antipyretics.
- Treat a fever with antipyretics when:
  - The fever is really hyperthermia.
  - The fever is dangerously high: >41°C (>105°F).
  - The patient is pregnant.
  - There is significant cardiopulmonary disease (increased oxygen demand may cause ischemia).
  - The patient wants symptomatic relief (chills, myalgias).

2. If the patient is not acutely ill, observation alone may be all that is necessary to arrive at a specific diagnosis.
3. In some cases of FUO, fevers may resolve spontaneously without ever being diagnosed.
4. The sense of urgency in determining the cause of the fevers should be in proportion to the severity of illness and the host's immune status.

Toxic Shock Syndrome

A. General characteristics

1. TSS is most commonly associated with menstruating women and tampon use, but can occur in patients of all ages, male and female.
2. Other risk factors include surgical wounds, burns, and infected insect bites.
3. It is caused by an enterotoxin of *S. aureus*, or less frequently an exotoxin of group A Streptococcus. **Note that it is the toxin rather than the bacteria that causes the pathology associated with TSS.**

B. Clinical features

1. The onset of symptoms is characteristically abrupt
2. Symptoms may include:
   a. Flu-like symptoms: high fevers, headache, myalgias
   b. Diffuse macular, erythematous rash
   c. Hyperemic mucous membranes, "strawberry tongue"
   d. Warm skin due to peripheral vasodilation (see Chapter 1, Shock)
   e. Hypotension
   f. Nausea, vomiting, and diarrhea may also be present
3. By definition, there must be involvement of at least three organ systems, which may include:
   a. GI—nausea, vomiting, and diarrhea; elevations of aminotransferases
   b. Renal—elevations of BUN and/or creatine, pyuria
   c. Hematologic—thrombocytopenia
   d. Musculoskeletal—elevations of creatine kinase levels
   e. CNS—confusion, disorientation (must be present when fever is absent)
4. Multisystem organ dysfunction or failure may occur
5. During the convalescent phase of illness, the **rash usually desquamates over the palms and soles**

C. Diagnosis

1. A high index of clinical suspicion is important.
2. Blood cultures are often negative.
3. Cultures may be taken from the suspected source, but the diagnosis is primarily clinical.

D. Treatment

1. Hemodynamic stabilization should be the first concern and may require aggressive fluids and even vasopressors. Patient is often treated in a burn intensive care unit.
2. The source of toxin (e.g., tampon) should be removed immediately. Wounds may require drainage or debridement.
3. Give antistaphylococcal therapy, such as nafcillin, oxacillin, or vancomycin, in a very ill patient. Clindamycin is sometimes used as adjunctive therapy.

> **Quick HIT**
> - The mortality rate for menstrual-related TSS is now <2% but is slightly higher (8%) for non–menstrual-related TSS.
> - Previous TSS does **not** confer immunity. In fact, patients with a history of TSS are at greater risk for recurrent TSS.

Catheter-related Sepsis

- Central venous catheters are a common cause of fever and sepsis in the hospital, especially in the ICU.
- The most common organisms are *S. aureus* and *Staphylococcus epidermidis.*
- Risk factors for catheter-related sepsis are emergent placement, femoral lines, and prolonged indwelling of the line.
- Only half of all patients with catheter-related sepsis have clinical evidence of infection **at the site of insertion** (i.e., erythema, purulence). Therefore, a high index of suspicion is required.

> **Quick HIT**
> Catheter-related sepsis almost always involves central IV catheters. Peripheral venous catheters and arterial catheters are rarely involved.

> **Quick HIT**
> - Neutropenia is defined by absolute neutrophil count (ANC) <1,500/mm^3 (ANC: combination of bands and mature neutrophils).
> - ANC <500/mm^3 corresponds to a severely increased risk of infection.

- If you suspect catheter-related sepsis, promptly remove the catheter and send the tip for culture. This alone typically leads to resolution of fever and a decrease in leukocytosis. Antibiotics are usually initiated. Narrow the spectrum once the organism is identified.

Neutropenic Fever

- Common causes include bone marrow failure (e.g., due to toxins, drugs), bone marrow invasion (e.g., from hematologic malignancy, metastatic cancer), and peripheral causes (e.g., hypersplenism, SLE, AIDS). Isolated neutropenia (agranulocytosis) is commonly caused by drug reactions.
- Because neutropenia severely compromises the patient's ability to mount an inflammatory response, fever may be the only manifestation of a raging infection.
- The most common infections seen in neutropenic individuals are septicemia, cellulitis, and pneumonia.
- Obtain the following for any neutropenic patient with a fever: CXR, panculture (blood, urine, sputum, line tips, wound), CBC, complete metabolic panel.
- Place the patient on reverse isolation precautions (positive-pressure room, masks, and strict handwashing for those entering the patient's room).
- Give broad-spectrum antibacterial agents immediately after cultures are drawn.
- If fever persists beyond 4 to 5 days despite broad-spectrum antibacterial therapy, give antifungal agents, such as IV amphotericin B. Consider G-CSF.

Miscellaneous Infections

Infectious Mononucleosis

A. General characteristics

1. Caused by the EBV (rarely by CMV which causes a similar clinical picture but is milder) (see also Table 10-14).
2. It is most commonly seen in adolescents and young adults, especially college students and military recruits (but may occur at any age). Infected children often experience milder symptoms or no symptoms.
3. Differential diagnosis in patients with fever, lymphadenopathy, and pharyngitis includes acute HIV infection, streptococcal infection, CMV, or toxoplasma infection.
   a. In pregnant patients, it is important to perform diagnostic tests as HIV, CMV, and toxoplasma infection can have adverse effects on the fetus.
4. Transmission
   a. The usual mode of transmission is through infected saliva (e.g., kissing, sharing food).
   b. Most adults (90%) have been infected with EBV and are carriers but infectious mononucleosis is uncommon in adults.
   c. One infection usually confers lifelong immunity.
   d. The incubation period is typically 2 to 5 weeks.

> **Quick HIT**
> Infectious mononucleosis includes fever, fatigue, tonsillar pharyngitis, and lymphadenopathy.

B. Clinical features

1. Symptoms
   a. Fever—temperatures may be as high as 40°C (104°F); fever usually resolves within 2 weeks
   b. Sore throat
   c. Malaise, myalgias, weakness—may linger for several months
2. Signs
   a. Lymphadenopathy—this is found in >90% of patients. Tonsillar or cervical (especially posterior cervical) lymph nodes may be quite enlarged, painful, and tender
   b. Pharyngeal erythema and/or exudate—frequently present
   c. Splenomegaly—present in half of patients
   d. Maculopapular rash—present in approximately 15% of patients, but much higher if ampicillin is given

> **Quick HIT**
> Common laboratory abnormalities include lymphocytosis, elevated aminotransferases.

Infectious Diseases

TABLE 10-14 Common Organisms in Various Infections

Pneumonia	Community-acquired	
	Typical	*S. pneumoniae, H. influenzae, Moraxella catarrhalis*
	Atypical	*Mycoplasma* spp., *Chlamydia* spp., *Legionella* spp.
	Nosocomial	*S. aureus*, gram-negative rods
	Aspiration pneumonia	Oral anaerobes, gram-negative rods, *S. aureus*
Urinary Tract Infection		*E. coli, S. saprophyticus, Enterococcus, Klebsiella, Proteus* spp., *Pseudomonas, Enterobacter*, yeast (*Candida* spp.)
Osteomyelitis, Septic Arthritis		*S. aureus, S. epidermidis, Streptococcus* spp., gram-negative rods Consider *N. gonorrhoeae* in septic arthritis in adolescents
Skin/soft Tissue	Surgical wound	*S. aureus*, gram-negative rods
	Diabetic ulcer	*S. aureus*, gram-negative rods, anaerobes
	Intravenous catheter site	*S. aureus, S. epidermidis*
	Cellulitis	*S. aureus*, group A streptococci
	Necrotizing fasciitis	*C. perfringens*, group A streptococci
Upper Respiratory	Pharyngitis	Viral, group A streptococci
	Acute bronchitis	Viral
	Acute sinusitis	Viral, *S. pneumoniae, H. influenzae, M. catarrhalis*
	Chronic sinusitis	*S. aureus*, anaerobes
Endocarditis	Subacute	*Streptococcus viridans*
	Acute	IV drug abuser: *S. aureus*, gram-negative rods, *Enterococcus* spp., yeast Prosthetic valve: *S. epidermidis*
Gastroenteritis		Viral, *Salmonella, Shigella, E. coli, C. botulinum, Giardia, Helicobacter* spp., *Campylobacter*
Intra-abdominal		*Enterococcus, Bacteroides fragilis, E. coli*
Meningitis		See Table 10-3.

e. Hepatomegaly—in 10% of cases
f. Palatal petechiae and eyelid (periorbital) edema—may occur in a minority of cases

C. Diagnosis

1. Serology
   a. Monospot test—for detection of heterophile antibody
      - Heterophile antibodies are positive within 4 weeks of infection with EBV mononucleosis and are undetectable by 6 months. Thus, a positive monospot test indicates acute infection with EBV mononucleosis
      - Heterophile antibodies do not form in CMV mononucleosis
      - Rapid heterophile tests are highly sensitive and specific, particularly in adolescents
   b. EBV-specific antibody testing—perform in cases in which diagnosis is not straightforward (usually done by indirect immunofluorescence microscopy or by ELISA)
2. Peripheral blood smear—usually reveals lymphocytic leukocytosis with large, atypical lymphocytes
3. Throat culture—perform if pharyngitis is present to rule out a secondary infection with β-hemolytic streptococci

Quick HIT

CMV Mononucleosis
- Most commonly seen in sexually active adolescents/young adults. Milder than EBV-associated IM.
- Characterized by fevers, chills, fatigue, headaches, and frequently, splenomegaly
- Cervical lymphadenopathy and pharyngitis usually absent
- Negative for heterophile antibodies

Quick HIT

If you suspect IM, order WBC count with differential and a monospot test. If monospot test is positive, no further testing needed. If negative and clinical suspicion is high, can repeat monospot test.

D. Complications

1. Hepatitis
2. Neurologic complications (rare): meningoencephalitis, Guillain–Barré syndrome, Bell palsy
3. Splenic rupture—rare
4. Thrombocytopenia, hemolytic anemia
5. Upper airway obstruction due to lymphadenopathy—rare

E. Treatment

1. Generally, no specific treatment is indicated (or available) as most people recover completely within 3 to 4 months. Supportive care includes:
   a. Rest, fluids
   b. Avoidance of strenuous activities until splenomegaly resolves to prevent splenic rupture
   c. Analgesics to reduce temperature and pharyngeal pain—NSAIDs or acetaminophen
2. Give a short course of steroids if there is airway compromise. Steroids have also been effective in patients with thrombocytopenia or hemolytic anemia. Steroids are not recommended for routine IM without complications
3. When to return to sports—concern is splenic rupture. Patients should wait 3 to 4 weeks from symptom onset before returning to sports as splenic rupture is very rare after 4 weeks

DISEASES OF THE SKIN AND HYPERSENSITIVITY DISORDERS

11

COMMON DERMATOLOGIC PROBLEMS

Inflammatory, Allergic, and Autoimmune Skin Conditions

Acne Vulgaris

A. General characteristics

1. Acne vulgaris is an inflammatory condition of the skin that is most prevalent during adolescence.
2. Severe acne is more common in men than in women due to higher levels of circulating androgens.
3. Pathogenesis
   a. Obstruction of sebaceous follicles (by sebum) leads to the proliferation of *Propionibacterium acnes* (an anaerobic bacterium) in the sebum.
   b. This obstruction can lead to either noninflammatory comedones ("pimples"), or, if severe, inflammatory papules or pustules.
   c. Both noninflammatory and inflammatory lesions are present in most patients with acne.
4. Risk factors are male sex, puberty, Cushing syndrome, oily complexion, androgens (due to any cause), and medications.
5. Classification
   a. Obstructive acne: closed comedones (whiteheads) or open comedones (blackheads).
   b. Inflammatory acne: Lesions progress from papules/pustules to nodules, then to cysts, then scars.

B. Treatment

1. General guidelines.
   a. Instruct patient to keep affected area clean (vigorous washing is unnecessary); reduce or discontinue acne-promoting agents (certain make-up, creams, oils, steroids, androgens).
   b. It takes about 6 weeks to notice the effects of medications (skin may get worse before it gets better). Start with one drug to assess its efficacy.
2. Mild to moderate acne.
   a. Begin with topical benzoyl peroxide (2.5%)—should be applied once or twice daily. It destroys acne-causing bacteria and prevents plugging of pores by drying the skin.
   b. Add topical retinoids if the above fails. They cause peeling of the skin, which prevents clogging of pores.
   c. Add topical erythromycin or topical clindamycin—both act to suppress *P. acnes*.
3. Moderate to severe nodular pustular acne.
   a. Prescribe systemic antibiotic therapy: tetracycline, minocycline, doxycycline, erythromycin, clindamycin, and TMP-SMX.

Quick HIT

Quick Hit: For definitions of common dermatologic terms, see the end of this chapter, page 435.

Quick HIT

- There is no proven link between acne and diet (e.g., chocolate, fatty foods).
- Oral contraceptives (especially some of the newer oral contraceptive pills) help some women with acne.

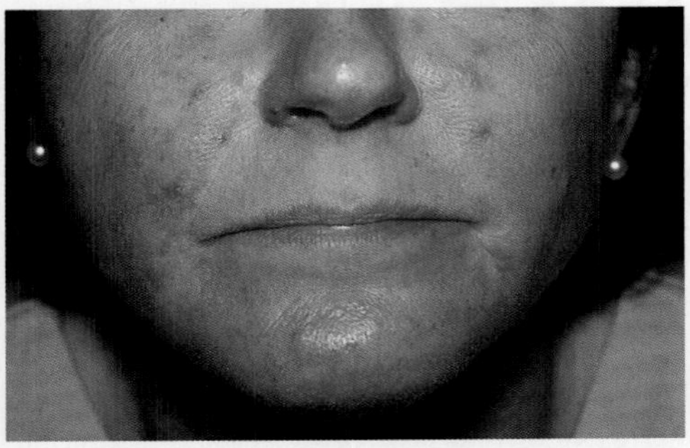

FIGURE 11-1 **Rosacea.**
(From Goodheart HP. *Goodheart's Photoguide of Common Skin Disorders.* 2nd ed. Philadelphia, PA: Lippincott Williams & Wilkins, 2003, Figure 1.14.)

Quick HIT

Do not give systemic antibiotics unless the patient is already on topical benzoyl peroxide, topical tretinoin, and topical antibiotics and the response is inadequate.

b. Add oral retinoids (e.g., isotretinoin) for severe, recalcitrant, nodular acne that is not responsive to the above treatments. Oral retinoids are extremely teratogenic. All female patients must have two negative pregnancy tests before starting oral isotretinoin. In addition, they should use two forms of birth control for 1 month before starting the medication through 1 month after stopping the medication.

Rosacea

- A chronic condition resulting in reddening of the face (mainly the forehead, nose, and cheeks). It often appears very similar to acne, but unlike acne it first starts in middle age.
- Mostly affects Caucasian women between 30 and 50 years of age.
- The most common skin findings include erythema, telangiectasia, papules, and pustules with redness, typically affecting the face. Unlike acne vulgaris, there are no comedones (Figure 11-1).
- In severe cases, skin can become thickened and greasy—on the nose, it creates a bulbous appearance; this is called rhinophyma (mostly seen in men).
- Symptoms may be reduced by avoiding alcoholic or hot beverages, as well as extremes of temperature, and by reducing emotional stressors.
- Treatment: Topical metronidazole (gel form) is effective and is applied twice per day for several months. Systemic antibiotics (e.g., tetracycline) are used for maintenance therapy. If the patient does not experience an appropriate response, prescribe isotretinoin for daily use.

Keratoacanthoma

- Epithelial tumors which clinically resemble squamous cell carcinoma (SCC). Current debate centers on whether this is a subtype of SCC or a separate entity altogether.
- Lesions grow **VERY** quickly. The lesions progress to the typical dome with central crater containing keratinous material over the course of several weeks. This type of growth is very rare for SCC.
- Treatment involves observation, as many of these will regress spontaneously over several months.

Tinea Versicolor

- A common superficial fungal infection which is likely caused by several species in the Malassezia group, which are part of the normal skin flora (Figure 11-2).
- Characteristic lesions are **well demarcated** and most commonly affect the trunk. As the name implies, lesions may be hyper- or hypopigmented and can range in color from brown to tan to white.
- Adolescents and young adults are most commonly affected, though almost any age can be affected.

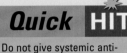

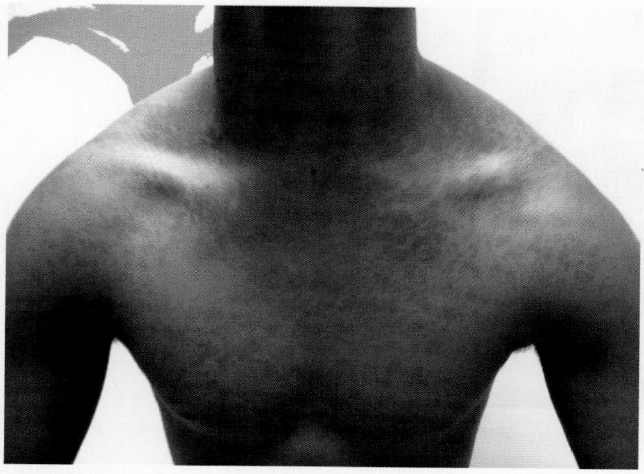

FIGURE 11-2 **Tinea versicolor.**
(Courtesy of Paul S. Matz, MD. *Visual Diagnosis and Treatment in Pediatrics.* Philadelphia, PA: Lippincott Williams & Wilkins, 2006.)

- Hot/humid weather, excessive sweating, and skin oils may contribute to transformation from normal skin flora to pathologic condition.
- Diagnosis should be made with KOH prep, which will show the "spaghetti and meatballs" pattern consistent with both hyphae and yeast balls.
- Treatment consists of oral or topical antifungals, depending on the severity of the disease. Selenium sulfide lotion may also be helpful.

Seborrheic Dermatitis

A. General characteristics

1. A chronic, idiopathic, inflammatory skin disorder which occurs in infants and adults.
2. Very common problem (affects 5% of the population), especially in patients with **oily** skin.
3. Exacerbating factors: anxiety, stress, fatigue, hormonal factors.
4. Common locations: scalp (dandruff), hairline, behind ears, external ear canal, folds of skin around nose, eyebrows, armpits, under breasts, groin area (skin folds).
5. May be complicated by secondary bacterial infection.

Quick HIT

Seborrheic dermatitis is a chronic condition with no cure. Therapy may be needed indefinitely for control of symptoms.

B. Clinical features

1. Mild cases manifest as dandruff.
2. Severe cases yellowish, oily, and thick flakes appear near eyelashes, in the ear canal, on the middle chest, behind the ears, and other skin folds.
3. Scaly patches with surrounding areas of mild to moderate erythema (Figure 11-3).
4. Usually asymptomatic, but pruritus, skin lesions, and hair loss can occur if left untreated.

C. Treatment

1. Sunlight exposure often helps.
2. Dandruff shampoo (over-the-counter) is usually adequate.
3. Topical ketoconazole (to decrease yeast count on skin) has been found to be effective.
4. Topical corticosteroids are appropriate in severe cases.

Contact Dermatitis

A. General characteristics

1. There are two forms of contact dermatitis: irritant and allergic.

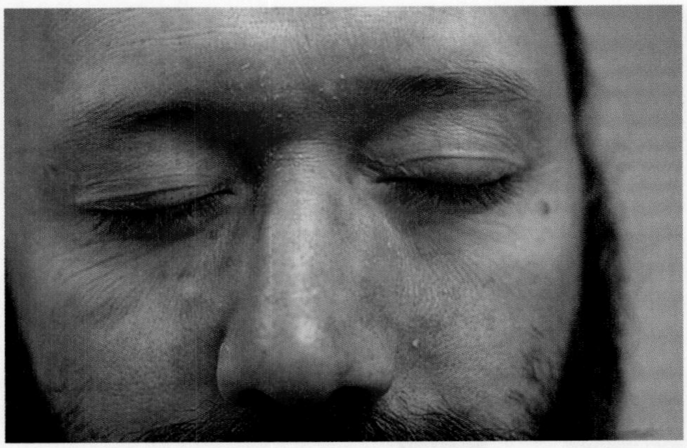

FIGURE
11-3 **Seborrheic dermatitis.**
(From Goodheart HP. *Goodheart's Same-Site Differential Diagnosis: A Rapid Method of Diagnosing and Treating Common Skin Disorders*. Philadelphia, PA: Lippincott Williams & Wilkins, 2010.)

2. Irritant contact dermatitis (more common than allergic type) results from a chemical or physical insult to the skin (e.g., contact with detergents, acids, or alkalis, or from frequent hand washing).
   a. A previous sensitizing event is not needed to produce the rash (i.e., it is not an immunologic reaction).
   b. The rash begins shortly after exposure to the irritant (in contrast to the allergic type, which begins several hours to a few days later).
3. Allergic contact dermatitis is **a delayed-type hypersensitivity (type IV) reaction.**
   a. No history of atopy is necessary for allergic contact dermatitis to occur. It can occur in anyone.
   b. Sensitization of the skin occurs 1 to 2 weeks after the first exposure to the allergen. Subsequent exposure leads to dermatitis hours to days after the reexposure. Therefore, dermatitis develops only in patients who have already been sensitized to the allergen. Common allergens include poison ivy, oak, and sumac; iodine; nickel; rubber; topical medications (e.g., neomycin, topical anesthetics); and cosmetics.

B. Clinical features

1. The appearance of the rash depends on the stage.
   a. Acute stage: erythematous papules and vesicles with oozing (Figure 11-4); edema may be present.
   b. Chronic stage: crusting, thickening, and scaling; lichenification.
2. The rash is usually very pruritic.
3. The interval between exposure and appearance of the rash varies, but is usually from several hours to as long as 4 to 5 days.
4. The rash is found only in exposed areas.

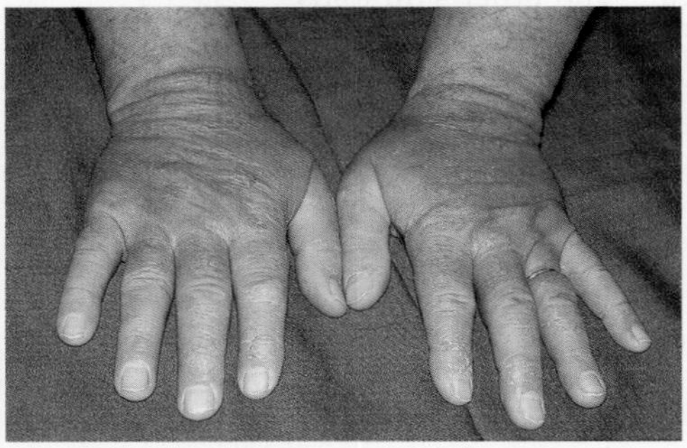

FIGURE
11-4 **Contact dermatitis.**
(From Goodheart HP. *Goodheart's Photoguide of Common Skin Disorders*. 2nd ed. Philadelphia, PA: Lippincott Williams & Wilkins, 2003, Figure 2.41.)

C. Diagnosis

1. Diagnosis is usually made clinically based on history and examination.
2. Patch testing (to identify the allergen that caused the allergic reaction) is indicated in any of the following cases:
   a. The diagnosis is in doubt.
   b. The rash does not respond to treatment.
   c. The rash recurs.

D. Treatment

1. Avoid the contact allergen!
2. Apply cool tap water compresses.
3. Apply topical corticosteroids.
4. Prescribe systemic corticosteroids (e.g., prednisone, 1 mg/kg/day) for severe cases. Continue for 10 to 14 days and then taper.

> **Quick HIT**
>
> Do not confuse allergic contact dermatitis with any of the following:
> - Irritant contact dermatitis—rash is usually identical to that seen in allergic contact dermatitis, except the rash begins very soon after exposure
> - Atopic dermatitis—onset is in infancy or childhood
> - Seborrheic dermatitis
> - Psoriasis

Pityriasis Rosea

- Papulosquamous eruption—Initially, "herald patches" that resemble a ring worm (multiple round/oval patches) appear, and then a generalized rash with multiple oval-shaped lesions appears. **The rash is classically described as having a Christmas tree-type appearance** (Figure 11-5).
- It is **not** contagious and is possibly related to herpes type 7.
- It is common on the trunk and upper arms and thighs, and is usually not found on the face. Pruritus is often present, and varies in severity.
- It spontaneously remits within a few (6 to 8) weeks without treatment. There is no treatment other than antihistamines for pruritus. Recurrences are rare.
- A commonly tested topic.

Erythema Nodosum

- Erythema nodosum appears as painful, red, subcutaneous, elevated nodules, typically located over the anterior aspect of the tibia (less commonly on the trunk or arms) (Figure 11-6). It is self-limited and usually resolves within a few weeks. Low-grade fever, malaise, and joint pain may precede the rash.
- It is much more common in women (especially young women) than in men.
- Many causes: *Streptococcus* infection, sarcoidosis, inflammatory bowel disease, Behçet disease, fungal infections, pregnancy, medications (e.g., oral contraceptives, sulfa drugs, amiodarone, antibiotics), syphilis, tuberculosis; many cases are idiopathic.
- Perform the following to help determine the underlying condition: chest radiograph (for sarcoidosis, tuberculosis); antistreptolysin-O titer; VDRL (serologic test for syphilis); CBC, erythrocyte sedimentation rate, and cultures, as appropriate. Skin biopsy may be helpful.
- Treat the underlying condition, if known.

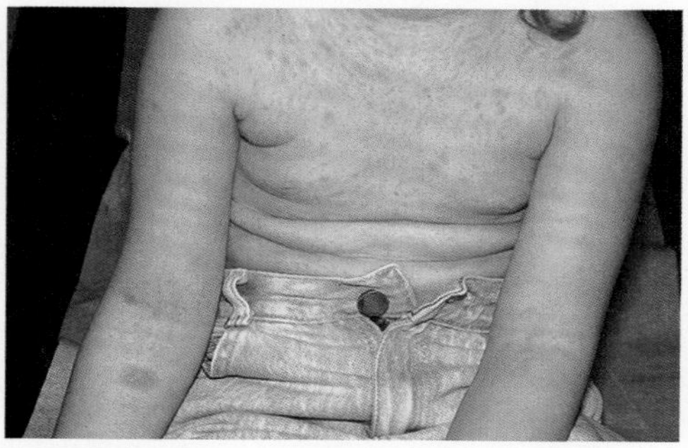

FIGURE 11-5 **Pityriasis rosea.**
(From Goodheart HP. *Goodheart's Photoguide of Common Skin Disorders.* 2nd ed. Philadelphia, PA: Lippincott Williams & Wilkins, 2003, Figure 4.3.)

Diseases of the Skin and Hypersensitivity Disorders

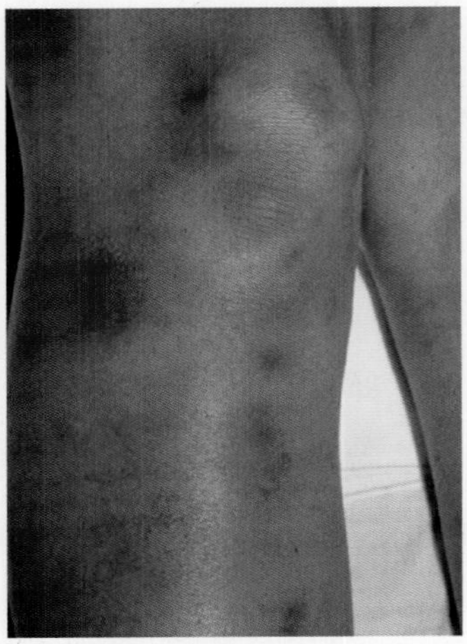

FIGURE **11-6** **Erythema nodosum.**
(From Goodheart HP. *Goodheart's Photoguide of Common Skin Disorders.* 2nd ed. Philadelphia, PA: Lippincott Williams & Wilkins, 2003, Figure 25.17.)

- Prescribe bed rest, leg elevation, NSAIDs, and heat for symptoms. Potassium iodide may help.

Erythema Multiforme

- Erythema multiforme (EM) is an inflammatory skin condition characterized by erythematous macules/papules that resemble target lesions (**"bull's-eye lesions"**) that can become bullous (Figure 11-7).
- Skin lesions may be pruritic and painful.
- EM can be caused by medications and may follow an infection by HSV. Many cases are idiopathic. EM due to HSV infection can recur.
- Medications implicated include sulfa drugs (most common), penicillin, and other antibiotics, phenytoin, allopurinol, and barbiturates.
- If initiated early when the first symptom of HSV infection appears, acyclovir can help to prevent HSV-associated EM. For recurrent and debilitating EM, acyclovir may be given prophylactically for prolonged periods.
- Antihistamines or analgesics for symptomatic relief.

Stevens–Johnson Syndrome and Toxic Epidermal Necrolysis

- No precise definition exists, but Stevens–Johnson syndrome (SJS) is considered the most severe form of EM. Toxic epidermal necrolysis (TEN) is considered to be the most severe form of SJS.

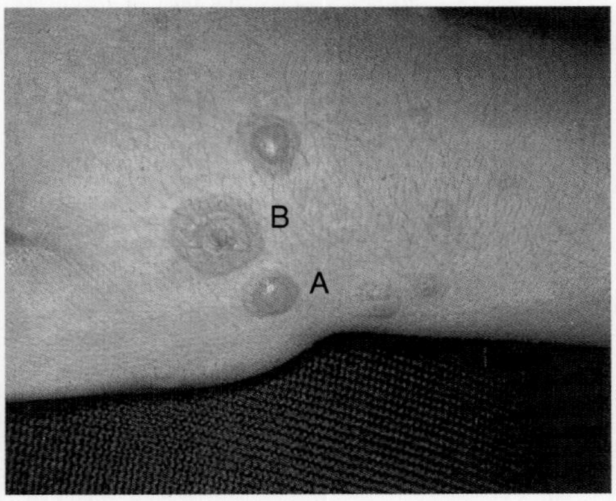

FIGURE **11-7** **Erythema multiforme. A: Bulla. B: Target (or iris) lesion.**
(From Bickley LS, Szilagyi P. *Bates' Guide to Physical Examination and History Taking.* 8th ed. Philadelphia, PA: Lippincott Williams & Wilkins, 2003, Table 4.8.)

- In SJS and TEN, skin involvement is extensive and severe, with possible detachment of areas of epidermis.
- The eyes and mouth may also be involved.
- Systemic manifestations include fever, difficulty eating, renal failure, and sepsis.
- **Potentially life-threatening** (mortality rate is 5% for SJS and 30% for TEN).
- Half of all cases are due to medications (e.g., sulfa drugs, penicillins, barbiturates, phenytoin, allopurinol, carbamazepine, vancomycin, rifampin). In many cases, no specific cause is identified.
- Admit patient to an ICU—The burn unit is often the most appropriate setting for these patients. Withdraw the suspected medication; aggressive rehydration and symptomatic management. Urgent dermatology and ophthalmology consultation is indicated.

Lichen Planus

- Chronic, inflammatory lesions of unknown etiology.
- (4 Ps): **P**ruritic, **p**olygonal, **p**urple, flat-topped **p**apules.
- Most commonly seen on wrists, shins, **oral mucosa**, and genitalia.
- Treat with glucocorticoids.

Bullous Pemphigoid

- Multiple subepithelial blisters on abdomen, groin, and extremities (Figure 11-8).
- Elderly people are most commonly affected.
- Blisters are less easily ruptured than in pemphigus vulgaris.
- Autoimmune condition; no malignant potential but may be persistent.
- Treat with systemic or topical glucocorticoids.

Pemphigus Vulgaris

- Autoimmune blistering condition resulting in loss of normal adhesion between cells (acantholysis) (Figure 11-9).
- Starts in oral mucosa; may become generalized.
- Blisters rupture, leaving painful erosions.
- Most commonly affects elderly people, **often fatal if untreated.**
- Autoantibodies (usually IgG) directed against the adhesion molecule desmoglein.
- Treat with systemic glucocorticoids and other immunosuppressants.
- Pemphigus may be the presenting symptoms of malignancies such as non-Hodgkin lymphoma, chronic lymphocytic leukemia, and Castleman disease.

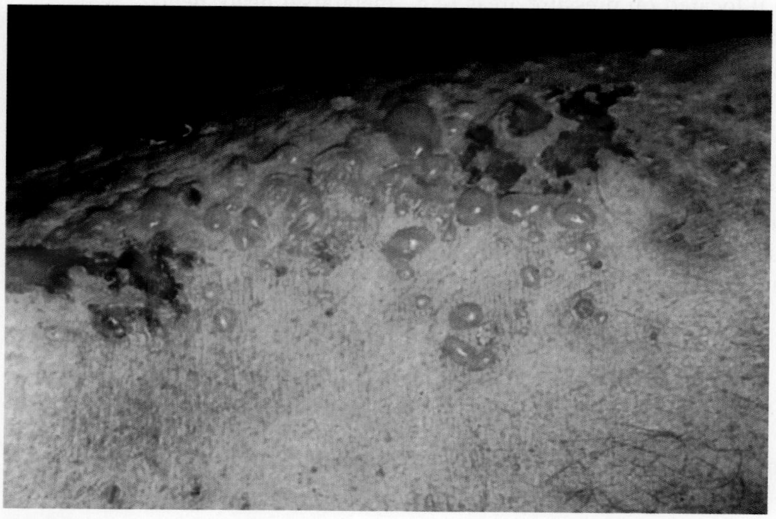

FIGURE **11-8** **Bullous pemphigoid.**

(From Elder D, Rubin A, Ioffreda M, et al. *Atlas and Synopsis of Lever's Histopathology of the Skin.* Philadelphia, PA: Lippincott Williams & Wilkins, 2012.)

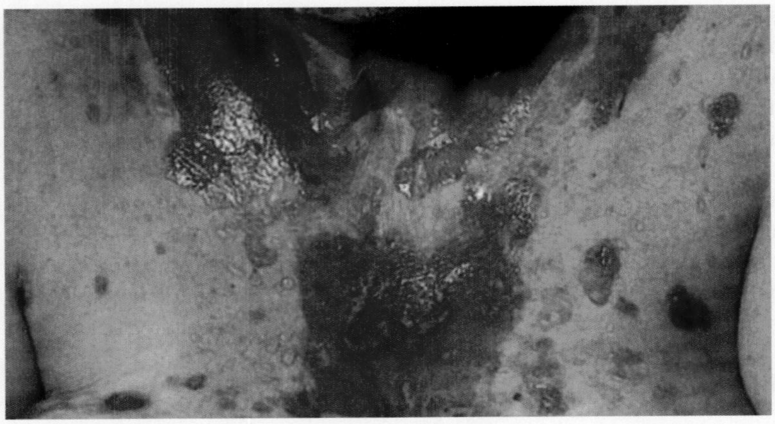

FIGURE **11-9** **Pemphigus vulgaris.**
(From Elder D, Elenitsas R, Johnson B, et al. *Synopsis and Atlas of Lever's Histopathology of the Skin* [Clinical Figure IVD3.b]. Philadelphia, PA: Lippincott Williams & Wilkins, 1999.)

Skin Conditions Related to Microbial Infection

Warts

A. General characteristics

1. Warts are caused by HPV and are transmitted via skin-to-skin contact. For genital warts, transmission is via intimate sexual contact.
2. Types
   a. **The common wart (*Verruca vulgaris*)—most common type.**
      - May occur anywhere, but the most common sites include elbows, knees, fingers, and palms.
      - Appearance: flesh-colored or whitish with a hyperkeratotic surface.

   b. The flat wart (*Verruca plana*).
      - Common sites include the chin/face, dorsum of hands, and legs.
      - Appears flesh-colored with smooth papules and a flat surface.

   c. The plantar wart (*Verruca plantaris*).
      - Solitary or multiple warts found on the plantar side of the foot; can cause foot pain if located on pressure areas (e.g., metatarsal head, heel).
      - Appearance: flesh-colored with a rough, hyperkeratotic surface.

   d. Anogenital wart (*Condyloma acuminatum*).
      - **Most common STD**, commonly associated with HPV 6 and 11 (Figure 11-10).
      - HPV (types 16, 18) infection can lead to cervical cancer in women (Pap smear is important). Vaccines which protect against HPV 16 and 18 are now available. These vaccines have been shown to prevent HPV infection by serologic/DNA testing as well as adenocarcinoma and precancerous lesions associated with these HPV subtypes. This is the first vaccine approved to prevent cancer.
      - Appearance: single or multiple soft, fleshy growths on the genitalia, perineum, and anus.

Quick HIT

Most warts disappear spontaneously within 1 to 2 years. However, if the condition is left untreated, more warts can appear.

B. Clinical features

1. Most warts are asymptomatic unless "bumped." Plantar warts can be painful during walking.
2. Some warts may bleed.
3. Warts are unsightly and can be disfiguring.

C. Treatment

1. Freezing lesion with liquid nitrogen (applied on a cotton swab)—multiple treatments may be necessary.

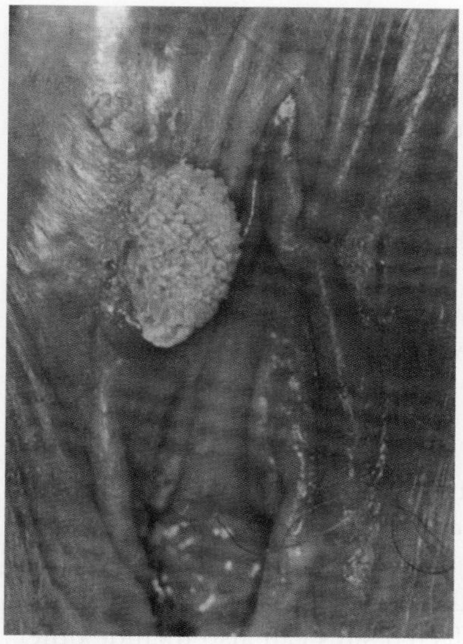

FIGURE **11-10** **Human papilloma virus (genital wart).**
(From Wilkinson EJ, Stone IK. *Atlas of Vulvar Disease*. Baltimore: Williams & Wilkins, 1994, Figure 17.9a.)

2. Salicylic acid (Compound W)—applied daily for several weeks.
3. 5-FU cream or retinoic acid cream for flat warts.
4. Surgical excision or laser therapy.
5. Podophyllin for genital warts.

Quick HIT
Warts can be recurrent and may require multiple treatments (despite the method of therapy chosen).

••• Molluscum Contagiosum

- A common, self-limited viral infection caused by a **poxvirus**; common in sexually active young adults and in children.
- It manifests as small papules (2 to 5 mm) with central umbilication. Lesions are asymptomatic. In HIV-positive patients, lesions can be extensive (Figure 11-11).
- It is transmitted via skin-to-skin contact (sexual contact can lead to genital involvement) and is **highly contagious.** Child abuse should always be ruled out when a young child presents with molluscum.
- It persists up to 6 months, but spontaneously regresses with time. In immunosuppressed individuals (HIV-positive patients), the lesions can progress to grow quite large and often are refractory to treatment.
- Multiple treatment modalities are effective (e.g., curettage, drops containing podophyllin and cantharidin, cryosurgery), but scarring is always a risk.

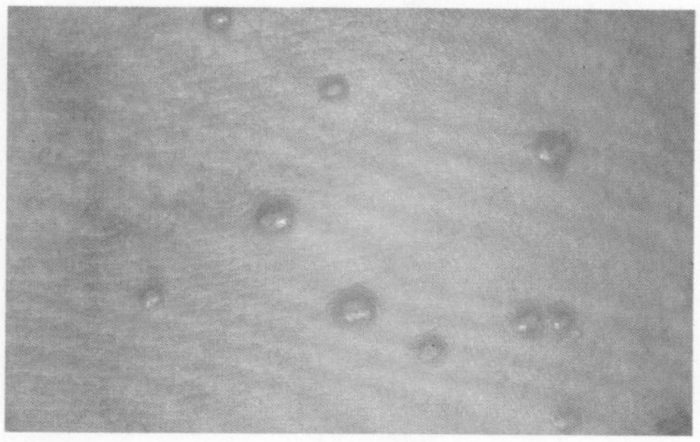

FIGURE **11-11** **Molluscum contagiosum.**
(From Goodheart HP. *Goodheart's Photoguide of Common Skin Disorders*. 2nd ed. Philadelphia, PA: Lippincott Williams & Wilkins, 2003, Figure 6.13.)

Quick HIT

Complications of zoster
- Postherpetic neuralgia
- Occurs most frequently in patients older than 50 years
- Manifests as excruciating pain that persists after the lesions have cleared, and does not respond to analgesics
- Can be chronic and debilitating
- Uveitis
- Dissemination
- Meningoencephalitis, deafness

Herpes Zoster (Shingles)

A. General characteristics

1. Caused by reactivation of the varicella-zoster virus, which remains dormant in the dorsal root ganglia and is reactivated in times of stress, infection, or illness; only occurs in those who have previously had chickenpox.
2. It is typically seen in patients over 50 years of age. In patients less than 50 years of age, suspect an immunosuppressed state.
3. Contagious when open vesicles present and only for those who have never had chickenpox or are immunocompromised (or newborns). Zoster is not as contagious as chickenpox.

B. Clinical features

1. **Severe pain and rash in a dermatomal distribution.** Pain comes before the rash. Rash is characterized by grouped vesicles on an erythematous base. If severe, low-grade fever and malaise may be present.
2. The most common sites of involvement are the thorax (most cases) and trigeminal distribution (especially ophthalmic division). Affected sites can also include other cranial nerves, as well as arms and legs (Figure 11-12).
3. Rarely life-threatening, even if dissemination occurs. Herpes zoster is more severe, however, in immunocompromised patients.

C. Treatment

1. Keep the lesions clean and dry.
2. Prescribe analgesics for pain relief (aspirin or acetaminophen; codeine if needed). In severe cases, administer a local injection of triamcinolone in lidocaine.
3. Prescribe antiviral agents (acyclovir, famciclovir, valacyclovir) to reduce the pain, decrease the length of illness, and reduce the risk of postherpetic neuralgia.
4. The use of corticosteroids to decrease the incidence of postherpetic neuralgia remains controversial.
5. Live vaccine has been shown to be effective in reducing the number of cases of shingles in patients over the age of 60 in addition to reducing the severity and duration of postherpetic neuralgia in patients who do end up with the disease. The vaccine should be recommended to all patients over 60 who do not have contraindications.

Dermatophytes

- Dermatophytes are superficial fungi that infect cutaneous epithelium, nails, and hair.
- The three main genera of dermatophytes are *Trichophyton*, *Microsporum*, and *Epidermophyton*.

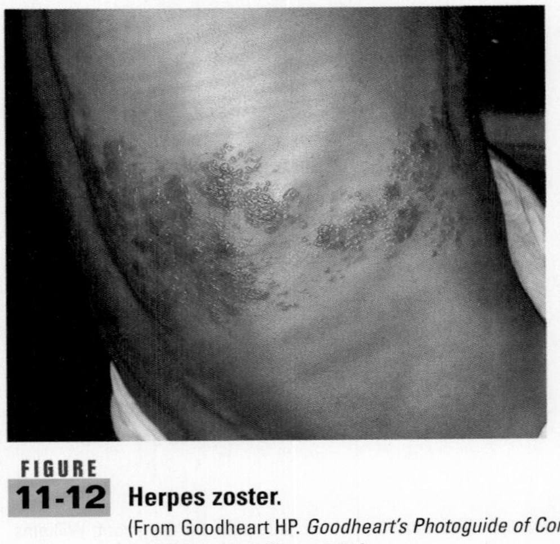

FIGURE 11-12 Herpes zoster.
(From Goodheart HP. *Goodheart's Photoguide of Common Skin Disorders*. 2nd ed. Philadelphia, PA: Lippincott Williams & Wilkins, 2003, Figure 6.33.)

TABLE 11-1 Important Dermatophyte Infections

Fungal Infection	Location	Age Group	Findings	Diagnosis	First-line Treatment
Tinea corporis ("ringworm")	Body/trunk	All ages	Pinkish, annular lesions	Direct microscopy: visualization of hyphae from skin scrapings with KOH preparation	Topical antifungals (e.g., ketoconazole, miconazole)
Tinea capitis	Scalp	Children	Areas of scaling with hair loss ± pruritus	• Direct microscopy • Wood lamp: if hairs fluoresce, *Microsporum* spp. is the cause. If not, *Trichophyton* spp. is the cause.	Oral griseofulvin (antifungal)
Tinea unguium (onychomycosis)	Nails	Elderly people	Thick, opacified nails	Direct microscopy (nail scrapings)	Oral griseofulvin (antifungal)
Tinea pedis ("athlete's foot")	Feet—web spaces of toes	Young adults	Scaling, erythema, pruritus	Direct microscopy	Topical antifungals, good foot hygiene
Tinea cruris ("Jock itch")	Groin, inner thighs	Adults: males > females	Areas of scaling, erythema: spares scrotum	Direct microscopy	Topical antifungals, good hygiene

- Important dermatophyte infections are covered in Table 11-1.
- Scrape lesions and use KOH preparation to visualize the fungus.

Quick HIT

Treat tinea capitis and onychomycosis with oral antifungal agents. Others are treated with topical antifungals.

Scabies

A. General characteristics

1. Caused by the human skin mite *Sarcoptes scabiei* var *hominis*
2. Highly contagious—transmitted via skin-to-skin contact or through towels, bed linens, or clothes
3. Pathogenesis—The mites tunnel into the epidermis, lay eggs, and deposit feces (called scybala). A delayed type IV hypersensitivity reaction develops toward the mites, eggs, and feces, causing intense pruritus.
4. Common locations.
   a. **Fingers, interdigital areas, and wrists.**
   b. Elbows, feet, ankles, penis, scrotum, buttocks, and axillae.
   c. Head, neck, palms, and soles are typically spared (except in infants, the elderly, or immunosuppressed people).

B. Clinical features

1. Severe pruritus—this is often the most severe during the night. The head and neck are usually spared.
2. Burrows—Linear marks (several millimeters in length) represent the tunneled path of the mite. There is typically a dark dot at one end, representing the female mite.
3. Scratching may lead to excoriations.
4. Eczematous plaques, crusted papules, or secondary bacterial infection may develop (Figure 11-13).

Quick HIT

Suspect scabies in any patient who has persistent, generalized, severe pruritus.

C. Diagnosis

1. Look for characteristic burrows on hands, wrists, and ankles, and in the genital region.
2. Confirm the diagnosis by scraping the burrow with a scalpel and examining it under a microscope to detect the presence of mites, ova, or scybala.

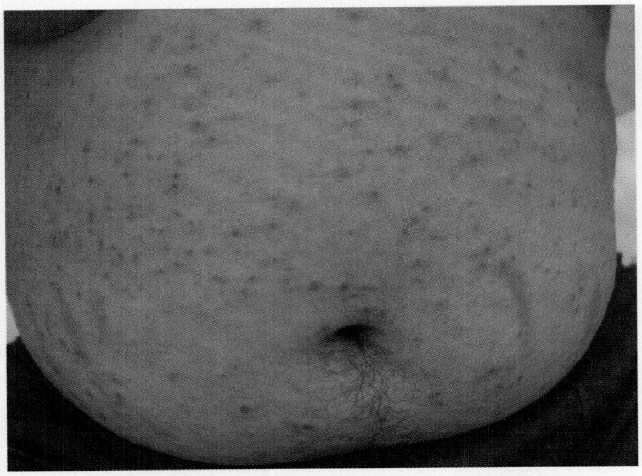

FIGURE **11-13** **Scabies.**
(Image provided by Stedman's.)

D. Treatment

1. Specific medications.
   a. Permethrin 5% cream (Elimite).
      - First-line treatment; causes paralysis of the parasite (acts on nerve cell membrane).
      - Should be applied to **every area of the body** (head to toe), even under fingernails and toenails, around the genital area, and in the cleft of the buttocks.
      - Patients should leave cream on overnight (>8 to 10 hours) and wash it off the next morning.

   b. Lindane (γ-benzene-hexachloride) lotion.
      - Second-line treatment which should not be used unless Permethrin is not available, is contraindicated, or has failed.
      - Contraindicated in children under 2 years of age, as well as in pregnant or lactating women, due to the possibility of severe seizures.
2. General recommendations.
   a. Treat all close contacts of the patient simultaneously (even if asymptomatic) with Permethrin 5% cream.
   b. The patient is no longer contagious after one treatment, although pruritus may continue for a few weeks as dead mites are shed from the skin. Use topical corticosteroids and oral antihistamines to control pruritus during this time.
   c. Thoroughly wash all underwear and bed linens.

Precancerous and Cancerous Diseases of the Skin

Actinic Keratosis (Also Called Solar Keratosis)

- Small, rough, scaly lesions due to prolonged and repeated sun exposure (Figure 11-14).
- Most commonly seen in fair-skinned people. Lesions are typically on the face.
- Prevention: advise patients to avoid excessive sun exposure and to use sunscreen.
- Although the risk of malignant transformation is low (1 in 1,000), biopsy is still recommended for hyperkeratotic actinic keratosis lesions to exclude SCC. Additionally, lesions which become indurated, tender, or bleed spontaneously must be biopsied to exclude SCC.
- Treatment options include surgical removal (scraping), freezing with liquid nitrogen, or application of topical 5-FU for multiple lesions (destroys sun-damaged skin cells).

Quick HIT

Once a patient has developed actinic keratosis with excessive sun exposure, other lesions may develop, even without further sun exposure.

Basal Cell Carcinoma

- **Basal cell carcinoma (BCC) is the most common skin cancer** (accounts for 60% to 75% of all skin cancers).

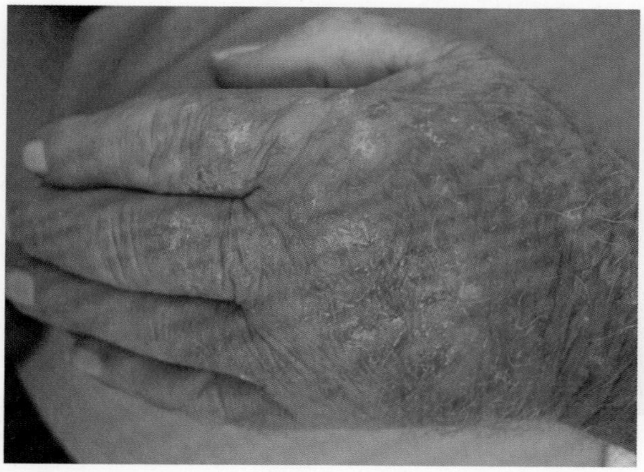

FIGURE
11-14 **Actinic keratosis.**
(Image provided by Stedman's.)

- It arises from the basal layer of cells in the epidermis.
- The most important risk factor is sun exposure.
- It occurs most frequently in fair-skinned individuals who burn easily and involves sun-exposed areas, such as the head and neck (the nose is the most common site).
- The classic appearance is a pearly, smooth papule with rolled edges and surface telangiectases (3 Ps: pearly, pink, papule) (Figure 11-15).
- Metastasis is extremely rare, but can be locally destructive.
- Surgical resection is curative.

●●● Squamous Cell Carcinoma

- SCC is less common than BCC. (SCC accounts for less than 20% of all skin cancers.)
- It arises from epidermal cells undergoing keratinization.
- Sunlight exposure is the most important risk factor. Concomitant actinic keratoses, chronic skin damage, and immunosuppressive therapy are also risk factors.
- It is typically described as a crusting, ulcerated nodule or erosion (Figure 11-16).
- The likelihood of metastasis is higher than with BCC, but much lower than with melanoma.
- The prognosis is excellent if it is completely excised (95% cure rate). Lymph node involvement, however, carries a poor prognosis.

Quick HIT
Marjolin ulcer: a SCC arising from a chronic wound such as a previous burn scar (tends to be very aggressive)

Quick HIT
Women with malignant melanoma have a better prognosis than men (with equivalent lesions).

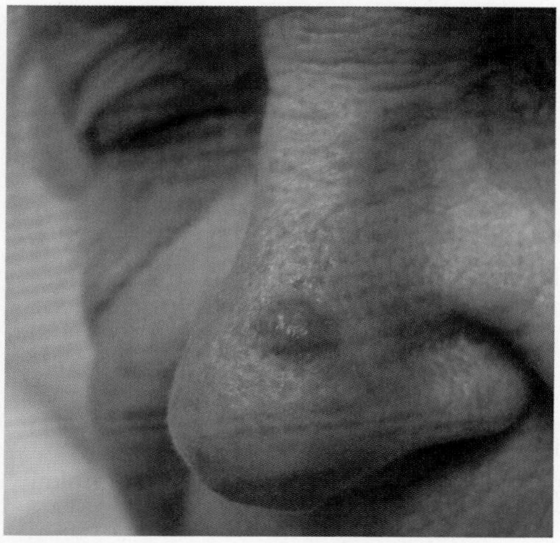

FIGURE
11-15 **Basal cell carcinoma.**
(Image provided by Stedman's.)

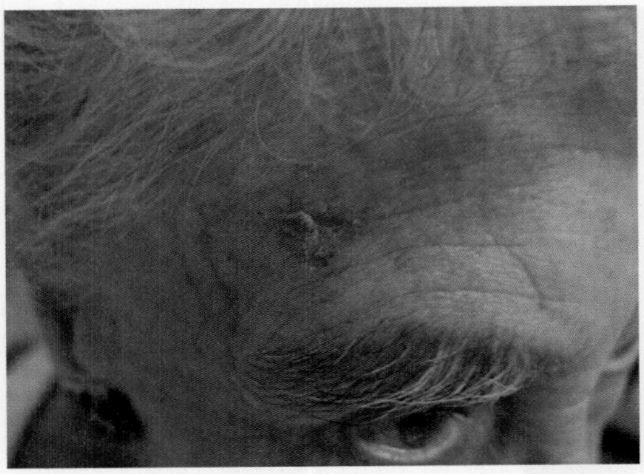

FIGURE 11-16 **Squamous cell carcinoma.**
(Image provided by Stedman's.)

Melanoma

A. General characteristics

1. Most aggressive form of skin cancer and **the number one cause of death due to skin cancer**
2. Increasing incidence worldwide
3. Risk factors
   a. Fair complexion; primarily affects Caucasian patients, especially those with any of the following:
      - Inability to tan
      - Easily sunburned
      - Red hair and/or freckles
      - Numerous moles
   b. Sun exposure, especially for:
      - Patients with a history of severe sunburn before age 14
      - Patients living in a sunny climate
   c. Family history of melanoma (e.g., first-degree relative)
   d. Genodermatoses (e.g., xeroderma pigmentosa)
   e. Increasing age
   f. Large numbers of nevi (moles)
      - Although most melanomas arise de novo, they may arise from pre-existing nevi in up to 50% of cases
      - Any change in a nevus is concerning because it may indicate malignancy or malignant transformation. Look for color change, bleeding, ulceration, or a papule arising from the center of an existing nevus
   g. Dysplastic nevus syndrome
      - Numerous, atypical moles—These tend to be large with indistinct borders and variations in color. The chances of **a single** dysplastic nevus becoming a melanoma are small
      - If dysplastic nevus syndrome **and** a family history of melanoma are present, the risk of developing melanoma approaches 100%
   h. Giant congenital nevi—The risk of melanoma is about 5% to 8%. Prophylactic excision is recommended
4. Growth phases
   a. Radial (initial) growth phase
      - Growth is predominantly lateral within the epidermis
      - There is a good prognosis with surgical resection because metastasis is unlikely
   b. Vertical (later) phase
      - Growth extends into the reticular dermis or beyond
      - Lymphatic or hematogenous metastasis may occur
      - **Depth of invasion is the most important indicator of prognosis**

Quick HIT

Spitz Nevi
- Well-circumscribed, raised lesion commonly confused with melanoma; color varies.
- Complete excision is recommended.

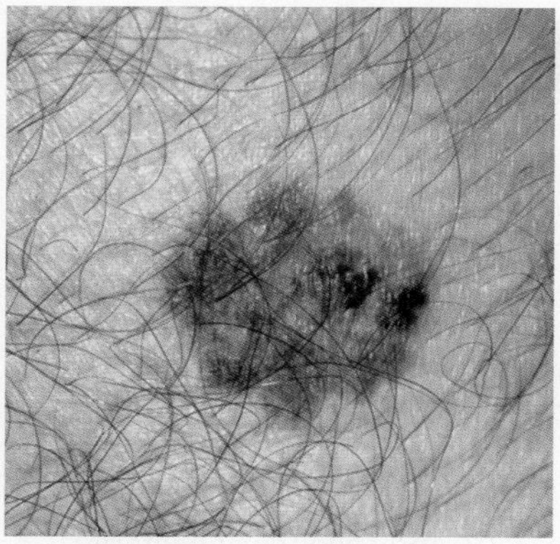

FIGURE **11-17** **Malignant melanoma.**
(From Goodheart HP. *Goodheart's Photoguide of Common Skin Disorders.* 2nd ed. Philadelphia, PA: Lippincott Williams & Wilkins, 2003, Figure 21.20.)

B. Clinical features

1. A melanoma may present with some or all of the following features:
   a. **A**symmetry
   b. **B**order irregularity
   c. **C**olor variegation—ranging from pink to blue to black
   d. **D**iameter greater than 6 mm
   e. **E**levation—typically has a raised surface (Figure 11-17)
2. Changing mole—most common presentation of melanoma
3. The most common site is the back
4. Advanced lesions often present with itching and bleeding

C. Diagnosis

1. Excision biopsy is the standard of care for diagnosis of any suspicious lesion.
   a. Shave biopsy and punch biopsy are less accurate than excision biopsy in assessing the depth of invasion.
   b. Acceptable skin margins are 1 to 3 cm for most lesions, as determined by depth of invasion.
2. Lymph node dissection is appropriate if nodes are palpable.

D. Treatment

1. Early detection is the most important way to prevent death, because prognosis is directly related to depth of invasion.
2. Perform lymph node dissection if nodes are involved. This is controversial because of the risk of lymphedema and the little benefit gained in patients with distant metastasis.

Quick HIT

Sites of Metastases
- Lymph nodes, skin, subcutaneous (59%)
- Lung (36%)
- Liver (20%)
- Brain (20%)—common cause of death
- Bone (17%)
- GI tract (7%)

Miscellaneous Skin Conditions

Decubitus Ulcers

- Decubitus ulcers are also called pressure sores (see also Clinical Pearl 11-1). They result from necrosis of tissue that becomes ischemic and ulcerates, and they are caused by prolonged pressure from the weight of the patient.
- Risk factors include immobilization for any reason, peripheral vascular disease, and dementia. Those at increased risk include debilitated or paraplegic people, nursing-home residents, and people with neurologic disorders.
- They typically occur over bony prominences. The sacrum, greater tuberosity, and ischial tuberosity are the most common sites. Other sites include the calcaneus, malleoli occiput, elbows, and back.

CLINICAL PEARL 11-1

Stages of Decubitus Ulcers

- Stage 1: skin is intact; nonblanching erythema, signs of impending ulceration may be present
- Stage 2: partial-thickness skin loss—epidermis and varying amounts of dermis (abrasion, blister, superficial ulcer or crater)
- Stage 3: full-thickness skin loss—extends into subcutaneous tissue, but not through underlying fascia
- Stage 4: full-thickness skin loss—extends into muscle, bone, joints, tendons; severe tissue necrosis is present; osteomyelitis, pathologic fractures, sinus tracts may be present

- If unrecognized and untreated, tissue can become necrotic and secondary bacterial infection can occur: Cellulitis, osteomyelitis, sepsis, necrotizing fasciitis, gangrene, tetanus, and wound botulism are all potential consequences.
- Prevention is most important; patients should be turned and repositioned every 2 hours. Special mattresses and beds are designed to reduce local tissue pressure by distributing it more evenly.
- Treatment
  - Local wound care (e.g., for more superficial ulcers).
  - Wet-to-dry dressings or wound gel for deeper ulcers.
  - Surgical débridement of necrotic tissue.
  - Antibiotics if evidence of infection (e.g., surrounding cellulitis).

Psoriasis

A. General characteristics

1. Psoriasis is due to abnormal (markedly accelerated) proliferation of skin cells. Because of this, the skin does not have time to mature normally. This leads to defective keratinization, which causes the scaling.
2. The cause is unknown, but genetics are believed to be important.
3. This is a chronic condition characterized by exacerbations and remissions—it improves during the summer (sun exposure) and worsens in the winter (dries skin).
4. Trauma to the skin in any form (e.g., infection, abrasion) can cause exacerbations, as can psychosocial stress.
5. Up to three-fourths of patients have somewhat localized disease (<20% to 25% of body surface area). Nevertheless, clinical features vary, and some patients have generalized skin involvement.
6. **Less than 10% of patients develop psoriatic arthritis** (see Chapter 6).

Quick HIT

There is no cure for psoriasis, but the disease can be managed.

B. Clinical features

1. Well-demarcated, erythematous papules or plaques that are covered by a thick, *silvery scaling;* pruritus is rarely present (Figure 11-18).
2. *Auspitz sign*—Removal of the scale causes pinpoint bleeding.
3. It can involve any part of the body, but the most common areas are the **extensor surfaces of extremities (knees, elbows)**, scalp, intergluteal cleft, palms, and soles.
4. Pitting of the surface of nails, or onycholysis (distal separation of the nail from the nail bed).

C. Treatment

1. Topical therapy
   a. Corticosteroids are the most commonly prescribed first-line agents, but they have adverse side effects with prolonged use
   b. Calcipotriene and calcitriol are vitamin D derivatives that have become first- or second-line agents. They are very effective in most patients
   c. Tars have an unpleasant odor, so they are less desirable to use. Patients should use tars for 4 to 6 weeks before expecting to see a benefit. Tars are more effective in combination therapy and are associated with an 80% to 90% remission rate

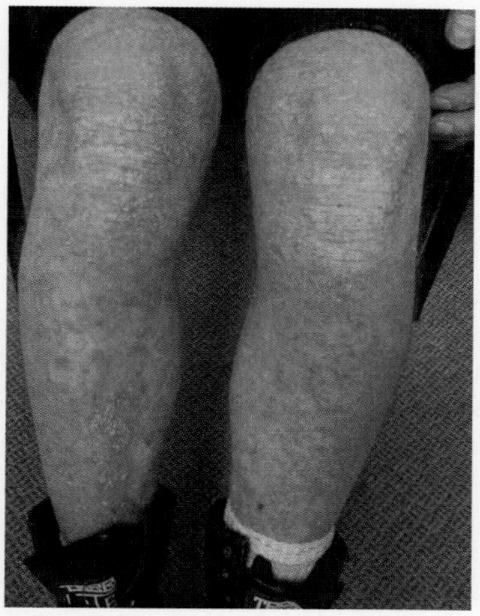

FIGURE
11-18 Psoriasis.
(Image provided by Stedman's.)

   d. Other options include tazarotene (a vitamin A derivative) and anthralin
   e. Combination therapy (e.g., steroids and calcipotriene) is more effective than either agent alone
2. Systemic treatment is indicated in patients with severe psoriasis. Options include:
   a. Immune-modulating therapy—for example, methotrexate, infliximab, cyclosporine
   b. Photochemotherapy
   c. Acitretin (a systemic retinoid)
   d. Acitretin plus phototherapy
3. Ultraviolet light has been shown to be very effective in some patients

Seborrheic Keratosis

- These are very common skin lesions that begin to appear after age 30. Hereditary—they probably are autosomal dominant, and are harmless growths with no malignant potential.
- There is no association with sunlight.
- They can be located anywhere, but are common on the face and trunk. They increase in number with time, and some patients have many of them.
- They are slightly elevated plaques, gradually turning darker in color, and appear as if they were "stuck" on the skin (Figure 11-19).
- Treatment is not necessary and is only for cosmetic reasons: Liquid nitrogen cryotherapy or curettage is effective and easily performed in the office setting.

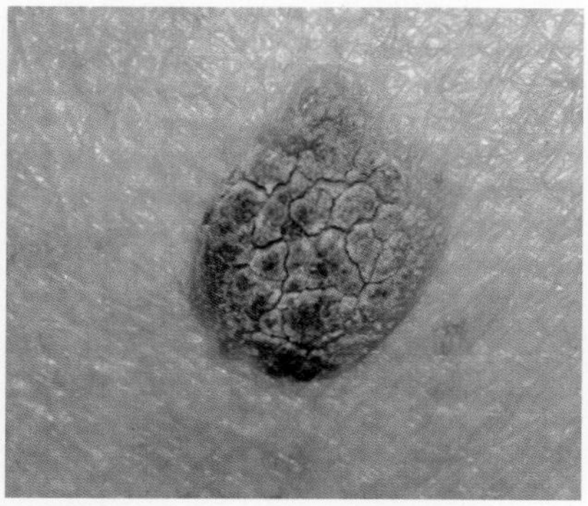

FIGURE
11-19 Seborrheic keratosis.
(From Goodheart HP. *Goodheart's Photoguide of Common Skin Disorders.* 2nd ed. Philadelphia, PA: Lippincott Williams & Wilkins, 2003, Figure 21.13.)

Vitiligo

- Chronic, depigmenting condition due to unknown cause; hereditary component is suspected
- Sharply demarcated areas of skin become amelanotic—most common on the face
- Associated with diabetes mellitus, hypothyroidism, pernicious anemia, and Addison disease
- Topical glucocorticoids and photochemotherapy are used to promote repigmentation with varying degrees of success

Allergic Reactions

Urticaria (Hives)

- Urticaria is caused by the release of mediators from mast cells, with a resultant increase in vascular permeability. There are different types of urticaria.
- Urticaria can be precipitated by foods, drugs, latex allergy, animal dander, pollen, dust, plants, an infection, or cold/heat. It can also be idiopathic.
- Findings—edematous wheals (hives) that are fleeting in nature, that is, they disappear within hours only to return in another location. They blanch with pressure, and may cause intense pruritus or stinging. Lesions get worse with scratching (Figure 11-20).
- Treatment involves removal of the offending agent. Antihistamines are effective for symptomatic relief. Systemic corticosteroids may help in more severe cases.

Quick HIT

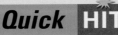

Hereditary angioedema: autosomal dominant condition caused by C1 esterase inhibitor deficiency, characterized by recurrent episodes of angioedema; can be life-threatening

Angioedema

- The mechanism is similar to that in urticaria, though angioedema occurs deeper in the skin (i.e., fluid extravasation occurs in deeper layers of skin/subcutaneous tissue). Angioedema and urticaria can occur simultaneously or independently.
- Angioedema can be caused by any of the precipitants of urticaria. **ACE inhibitors** are a specific cause of angioedema (reaction usually occurs within 1 week of initiating the drug).
- Unlike urticaria, which can occur anywhere, angioedema usually affects the eyelids, lips and tongue, genitalia, hands, or feet.
- Angioedema is characterized by localized edema of deep subcutaneous tissue, resulting in nonpitting, puffy skin with firm swelling that is more tender and "burning" than pruritic (because there are fewer mast cells/sensory nerve endings in deeper tissues) (Figure 11-21).
- **Severe angioedema can lead to potentially life-threatening airway obstruction.**
- Angioedema can even involve the GI tract, causing nausea/vomiting and abdominal pain (can be so severe as to mimic acute abdomen).
- Treatment is similar to treatment of urticaria. Give SC epinephrine for laryngeal edema or bronchospasm.

Quick HIT

Angioedema usually resolves in a few days, but can persist longer in some cases. (Although the swelling at any one spot resolves in a few days, the swelling can move from one location to another.)

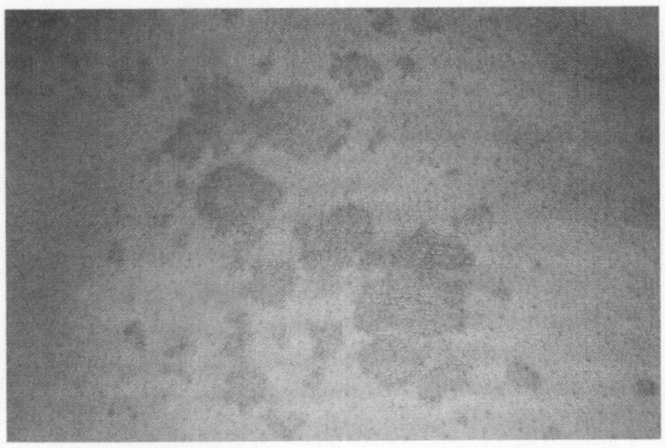

FIGURE 11-20 Urticaria.
(From Goodheart HP. *Goodheart's Photoguide of Common Skin Disorders.* 2nd ed. Philadelphia, PA: Lippincott Williams & Wilkins, 2003, Figure G.11.)

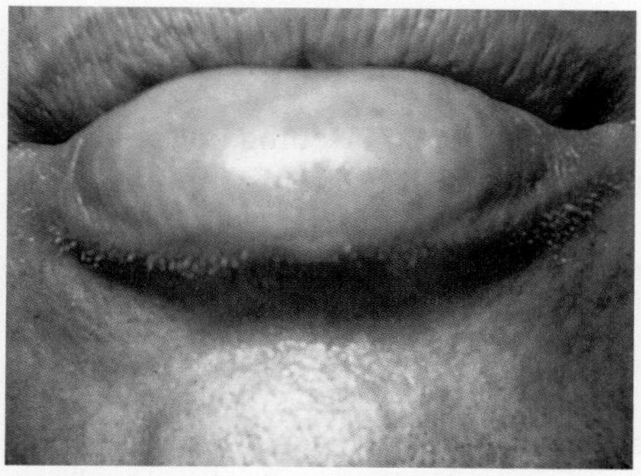

FIGURE **11-21** **Angioedema.**
(From Goodheart HP. *Goodheart's Photoguide of Common Skin Disorders*. 2nd ed. Philadelphia, PA: Lippincott Williams & Wilkins, 2003, Figure 20.1.)

Drug Allergy

- An adverse drug reaction is not necessarily an allergic drug reaction (see also Clinical Pearl 11-2). Adverse drug reactions include drug side effects, drug–drug interactions, drug toxicity and associated illnesses, and drug allergy. Most cases of adverse drug reactions are **not** related to allergy (only 10% have a true allergic basis).
- Many patients who state they are "allergic" to a medication believe themselves to be allergic because they have been incorrectly labeled without direct immunologic evidence. However, given the serious risks of a true drug allergy, one should avoid the suspected medication.
- All four types of hypersensitivity reactions may serve as the underlying mechanism of drug allergies. In many cases, however, the mechanism is unknown.
- *β*-Lactam antibiotics (penicillins), aspirin, NSAIDs, and sulfa drugs account for more than 80% of all cases of drug allergy. Other drugs implicated include insulin, local anesthetics, ACE inhibitors, and radiocontrast agents.
- Drug-induced hypersensitivity reactions can affect multiple organ systems and can manifest in a variety of forms, including:
  - **Dermatologic eruptions** (most common) (e.g., urticaria or angioedema, allergic contact dermatitis, EM-like eruptions, erythema nodosum).
  - **Pulmonary findings** (e.g., asthma, pneumonitis).
  - **Renal manifestations** (e.g., interstitial nephritis, nephrotic syndrome).
  - **Hematologic manifestations** (e.g., thrombocytopenia, hemolytic anemia, eosinophilia, agranulocytosis).
- If a drug allergy is suspected, inquire about any recent changes in the patient's medications. **Allergic reactions typically appear within 1 month of initiating the drug.** It is uncommon for a drug reaction to occur within less than 1 week of initiating the drug.
- Treatment: Discontinue the drug (if known). Give antihistamines for symptomatic relief. Treat as for anaphylaxis if severe.

CLINICAL PEARL 11-2

Types of Hypersensitivity Reactions

- **Type I:** IgE-mediated (e.g., anaphylaxis, asthma)
- **Type II:** IgG- (or IgM-) and cytotoxic cell-mediated (e.g., Goodpasture disease, pemphigus vulgaris)
- **Type III:** antigen-antibody complexes (e.g., SLE, Arthus reaction, serum sickness)
- **Type IV:** T-cell–mediated (delayed hypersensitivity) (e.g., allergic contact dermatitis, tuberculosis, transplant rejection)

Food Allergy

- Adverse food reactions can be due to true food allergies, food poisoning, metabolic conditions (e.g., lactose intolerance, phenylketonuria), malabsorption syndromes (e.g., celiac disease), or pre-existing illnesses (e.g., ulcer).
- As with drug allergies, people generally tend to believe they are allergic to a food based on an adverse reaction, even when they may not have a true food allergy.
- Hypersensitivity reactions to foods are usually due to immunoglobulin (Ig) E-mediated reactions to food and/or additives.
- The most common foods responsible include eggs, peanuts, milk, soy, tree nuts, shellfish, wheat, chocolate, legumes, and some fruits (e.g., kiwi). There are others, and preservatives or additives may be responsible. The cause may never be found.
- Food allergy reactions have the following effects:
  - **Dermatologic manifestations (most common)** (e.g., pruritus, erythema, urticaria, angioedema).
  - **GI manifestations (second-most common)** (e.g., nausea, vomiting, abdominal cramps, diarrhea).
  - **Anaphylactic reactions**—can affect the respiratory system and can be fatal.
  - **Cutaneous manifestations** (e.g., angioedema, urticaria).
- Treatment for mild reactions is supportive, with administration of antihistamines to lessen symptoms. If the reaction is more severe, treat as for anaphylaxis. Avoid the offending agent.

Insect Sting Allergy

- Insects responsible include yellow jackets, honeybees, wasps, and yellow and bald-faced hornets.
- Local **(nonallergic)** reaction is localized swelling, pain, pruritus, and redness, all of which subside in several hours. This is the normal reaction to an insect sting.
- Large local **(allergic)** reaction is marked swelling and erythema over a large area around the sting site. **Can be confused with cellulitis.** It may last for several days, and sometimes presents with mild, systemic manifestations (malaise, nausea). Prescribe antihistamines and analgesics for symptoms (short course of prednisone for severe cases).
- Anaphylaxis may occur and can be fatal.
- Treatment: ice and oral antihistamines for mild local reactions; if severe, treat as for anaphylaxis.

Anaphylaxis

- Most severe form of allergy—This is a systemic allergic reaction (usually a type I IgE reaction) that may be life-threatening.
- It occurs within seconds to minutes after exposure to antigen. Numerous causes have been identified, including foods **(most common cause)**, medications, radiocontrast agents, blood products, venoms (e.g., from snakes), insect stings, latex, hormones, ragweed/molds, and various chemicals.
- It can progress within seconds to minutes to a life-threatening situation characterized by shock or respiratory compromise (airway obstruction, vascular collapse).
- Typically, the initial findings are cutaneous, followed by respiratory symptoms.
- Treatment of anaphylaxis.
  - ABCs—secure the airway; intubation may be necessary.
  - Give epinephrine immediately. Give IV if severe (1:10,000), SC if less severe (1:1,000).
  - Give antihistamines (both H1 and H2 blockers) and corticosteroids as well (although they have a minimal effect in hyperacute condition).
  - Supportive care—IV fluids, oxygen.

Quick HIT

Clinical Features of Anaphylaxis
- Cutaneous findings—pruritus, erythema, urticaria, angioedema
- Respiratory findings—dyspnea, respiratory distress, asphyxia
- Cardiovascular findings—hypotension, shock, arrhythmias
- GI findings—abdominal pain, nausea/vomiting, severe diarrhea

Dermatology-related Key Terms

Dermatosis: any cutaneous lesion/group of lesions; nonspecific term used to include any type of skin disease
Dermatitis: inflammation of the skin
Macule: circumscribed *flat* alterations in skin color <2 cm
Patch: Macule ≥2 cm
Wheal: rounded/flat-topped edematous elevation in the skin; often erythematous
Papule: solid, **elevated** lesion with **no visible fluid** up to 0.5 cm
Nodule: Papule ≥0.5 cm
Plaque: Elevated area of skin ≥2 cm in diameter. A confluence of papules ≥1 cm
Vesicle: fluid-filled (serous/seropurulent fluid) elevated cyst ≤1 cm
Bullae: Vesicle ≥1 cm
Pustule: fluid-filled (cloudy/purulent material of necrotic inflammatory cells)

12 AMBULATORY MEDICINE

Cardiovascular Diseases

Hypertension

A. General characteristics

1. **Essential hypertension (HTN)** (i.e., there is no identifiable cause) **applies to more than 95% of cases of HTN.**
2. Secondary HTN has many identifiable causes.
   a. **Renal/renovascular disease—renal artery stenosis (most common cause of secondary HTN)**, chronic renal failure, polycystic kidneys.
   b. Endocrine causes—hyperaldosteronism, thyroid or parathyroid disease, Cushing syndrome, pheochromocytoma, hyperthyroidism, acromegaly.
   c. Medications—oral contraceptives, decongestants, estrogen, appetite suppressants, chronic steroids, tricyclic antidepressants (TCAs), nonsteroidal anti-inflammatory drugs (NSAIDs).
   d. Coarctation of the aorta.
   e. Cocaine, other stimulants.
   f. Obstructive sleep apnea (OSA).

Quick HIT

Birth control pills are the most common secondary cause of HTN in young women.

Quick HIT

Pathophysiology of the Effects of HTN on the Heart
- Increased systemic vascular resistance (afterload) → concentric LVH → decreased LV function. As a result, the chamber dilates → symptoms and signs of heart failure.
- HTN accelerates atherosclerosis, leading to a higher incidence of CAD (as well as peripheral vascular disease and stroke).

B. Risk factors

1. Age—both systolic and diastolic BP increase with age.
2. Gender—more common in men (gap narrows over age 60); men have higher complication rates.
3. Race—it is twice as common in African-American patients as in Caucasian patients; African-American patients have higher complication rates (stroke, renal failure, heart disease).
4. Obesity, sedentary lifestyle, dyslipidemia.
5. Family history.
6. Increased sodium intake—this correlates with increased prevalence in large populations, although not in individuals; individual susceptibility to the effects of high salt intake varies.
7. Alcohol—intake of more than 2 oz (8 oz of wine or 24 oz of beer) per day is associated with HTN.

Quick HIT

Target organ damage
- Heart—LVH, MI, CHF
- Brain—stroke, TIA
- Chronic kidney disease
- Peripheral arterial disease, AAA, aortic dissection
- Retinopathy

C. Definitions

1. **Classification**
   a. **Normal—Systolic BP <120 and diastolic BP <80**
   b. **Prehypertension—Systolic BP 120 to 139 or diastolic BP 80 to 89**
   c. **Stage I—Systolic BP 140 to 159 or diastolic BP 90 to 99**
   d. **Stage II—Systolic BP ≥160 or diastolic BP ≥100**
2. **Hypertensive urgency—Severe HTN (typically systolic BP ≥180 or diastolic BP ≥120) in an asymptomatic patient**

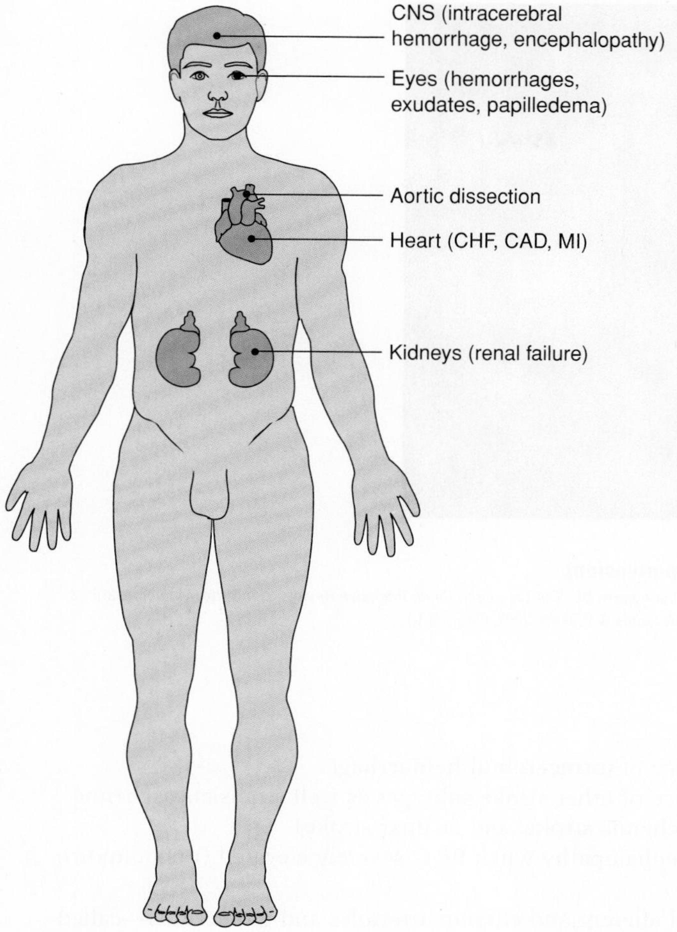

FIGURE 12-1 **Complications of uncontrolled hypertension.**

3. **Hypertensive emergency—Severe HTN with end organ damage (e.g., neurologic changes, myocardial ischemia, aortic dissection, etc.)**

D. Complications

1. **The major complications of HTN are cardiac complications (coronary artery disease [CAD], CHF with left ventricular hypertrophy [LVH]), stroke, and renal failure** (Figure 12-1). These account for the majority of deaths associated with untreated HTN.
2. HTN has effects on the following organs (target organ damage):
   a. Cardiovascular system.
      - Effects on the heart are most important. **HTN is a major risk factor for CAD**, with resultant angina and MI.
      - **CHF is a common end-result of untreated HTN** as LVH occurs.
      - Most deaths due to HTN are ultimately due to MI or CHF.
      - HTN predisposes the patient to peripheral artery disease (PAD).
      - HTN is associated with increased incidence of abdominal aortic aneurysm (AAA) and **aortic dissection.**

   b. Eyes (retinal changes).
      - Early changes—arteriovenous nicking (discontinuity in the retinal vein secondary to thickened arterial walls) and cotton wool spots (infarction of the nerve fiber layer in the retina) can cause visual disturbances and scotomata (Figure 12-2).
      - More serious disease—hemorrhages and exudates.
      - **Papilledema**—an ominous finding seen with severely elevated BP.

Quick HIT

HTN is an asymptomatic disease ("silent killer")—it causes insidious damage to the following target organs: heart, eyes, CNS, kidneys.

Quick HIT

Patients with a systolic BP of 120 to 139 or a diastolic BP of 80 to 89 are considered prehypertensive and require lifestyle modifications to prevent cardiovascular disease.

Quick HIT

Goals in evaluating a patient with HTN
- Look for secondary causes (may be treatable).
- Assess damage to target organs (heart, kidneys, eyes, CNS).
- Assess overall cardiovascular risk.
- Make therapeutic decisions based on the above.

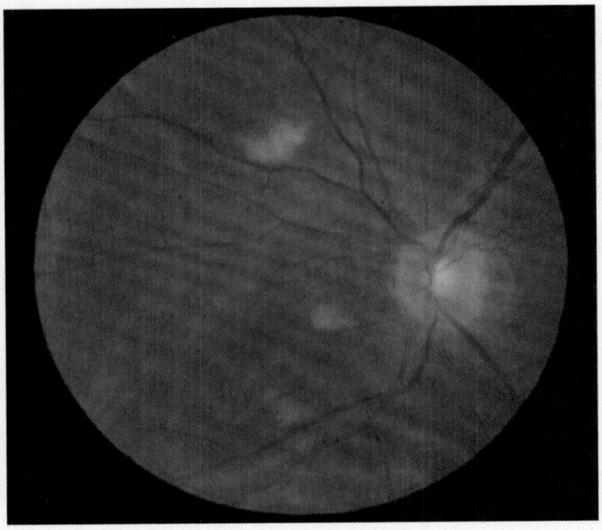

FIGURE 12-2 **Cotton wool spots (hypertension).**
(From Stoller JK, Ahmad M, Longworth DL. *The Cleveland Clinic Intensive Review of Internal Medicine.* 3rd ed. Philadelphia, PA: Lippincott Williams & Wilkins, 2002, Figure 6.1.)

c. CNS
- Increased incidence of **intracerebral hemorrhage.**
- Increased incidence of other stroke subtypes as well (transient ischemic attacks [TIAs], ischemic stroke, and lacunar stroke).
- Hypertensive encephalopathy when BP is severely elevated (uncommon).

d. Kidney
- Arteriosclerosis of afferent and efferent arterioles and glomerulus—called nephrosclerosis.
- Decreased GFR and dysfunction of tubules—with eventual **renal failure.**

Quick HIT

Definition of HTN: BP >140/90 in general population (including patients with diabetes and renal disease)

E. Diagnosis

1. BP measurement
   a. Unless the patient has severe HTN or evidence of end-organ damage, never diagnose HTN on the basis of one BP reading. Establish the diagnosis on the basis of at least two readings over a span of 4 or more weeks
   b. Observe the following to obtain an accurate BP reading
   - The arm should be at heart level, and the patient should be seated comfortably
   - Have the patient sit quietly for at least 5 minutes before measuring BP
   - Make sure the patient has not ingested caffeine or smoked cigarettes in the past 30 minutes (both elevate BP temporarily)
   - Use a cuff of adequate size (a cuff that is too small can falsely elevate BP readings). The bladder within the cuff should encircle at least 80% of the arm
2. Order the following laboratory tests to evaluate target organ damage and assess overall cardiovascular risk
   a. Urinalysis
   b. Chemistry panel: serum K^1, BUN, Cr
   c. Fasting glucose (if patient is diabetic, check for microalbuminuria)
   d. Lipid panel
   e. ECG
3. If the history and physical examination (H&P) or laboratory tests suggest a secondary cause of HTN, order appropriate tests

F. Treatment

1. Management goals (Table 12-1).

TABLE 12-1 Management Goals of Hypertension

Patient Classification	Blood Pressure Goal	Recommended Management
General population ≥60 yrs	<150/<90	• Nonblack: thiazide, ACEI/ARB, or CCB, alone or in combination • Black: thiazide or CCB, alone or in combination
General population <60 yrs	<140/<90	
Diabetic, no CKD	<140/<90	
CKD, ± diabetes	<140/<90	ACEI or ARB

Modified from James PA, Oparil S, Carter BL, et al. 2014 Evidence-based guideline for the management of high blood pressure in adults. Report from the panel members appointed to the Eighth Joint National Committee (JNC 8). *JAMA*. 2014;311(5):507–520.

2. Lifestyle changes, listed in order of effect on BP reduction:
   a. Weight loss lowers BP significantly. In patients with central obesity (who often have coexisting diabetes, hyperlipidemia, and other risk factors), weight loss is particularly important because multiple risk factors are reduced concomitantly.
   b. Follow a low-saturated-fat diet rich in fruits, vegetables, and low-fat dairy products (DASH diet).
   c. Exercise regularly. Regular aerobic exercise can lower BP (and reduces overall cardiovascular risk).
   d. Reduce salt intake. Reduction in dietary salt has been shown to reduce BP. Recommend either a no-added-salt diet (4 g sodium/day) or a low-sodium diet (2 g/day).
   e. Avoid excessive alcohol consumption. Alcohol has a pressor action, and excessive use can increase BP.
   f. Others—stop unnecessary medications that may contribute to HTN. Engage in appropriate stress management practices.
3. Pharmacologic treatment (seven classes of drugs) (Table 12-2).
   a. Thiazide diuretics.
      - Because "salt-sensitive" HTN is more common in African-American patients, diuretics are a good initial choice for these patients (though a calcium channel blocker is equally recommended as a first-line option).
      - A good option in patients with osteoporosis (increases calcium reabsorption in the nephron).
   b. β-Blockers—decrease HR and cardiac output and decrease renin release.
      - A good option in patients with CHF, CAD, or atrial fibrillation; a poor option in patients with obstructive lung disease, heart block, or depression.
   c. ACE inhibitors.
      - Inhibit the renin–angiotensin–aldosterone system by inhibiting the conversion of angiotensin I to angiotensin II. Angiotensin II normally causes vasoconstriction, aldosterone release, and ventricular remodeling.
      - ACE also acts to degrade bradykinin, so inhibition results in excess levels in the lung that can cause a chronic dry cough.
      - **Preferred in all diabetic patients** because of their protective effect on kidneys; also a good option for patients with CHF, CAD.
   d. Angiotensin II receptor blockers (ARBs).
      - Also inhibit renin–angiotensin–aldosterone system.
      - ARBs have the same beneficial effects on the kidney in diabetic patients as ACE inhibitors and do not cause a chronic cough; ACE inhibitors and ARBs should not be used in combination.
   e. Calcium channel blockers—cause vasodilation of arteriolar vasculature.

Quick HIT

Always obtain a pregnancy test in reproductive age women before starting an antihypertensive medication. Thiazides, ACE inhibitors, calcium channel blockers, and ARBs are contraindicated in pregnancy. β-Blockers and hydralazine are safe.

Quick HIT

If a patient presents with moderate-to-severe HTN, consider initiating therapy right away instead of waiting 1 to 2 months to confirm diagnosis and start treatment.

Quick HIT

Unless there is a compelling indication to use a specific drug class, it makes little difference whether the initial drug is a thiazide diuretic, calcium channel blocker, ACE inhibitor, or ARB.

TABLE 12-2 Side Effects of Antihypertensive Medications

Medication	Side Effects
Thiazide diuretics	**Hypokalemia,** hyperuricemia, hyperglycemia, elevation of cholesterol and triglyceride levels, metabolic alkalosis, hyperuricemia, hypomagnesemia
β-Blockers	Bradycardia, bronchospasm, sleep disturbances (insomnia), fatigue, may increase TGs and decrease HDL, depression, sedation, may mask hypoglycemic symptoms in diabetic patients on insulin
Ace inhibitors	Acute renal failure, hyperkalemia, dry cough, angioedema, skin rash, altered sense of taste
Calcium channel blockers	Dihydropyridines (e.g., amlodipine): peripheral edema Nondihydropyridines (e.g., verapamil, diltiazem): heart block

Quick HIT

Treatment with ACE inhibitors and ARBs is associated with decreased risk of new-onset diabetes in patients with HTN.

Quick HIT

Most patients eventually need more than one drug to attain goal BP (especially diabetics, obese patients, and those with renal failure).

Quick HIT

If "white coat hypertension" is suspected, there are two options for determining whether the increased BP persists outside the office.
- Twenty-four–hour ambulatory blood pressure monitoring is the most effective.
- Home blood pressure monitoring is an alternative.

Quick HIT

Cardiovascular risk factors: smoking, diabetes, hypercholesterolemia, age over 60, family history, male sex (higher than for female only until menopause)
Clinical risk factors: presence of CAD, PAD, or prior MI; any manifestations of target organ disease—LVH, retinopathy, nephropathy; stroke or TIA

Ambulatory Medicine

f. α-Blockers—decrease arteriolar resistance.
   - May be of benefit if the patient has concurrent benign prostatic hyperplasia (BPH) but these are not considered first- or second-line agents.

g. Vasodilators (hydralazine and minoxidil)—not commonly used; typically given in combination with β-blockers and diuretics to patients with refractory HTN.

4. General principles of treatment.
   a. BP should be lowered to <140/90 mm Hg for patients <60 years old, and <150/90 mm Hg for patients ≥60 years old. If patients ≥60 years old previously tolerated a BP goal <140/90 mm Hg, their treatment does not need to be changed.
   b. Each of the antihypertensive agents is roughly equally effective in lowering BP. But there is great variability in how patients respond to each drug. The three classes of drugs that are used for initial monotherapy are thiazide diuretics, long-acting calcium channel blockers (most often a dihydropyridine), and ACE inhibitors or ARBs. β-Blockers are not commonly used as initial monotherapy in the absence of a specific indication because of adverse effects on some cardiovascular outcomes especially in elderly patients.
   c. Drug treatment is often lifelong. However, patients with very mild HTN may be able to be weaned off medication if their BP can be lowered and controlled with nonpharmacologic measures. However, these patients need frequent BP checks.
   d. ALLHAT trial compared chlorthalidone, amlodipine, lisinopril, and doxazosin in patients with essential HTN and at least one CAD risk factor. The doxazosin arm was terminated early because of an increased risk of CHF compared to chlorthalidone. The other three agents were similar in regards to rates of fatal CAD and nonfatal MI, however chlorthalidone reduced rates of CAD, stroke, CHF, and angina when compared to lisinopril.
   e. ACCOMPLISH trial showed that treatment with antihypertensive combination therapy—the ACE inhibitor benazepril plus the calcium channel blocker amlodipine—was more effective than treatment with the ACE inhibitor plus diuretic. Based on this trial, it makes sense to start monotherapy with either a calcium channel blocker or an ACE inhibitor, so that the other can be added if combination therapy is needed. **Despite the findings of this trial, thiazide diuretics remain a common initial drug choice.**
   f. If the patient's response to one agent is not adequate, there are two options:
      - Increase the dose of the first agent to the maximum dose.
      - Add a second medication (thiazide, calcium channel blocker, ACE inhibitor, or ARB); if target BP not achieved, increase the dose of each as necessary until the maximum dose is achieved.
   g. If a patient's response is still inadequate with two agents, consider a third agent and referral to a HTN specialist.
   h. When to start treatment.
      - The decision of when to start pharmacologic treatment is based on the patient's total cardiovascular risk, not just the elevation in BP.

CLINICAL PEARL 12-1

Risk Factors for CAD in Evaluation of Patients With Hyperlipidemia

- Current cigarette smoking (dose-dependent risk)
- HTN
- Diabetes mellitus
- Low HDL cholesterol (<35 mg/dL); high HDL (>60 mg/dL) is a negative risk factor (subtract 1 from total)
- Age
  - Male: >45 years of age
  - Female: >55 years of age
- Male gender—if you count as a risk factor, do not count age
- Family history of premature CAD
  - MI/sudden death in male first-degree relative <55 years of age
  - MI/sudden death in female first-degree relative <65 years of age

- For any level of BP elevation, the presence of cardiovascular risk factors and/or comorbid conditions dramatically accelerates the risk from HTN, and therefore modifies the treatment plan. Estimation of overall risk depends on **cardiovascular risk factors** and **clinical risk factors** (see Clinical Pearl 12-1).

Quick HIT

All people should be screened with fasting lipid profile every 5 years starting at age 20. Earlier and more frequent screening is recommended for a strong family history and/or obesity.

Hyperlipidemias

A. General characteristics

1. Hyperlipidemia is one of the most important (and modifiable) risk factors for CAD. It causes accelerated atherosclerosis.
2. Hyperlipidemia may be a primary disorder, such as a familial dyslipidemia syndrome, or secondary to another cause.
3. Classification of dyslipidemia syndromes—types IIA, IIB, and IV account for over 80% of all of familial dyslipidemias (Table 12-3)
4. Secondary causes of hyperlipidemia
   a. Endocrine disorders—hypothyroidism, DM, Cushing syndrome
   b. Renal disorders—nephrotic syndrome, uremia
   c. Chronic liver disease

TABLE 12-3 Dyslipidemia Syndromes

Class	Name	Lipoprotein Elevated	Treatment
Type I	Exogenous hyperlipidemia	Chylomicrons	Diet
Type IIa	Familial hypercholesterolemia	LDL	Statins Niacin Cholestyramine
Type IIb	Combined hyperlipoproteinemia	LDL + VLDL	Statins Niacin Gemfibrozil
Type III	Familial dysbetalipoproteinemia	IDL	Gemfibrozil Niacin
Type IV	Endogenous hyperlipidemia	VLDL	Niacin Gemfibrozil Statins
Type V	Familial hypertriglyceridemia	VLDL + chylomicrons	Niacin Gemfibrozil

IDL, intermediate density lipoprotein.

d. Medications—glucocorticoids, estrogen, thiazide diuretics, β-blockers
e. Pregnancy

5. Risk factors
   a. Diet
      - Saturated fatty acids and cholesterol cause elevation in LDL and total cholesterol
      - High-calorie diets do not increase LDL or cholesterol levels (are "neutral") but do increase triglyceride (TG) levels
      - Alcohol increases TG levels and HDL levels but does not affect total cholesterol levels
   b. Age—cholesterol levels increase with age until approximately age 65. The increase is greatest during early adulthood—about 2 mg/dL per year
   c. Inactive lifestyle, abdominal obesity
   d. Family history of hyperlipidemia
   e. Gender—men generally have higher cholesterol levels than do women; when women reach menopause, cholesterol levels then equalize and may even be higher in women than in men
   f. Medications
      - Thiazides—increase LDL, total cholesterol, TG (VLDL) levels
      - β-Blockers (propranolol)—increase TGs (VLDL) and lower HDL levels
      - Estrogens—TG levels may further increase in patients with hypertriglyceridemia
      - Corticosteroids and HIV protease inhibitors can elevate serum lipids
   g. Genetic mutations that predispose to the most severe hyperlipidemias
   h. Secondary causes of dyslipidemia (see above)
6. Role of lipids in CAD risk
   a. LDL cholesterol
      - Accounts for two-thirds of total cholesterol. **CAD risk is primarily due to the LDL component** because LDL is the most atherogenic of all lipoproteins
      - LDL cholesterol is not directly measured. It is calculated as follows: LDL = total cholesterol − HDL − TG/5
   b. Total cholesterol
      - The risk of CAD increases sharply when total cholesterol is above 240 mg/dL
   c. HDL cholesterol
      - Its protective effect (removes excess cholesterol from arterial walls) is at least as strong as the atherogenic effect of LDL
      - For every 10 mg/dL increase in HDL levels, CAD risk decreases by 50%
      - High HDL (>60 mg/dL) is a "negative" risk factor (counteracts one risk factor) for CAD
   d. **The total cholesterol-to-HDL ratio**—The lower the total cholesterol-to-HDL ratio, the lower the risk of CAD
      - Ratio of 5.0 is average (standard) risk
      - Ratio of 10 is double the risk
      - Ratio of 20 is triple the risk
      - Ratio of <4.5 is desirable
   e. TGs—Elevated TGs are associated with coronary risk, but it is unknown whether this association is causal. It is uncertain whether lowering TG level reduces coronary risk.

Quick HIT

Estrogen Replacement Therapy in Postmenopausal Women
Recent HERS trial showed no benefit of hormone replacement therapy on cardiovascular outcomes in women with established CHD. However, the study did not address the issue in women without CHD. The results are somewhat controversial.

Quick HIT

Statins and fibrates can induce transient elevation in serum transaminases. LFT must be monitored.

B. Clinical features

1. Most patients are asymptomatic.
2. The following may be manifestations of severe hyperlipidemia:
   a. *Xanthelasma*—yellow plaques on eyelids.
   b. *Xanthoma*—hard, yellowish masses found on tendons (finger extensors, Achilles tendon, plantar tendons).
3. Pancreatitis can occur with severe hypertriglyceridemia.

C. Diagnosis

1. Lipid screening (see Health Maintenance section)—measure total cholesterol and HDL levels (nonfasting is acceptable). If either is abnormal, then order a full fasting lipid profile.

2. A full fasting lipid profile includes TG levels and calculation of LDL levels.
3. Consider checking laboratory tests to exclude secondary causes of hyperlipidemia.
   a. TSH (hypothyroidism).
   b. LFTs (chronic liver disease).
   c. BUN and Cr, urinary proteins (nephrotic syndrome).
   d. Glucose levels (diabetes).

D. Treatment

1. New guidelines issued by the ACC/AHA in 2013 have dramatically changed lipid management.
   a. The long-term goal is the same: to reduce morbidity and mortality from CAD.
   b. Key differences of the new guidelines compared to the previous guidelines (Adult Treatment Panel III):
      - Targeting specific cholesterol goals is no longer recommended.
      - The use of nonstatin medications to lower LDL is generally not recommended.
      - The use of a new risk calculator to calculate a patient's 10-year risk of atherosclerotic cardiovascular disease (ASCVD) (found online at http://my.americanheart.org/cvriskcalculator).
2. Therapy for ASCVD risk reduction.
   a. Statin therapy is recommended for four categories of patients (Table 12-4).
   b. Dietary therapy is important before and during statin therapy. Lowering fat intake (especially saturated fats) reduces serum cholesterol more than lowering cholesterol intake. Foods rich in omega-3 fatty acids (such as fish) are particularly beneficial. With an intensive diet, LDL can be reduced by an average of 10%, as follows: <30% of total calories from fat; with fewer than 10% from saturated fat; <300 mg/day of cholesterol.
   c. Exercise and weight loss—reduce risk of CAD.
      - Exercise increases HDL and reduces other CAD risk factors by lowering BP and enhancing the efficiency of peripheral oxygen extraction.
      - Weight loss reduces myocardial work as well as the risk of diabetes.
   d. Smoking cessation.
   e. Drug therapy—See Table 12-5. Available agents include HMG CoA reductase inhibitors (statins), niacin, bile-acid sequestrants, and gemfibrozil.
      - Patients given drug therapy should almost always be treated with a statin. Statins can reduce relative cardiovascular risk by about 20% to 30% regardless of baseline LDL levels.

Quick HIT

Statins have been shown to significantly reduce rates of MI, stroke, and coronary and all-cause mortality in prospective placebo-controlled trials.

Quick HIT

Potency of HMG CoA reductase inhibitors ("statins"):
- High-intensity: atorvastatin 40 to 80 mg, rosuvastatin 20 to 40 mg
- Moderate-intensity: atorvastatin 10 to 20 mg, rosuvastatin 5 to 10 mg, simvastatin 20 to 40 mg, lovastatin 40 mg, pravastatin 40 to 80 mg, fluvastatin XL 80 mg (or 40 mg twice daily), pitavastatin 2 to 4 mg
- Low-intensity: simvastatin 10 mg, pravastatin 10 to 20 mg, lovastatin 20 mg, fluvastatin 20 to 40 mg, pitavastatin 1 mg

Quick HIT

All patients should have their AST and ALT measured before starting a statin and after starting a statin if symptoms of hepatotoxicity are evident. About 1% of patients on statins will develop such elevations in AST and ALT that the statin will need to be discontinued.

TABLE 12-4 Updated Cholesterol Treatment Guidelines

Four Categories of Patients Aged >21 yrs That Benefit From Statin Therapy[a]

Category	Recommended Therapy
Clinical ASCVD[b,c]	High-intensity statin
LDL cholesterol ≥190 mg/dL	High-intensity statin
Diabetic patients aged 40–75 yrs with LDL cholesterol 70–189 mg/dL	– ASCVD risk score <7.5%, moderate-intensity statin – ASCVD risk score ≥7.5%, high-intensity statin
Nondiabetic patients aged 40–75 yrs with LDL cholesterol 70–189 mg/dL	ASCVD risk score ≥7.5%, moderate- to high-intensity statin

[a]The new guidelines do not make recommendations due to insufficient evidence from randomized controlled trials for patients aged >75 yrs, with NYHA class II–IV heart failure, or with end-stage renal disease undergoing hemodialysis.

[b]ASCVD, atherosclerotic cardiovascular disease

[c]Includes patients with acute coronary syndromes or a history of MI, stable or unstable angina, coronary or other arterial revascularization, stroke, TIA, or peripheral arterial disease from atherosclerosis.

Modified from Stone NJ, Robinson J, Lichtenstein AH, et al. 2013 ACC/AHA Guidelines on the treatment of blood cholesterol to reduce atherosclerotic cardiovascular risk in adults: A Report of the American College of Cardiology/American Heart Association Task Force on Practice Guidelines. *Circulation.* 2014;129:S1–S45.

TABLE 12-5 Drug Therapy for Hyperlipidemia

Drug	Effects	Comments	Side Effects
HMG CoA reductase inhibitors (statins)	Lower LDL levels (most potent for lowering LDL) Minimal effect on HDL and TG levels	Have been shown to reduce mortality from cardiovascular events and significantly reduce total mortality Drugs of choice for ASCVD risk reduction	Monitor LFTs. Harmless elevation in muscle enzymes (CPK) may occur
Niacin	Lowers TG levels Lowers LDL levels Increases HDL levels	Do not use in diabetic patients (may worsen glycemic control) Most potent agent for increasing HDL levels and lowering TG levels	Flushing effect (cutaneous flushing of face/arms; pruritus may be present) Check LFTs and CPK levels as with statin drugs
Bile acid-binding resins (cholestyramine, colestipol)	Lowers LDL Increases TG levels	Effective when used in combination with statins or niacin to treat severe disease in high-risk patients	Adverse GI side effects, poorly tolerated
Fibrates (gemfibrozil)	Lower VLDL and TG Increase HDL	Primarily for lowering TG levels	GI side effects (mild) Mild abnormalities in LFTs Gynecomastia, gallstones, weight gain, and myopathies are other side effects

CPK, creatine phosphokinase.

Quick HIT

Statins are the most common drugs used, and can reduce LDL by 20% to 60%.

Quick HIT

Emergency evaluation of headache
- Obtain a noncontrast CT scan to first rule out any type of intracranial bleed.
- However, small bleeds (subarachnoid hemorrhage) may be missed by CT scan, so a lumbar puncture may be necessary.

- The other classes of drugs should only be used if a patient does not tolerate statin therapy.

3. Therapy for high TG levels—the data is fairly limited regarding which patients should be treated and which medication to use.
   a. First-line therapy is weight loss, aerobic exercise, glycemic control in diabetics, and low-fat diet.
   b. Medications include fibrates, nicotinic acid, and fish oil.
   c. Statins should be considered even in patients with high TG levels because of their cardioprotective effects.

Headache

Tension Headache

A. General characteristics

1. Cause is unknown; may be similar to that of migraines (see below) (see also Clinical Pearls 12-2 and 12-3)
2. Usually worsens throughout the day; precipitants include anxiety, depression, and stress
3. Mild migraine can easily be confused with tension headache and vice versa

CLINICAL PEARL 12-2

Differential Diagnosis of Headache

- Primary headache syndromes—migraines, cluster headache, tension headache
- Secondary causes of headache ("VOMIT")
  - **V**ascular—subarachnoid hemorrhage, subdural hematoma, epidural hematoma, intraparenchymal hemorrhage, temporal arteritis
  - **O**ther causes—malignant HTN, pseudomotor cerebri, postlumbar puncture, pheochromocytoma
  - **M**edication/drug related—nitrates, alcohol withdrawal, chronic analgesic use/abuse
  - **I**nfection—meningitis, encephalitis, cerebral abscess, sinusitis, herpes zoster, fever
  - **T**umor

CLINICAL PEARL 12-3

Headache Red Flags

- Sudden onset within seconds to minutes.
- Worst headache of the patient's life.
- New-onset headache that the patient has never experienced before, especially over the age of 50 years.
- Headache pattern: increase in severity and frequency over time, worse after lying down.
- Mental status change or any focal neurologic symptoms/signs.
- New-onset headache associated with heavy exertion or head trauma.
- New-onset headache associated with fever, stiff neck, or rash.
- New-onset headache in a patient with HIV infection or cancer.

B. Clinical features

1. Pain is steady, aching, "vise-like," and encircles the entire head (tight band-like pain around the head).
   a. Usually generalized, but may be the most intense around the neck or back of head.
   b. Can be accompanied by tender muscles (posterior cervical, temporal, frontal).
2. Tightness in posterior neck muscles.

C. Treatment

1. Attempt to find the causal factor(s). Evaluate the patient for possible depression or anxiety. Stress reduction is important.
2. NSAIDs, acetaminophen, and aspirin are the standard treatment for mild/moderate headaches.
3. If headaches are severe, medications that are used for migraines may be appropriate, given the difficulty in distinguishing between these two entities.

Cluster Headaches

A. General characteristics

1. Very rare—thought by some to be a variant of migraine headache
2. Usually occurs in middle-aged men
3. Subtypes
   a. Episodic cluster headaches (90% of all cases)—last 2 to 3 months, with remissions of months to years
   b. Chronic cluster headaches (10% of all cases)—last 1 to 2 years; headaches do not remit

B. Clinical features

1. Excruciating periorbital pain ("behind the eye")—**almost always unilateral**
2. Cluster headache is described as a "deep, burning, searing, or stabbing pain." Pain may be so severe that the patient may even become suicidal
3. Accompanied by ipsilateral lacrimation, facial flushing, nasal stuffiness/discharge
4. Usually begins a few hours after the patient goes to bed and lasts for 30 to 90 minutes; awakens patient from sleep (but daytime cluster headaches also occur)
5. Attacks occur nightly for 2 to 3 months and then disappear. Remissions may last from several months to several years
6. Worse with alcohol and sleep

C. Treatment

1. Acute attacks
   a. **Sumatriptan** (Imitrex) and inhaled O_2 are the first-line treatments
2. Prophylaxis
   a. Of all the headache types, cluster headaches are the most responsive to prophylactic treatment. Offer all patients prophylactic medication. **Verapamil** taken daily is the drug of choice

Quick HIT

Visual Aura in Migraine
- The classic presentation is a bilateral homonymous scotoma. Bright, flashing, crescent-shaped images with jagged edges often appear on a page, obscuring the underlying print. The aura usually lasts 10 to 20 minutes.
- A patient may have isolated visual migraines (as above) without headaches.

b. Ergotamine, methysergide, lithium, and corticosteroids (prednisone) are alternative agents
c. These agents cause resolution (or marked reduction) of the number of headaches within 1 week

Migraine

A. General characteristics

1. An inherited disorder (probably an autosomal dominant trait with incomplete penetrance)
2. The pathogenesis is not clearly defined, but serotonin depletion plays a major role
3. More common in women than men; more common in those with a family history; typically occurs one to two times per month
4. Types
   a. Migraine with aura (15% of cases)—"classic migraine." Aura is usually visual (flashing lights, scotomata, visual distortions), but can be neurologic (sensory disturbances, hemiparesis, dysphasia)
   b. Migraine without aura (85% of cases)—"common migraine"
   c. Menstrual migraine
      - Occurs between 2 days before menstruation and the last day of menses; linked to estrogen withdrawal
      - Treatment is similar to that of nonmenstrual migraine except that estrogen supplementation is sometimes added
   d. Status migrainosus—lasts over 72 hours and does not resolve spontaneously
5. The following can provoke a migraine:
   a. Hormonal alteration (menstruation)
   b. Stress, anxiety
   c. Sleeping disturbances (lack of sleep)
   d. Certain drugs/foods—chocolate, cheese, alcohol, smoking, oral contraceptive pills
   e. Weather changes and other environmental factors

Quick HIT

Many patients who are labeled as having migraines actually have **rebound analgesic headaches.** These occur more frequently (every 1 to 2 days) than migraines. These headaches do not respond to drugs used to treat migraines. Wean patient from analgesics. Do not use narcotics!

B. Clinical features

1. Prodromal phase (occurs in 30% of patients)
   a. Consists of symptoms of excitation or inhibition of the CNS: elation, excitability, increased appetite and craving for certain foods (especially sweets); alternatively, depression, irritability, sleepiness, and fatigue may be manifested
   b. May precede the actual migraine attack by up to 24 hours
2. Severe, throbbing, unilateral headache (not always on the same side)
   a. Lasts 4 to 72 hours
   b. At times, it may be generalized over the entire head and may last for days if not treated
   c. Pain is aggravated by coughing, physical activity, or bending down
   d. Variable pain quality—"throbbing" or "dull and achy"
3. Other symptoms include nausea and vomiting (in as many as 90% of cases), photophobia, and increased sensitivity to smell

Quick HIT

Most patients experience a decrease in the number and intensity of headaches as they age.

C. Treatment

1. Acute attacks of migraine
   a. If migraines are mild, analgesics such as NSAIDs or acetaminophen may be effective. If they are not effective, try either dihydroergotamine (DHE) or a triptan
   b. DHE—a serotonin (5-HT1) receptor agonist
      - This is highly effective in terminating the pain of migraines. It is available for SC, IM, IV, or nasal administration
      - Contraindications—CAD, pregnancy, TIAs, PAD, sepsis
   c. Sumatriptan—a more selective 5-HT1 receptor agonist than DHE or other triptans
      - Acts rapidly (within 1 hour) and is highly effective
      - Should not be used more than once or twice per week
      - Contraindications—CAD, pregnancy, uncontrolled HTN, basilar artery migraine, hemiplegic migraine, use of MAOI, SSRI, or lithium

   d. If none of the available migraine medications work, it is unlikely that the patient is suffering from a migraine headache
2. Prophylaxis (must be taken daily)
   a. Consider prophylaxis for patients with weekly episodes that are interfering with activities. Before initiating prophylactic medications, the patient should make attempts to avoid any known precipitants of the migraines
   b. First-line agents include TCAs (amitriptyline) and propranolol (β-blocker). Propranolol is most effective of the prophylactic medications for migraines
   c. Second-line agents include verapamil (calcium channel blocker), valproic acid (anticonvulsant), and methysergide
   d. NSAIDs are effective for menstrual migraines

Quick HIT

Beware of the patient with "migraine headache" for whom no medications work. The probability of that patient having migraine headache as the primary headache is very low.

Upper Respiratory Diseases

Cough

A. General characteristics

1. Cough can be divided into acute (less than 3 weeks duration) and chronic (more than 3 weeks duration)
2. If the cause is benign, cough usually resolves in a few weeks. If a cough lasts for longer than 1 month, further investigation is appropriate
3. Causes
   a. Conditions that are usually associated with other symptoms and signs
      - Upper respiratory infections (URIs)—this is probably the most common cause of acute cough
      - Pulmonary disease—pneumonia, chronic obstructive pulmonary disease (COPD), pulmonary fibrosis, lung cancer, asthma, lung abscess, tuberculosis
      - CHF with pulmonary edema
   b. Isolated cough in patients with normal chest radiograph
      - Smoking
      - Postnasal drip—may be caused by URIs (viral infections), rhinitis (allergic or nonallergic), chronic sinusitis, or airborne irritants
      - Gastroesophageal reflux disease (GERD)—especially if nocturnal cough (when lying flat, reflux worsens due to position and decreased lower esophageal sphincter [LES] tone)
      - Asthma—cough may be the only symptom in 5% of cases
      - ACE inhibitors—may cause a dry cough (due to bradykinin production)

Quick HIT

Postnasal Drip
The mucosal receptors in the pharynx and larynx are stimulated by secretions of the nose and sinuses that drain into the hypopharynx.

B. Diagnosis

1. Usually no tests are indicated in a patient with acute cough.
2. CXR is indicated only if a pulmonary cause is suspected, if the patient has hemoptysis, or if the patient has a chronic cough. It also may be appropriate in a long-term smoker in whom COPD or lung cancer is a possibility.
3. CBC if infection is suspected.
4. Pulmonary function testing if asthma is suspected or if cause is unclear in a patient with chronic cough.
5. Bronchoscopy (if there is no diagnosis after above workup) to look for tumor, foreign body, or tracheal web.

Quick HIT

Causes of Chronic Cough in Adults
- **Smoking**
- Postnasal drip
- GERD
- Asthma

C. Treatment

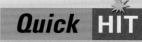

1. Treat the underlying cause, if known
2. Smoking cessation, if smoking is the cause
3. Postnasal drip—treat this with a first-generation antihistamine/decongestant preparation. If sinusitis is also present, consider antibiotics. For allergic rhinitis, consider a nonsedating long-acting oral antihistamine (loratadine)
4. Nonspecific antitussive treatment
   a. Unnecessary in most cases, because cough usually resolves with specific treatment of the cause

Quick HIT

It is often difficult to distinguish between a viral and a bacterial infection.

Common Features of Viral Versus Bacterial URIs

Feature	Viral	Bacterial
Rhinorrhea	X	—
Myalgias	X	—
Headache	X	—
Fever	X	X
Cough	X	X
Yellow sputum	—	X

b. May be helpful in the following situations:
- If cause is unknown (and thus specific therapy cannot be given)
- If specific therapy is not effective
- If cough serves no useful purpose, such as clearing excessive sputum production or secretions

c. Medications
- Codeine
- Dextromethorphan
- Benzonatate (Tessalon Perles) capsules

d. Agents used to improve the effectiveness of antitussive medications include expectorants such as guaifenesin and water

●●● Acute Bronchitis

A. General characteristics

1. Viruses account for the majority of cases.
2. Laboratory tests are not indicated. Obtain a chest radiograph only if you suspect pneumonia; there is no infiltrate or consolidation in acute bronchitis (presence of fever, tachypnea, crackles, egophony on auscultation, or dullness to percussion suggests pneumonia).

B. Clinical features

1. **Cough (with or without sputum) is the predominant symptom**—it lasts 1 to 2 weeks. In a significant number of patients, the cough may last for 1 month or longer.
2. Chest discomfort and shortness of breath may be present.
3. Fever may or may not be present.

C. Treatment

1. Antibiotics are usually **not** necessary—most cases are viral.
2. Cough suppressants (codeine-containing cough medications) are effective for symptomatic relief.
3. Bronchodilators (albuterol) may relieve symptoms.

Quick HIT

- The common cold is synonymous with acute rhinosinusitis—inflammation and congestion of mucous membranes of nasal and sinus passages.
- In most cases, it is very difficult to distinguish between the common cold (viral rhinosinusitis) and acute bacterial sinusitis on the basis of clinical features.
- Sneezing/rhinorrhea, nasal discharge (whether clear, purulent, or colored), nasal obstruction, and facial pain/headaches occur in both.

●●● The Common Cold

A. General characteristics

1. The "common cold" is the most common upper respiratory tract infection. Children are more frequently affected than adults. Susceptibility depends on pre-existing antibody levels.
2. Caused by viruses (identification of virus is not important).
   a. Rhinoviruses are the most common (at least 50% of cases)—there are more than 100 antigenic serotypes, so reinfection with another serotype can lead to symptoms (no cross-immunity among the serotypes).
   b. Other viruses include coronavirus, parainfluenza viruses (types A, B, and C), adenovirus, coxsackievirus, and RSV.
3. **Hand-to-hand transmission** is the most common route.
4. Complications include secondary bacterial infection (bacterial sinusitis or pneumonia). These secondary infections (especially pneumonia) are very rare.
5. Most resolve within 1 week, but symptoms may last up to 10 to 14 days.

B. Clinical features

1. Rhinorrhea, sore throat, malaise, nonproductive cough, nasal congestion.
2. Fever is uncommon in adults (suggests a bacterial complication or influenza), but is not unusual in children.

C. Treatment (symptomatic)

1. Adequate hydration
   a. Loosens secretions and prevents airway obstruction
   b. Can be achieved by increasing fluid intake and inhaling steam

2. Rest and analgesics (aspirin, acetaminophen, ibuprofen)—for relief of malaise, headache, fever, aches
3. Cough suppressant (dextromethorphan, codeine)
4. Nasal decongestant spray (Neo-Synephrine) for less than 3 days
5. Oral first-generation antihistamines for rhinorrhea/sneezing

Quick HIT

Many of the symptoms seen with the common cold are also seen in influenza, but are more severe in the latter. Fever, headache, myalgias, and malaise are much more pronounced with influenza.

Sinusitis

A. General characteristics

1. There is inflammation of the lining of the paranasal sinuses, often due to infection. Mucosal edema obstructs the sinus openings (ostia), trapping sinus secretions
2. Most cases of acute sinusitis occur as a complication of the common cold or other URIs. (However, fewer than 1% of URIs lead to acute sinusitis.) May also be caused by nasal obstruction due to polyps, deviated septum, or foreign body
3. Classification
   a. Acute bacterial sinusitis—usually due to *Streptococcus pneumoniae, Haemophilus influenzae,* or anaerobes
   b. Other types—viral, fungal, or allergic
4. The most common sinuses involved are the **maxillary sinuses**

Quick HIT

Sinusitis is usually self-limited, but **can be associated with high morbidity.** It can be life-threatening if the infection spreads to bone or to the CNS.

B. Clinical features

1. Acute sinusitis
   a. Nasal stuffiness, purulent nasal discharge, cough
   b. Sinus pain or pressure (location depends on which sinus is involved)—pain worsens with percussion or bending head down
      - Maxillary sinusitis (most common)—pain over the cheeks that **may mimic pain of dental caries**
      - Frontal sinusitis—pain in the lower forehead
      - Ethmoid sinusitis—retro-orbital pain, or pain in the upper lateral aspect of the nose
   c. Fever in 50% of cases
2. Chronic sinusitis
   a. Nasal congestion, postnasal discharge
   b. Pain and headache are usually mild or absent; fever is uncommon
   c. By definition, symptoms should be present **for at least 2 to 3 months**
   d. In addition to the organisms listed for acute sinusitis, patients with a history of multiple sinus infections (and courses of antibiotics) are at risk for infection with *S. aureus* and gram-negative rods.

Quick HIT

If a patient has a cold beyond 8 to 10 days, or if the cold symptoms improve and then worsen after a few days ("double-sickening"), consider acute bacterial sinusitis (may be a secondary bacterial infection after a primary viral illness).

C. Diagnosis

1. Diagnosis is based on clinical findings. Consider acute bacterial sinusitis if a patient has a cold for more than 8 to 10 days or has prolonged nasal congestion.
2. Physical examination.
   a. Look for purulent discharge draining from one of the turbinates.
   b. Perform transillumination of maxillary sinuses (note impaired light transmission)—the room must be completely dark with a strong light source.
   c. Palpate over the sinuses for tenderness (not a reliable finding).
3. Imaging studies—usually not indicated in routine community-acquired infections.
   a. Conventional sinus radiographs—look for air–fluid levels in acute disease.
   b. A CT scan (coronal view) is superior to a plain radiograph. It should be performed in complicated disease or if surgery is being planned.

Quick HIT

Treat with antibiotics and decongestants for 1 to 2 weeks, depending on severity. If there is no improvement after 2 weeks of therapy, then sinus films and a penicillinase-resistant antibiotic are appropriate. Consider ENT consultation. Because of the anatomic difficulties in drainage, the course of acute sinusitis takes longer to resolve than other URIs.

D. Complications

1. Mucocele, polyps
2. Orbital cellulitis—usually originating from ethmoid sinusitis
3. Osteomyelitis of the frontal bones or maxilla
4. Cavernous sinus thrombosis (rare)
5. Very rare—epidural abscess, subdural empyema, meningitis, and brain abscess—due to contiguous spread through bone or via venous channels

Quick HIT

Antihistamines have a drying effect (making secretions thicker) and can sometimes worsen congestion. If this occurs, avoid decongestants with antihistamines.

E. Treatment

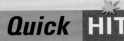

1. Acute purulent sinusitis
   a. General measures/advice for the patient
      - Saline nasal spray aids drainage
      - Avoid smoke and other environmental pollutants

   b. Decongestants (pseudoephedrine or oxymetazoline)
      - **Facilitate sinus drainage** and relieve congestion
      - Available in both topical and systemic preparations
      - Give for no more than 3 to 5 days

   c. Antibiotics
      - Amoxicillin, amoxicillin-clavulanate, TMP/SMX, levofloxacin, moxifloxacin, and cefuroxime are good choices.

   d. Antihistamines
      - Reserve for patients with allergies; use discriminately because of the "drying effect"
      - Loratadine (Claritin), fexofenadine (Allegra), chlorpheniramine (Chlor-Trimeton)

   e. Nasal steroids (fluticasone, beclomethasone)—may be worth a trial if sinusitis is secondary to allergic rhinitis or if there is concurrent allergic rhinitis
2. Chronic sinusitis
   a. Treat with a broad-spectrum penicillinase-resistant antibiotic
   b. Refer to an otolaryngologist—endoscopic drainage may be necessary

●●● Laryngitis

- Usually viral in origin; may also be caused by *Moraxella catarrhalis* and *H. influenzae*
- Common cause of hoarseness; cough may be present along with other URI symptoms
- Typically self-limiting
- Patient should rest voice until laryngitis resolves to avoid formation of vocal nodules

●●● Sore Throat

Quick HIT

Think of the following if a patient has a sore throat:
- Viral infection
- Tonsillitis (usually bacterial)
- **Strep throat**
- Mononucleosis

Quick HIT

Only 50% of patients with pharyngeal exudates have strep throat, and only 50% of patients with strep throat have exudates.

A. General characteristics

1. Causes of sore throat
   a. Viruses are by far the most common cause (adenovirus, parainfluenza and rhinovirus, Epstein–Barr virus, herpes simplex)
   b. **The main concern is infection with group A β-hemolytic streptococcus due to the possibility of rheumatic fever**
   c. Other organisms
      - Chlamydia, mycoplasma
      - Gonococci (oral sex)
      - *Corynebacterium diphtheriae*—pseudomembrane covering pharynx
      - *Candida albicans* (if immunosuppressed, on antibiotics, or severely ill)
2. Viral versus bacterial infection—often difficult to distinguish, but if patient has a cough and runny nose, virus is more likely

B. Diagnosis

1. Throat culture—takes 24 hours, but is more accurate than rapid strep test
2. Rapid strep test—results within 1 hour, but will not indicate whether sore throat is caused by a bacterium other than *Streptococcus* or a virus
   a. Centor criteria: helps predict the likelihood of Strep throat and the appropriate management
      - One point each for history of fever, tonsillar exudates, tender anterior cervical lymphadenopathy, absence of cough, age <15; age >44 subtracts one point
      - -1, 0, or 1 point: No antibiotic, no throat culture
      - 2 or 3 points: Throat culture, treat with antibiotic if throat culture is positive
      - 4 or 5 points: Treat empirically with an antibiotic
3. If mononucleosis is suspected, obtain the appropriate blood tests (Monospot)

Ambulatory Medicine

C. Treatment

1. If strep throat—penicillin for 10 days (erythromycin if patient has penicillin allergy)
2. If viral—symptomatic treatment (see below)
3. If mononucleosis—advise rest and acetaminophen/ibuprofen for symptoms; avoid contact sports since there is splenomegaly and a risk of splenic rupture
4. Symptomatic treatment of sore throat
   a. Acetaminophen or ibuprofen
   b. Gargling with warm salt water
   c. Use of a humidifier
   d. Sucking on throat lozenges, hard candy, flavored frozen desserts (such as Popsicles)

Quick HIT

Most cases (up to 90%) of dyspepsia/heartburn are due to PUD, GERD, gastritis, or nonulcer dyspepsia.

Gastrointestinal Diseases

Dyspepsia

A. General characteristics

1. "Dyspepsia" refers to a spectrum of epigastric symptoms, including heartburn, "indigestion," bloating, and epigastric pain/discomfort.
2. Dyspepsia is extremely common, and sometimes is confused with angina.
3. Etiology
   a. GI causes—**peptic ulcer disease (PUD)**, **GERD**, **nonulcer dyspepsia (functional dyspepsia)**, **gastritis**, hepatobiliary disease (cholecystitis, biliary colic), malignancy (gastric, esophageal), pancreatic disease (pancreatitis, pseudocyst, cancer), esophageal spasm, hiatal hernia.
   b. Other causes include lactose intolerance, malabsorption, DM (gastroparesis), and irritable bowel syndrome (IBS).

Quick HIT

Nonulcer dyspepsia
- A diagnosis of exclusion after appropriate tests (including endoscopy) does not reveal a specific cause.
- Dyspepsia symptoms must be present for at least 4 weeks to make the diagnosis of nonulcer dyspepsia.

B. Diagnosis

1. Base the decision to perform tests on clinical presentation and response to empiric therapy.
2. **Endoscopy** is the test of choice for evaluation of dyspepsia.
   a. It can identify an esophageal stricture or ulcer, cancer, and reflux esophagitis.
   b. It should **not** be routinely performed in all patients with dyspepsia. Some general indications include:
      - Patients with alarming symptoms—weight loss, anemia, dysphagia, or obstructive symptoms.
      - Patients >55 years of age with new-onset dyspepsia.
      - Patients with recurrent vomiting or any evidence of upper GI bleeding.
      - Patients who do not respond to empiric therapy (see below).
      - Patients with signs of complications of PUD.
      - Patients with recurrent symptoms.
      - Patients with evidence of systemic illness.
3. Noninvasive testing for *Helicobacter pylori:* an option if the patient does not require an EGD.
   a. Urea breath test: detects active infection.
   b. Serology: cannot reliably determine active infection (antibodies may persist after *H. pylori* is cleared).
   c. Stool antigen test: detects active infection.
   d. Results
      - If positive, treat empirically for *H. pylori.*
      - If negative, PUD is unlikely and the patient likely has either GERD or nonulcer dyspepsia (treat empirically—see below).

C. Treatment

1. Treat the cause if known

Quick HIT

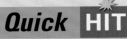

If GERD is associated with dysphagia, this suggests the development of **peptic stricture.** Alternatively, a motility disorder or cancer may be present.

Quick HIT

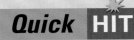

Diagnostic tests are usually not necessary for typical, uncomplicated cases of GERD, and therapy can be initiated. Tests are indicated in atypical, complicated, or persistent cases (despite treatment). Endoscopy should be performed if worrisome symptoms (anemia, weight loss, or dysphagia) are present.

Quick HIT

GERD is a chronic disorder. Regular follow-up is recommended to identify any complications (e.g., Barrett esophagus, stricture, esophagitis).

2. Advise the patient to:
   a. Avoid alcohol, caffeine, and other foods that irritate the stomach
   b. Stop smoking
   c. Raise the head of the bed when sleeping
   d. Avoid eating before sleeping
3. Use a proton pump inhibitor (PPI) trial for 8 weeks. Endoscopy is indicated if this fails to relieve symptoms
4. Eradication of *H. pylori* infection—See Chapter 3

Gastroesophageal Reflux Disease

A. General characteristics

1. GERD is a multifactorial problem. Inappropriate relaxation of the LES (**decreased LES tone**) is the primary mechanism, leading to retrograde flow of stomach contents into the esophagus. Other factors that may contribute include:
   a. Decreased esophageal motility to clear refluxed fluid
   b. A gastric outlet obstruction
   c. **A hiatal hernia (common finding in patients with GERD)**
   d. Dietary factors (e.g., alcohol, tobacco, chocolate, high-fat foods, coffee)—may decrease LES pressure and exacerbate the condition
2. GERD is a very common condition. Its prevalence increases with age

B. Clinical features

1. **Heartburn, dyspepsia**
   a. Retrosternal pain/burning shortly after eating (especially after large meals)
   b. Exacerbated by lying down after meals
   c. **May mimic cardiac chest pain** (which may lead to unnecessary workup for ischemic heart disease)
2. Regurgitation
3. Waterbrash—reflex salivary hypersecretion
4. Cough—due to either aspiration of refluxed material or a reflex triggered by acid reflux into the lower esophagus
5. Hoarseness, sore throat, feeling a lump in the throat
6. Early satiety, postprandial nausea/vomiting

C. Diagnosis

1. **Endoscopy with biopsy**—the test of choice but not necessary for typical uncomplicated cases.
   a. Indicated if heartburn is refractory to treatment, or is accompanied by dysphagia, odynophagia, or GI bleeding.
   b. A biopsy should also be performed to assess changes in esophageal mucosa.
2. Upper GI series (barium contrast study)—this is only helpful in identifying complications of GERD (strictures/ulcerations), but cannot diagnose GERD itself.
3. Twenty-four–hour pH monitoring in the lower esophagus—this is the most sensitive and specific test for GERD. It is the gold standard, but is usually unnecessary.
4. Esophageal manometry—use if a motility disorder is suspected.

D. Complications

1. Erosive esophagitis—These patients are at high risk of developing complications such as stricture, ulcer, or Barrett esophagus. These patients are candidates for long-term PPI therapy (see below).
2. Peptic stricture
   a. Consists of fibrotic rings that narrow the lumen and obstruct the passage of food
   b. Presents with dysphagia; may mimic esophageal cancer
   c. EGD can confirm the diagnosis. Dilation should be performed
3. Esophageal ulcer—possible cause of upper GI bleeding
4. Barrett esophagus—occurs in 10% of patients with chronic reflux
   a. The normal, stratified, squamous epithelium of the distal esophagus is replaced by columnar epithelium. Dysplastic changes may occur, with risk of adenocarcinoma

b. Patients who have had symptomatic GERD for at least 5 years (and can undergo surgery if cancer is found) should be screened for the possibility of Barrett esophagus
c. Endoscopy with biopsy is required. If the patient has documented Barrett esophagus without any dysplastic changes, periodic surveillance is appropriate (every 3 years)
d. Medical treatment—long-term PPIs

5. Recurrent pneumonia (due to recurrent pulmonary aspiration)—The cytologic aspirate finding on bronchoscopy that can diagnose aspiration of gastric contents is **lipid-laden macrophages** (from phagocytosis of fat)
6. Pitting of dental enamel (dental erosion); gingivitis
7. Laryngitis, pharyngitis

E. Treatment

1. Initial treatment:
   a. Behavior modification—diet (avoid fatty foods, coffee, alcohol, orange juice, chocolate; avoid large meals before bedtime); sleep with trunk of body elevated; stop smoking
   b. Antacids—after meals and at bedtime
2. Add an H_2 blocker—can be used instead of or in addition to antacids for mild and intermittent symptoms
3. If above treatment fails or patient has severe GERD (e.g., erosive esophagitis), switch to a PPI
4. Antireflux surgery for severe or resistant cases
   a. Indications for surgery
      - Intractability (failure of medical treatment)
      - Respiratory problems due to reflux and aspiration of gastric contents
      - Severe esophageal injury (ulcer, hemorrhage, stricture, Barrett esophagus)
   b. Types of surgery
      - Nissen fundoplication (may be done open or laparoscopically)—procedure of choice for a patient with normal esophageal motility
      - Partial fundoplication—when esophageal motility is poor
   c. Outcome of surgery—excellent results have been reported

Diarrhea

A. General characteristics

1. Most cases of diarrhea are acute, benign, and self-limited (see also Clinical Pearl 12-4). Some cases are chronic and may be associated with underlying disease.
2. Acute diarrhea is diarrhea that lasts less than 2 to 3 weeks; chronic diarrhea lasts more than 4 weeks.
3. Most common cause of acute diarrhea is viral infection (rotavirus and the Norwalk virus are the most common). Most severe forms of acute diarrhea are due to bacterial infections (*Shigella, Escherichia coli, Salmonella, Campylobacter, Clostridium*

CLINICAL PEARL 12-4

Diarrhea Pearls

- Acute diarrhea is usually due to infection (virus, bacteria, and parasite) or medications.
- If nausea and vomiting are present, suspect viral gastroenteritis or food poisoning.
- If food poisoning is the cause, diarrhea appears within hours of the meal.
- Remember that occult blood in the stool **may** be present in all types of acute infectious diarrhea, but it is much less common to have gross blood.
- A finding of fever and blood together is typical of infection with *Shigella, Campylobacter, Salmonella* (may also be without blood), enterohemorrhagic *E. coli.*
- No fever and no blood is typical of infection with viruses (rotavirus, Norwalk virus), enterotoxic *E. coli,* and food poisoning (*S. aureus, C. perfringens*).

perfringens, Clostridium difficile). Protozoa that may cause diarrhea include *Giardia lamblia, Entamoeba histolytica,* and *Cryptosporidium*.

4. Elderly and immunocompromised patients (e.g., with HIV, transplantation patients) are vulnerable to diarrheal illnesses due to impaired immunity. In patients with HIV, diarrhea can be caused by *Mycobacterium avium-intracellulare, Cryptosporidium, Cyclospora,* or CMV.

B. Causes

1. Acute diarrhea
    a. **Infection**—viruses most common (viral gastroenteritis), followed by bacteria, then parasites
    b. **Medications**
        - Antibiotics (most common cause)—antibiotic-associated diarrhea is caused by *C. difficile* toxin in 25% of cases (see Chapter 3)
        - Others include laxatives, prokinetic agents (cisapride), antacids, digitalis, colchicine, antibiotics, alcohol, magnesium-containing antacids, and chemotherapeutic agents
    c. Malabsorption (e.g., lactose intolerance)
    d. Ischemic bowel in elderly patients with history of PAD and bloody diarrhea, along with abdominal pain
    e. Intestinal tumors (very rare)
2. Chronic diarrhea
    a. IBS (most common cause, but is a diagnosis of exclusion)
    b. Inflammatory bowel disease (IBD)
    c. Medications—see above
    d. Infection—see above, bacterial enterocolitis (*Shigella, Salmonella, Campylobacter,* enteroinvasive *E. coli*)
    e. Colon cancer
    f. Diverticulitis
    g. Malabsorption syndromes—pancreatic insufficiency, celiac disease, short bowel syndrome, ischemic bowel, bacterial overgrowth
    h. Postsurgical (e.g., gastrectomy, vagotomy)
    i. Endocrine causes (hyperthyroidism, Addison disease, diabetes, gastrinoma, VIPoma)
    j. Fecal impaction—because only liquid stool can pass around the impaction
    k. Laxative abuse (factitious diarrhea)
    l. Immunocompromised patients with acute infectious diarrhea

C. Diagnosis

1. Laboratory tests are usually unnecessary in acute diarrhea (see also Clinical Pearl 12-5 and Figure 12-3)
2. Some indications for diagnostic studies
    a. Chronic diarrhea or diarrhea that is prolonged
    b. Severe illness or high fever
    c. Presence of blood in the stool/high suspicion for IBD

CLINICAL PEARL 12-5

Important Parts of the History in a Patient With Diarrhea

- Is the stool bloody or melanotic?
- Are there any other symptoms (e.g., fever, abdominal pain, vomiting)?
- Is there anyone in the family or group with a similar illness?
- Has there been any recent travel outside the United States, or any hiking trips? (parasitic infections)
- Are symptoms linked to ingestion of certain foods (e.g., milk)?
- Are there any medical problems (e.g., AIDS, hyperthyroidism)?
- Have there been recent changes in medications (e.g., antibiotics within the past few weeks)?

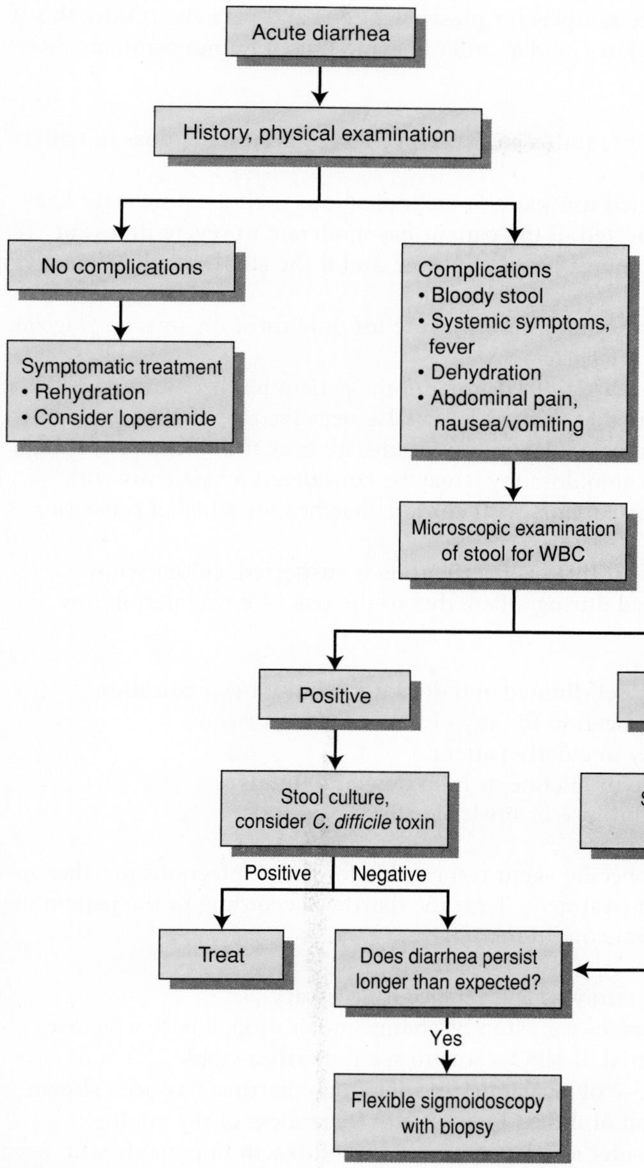

FIGURE 12-3 Approach to the patient with acute diarrhea.
(Adapted from Humes DH, Dont HL, Gardner LB, et al. *Kelley's Textbook of Internal Medicine.* 4th ed. Philadelphia, PA: Lippincott Williams & Wilkins, 2000:748, Figure 99.1.)

d. Severe abdominal pain
e. Immunodeficiency
f. Signs of volume depletion

3. Laboratory tests to order
   a. CBC—look for anemia, WBC elevation
   b. Stool sample—for presence of fecal leukocytes
      - If fecal leukocytes are absent, there is no need to order stool cultures because they are unlikely to grow pathogenic organisms (unless invasive bacterial enteritis is suspected or the patient has bloody diarrhea)
      - If fecal leukocytes are present and the patient has moderate to severe diarrhea, consider sending stool for culture and/or *C. difficile* toxin assay, and consider empiric treatment with an antibiotic
      - Fecal leukocytes are present in *Campylobacter, Salmonella, Shigella,* enteroinvasive *E. coli* infection, and *C. difficile;* absent in staphylococcal or clostridial food poisoning; and absent in viral gastroenteritis

Quick HIT

Assess volume status (dehydration is a concern), perform an abdominal examination, and check stool for occult blood in patients with diarrhea. In mild to moderate cases of acute diarrhea, further workup is unnecessary.

Quick HIT

Laboratory tests to consider:
- Stool WBCs
- Stool for ova and parasites
- Stool culture
- Stool for *C. difficile* culture
- Stool for *C. difficile* toxin assay
- Stool for *Giardia* antigen

Quick HIT

Salmonella, Campylobacter, Shigella, and enteroinvasive *E. coli* cause diarrhea with fecal leukocytes and often blood.

Quick HIT

The most common electrolyte/acid–base abnormality seen with severe diarrhea is **metabolic acidosis** and **hypokalemia.**

c. Stool sample—test three samples for presence of ova and parasites. Order this if a parasite is suspected. For *Giardia,* order enzyme-linked immunosorbent assay test for antigen

d. Bacterial stool culture
   - This has low sensitivity (and is an expensive test), and usually does not affect treatment or outcome
   - It should not be ordered routinely. Some indications include: if invasive bacterial enteritis is suspected, if the patient has moderate to severe illness or fever, if the patient requires hospitalization, and if the stool sample is positive for fecal leukocytes
   - Most laboratory tests examine stool culture for only three organisms: *Shigella, Salmonella,* and *Campylobacter*

e. Stool sample—Measure for *C. difficile* toxin if the patient has been treated with antibiotics recently. Note that this test has a false-negative rate of 10%. Treat the patient empirically even before laboratory results are back if the suspicion is high

f. Colonoscopy/flexible sigmoidoscopy—may be considered for patients with blood in the stool or for patients with chronic diarrhea for which a cause cannot be identified

g. CT scan may be helpful if IBD or diverticulitis is suspected; colonoscopy should not be performed during a flare due to the risk of bowel perforation

D. Treatment

1. Acute diarrhea is typically self-limited and does not require hospitalization. However, consider hospitalization for any of the following reasons:
   a. Dehydration (especially in elderly patients)
   b. Patients initially unable to tolerate or hold down PO fluids
   c. Bloody diarrhea (with profuse or brisk bleeding)
   d. High fever, toxic appearance
2. The identification of the specific agent responsible for acute infectious diarrhea is not critical with regard to treatment. Treat the diarrhea according to the patient's medical history and clinical condition
3. Specific therapy
   a. Rehydrate; monitor electrolytes and replace if necessary
   b. Treat the underlying cause (e.g., stop or change medication, advise a lactose-free diet). Consider a trial of NPO status to see if diarrhea stops
   c. Consider antibiotics. Use of antibiotics in **infectious** diarrhea has been shown to decrease the duration of illness by 24 hours (regardless of the etiologic agent). Therefore, consider a 5-day course of ciprofloxacin in patients who have moderate to severe disease. Antibiotics are definitely recommended in the following situations:
      - Patient has high fever, bloody stools, or severe diarrhea—quinolones are appropriate
      - Stool culture grows one of the pathogenic organisms (see Table 12-6)
      - Patient has traveler's diarrhea
      - *C. difficile* infection—metronidazole
4. Loperamide (Imodium) is an antidiarrheal agent that should only be given if diarrhea is mild to moderate and is not recommended in patients with fever or with blood in their stool

Constipation

A. Causes

1. Diet—lack of fiber
2. Medications—anticholinergic drugs (antipsychotics), antidepressants, **narcotic analgesics,** iron, calcium channel blockers, aluminum- or calcium-containing antacids, laxative abuse and dependence
3. IBS
4. Obstruction—colorectal cancer (CRC) (always keep this in mind!), anal stricture, hemorrhoids, anal fissure

TABLE 12-6 Common Pathogens Responsible for Acute Infectious Diarrhea

Pathogen	Symptoms	Fever?	Fecal Leukocytes	Duration of Illness	Transmission	Comments
Acute viral gastroenteritis (rotavirus, Norwalk virus)	**Myalgias, malaise,** headache, watery diarrhea, abdominal pain, **nausea/vomiting**	Possible, low-grade	No	48–72 hrs, symptoms may linger for up to 1 wk	Fecal–oral route	Most common cause of acute diarrhea in the United States Look for similar illness in family members
Salmonella	Abdominal pain, diarrhea, nausea, and vomiting	Possible	Yes	Resolves within 1 wk (rarely longer)	Food (domestic fowl and their eggs—most common); fecal–oral route as well	Symptoms appear 24–48 hrs after ingesting food. No treatment is required except in immunocompromised patients or in cases of enteric fever (caused by *Salmonella typhi*)—rare in the United States. Ciprofloxacin (Cipro) is the preferred agent
Shigella	Diarrhea, abdominal pain, **tenesmus;** nausea, vomiting less common	Possible	Yes	Resolves within 1 wk (4–5 days)	Fecal–oral route more common than food	Treat with a fluoroquinolone
Staphylococcus food poisoning	Abdominal pain, nausea and vomiting, diarrhea	No	No	**Within 24 hrs**	Food (e.g., ham, poultry, potato salad, any food containing mayonnaise)	Exposed people become ill **within 1–6 hrs** (e.g., after a picnic). Can be quite severe and may require hospitalization
Campylobacter jejuni	Headache, fatigue followed by diarrhea and abdominal pain	Yes	Yes	Less than 1 wk	Food (e.g., contaminated meat, especially poultry), animals (e.g., puppies, kittens)	Most common cause of acute bacterial diarrhea. Can be severe: blood appears in stool in 50% of cases. Treat with fluoroquinolone or azithromycin. Relapses may occur
C. perfringens	Diarrhea; **crampy abdominal pain is prominent;** vomiting and fever are rare	No	No	Within 24 hrs	Food (poultry, gravy)	Illness begins soon after ingesting food (within 12–24 hrs)
Enterotoxic *E. coli* ("travelers' diarrhea")	Watery diarrhea, nausea, abdominal pain	No	No	Few days	Contaminated food and water	Self-limiting disease is common in developing countries.
E. coli 0157:H7	Bloody diarrhea; patient can appear very sick	Yes	Yes		Food (undercooked meat, raw milk)	Hemorrhagic colitis that is usually self-limited, but has been associated with hemolytic-uremic syndrome (HUS) and thrombotic thrombocytopenic purpura (TTP); supportive treatment, do not give antibiotics (induces the release of Shiga toxin, increasing the risk of HUS/TTP)
Giardiasis	Watery, foul-smelling diarrhea; abdominal bloating	No	No	5–7 days, sometimes longer	Fecal–oral route, food, or contaminated water	Treat with metronidazole; can become chronic
Vibrio cholerae	Voluminous diarrhea ("rice water" stools), abdominal pain, vomiting	Low-grade	No			Rare in the United States, but common in developing countries

5. Ileus, pseudo-obstruction
6. Anorectal problems—hemorrhoids, fissures
7. Endocrine/metabolic causes—hypothyroidism, hypercalcemia, hypokalemia, uremia, dehydration
8. Neuromuscular disorders—Parkinson disease, multiple sclerosis, CNS lesions, scleroderma, DM (autonomic neuropathy)
9. Congenital disorders—Hirschsprung disease

Quick HIT

Complications of Chronic Constipation
- Hemorrhoids
- Rectal prolapse
- Anal fissures
- Fecal impaction

B. Diagnosis

1. Laboratory tests that **may** be necessary include TSH, serum calcium levels, CBC (if colon cancer is suspected), and electrolytes (if obstruction is suspected).
2. Always attempt to rule out obstruction.
   a. If H&P is suggestive of obstruction, order abdominal films.
   b. Consider flexible sigmoidoscopy in select cases (if an obstructing colorectal mass is suspected).
3. A rectal examination may help identify fissures, hemorrhoids, fecal impaction, or masses.
4. If no cause is found after the above measures, and conservative treatment does not help, more specialized tests are available—for example, radiopaque marker transit study, anorectal motility study.

C. Treatment

1. Diet and behavioral modification are the most important aspects of treatment. Advise the patient to:
   a. Increase physical activity.
   b. Eat high-fiber foods.
   c. Increase fluid intake.
2. Bulk laxatives are preferred over osmotic laxatives in patients that do not respond to diet and lifestyle changes.
3. Use an enema, such as a disposable Fleet enema, for temporary relief if no bowel movement occurs despite the above measures or if the patient is bedridden.
4. If obstruction is present, urgent surgery consultation is indicated.

Irritable Bowel Syndrome

A. General characteristics

1. IBS refers to an idiopathic disorder associated with an intrinsic bowel motility dysfunction (abnormal resting activity of GI tract) that affects 10% to 15% of all adults.
2. Common associated findings include depression, anxiety, and somatization. Psychiatric symptoms often precede bowel symptoms. **Symptoms are exacerbated by stress and irritants in the intestinal lumen.**
3. All laboratory test results are normal, and no mucosal lesions are found on sigmoidoscopy. IBS is a benign condition and has a favorable long-term prognosis.
4. Symptoms should be present for **at least 3 months** to diagnose IBS.

Quick HIT

Differential Diagnosis of IBS
Colon cancer, IBD, drugs, mesenteric ischemia, celiac disease, ischemic colitis, giardiasis, pseudo-obstruction, depression, somatization, intermittent sigmoid volvulus, megacolon, bacterial overgrowth syndrome, endometriosis.

B. Clinical features

1. Change in frequency/consistency of stool—diarrhea, constipation (or alternating diarrhea and constipation)
2. Cramping abdominal pain (relieved by defecation)—location varies widely, but sigmoid colon is the common location of pain
3. Bloating or feeling of abdominal distention

C. Diagnosis

1. This is a clinical diagnosis, and a diagnosis of exclusion.
2. Rome III diagnostic criteria: recurrent abdominal pain/discomfort ≥3 days per month in the last 3 months, and ≥2 of the following:
   a. Pain/discomfort improves with defecation.
   b. Symptom onset is associated with a change in the frequency of the stool.
   c. Symptom onset is associated with a change in the form of the stool.

3. Initial tests that may help exclude other causes include CBC, renal panel, fecal occult blood test, stool examination for ova and parasites, erythrocyte sedimentation rate, and possibly a flexible sigmoidoscopy. Order these tests only if there is suspicion of other causes for the symptoms.

D. Treatment

1. For mild symptoms, diet and lifestyle changes (e.g., avoiding dairy products, excess caffeine). Manage the symptoms below as indicated:
   a. Diarrhea—diphenoxylate, loperamide.
   b. Constipation—colace, psyllium, cisapride.
   c. Abdominal pain—antispasmodics (e.g., pinaverium, trimebutine, peppermint oil, cimetropium/dicyclomine), antidepressants, rifaximin.

Quick HIT

The following must be frequently excluded in diagnosing IBS:
- Obstruction (plain abdominal film)
- IBD
- Lactose or sorbitol intolerance
- Malignancy (in older patients or those with family history)—colonoscopy, occult blood in stool

Nausea and Vomiting

A. General characteristics

1. The most common causes are viral gastroenteritis and food poisoning. However, other more emergent diseases must be kept in mind.
2. Many conditions present with other prominent symptoms (e.g., abdominal pain, diarrhea, fever) in addition to nausea/vomiting.

Quick HIT

Gastroenteritis
- Typically caused by an enterovirus, and is seen in groups among family members, colleagues, and so on.
- Diarrhea is often present as well, but may appear later.

B. Causes

C. Approach

1. Questions to ask when taking the history: Ask about recent food intake (Unusual foods? Time of onset of vomiting in relation to food intake? Did anyone else eat that food?) (Clinical Pearl 12-6). Are symptoms related to meals? Ask about medications and recent changes/additions. Is there a history of abdominal surgery (obstruction) or recent surgery? Are there family members with similar illness?
2. Define the vomitus
   a. Bilious—obstruction is distal to ampulla of Vater
   b. Feculent—distal intestinal obstruction, bacterial overgrowth, gastrocolic fistula
   c. Vomiting of undigested food—esophageal problem more likely (achalasia, stricture, diverticulum)
   d. Projectile vomiting—increased intracranial pressure or pyloric stenosis
   e. Coffee-ground material or blood—GI bleeding
3. Accompanying symptoms
   a. Diarrhea and fever point to an infectious process (gastroenteritis)
   b. Abdominal pain points to obstruction, acute inflammatory conditions (e.g., peritonitis, cholecystitis)
   c. Headache, visual disturbances, and other neurologic findings point to increased intracranial or intraocular pressure (IOP).

CLINICAL PEARL 12-6

Causes of Acute Nausea/Vomiting

- Pregnancy (normal pregnancy, hyperemesis gravidarum)
- Metabolic: diabetic ketoacidosis, Addison disease, uremia, electrolyte disturbance (hypercalcemia, hypokalemia), hyperthyroidism
- GI: gastroenteritis (viral, food poisoning), PUD, GERD, gastroparesis (diabetics), gastric outlet obstruction, intestinal obstruction (SBO, pseudo-obstruction), ileus, peritonitis
- Acute visceral conditions: pancreatitis, appendicitis, pyelonephritis, cholecystitis, cholangitis
- Neurologic: increased intracranial pressure, vestibular disturbance (vertigo), migraine
- Acute MI
- Drugs: chemo, digoxin, ASA/NSAIDs, narcotics, antibiotics, excessive alcohol intake
- Psychiatric: eating disorder (bulimia nervosa, anorexia nervosa), anxiety
- Miscellaneous: motion sickness, systemic illness, radiation therapy, postoperatively

Quick HIT

Possible Complications of Severe or Prolonged Vomiting
- Fluid/electrolytes—dehydration, metabolic alkalosis, hypokalemia
- Dental caries
- Aspiration pneumonitis
- GI: Mallory–Weiss tears, Boerhaave syndrome, Mallory–Weiss syndrome

Quick HIT

The most common electrolyte abnormality seen after severe vomiting is **hypokalemia with metabolic alkalosis.**

D. Diagnosis

1. Order routine laboratory tests such as CBC, electrolytes, glucose levels, LFTs, if appropriate, based on history and examination findings.
2. Order a pregnancy test in women of child-bearing age.
3. Abdominal films—Order upright and supine films in patients with acute vomiting if obstruction or perforation is suspected.
4. Order other diagnostic tests depending on clinical findings (e.g., upper GI endoscopy for ulcer disease or outlet obstruction, ultrasound for biliary disease, CT scan of head for neurologic findings).
5. In at least 50% of patients, the above tests do not reveal a cause. Special tests for GI motility may be indicated if there is suspicion of a motility disorder.

E. Treatment

1. Most causes are self-limiting. If vomiting is severe it may cause dehydration, requiring hospitalization.
2. Assess hydration status—Fluid replacement is the first step in management, NS is used in most cases (but type of fluid and electrolyte repletion based on laboratory findings).
3. Identify and treat the underlying cause if possible.
4. Medications—Choice of drug depends on the suspected cause (e.g., promethazine for hyperemesis gravidarum),
   a. Prochlorperazine, promethazine, metoclopramide, ondansetron (especially with chemotherapy), erythromycin (prokinetic).

Hemorrhoids

A. General characteristics

1. Varicose veins of anus and rectum
2. Two types
   a. External hemorrhoids—dilated veins arising from inferior hemorrhoidal plexus; distal to dentate line (sensate area)
   b. Internal hemorrhoids—dilated submucosal veins of superior rectal plexus; above dentate line (insensate area)

B. Risk factors

1. Constipation/straining
2. Pregnancy
3. Portal HTN
4. Obesity
5. Prolonged sitting (especially truck drivers and pilots) or prolonged standing
6. Anal intercourse

C. Clinical features

1. Bleeding and rectal prolapse (main symptoms)
   a. Bright red blood per rectum
   b. This is usually harmless, but look for iron deficiency anemia (rare). Occult rectal bleeding should prompt an investigation into more serious causes and should never be attributed to hemorrhoids until other conditions are ruled out
   c. Bleeding is usually painless
2. External hemorrhoids are usually asymptomatic unless thrombosed, in which case they present as sudden painful swelling (may ulcerate, bleed). Pain lasts for several days, and then gradually subsides. The response to surgery is rapid
3. Internal hemorrhoids usually do not cause pain. A mass is present when they prolapse

D. Treatment

1. General measures to ease symptoms
   a. Sitz bath
   b. Application of ice packs to anal area and bed rest

c. Stool softeners to reduce strain
d. High-fiber, high-fluid diet
e. Topical steroids
2. Rubber band ligation for internal hemorrhoids—rubber bands applied to hemorrhoidal bundle(s) leads to necrosis and sloughing of lesion
3. Surgical (hemorrhoidectomy)—Perform surgery if the condition does not respond to conservative methods, or if severe prolapse, strangulation, very large anal tags, or fissure is present. Surgery can be performed in an ambulatory setting

MUSCULOSKELETAL PROBLEMS

Overview of Musculoskeletal Examination Maneuvers

Low Back Pain

A. General Characteristics

1. Second most common reason for medical office visits in the United States (Table 12-7).
2. Acute low back pain (LBP) refers to symptoms present for less than 4 weeks, subacute is 4 to 12 weeks, and chronic LBP refers to pain lasting more than 12 weeks. The natural history of acute and subacute LBP is very favorable. Management of chronic back pain is very challenging.
3. Risk factors for chronic LBP: smoking, obesity, older age, sedentary work, physically strenuous work, psychologically strenuous work, low educational attainment, worker's compensation insurance, job dissatisfaction, psychological factors (depression, anxiety, etc.)
4. Majority of patients present with "nonspecific" or mechanical back pain, meaning there is no significant underlying cause such as neoplasm or infection or spine pathology.
5. If patient has significant radicular leg pain, nerve compression is likely. If leg symptoms are severe, or if objective weakness is present, an MRI of lumbar spine is obtained. An MRI is unnecessary in most patients who present with an acute episode of pain.

B. Causes

1. There are many causes of LBP. Most patients who present with back pain do not have a specific spine pathology, which is referred to as "nonspecific" LBP.
2. The following conditions can all cause LBP. Note that many patients with these imaging findings do not have back pain. Therefore, imaging findings do not necessarily correlate with symptoms. For example, many patients with degenerative disc disease or spondylolisthesis have no back pain.
   a. Degenerative disc disease (osteoarthritis)—many people with severe degenerative disc disease do not have back pain. Surgery is controversial for this indication.
   b. Spondylolisthesis—forward slippage of cephalad vertebra on the caudal vertebra. Most common at L4-L5 and L5-S1. Spinal stenosis often coexists, leading to neurogenic claudication.
   c. Lumbar disc herniation—radicular leg pain (commonly referred to as sciatica) is the predominant finding, although some patients have back pain as well. Back pain without any radicular pain is uncommon but can occur. Most common at L4-L5 and L5-S1. Treatment is anti-inflammatory medication, physical therapy, and epidural steroid injections. Surgery indicated when conservative treatment fails or if patient has progressive neurologic deficit.
   d. Spinal stenosis—narrowing of spinal canal due to degenerative changes which causes neurogenic claudication. Back pain may coexist, but predominant finding is neurogenic claudication.

Quick HIT

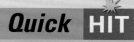

Most Common Causes of LBP
- Musculoligamentous strain
- Degenerative disc disease
- Facet arthritis

Quick HIT

Factors that Exacerbate Pain in Disc Herniation
- Maneuvers that increase intraspinal pressure, such as coughing or sneezing
- Forward flexion—sitting, driving, or lifting; worsens leg pain

Quick HIT

Majority of patients with lumbar disc herniation and sciatica improve with conservative care. Only about 10% will require surgical intervention.

Quick HIT

Patients with spinal stenosis have leg pain on back extension—pain worsens with standing or walking (relief with bending or sitting).

Quick HIT

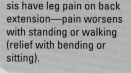

Pathology in other organ systems cause back pain and should be ruled out:
- Vascular disease (aortic aneurysm, aortic dissection)
- Pancreatic disease
- Urologic disease (prostate infection, renal calculi)
- Gynecologic/obstetric disease (endometriosis, ectopic pregnancy, pelvic inflammatory disease)

TABLE 12-7 Important Musculoskeletal Physical Examination Maneuvers

General	
Important aspects include observation (asymmetry, atrophy, etc.), palpation of important landmarks (joint line, surrounding muscles and tendons, etc.), active and passive range of motion, assessment of muscle strength, and special testing (below) when a diagnosis is suspected.	
Neck	
Spurling maneuver	• Technique: patient asked to extend neck, rotate and tilt to side of pain • High specificity but low sensitivity for cervical root compression, which is suggested by reproduction of the pain below the shoulder joint (radicular pain)
Shoulder	
Empty can test	• Technique: arms held out in front of the patient parallel to the ground with thumbs pointed downward. Resistance is applied by the examiner and the patient tries to maintain the position • Pain with resistance may indicate a supraspinatus defect
External rotation	• Technique: arm is held at patient's side with elbow flexed at 90 degrees. Patient is asked to externally rotate the forearm against resistance. • Pain with resistance may indicate an infraspinatus defect.
Lift-off test	• Technique: patient's hand is placed behind their back with the dorsum of the hand against the back. They are asked to lift their hand off their back. • An inability to bring their hand off their back indicates a defect in internal rotation, which may indicate a subscapularis defect.
Neer test	• Technique: the patient's arm is fully pronated (thumb pointed downward) and forcibly flexed above their head. • Pain with this maneuver may indicate rotator cuff impingement.
Hawkins test	• Technique: patient's arm is abducted to 90 degrees with the elbow bent (as if holding the arm out to catch a *hawk*), and the examiner internally rotates the shoulder. • Pain with this maneuver may indicate rotator cuff impingement.
Cross-arm test	• Technique: patient's arm is held in front of them to 90 degrees and the patient actively adducts the arm (crosses it in front of them). • Pain at the acromioclavicular (AC) joint indicates AC joint dysfunction (which can be confused with rotator cuff pathology).
Knee	
Varus/valgus stress test	• Technique: examiner stabilizes the knee joint with one hand and uses the other hand to grab the lower leg and apply a lateral force. A varus stress is when the force on the knee is applied toward the body (in a lateral to medial), and a valgus stress is the opposite. • Laxity with a varus stress implies a defect in the lateral collateral ligament (LCL), and laxity with a valgus stress implies a defect in the medial collateral ligament (MCL).
Lachman and anterior drawer	• Technique: the Lachman test is performed with the knee flexed at 30 degrees whereas the anterior drawer is performed with the knee flexed at 90 degrees. In both examinations, the proximal tibia is pulled anteriorly, away from the femur. • Excessive anterior translation of the tibia suggests an anterior cruciate ligament (ACL) tear.
Posterior drawer	• Technique: The patient is placed supine and the knee flexed at 90 degrees. The proximal tibia is pushed posteriorly toward the femur. • Excessive posterior translation of the tibia suggests a posterior cruciate ligament (PCL) tear.
McMurray test	• Technique: the knee is passively flexed by the examiner, then externally rotated with a varus stress as the knee is extended. This is repeated with internal rotation. • A painful click or joint line tenderness suggests a meniscal injury.

- Neurogenic claudication refers to radicular leg or buttock pain that is caused by spinal stenosis. It can manifest as pain, cramping, numbness or paresthesias, particularly worse with walking and relieved with sitting. Forward flexion of spine improves symptoms (patients lean on shopping cart).

- Treat with epidural steroid injections if it is affecting patient's quality of life. Surgery is very effective if conservative treatment fails.

e. Musculoligamentous strain—usually after an episode of bending/twisting, patient feels the back "give way," often when lifting a heavy object, with immediate onset of back pain. Radiation of pain may occur to buttock/upper posterior thigh to knee level—this is called "referred pain" from muscle spasm. Pain typically does not radiate distal to the knee because no nerve root compression is present.

f. Vertebral compression fracture—acute back pain caused by minor stress in elderly or in patients on long-term steroid treatment. Pain is at the level of the fracture with local radiation across the back and around the trunk (rarely into legs).
- Can occur with minimal or no trauma in patients with osteoporosis.
- Multiple compression fractures can lead to severe kyphosis in the thoracic spine.
- Treatment options include bracing (if patient's body habitus allows), analgesics, and giving the fracture time to heal. Most fractures heal in 6 to 8 weeks and symptoms gradually improve. Interventional options include kyphoplasty/vertebroplasty (injection of cement into vertebral body). Recent randomized controlled trials have brought the efficacy of these interventions into question.

g. Neoplasms—most common spinal tumor by far is metastatic carcinoma—common primary neoplasms that metastasize to spine include breast, lung, prostate, kidney, and thyroid.

h. Infection—discitis or osteomyelitis.
- Suspect in patients with history of IV drug use, dialysis, indwelling catheter; most common organism is *S. aureus*.
- Laboratory tests to order include CBC with differential, ESR, and CRP.
- If suspicion is high, MRI should be obtained.
- Epidural abscess in the cervical and thoracic spine can lead to rapid neurologic deterioration and in most cases requires surgical decompression; epidural abscess in the lumbar spine can often be medically managed with antibiotics if there are no neurologic deficits and patient is not septic.

> **Quick HIT**
> Chronic LBP: Imaging findings on MRI do not necessarily correlate with presence or severity of pain. Psychosocial variables are much stronger predictors of pain and disability.

C. Back examination

1. The main goal of the history and physical examination is to rule out any structural or systemic conditions that can be the source of back pain. The neurologic examination is very important, and any weakness should be documented.
2. The straight leg raise can suggest nerve root compression. The test is positive if radiculopathy is reproduced when the leg is elevated 30 to 60 degrees with the patient supine. If patient is in severe pain and cannot tolerate even a slight elevation of the leg during this test, it is highly suggestive of nerve root compression.

> **Quick HIT**
> **Major Segmental Innervation of the Lower Limb**
> - Hip flexion—L2
> - Knee extension—L3
> - Ankle dorsiflexion—L4 and L5
> - Great toe dorsiflexion—L5
> - Ankle plantar flexion—S1

D. Diagnostic tests

1. Imaging is not necessary during the first 4 to 6 weeks in the absence of any of the following—**progressive neurologic deficits or disabling symptoms, osteoporosis or prolonged steroid use, constitutional symptoms (unexplained fever or weight loss), history of malignancy, recent trauma, IV drug use** (see also Clinical Pearl 12-7).
2. MRI is indicated if patient has failed a course of conservative treatment (rest, physical therapy, NSAIDs) for at least 3 months. Patients with neurologic signs or symptoms should have an MRI sooner, depending on the severity and acuteness of clinical findings.

> **Quick HIT**
> In general, radiologic imaging is unnecessary in evaluation of LBP. Imaging is appropriate if symptoms do not resolve within 1 month or if there are neurologic signs/symptoms.

E. Treatment

1. Most patients with acute LBP have improvement or resolution within 3 to 6 weeks and are managed with NSAIDs, acetaminophen, activity modification, and gradual return to activities. Narcotic analgesics and muscle relaxants should be used judiciously if at all. Patients should be advised to continue ordinary activities within the limits permitted by pain. If symptoms do not improve in 4 to 6 weeks, a course of physical therapy for core-strengthening exercises may be helpful.

CLINICAL PEARL 12-7

Cauda Equina Syndrome

- Caused by severe stenosis in the lumbar spine, most commonly due to an acute disc herniation.
- Patients present with severe back or leg pain (uni- or bilateral), with or without weakness in the legs. The key findings are bladder dysfunction (retention, incontinence) and saddle anesthesia (numbness in perineal or buttock region).
- Symptoms can have acute onset, or start with leg pain initially and over the ensuing days progress to weakness and bladder dysfunction.
- This is a surgical emergency. An MRI should be obtained immediately.

Quick HIT

It is helpful to differentiate patients with predominantly LBP from those with predominantly leg pain. When conservative treatment has failed, surgery is often effective for leg pain, but results for LBP are less predictable.

Quick HIT

Management of LBP
Avoid prolonged inactivity (leads to deconditioning).
In the first week, attempt a walking routine (20 minutes, three times per day, interspersed with bed rest).

2. If neurologic deficits present, particularly if these deficits are progressive, a more aggressive approach is indicated. An MRI should be obtained, and if nerve root or spinal cord compression is present, evaluation by a spine specialist is recommended.
3. The treatment of chronic nonspecific LBP is challenging. Most patients with **chronic** LBP with or without radiculopathy are treated conservatively (with physical therapy, NSAIDs, injections).
   a. Physical therapy is focused on core-strengthening exercises and aerobic conditioning.
   b. There is some evidence that massage therapy, chiropractic, and acupuncture may be helpful in the short term, but studies have not been able to show long-lasting benefits.
   c. If conservative measures fail and symptoms persist for at least 1 year, surgery can be considered, depending on findings on imaging studies and degree of disability. In general, outcomes from surgery are more predictable and successful when surgery is done for radiculopathy (to decompress nerve roots) than for LBP per se. Surgery (fusion) for degenerative disc disease and chronic LBP is controversial, and randomized controlled trials have NOT shown significant benefits. A very small percentage of patients may benefit from surgery but careful patient selection is critical and informed consent about expected outcomes is recommended.

Common Disorders of the Cervical Spine

A. General characteristics

1. Spondylosis (osteoarthritis) of the cervical spine is very common and is not necessarily a source of neck pain. Patients with spondylosis of the cervical spine present with axial neck pain, cervical radiculopathy, or cervical myelopathy.
2. Chronic axial neck pain (without radiating arm pain) is common and just like chronic LBP can be difficult to treat. Many of the principles discussed above for nonspecific LBP apply to nonspecific neck pain as well. Surgery is not a good option for patients with neck pain without radicular arm symptoms.
3. The most common cause of acute neck pain is cervical strain which is usually self-limiting and resolves with time. Physical therapy can be helpful if symptoms last longer than 2 to 4 weeks.

B. Cervical radiculopathy

1. Compression of a spinal nerve leads to arm pain, numbness, tingling, or weakness. Most common complaint is unilateral neck pain radiating to the arm in a dermatomal pattern.
2. The most common cause is cervical spondylosis (osteoarthritis) and disc herniation. Differential diagnosis includes shoulder pathology (impingement syndrome, rotator cuff disease), peripheral nerve entrapment (carpal tunnel or cubital tunnel syndrome), thoracic outlet syndrome, zoster, and Pancoast tumor (can present with brachial plexus symptoms).

3. The best test to diagnose nerve root compression is MRI of cervical spine.
4. Most patients can be treated conservatively (NSAIDs, time, physical therapy, epidural injections). Surgery is helpful in patients who do not respond to conservative management or who have significant weakness in one or more muscle groups.
5. It is very unusual for a patient with cervical radiculopathy to progress to myelopathy. It appears that these are two distinct entities.

C. Cervical myelopathy

1. Neurologic dysfunction secondary to spinal cord compression (cervical stenosis) in the cervical spine. Diagnosis made by MRI of cervical spine.
2. Earliest symptom is gait disturbance. Patients feel unsteady when ambulating. Other symptoms include loss of hand dexterity (clumsiness, difficult with buttoning shirts, changes in handwriting), bowel and bladder dysfunction are late findings.
   a. Pain is not a common finding so patients may go undiagnosed until the myelopathy is severe.
3. Patients often start relying on a cane or walker (due to unsteady gait), and if untreated may eventually lose the ability to walk. Frank weakness is a late finding. In its most advanced stage, patients become nonambulatory, without functional use of upper extremities and with loss of bowel and bladder function.
4. Natural history is gradual deterioration. Treatment is surgery to decompress the spinal cord when diagnosis is made. Conservative treatment does not play a role in the treatment of cervical stenosis with myelopathy. Main goal of surgery is to prevent further neurologic worsening which is why it is important to make the diagnosis early. Once the patient loses ability to ambulate, it is unlikely to return even with surgery.

Quick HIT

Shoulder impingement syndrome is often confused with cervical radiculopathy involving the C5 nerve root. If in doubt, inject the shoulder (subacromial space) with cortisone to see if symptoms resolve.

Quick HIT

Gait unsteadiness in elderly patients is often not investigated and attributed to "old age." Whenever an elderly patient is beginning to rely more on assistive devices for walking, consider cervical stenosis and order an MRI. Refer for surgical consultation if stenosis is present.

Knee Pain

A. Causes

1. Osteoarthritis—most common cause of knee pain in older patients (see below) (see Clinical Pearl 12-8).
2. Patellofemoral pain—very common cause of anterior knee pain; worse with climbing and descending stairs. Physical therapy aimed at quadriceps/hamstrings rehabilitation (stretching/strengthening) is very effective.
3. Degeneration or tear of a meniscus—meniscus tear may be due to a specific injury or secondary to a degenerative process (the latter being a common cause of knee pain in older patients). Key features include recurrent knee effusions, tenderness along medial or lateral joint lines, and a positive McMurray test. If no arthritic changes present, surgery (arthroscopic meniscectomy or repair) is effective. Surgery is less effective when concomitant arthritic changes are present and results are less predictable.
4. Rheumatoid arthritis, psoriatic arthritis, SLE.

Quick HIT

Patellofemoral pain is a very common cause of anterior knee pain. Send these patients to physical therapy to strengthen/stretch quadriceps and hamstrings.

CLINICAL PEARL 12-8

Causes of Arthritis

- Osteoarthritis (most common cause)
- Systemic immune disease—rheumatoid arthritis, SLE, seronegative spondyloarthropathies (e.g., reactive arthritis, ankylosing spondylitis, IBD)
- Crystal disease—gout, pseudogout
- Infectious—septic arthritis, Lyme disease
- Trauma
- Charcot joint (diabetes)
- Pediatric orthopedic conditions such as congenital hip dysplasia, Legg–Calvé–Perthes disease, slipped capital femoral epiphysis
- Hematologic—sickle cell disease (avascular necrosis of femoral head), hemophilia (recurrent hemarthrosis)
- Deposition diseases—Wilson disease, hemochromatosis

5. Acute monoarticular arthritis—septic arthritis, disseminated gonorrhea, gout, pseudogout, rheumatic fever, seronegative spondyloarthropathy, Lyme disease.
6. Osteochondritis dissecans (OCD)—an area of necrotic bone and degenerative changes in the overlying cartilage. The bone/cartilage piece may separate from the underlying bone and become a loose body in the joint, causing symptoms of pain, catching, and popping. Treatment options are limited but arthroscopic surgery can help. If the loose fragment is in the joint, arthroscopic removal of fragment is indicated.
7. Iliotibial (IT) band syndrome—pain over the lateral knee (where the IT band attaches to the proximal tibia) primarily in runners and cyclists.
8. Osgood–Schlatter disease in adolescents—resolves with skeletal maturity.
9. Baker cyst—caused by intra-articular pathology (e.g., meniscus tear).
   a. Rupture can cause pain/swelling, and if it extends into the calf, may mimic thrombophlebitis or acute deep venous thrombosis.
   b. Majority resolve spontaneously.
10. Patellar tendinitis ("jumper's knee").
   a. Common cause of anterior knee pain (at inferior pole of patella).
   b. Running and jumping sports—an "overuse" injury.
   c. Treatment is activity modification and quadriceps/hamstring rehabilitation (stretching/strengthening program).
11. Plica Syndrome—a diagnosis of exclusion, typically seen in athletes or with overuse injuries, sometimes after trauma. MRI and examination findings are unreliable. Patients have pain along the medial patella and a feeling of snapping of the knee with walking, with or without intermittent effusion. Treatment is conservative (physical therapy), anti-inflammatory medications, steroid injections. If conservative treatment fails, arthroscopic release of plica can be helpful.

Quick HIT

Recurrent knee effusion is a sign of intra-articular pathology and further investigation is warranted.

B. Diagnosis

1. Radiographs—if degenerative disease is suspected or if there is a history of trauma or acute injury.
2. MRI—if any ligamentous instability is apparent or a meniscus tear is suspected.
3. Knee aspiration ("tap")—use this for analysis of synovial fluid if septic joint is suspected. In general, synovial fluid examination is recommended for monoarticular joint swelling. It may relieve symptoms.

Ankle Sprains

A. General characteristics

1. The lateral side of the ankle consists of three ligaments: anterior talofibular ligament (ATFL), calcaneofibular ligament (CFL), and posterior talofibular ligament. The ATFL is most commonly injured.
2. The medial side ligaments (deltoid ligaments) are typically not injured in a classic inversion ankle sprain.
3. Classification into three grades is based on severity.
   a. Grade 1: partial rupture of ATFL.
   b. Grade 2: complete rupture of ATFL and partial rupture of CFL.
   c. Grade 3: complete rupture of both ATFL and CFL.

Quick HIT

By following the Ottawa rules, unnecessary radiographs of the ankle are avoided and clinically significant fractures are not missed.

B. Diagnosis

1. Patients typically have tenderness directly over the injured ligament. ATFL is located just at the anterior tip of the distal fibula.
2. Ankle radiographs are not necessary if the following conditions are met (Ottawa rules):
   a. Patient is able to walk four steps at the time of injury and at the time of evaluation.
   b. There is no bony tenderness over distal 6 cm of either malleolus.

C. Treatment

1. Rest, ice, compression, elevation (RICE) in the acute period, then controlled pain-free range of motion exercises with gradual return to weight bearing.

Quick HIT

Treatment of all acute ankle sprains (even severe sprains) involves RICE and physical therapy. Surgery is rarely, if ever, needed acutely. Recurrent ankle sprains, however, require evaluation for possible surgery.

2. Physical therapy after the acute phase of swelling has subsided to regain full range of motion, strength, and proprioception. Physical therapy involves peroneal tendon strengthening and proprioceptive training.
3. Surgery is rarely necessary acutely, even for grade 3 sprains.
4. Chronic ankle instability (recurrent ankle sprains) needs further evaluation by an orthopedic surgeon.

Tendinitis and Bursitis

A. Tendinitis

1. Supraspinatus (rotator cuff) tendinitis—impingement syndrome.
   a. Most common cause of shoulder pain.
   b. Pain occurs subacromially and on the lateral aspect of the shoulder with arm abduction; pain is poorly localized (difficult for patient to pinpoint) with an insidious onset. It is generally located over the lateral deltoid.
   c. This is seen in elderly patients (degeneration of tendons) and in young patients who do a lot of overhand lifting/throwing (sports or work-related).
   d. Pain may be referred to the lateral arm.
   e. If weakness is present on shoulder abduction, a rotator cuff tear should be suspected. (MRI is the best test for diagnosis of rotator cuff tear.)
   f. Treatment: physical therapy (strengthen shoulder musculature), subacromial steroid injection. Arthroscopic surgery is helpful if conservative treatment fails.
2. Lateral epicondylitis at the elbow ("tennis elbow").
   a. Caused by inflammation/degeneration of the extensor tendons of the forearm, which originate from the lateral epicondyle; results from excessive/repetitive supination/pronation.
   b. Splinting the forearm (counterforce brace) is the initial treatment (do not splint or wrap the elbow itself).
   c. Physical therapy is often helpful—strengthening/stretching extensors of forearm. This, along with activity modification, typically leads to resolution of pain.
   d. Injections only if physical therapy fails. Surgery is effective but only used if all conservative measures have been exhausted. Surgery is rarely necessary for this condition.
3. Medial epicondylitis ("golfer's elbow").
   a. Pain distal to medial epicondyle (origin of flexor muscles of the forearm).
   b. Exacerbated by wrist flexion; caused by overuse of the flexor pronator muscle group. Treatment similar to lateral epicondylitis (physical therapy, activity modification).
4. De Quervain disease
   a. Pain at the radial aspect of the wrist (especially with pinch gripping) in region of radial styloid; common for pain to radiate to elbow or into thumb.
   b. Due to inflammation of the abductor pollicis longus and extensor pollicis brevis tendons.
   c. Positive Finkelstein test—have the patient clench the thumb under the other fingers when making a fist. Then ulnarly deviate the wrist. The test is positive if pain is reproduced.
   d. Treatment is thumb spica splint and NSAIDs. Local cortisone injections can be helpful. Surgery done if conservative measures fail and is usually effective.

B. Bursitis

1. Olecranon bursitis—swelling (and perhaps pain) at point of elbow; spongy "bag of fluid" over olecranon (due to effusion into the olecranon bursa).
   a. Treatment is conservative.
   b. If infection is suspected, drainage may be necessary.
2. Trochanteric bursitis—this is a very common cause of lateral hip pain. The greater trochanter is exquisitely painful on palpation.
   a. Causes include trauma, overuse injury, weakness of hip musculature. In many cases, no inciting event is present and the onset is insidious.

Quick HIT

Impingement Syndrome
- Common cause of shoulder pain
- Due to impingement of greater tuberosity on acromion
- Pain with overhead activity
- May lead to rotator cuff pathology over time
- Steroid injections give temporary relief
- Surgery (acromioplasty) is very effective

Quick HIT

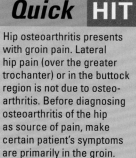

Hip osteoarthritis presents with groin pain. Lateral hip pain (over the greater trochanter) or in the buttock region is not due to osteoarthritis. Before diagnosing osteoarthritis of the hip as source of pain, make certain patient's symptoms are primarily in the groin.

Quick HIT

Differential diagnosis of hand numbness (as seen in carpal tunnel syndrome):
- Cervical radiculopathy (nerve root compression in the cervical spine)
- Peripheral neuropathy (diabetes)
- Median nerve compression in forearm

b. Treatment is NSAIDs and activity modification. If symptoms persist, local cortisone injections into the bursa are very effective in providing relief.

Carpal Tunnel Syndrome

Quick HIT

A negative Phalen test or Tinel sign does not exclude carpal tunnel syndrome.

A. General characteristics

1. Caused by **median nerve compression** within the tight confines of the carpal tunnel, causing numbness and pain in median nerve distribution. If long standing and severe, atrophy of thenar muscles may be seen.
2. Associated conditions include hypothyroidism, diabetes, repetitive use of hands in certain activities, pregnancy, recent trauma, or fracture of the wrist.

B. Clinical features

1. Numbness, pain, or tingling in the **median nerve distribution**—usually worse at night; sometimes patient has pain/numbness along the entire arm (as far as the shoulder).
2. Muscle weakness and thenar atrophy may develop later.

C. Diagnosis

1. Physical examination
   a. **Tinel sign**—tap over median nerve at wrist crease; causes paresthesias in median nerve distribution
   b. **Phalen test**—palmar flexion of the wrist for 1 minute; causes paresthesias in median nerve distribution
2. Electromyography (EMG) and nerve conduction velocity (NCV) study
   a. For definitive diagnosis
   b. Indicated if diagnosis is not clear from clinical findings or if patient develops weakness or persistent symptoms

D. Treatment

1. Wrist splints (volar carpal splint) should be worn at night during sleep. The purpose is to prevent wrist flexion during sleep (which compresses the nerve).
2. Anti-inflammatory medications (NSAIDs).
3. Local corticosteroid injection—relief can be long term in some patients.
4. Surgical release is very effective. Consider this option for patients who have persistent symptoms or if the symptoms are limiting the patient's activities or quality of life.

Osteoarthritis

A. General characteristics

1. Osteoarthritis is characterized by **degeneration of cartilage** (due to wear and tear) and by hypertrophy of bone at the articular margins.
2. By age 65, more than 75% of the population has radiographic evidence of osteoarthritis in weight-bearing joints (hips, knees, lumbar spine).
3. Any joint can be affected, but weight-bearing joints are most commonly involved (hips, knees, cervical, and lumbar spine).

B. Risk factors

1. Age
2. Obesity
3. Excessive joint loading (manual labor, athletes, etc.)
4. Trauma
   a. Repeated microtrauma—in many cases, a patient's occupation or athletic activities require repetitive motions (such as repeated knee bending) that predispose the patient to degenerative joint disease in later years
   b. Macrotrauma (fractures, ligament injuries)—fractures that are intra-articular can cause OA
5. Genetic predisposition

6. Altered joint anatomy or instability (developmental hip dysplasia, dislocation due to trauma, rheumatoid arthritis, gout, pseudogout)
7. Deposition diseases cause chondrocyte injury, or make the cartilage more stiff (hemochromatosis, ochronosis, alkaptonuria, Wilson disease, Gaucher disease, gout, CPPD)
8. Hemophilia (hemarthroses)

C. Clinical features

1. Joint pain (often monoarticular)
   a. This is caused by movement of one joint surface against another (bone on bone) because of cartilage loss. There are no pain fibers in cartilage, so its insidious destruction over time goes unnoticed. Once it is completely worn out, the bones (which do have pain fibers) start rubbing against each other, producing the pain of osteoarthritis
   b. Deep, dull ache that is relieved with rest and worsened with activity
   c. Insidious onset, with gradual progression over many years
2. Stiffness in the morning or after a period of inactivity (Note: morning stiffness lasting >30 minutes may suggest an inflammatory arthritis such as rheumatoid arthritis)
3. Limited range of motion (late stages) due to bony enlargement of joints (osteophytes); bony crepitus may be present
4. No systemic symptoms; no erythema or warmth. Swelling may be present and suggests inflammation

D. Diagnosis

1. Plain radiographs are the initial tests and should be obtained in all patients suspected of having osteoarthritis (Figure 12-4). Ideally, radiographs should be obtained in the standing position (for lower extremities). Findings include:
   a. **Joint space narrowing** (due to loss of cartilage)—key finding on radiographs
   b. **Osteophytes**
   c. **Sclerosis** of subchondral bony end-plates adjacent to diseased cartilage—most severe at points of maximum pressure
   d. **Subchondral cysts**—occur as a result of increased transmission of intra-articular pressure to the subchondral bone
2. All blood tests are normal
3. MRI of the spine if indicated (neurologic findings, before surgery)

E. Treatment

1. Nonpharmacologic treatment.
   a. Avoid activities that involve excessive use of the joint.
   b. Weight loss is very important.
   c. Physical therapy can be beneficial. Goals are to maintain range of motion and muscle strength. Swimming is an ideal exercise (involves minimal involvement of weight-bearing joints); avoid excessive walking.
   d. Use canes or crutches to reduce weight on the joint.
2. Pharmacologic treatment.
   a. Acetaminophen is the first-line agent.
   b. NSAIDs are just as effective as acetaminophen (but GI bleeding is a concern with long-term use). Of selective COX-2 inhibitors, only celecoxib remains on the market but is rarely used. All the others have been removed from the market due to increased risk of cardiovascular events. Main benefit of selective COX-2 inhibitors is a decrease in gastric/duodenal ulcers and a decrease in GI symptoms, with the same (not superior) analgesic and anti-inflammatory effects of the nonselective NSAIDs.
   c. Intra-articular injections of corticosteroids are very helpful, but more than three to four injections per year is not recommended. Patients may have up to 3 months of pain relief with each injection. In elderly patients with severe OA who are not good surgical candidates for joint replacement, more frequent injections are justified if it provides good pain control.

Quick HIT

The following can contribute to or exacerbate forces to the cartilage:
- Compromised pain sensation or proprioception
- Ligamental laxity
- Falls of very short distances (because they do not provide ample opportunity for compensatory movements to decrease the impact load)

Quick HIT

If the spine is involved, nerve roots may become compressed and lead to radicular pain.

Quick HIT

Hip osteoarthritis causes pain in the groin (not lateral hip or buttock). If patient is tender over the lateral aspect of hip, suspect greater trochanteric bursitis.

Quick HIT

Radiographic findings in osteoarthritis: joint space narrowing, osteophytes, subchondral sclerosis, subchondral cysts.

Quick HIT

Common (but Useless) "pimp" Information
- *Bouchard nodes:* Bony overgrowth and significant osteoarthritic changes (i.e., osteophytes) at the PIP joints
- *Heberden nodes:* Bony overgrowth and significant osteoarthritic changes (i.e., osteophytes) at the DIP joints

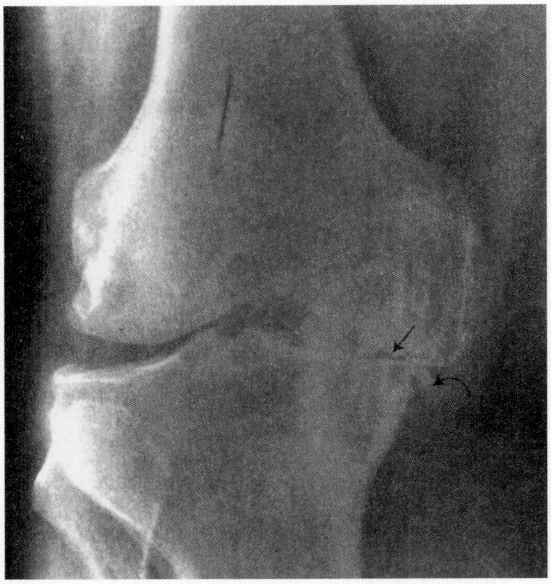

A

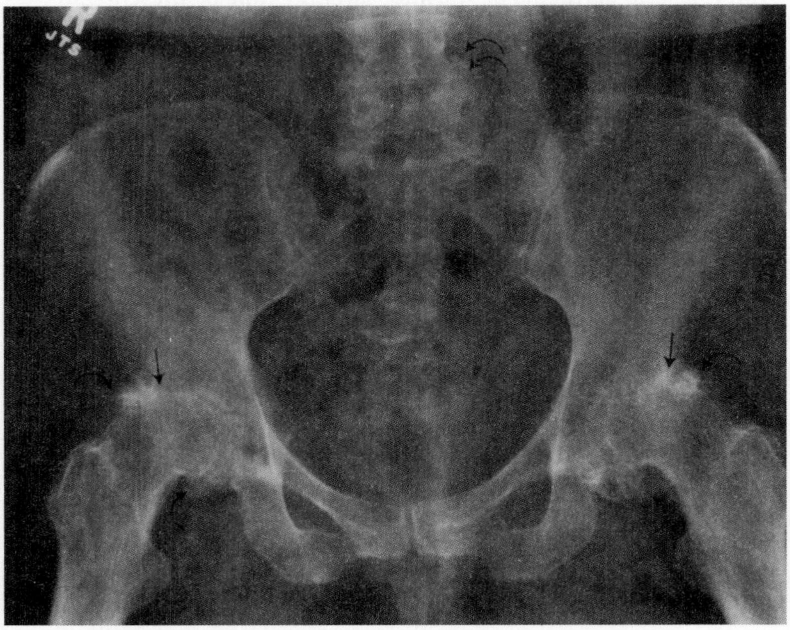

B

FIGURE 12-4 **A: Right knee AP radiograph showing osteoarthritis. Note medial joint space narrowing, osteophyte formation (*curved arrow*), and irregular articular surfaces (*straight arrow*). B: Pelvic AP radiograph. Bilateral osteoarthritis of the hip. Note narrowing of hip joint spaces, osteophytes (*curved arrows*), and osteophytes in the lumbar spine (*double curved arrows*). Also note subchondral cysts and sclerosis of the femoral heads.**

(**A** from Erkonen WE, Smith WL. *Radiology 101: The Basics and Fundamentals of Imaging.* Philadelphia, PA: Lippincott Williams & Wilkins, 1998:287, Figure 11-72.) (**B** from Erkonen WE, Smith WL. *Radiology 101: The Basics and Fundamentals of Imaging.* Philadelphia, PA: Lippincott Williams & Wilkins, 1998:288, Figure 11-73A.)

Quick HIT

With osteoarthritis of the hips, the pain is in the **groin region** and sometimes radiates to the anterior thigh.

Quick HIT

For **left** knee or hip pain, the cane should be held in the **right** hand.

d. Viscosupplementation—recent studies show good pain relief, but results are variable. Hyaluronic acid is injected into the knee joint and augments the viscoelastic properties of normal synovial fluid.

3. Surgery for serious disability.
   a. Total joint replacement may be performed if conservative therapy fails to control pain. It should be delayed as long as possible because a revision may be

needed 15 to 20 years after surgery. Total hip and knee replacements are among the most successful procedures in orthopedics with reliable pain relief.

4. Nutritional products—glucosamine and chondroitin sulfate.
   a. Over-the-counter products that many patients claim to improve arthritis symptoms, although high-quality randomized trials have not shown any meaningful benefit.

Osteoporosis

A. General characteristics

1. Decreased bone mass/quality causes increased bone fragility and fracture risk. In osteoporosis, the bone mineral density is at least 2.5 standard deviations below that of young, normal individuals.
2. Mechanism: failure to attain optimal (peak) bone mass before age 30, or rate of bone resorption exceeds rate of bone formation after peak bone mass is attained
3. Most osteoporotic patients are postmenopausal women and elderly men
4. Classification
   a. Primary osteoporosis (two types that are impractical clinically)
      - Type I (most often in postmenopausal women 51 to 75 years of age)—excess loss of trabecular bone; vertebral compression fractures and Colles fractures are common
      - Type II (most often in men and women over 70 years of age)—equal loss of both cortical and trabecular bone; fractures of femoral neck, proximal humerus, and pelvis most common

   b. Secondary osteoporosis—An obvious cause is present, such as excess steroid therapy/Cushing syndrome, immobilization, hyperthyroidism, long-term heparin, hypogonadism in men, and vitamin D deficiency

B. Risk factors

1. Estrogen depletion
   a. Postmenopausal state—all women are estrogen deficient after menopause; however, osteoporosis does not develop in all women
   b. History of athletic amenorrhea, eating disorders, oligomenorrhea
   c. Early menopause
2. Female gender—women have a lower peak bone mass and smaller vertebral end plates
3. Calcium deficiency/vitamin D deficiency
4. Decreased peak bone mass
5. Heritable risk factors—family history, European or Asian ancestry, thinness/slight build
6. Decreased physical activity (prolonged immobility)
7. Endocrine—hypogonadism in men (with low testosterone), hyperthyroidism, vitamin D deficiency (see Clinical Pearl 12-9)

CLINICAL PEARL 12-9

Osteoporotic Fracture Risk Assessment

Validated risk factors for osteoporotic fracture risk that are independent of bone mineral density are:

- Advanced age
- Previous osteoporotic fracture
- Long-term steroid therapy
- Cigarette smoking
- Low body weight (<58 kg)
- Family history of hip fracture
- Excess alcohol intake
- Rheumatoid arthritis
- Secondary osteoporosis

Quick HIT

Although x-rays are diagnostic of OA, not all patients with x-ray findings of OA have symptoms. There is no consistent correlation between symptoms and severity of x-ray findings.

Quick HIT

It is often difficult to differentiate between primary and secondary osteoporosis, and the two may coexist. It is best to attempt to identify any predisposing conditions and eliminate them if possible.

Quick HIT

Some elderly patients have progressive kyphosis (hunchback deformity) because they have multiple vertebral compression fractures.

Quick HIT

Osteoporosis is a "silent" disease. It is asymptomatic until a fracture occurs.

Quick HIT

An exercise program with calcium and vitamin D supplements is the mainstay of the therapy for prevention or treatment of osteoporosis.

Quick HIT

The **PROOF trial** showed the following regarding **calcitonin:**
- No effect at hip
- Shown to decrease risk of vertebral fractures by as much as 40%
- Slight increase in bone density at lumbar vertebrae

8. Smoking and alcohol abuse
9. Medications—corticosteroids, prolonged heparin use

C. Clinical features

1. Vertebral body compression fractures (of the middle and lower thoracic and upper lumbar spine) are the most common. Very rare in cervical spine
   a. Result in pain and deformity, including kyphosis
   b. Severe back pain after minor trauma
   c. Restricted spinal movement, loss of height
2. Colles fracture (distal radius fracture)—usually due to fall on outstretched hand; more common in postmenopausal women
3. Hip fractures—femoral neck, intertrochanteric fractures
4. Increased incidence of long bone fractures—humerus, femur, tibia

Quick HIT

Recommend the following to all patients with osteoporosis:
- Daily calcium
- Daily vitamin D
- Weight-bearing exercise
- Smoking cessation

D. Diagnosis

1. DEXA (dual-energy x-ray absorptiometry) scan is the gold standard.
   a. Very precise for measuring bone density.
   b. Indications for bone mineral density measurement:
      - All women 65 and older.
      - Postmenopausal women <65 with one or more risk factors for fracture.
      - Men with risk factors for fracture.
   c. Sites selected are femoral neck and lumbar spine. Compare the density of bone with a standard control, which is the bone density of a healthy 30-year-old person.
   d. Can range from normal to osteopenia to osteoporosis. T-scores are used according to WHO classification (see Table 12-8).
      - WHO classification (T-scores) are used in all postmenopausal and perimenopausal women, and in men over age 50. In all other patients (including premenopausal women), z-scores are used.
2. Rule out secondary causes—check calcium, phosphorus, alkaline phosphatase, TSH, vitamin D, free PTH, creatinine, CBC.

Quick HIT

Of all fragility fractures, hip fractures have highest morbidity and mortality.

Quick HIT

If DEXA scan is normal and no risk factors, repeat DEXA in 3 to 5 years.

E. Treatment

1. Nonpharmacologic therapy
   a. Diet—adequate calorie intake, avoid malnutrition
      - Supplemental elemental calcium (1,200 mg/day)
      - 800 international units of vitamin D daily
   b. Exercise—weight-bearing exercise for 30 minutes, at least 3 times a week, to stimulate bone formation
   c. Smoking cessation is critical—smoking accelerates bone loss
   d. Eliminate or reduce alcohol intake

Quick HIT

Unfortunately, most patients with fragility fractures do not subsequently receive osteoporosis therapy, despite data showing a beneficial effect in reducing the risk of a second fracture.

Ambulatory Medicine

TABLE 12-8 Bone Mineral Density T-score Criteria for Osteopenia and Osteoporosis

Diagnosis	T-score
Normal	Greater than or equal to 1.0
Osteopenia	Between −1.0 and −2.5
Osteoporosis	Less than or equal to −2.5
Severe osteoporosis	Less than or equal to −2.5 and fragility fracture

Adapted from World Health Organization: http://www.shef.ac.uk/FRAX/pdfs/WHO_Technical_Report.pdf

2. Pharmacologic therapy
   a. Indicated in the following patients:
      - Postmenopausal women with established osteoporosis (T-score 2.5 or less) or fragility fracture (hip or vertebral)
      - High-risk postmenopausal women with T-score between −1.0 and −2.5
   b. Bisphosphonates inhibit bone resorption and are first-line treatment
      - They decrease osteoclastic activity (via binding to hydroxyapatite) and decrease the risk of fractures
      - Oral bisphosphonates (alendronate, risedronate) are preferred in most patients
      - Side effects include reflux, esophageal irritation, and ulceration
      - If patient cannot tolerate oral bisphosphonates, IV bisphosphonates (IV zoledronic acid)
   c. PTH therapy or human recombinant PTH therapy
      - PTH is an effective drug that increases bone mineral density and reduces fracture risk. Due to high cost, subcutaneous administration, and long-term safety concerns, it is not a first-line drug
      - Indicated in patients with severe osteoporosis (T-score less than 2.5) who cannot tolerate bisphosphonates, or who continue to fracture despite being on bisphosphonates for 1 year
      - Maximum duration of treatment is 24 months, because of concern for osteosarcomas, which have been observed in rats. After stopping PTH, can restart bisphosphonates
   d. Calcitonin (can be administered by nasal spray)—long-term benefits are minimal, but it is useful as short-term therapy, especially in elderly female patients with vertebral compression fracture. It is less popular and not commonly used
   e. Estrogen–progestin therapy is no longer a first-line approach for the treatment of osteoporosis in postmenopausal women because of increased risk of breast cancer, stroke, venous thromboembolism, and perhaps CAD

Diseases of the Eye

Age-related Macular Degeneration

- Most common cause of vision loss in people over 65 years of age in developed countries.
- Age-related macular degeneration (ARMD) is characterized by loss of central vision (because the macula is affected). Blurred vision, distortion, and scotoma are common. Complete loss of vision almost never occurs. Peripheral vision is preserved.
- The main risk factor is advanced age. Other risk factors are female gender, Caucasian race, smoking, HTN, and family history.
- Two categories: exudative ("wet") and nonexudative ("dry") macular degeneration.
- Exudative ARMD causes sudden visual loss due to leakage of serous fluid and blood as a result of abnormal vessel formation (neovascularization) under the retina.
- Nonexudative ARMD is characterized by atrophy and degeneration of the central retina. Yellowish-white deposits called **drusen** form under the pigment epithelium and can be seen with an ophthalmoscope.
- Intraocular injections of medications (anti-VEGF inhibitors) have supplanted laser photocoagulation and other therapies for wet ARMD.
- Over-the-counter formulations of vitamins are recommended for dry and wet ARMD.

Glaucoma

A. General characteristics

1. Glaucoma is **one of the most important causes of blindness worldwide**. It is a complex disease typically characterized by increased IOP, damage to the optic nerve, and irreversible vision loss.
2. The pathogenesis of optic nerve damage in glaucoma is not fully understood. Ischemia may play a major role. Over time there is a loss of ganglion cells, leading to atrophy of the optic disc (and enlargement of the optic cup, called "**cupping**").

Quick HIT

Most common causes of visual impairment/loss in developed countries:
- Diabetic retinopathy (most common cause in adults <65 years)
- ARMD (most common cause in adults >65 years)
- Cataracts
- Glaucoma

Quick HIT

Age-related Macular Degeneration
- The "wet" form of ARMD can develop at any time, so patients with "dry" ARMD must be monitored closely.
- Supplements of certain vitamins containing antioxidants are thought to be beneficial, but a preventative or therapeutic effect has not been proven.
- **Ranibizumab (and several other related drugs), given as repeated intraocular injections,** have been shown to be effective in treating "wet" ARMD.

Quick HIT

Glaucoma is the most common cause of irreversible blindness in African Americans.

3. There are many types of glaucoma, but they generally fall into the following two categories:
   a. Open-angle glaucoma—accounts for 90% of all cases.
      - Characterized by impaired outflow of aqueous humor from the eye.
      - Absence of symptoms early in the course can lead to delay in diagnosis and "silent" progression.
   b. Closed-angle glaucoma.
      - Acute angle-closure glaucoma—characterized by very rapid increase in IOP due to occlusion of **the anterior chamber angle (between the cornea and the iris where the trabecular meshwork is located)** and obstruction of outflow of aqueous humor.
      - **This is an ophthalmologic emergency that can lead to irreversible vision loss within hours if untreated.**
      - May be precipitated by dilation of the iris in a patient with a pre-existing anatomically narrow anterior chamber angle.

B. Risk factors

1. Older age (over 50 years)
2. African-American race (increased incidence of open-angle glaucoma)
3. Asian or Eskimo ancestry (increased incidence of acute angle-closure glaucoma)
4. Family history of glaucoma
5. History of significant eye trauma or intraocular inflammation
6. Steroid medications

Quick HIT

Patients with acute angle-closure glaucoma may have severe abdominal pain and nausea, and they are occasionally misdiagnosed as having an acute surgical abdomen (e.g., appendicitis).

C. Clinical features

1. Open-angle glaucoma
   a. Painless, increased IOP (may be the only sign), characteristic changes in optic nerve
   b. Progressive and insidious visual field loss (usually sparing central vision until end-stage disease)
2. Closed-angle glaucoma
   a. Red, painful eye
   b. Sudden decrease in visual acuity (blurred vision), seeing "halos," markedly elevated IOP
   c. Nausea and vomiting (common), headache
   d. Involved pupil is dilated and nonreactive (in mid-dilation)

D. Diagnosis

1. Tonometry measures IOP; should be performed regularly in patients with or at risk for glaucoma.
2. Ophthalmoscopy—evaluate the optic nerve for glaucomatous damage.
3. Gonioscopy is used to visualize the anterior chamber and helps determine the cause of glaucoma. It requires skill to perform.
4. Visual field testing should be performed in all patients in whom glaucoma is suspected and regularly in everyone with glaucoma to monitor disease progression.
5. Imaging (OCT) of the optic nerve also is helpful in assessing and monitoring progression of axonal loss of the optic nerve in glaucoma patients.

Quick HIT

The goal of treatment is to control IOP, and thereby prevent further damage to the optic nerve and visual field loss.

E. Treatment

1. Chronic open-angle glaucoma (in escalating order).
   a. Topical medications—Most patients are first treated topically with a β-blocker, α-agonist, carbonic anhydrase inhibitor, and/or prostaglandin analogue singly or in combination to reach the target pressure.
   b. Laser or surgical treatment for refractory cases.
2. Acute angle-closure glaucoma.
   a. An ophthalmic emergency—refer to an ophthalmologist immediately. Emergently lower the IOP. Medical treatment includes timolol, a brimonidine, dorzolamide, pilocarpine, and/or prednisolone drops, IV acetazolamide, and oral mannitol if IOP is still elevated after previous measures.
   b. Laser or surgical iridectomy is a definitive treatment.

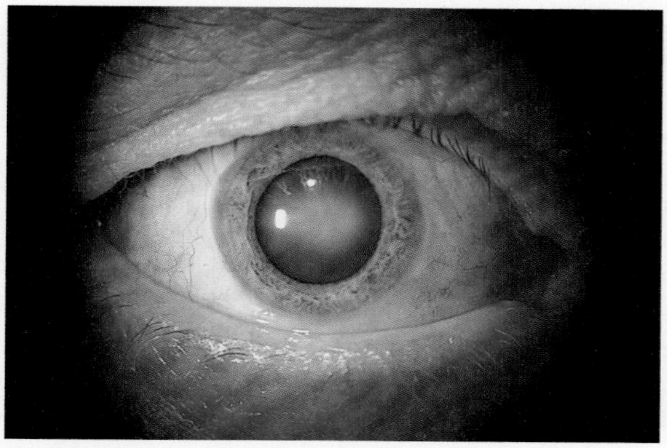

FIGURE 12-5 **Cataract.**
(From Tasman W, Jaeger E. *The Wills Eye Hospital Atlas of Clinical Ophthalmology.* 2nd ed. Philadelphia, PA: Lippincott Williams & Wilkins, 2001, Figure 12-2.)

Cataracts

- Opacifications of the natural lens of the eye: **half of people over age 75 have cataracts** (Figure 12-5).
- There is a **loss of visual acuity** that progresses slowly over many years. Patients may complain of glare and difficulty driving at night.
- Risk factors include old age, cigarette smoking, glucocorticoid use, prolonged UV radiation exposure, trauma, diabetes, Wilson disease, Down syndrome, and certain metabolic diseases.
- Surgery is the definitive treatment and is very effective in restoring vision. It is indicated if visual loss is significant to the patient and interferes with daily or occupational activities. It involves extraction of the cataract with implantation of an artificial intraocular lens.

Quick HIT

"Second sight"
- Some patients with cataracts become increasingly near-sighted and may no longer require reading glasses. This is referred to as "second sight."
- This phenomenon is due to increased refractive power of the lens of the eye caused by the cataract.

Red Eye

A. General characteristics

1. Many causes of red eye are benign, but the initial goal in evaluation should be to identify conditions that require referral (emergent or nonemergent) to an ophthalmologist.
2. Conjunctivitis is the most common cause of red eye, but always attempt to exclude other, more serious causes.
3. The following conditions require a referral to an ophthalmologist:
   a. Eye pain that does not respond to therapy.
   b. Flashers, floaters, or a sudden decrease in visual acuity.
   c. History of recent eye surgery—especially if infection is suspected.
   d. Corneal opacification, corneal ulcer, or corneal foreign body that cannot be removed.
   e. History of penetrating trauma or significant blunt trauma.
   f. History of chemical exposure (especially alkali agents).
   g. Orbital cellulitis.
   h. Presence of hypopyon or ciliary flush (suggests acute glaucoma, corneal inflammation, or iridocyclitis)
   i. Asymmetric or unreactive pupils.
4. Always check visual acuity, pupil size, and reactivity. Evert lids to look for a foreign body.

Quick HIT

In general, steroid eye drops should be given by an ophthalmologist.

B. Differential diagnosis

1. Conjunctivitis—see below
2. Subconjunctival hemorrhage
   a. Caused by rupture of small conjunctival vessels; induced by Valsalva maneuver trauma; or, less commonly, coagulopathies or HTN

b. Causes focal unilateral blotchy redness of the conjunctiva (looks worse than it is)
c. Usually self-limiting and resolves in a few weeks

3. Keratoconjunctivitis sicca (dry eye)
   a. Very long differential diagnosis, including medications (e.g., anticholinergics or antihistamines), autoimmune diseases (e.g., Sjögren), CN V or VII lesions
   b. The eye may appear normal, or may be mildly injected
   c. Patients may complain of a foreign body sensation
   d. Treat with artificial tears during the day. Consider a lubricating ointment at night. Many other treatments are available
4. Acute angle-closure glaucoma (see above)—consult an ophthalmologist immediately
5. Blepharitis
   a. Inflammation of the eyelid; often associated with infection with *Staphylococcus* spp.
   b. Usually diagnosed by careful examination of the eyelid margins, which are red and often swollen with crusting that sticks to the lashes
   c. Treat with lid scrubs and warm compresses. Give topical antibiotics for severe cases
6. Episcleritis
   a. Inflammation of vessels lining the episclera (the lining just beneath the conjunctiva)
   b. Thought to be an autoimmune process—may be seen with connective tissue diseases, but usually idiopathic
   c. Causes redness, irritation, dull ache, and possible watery discharge
   d. The sclera may appear blotchy with areas of redness over the episcleral vessels
   e. It is usually self-limited; NSAIDs may provide symptomatic relief
   f. Refer the patient for evaluation by an ophthalmologist
7. Scleritis
   a. Inflammation of the sclera is associated with systemic immunologic disease, such as rheumatoid arthritis
   b. It causes significant eye pain (severe, deep pain). On examination, there is ocular redness and pain on palpation of the eyeball. It can cause visual impairment
   c. Refer the patient for prompt evaluation by an ophthalmologist. Treatment involves topical and sometimes systemic corticosteroids
8. Acute anterior uveitis (also known as iritis or iridocyclitis)
   a. Inflammation of the iris and ciliary body; more common in the young and middle-aged
   b. Associated with connective tissue diseases (e.g., sarcoidosis, ankylosing spondylitis, Reiter syndrome, and IBD)
   c. Clinical findings: ciliary flush (redness most prominent around the cornea), blurred vision, pain and photophobia; constricted pupil compared with contralateral eye
   d. Refer the patient for prompt evaluation by an ophthalmologist
9. Herpes simplex keratitis
   a. Caused by HSV-1; may present similarly to viral conjunctivitis, except usually unilateral
   b. Presents with ocular irritation and photophobia. Pain may be absent
   c. Look for classic **dendritic ulcer on the cornea; can result in irreversible vision loss if untreated**
   d. Warrants semiurgent ophthalmology referral
   e. Treat with topical antiviral eye drops or ganciclovir gel. Consider oral acyclovir or valcylovir for those who cannot tolerate or administer topical therapy.

Quick HIT

Viral conjunctivitis is highly contagious! Patients should avoid any direct or indirect eye contact with others. Encourage strict personal hygiene and frequent handwashing. Clean all surfaces and equipment in contact with the patient as soon as the patient leaves the office.

Quick HIT

When a patient presents with red and itchy eyes, tearing, and nasal congestion, think allergic conjunctivitis.

Conjunctivitis

A. General characteristics

1. Conjunctivitis is the most common cause of red eye.
2. Conjunctivitis generally refers to inflammation of the transparent membrane that lines the inside of the eyelids (palpebral conjunctiva) and the globe (bulbar conjunctiva).

CLINICAL PEARL 12-10

Do Not Send a Patient Home Who Has a Rapid Onset of Copious, Purulent Exudate!

- This is consistent with **hyperacute bacterial conjunctivitis,** caused by *Neisseria gonorrhoeae.*
- The typical patient is a sexually active young adult.
- Symptoms progress rapidly to severe redness, swelling, and pain.
- **This warrants immediate attention from an ophthalmologist.**
- If untreated, it can lead to corneal scarring and blindness.

Quick HIT

Wearing contact lenses overnight dramatically increases a person's risk for developing corneal infection and ulceration.

B. Causes

1. Viral conjunctivitis (see also Clinical Pearl 12-10).
   a. The **most common** form of conjunctivitis. Adenovirus is the most common organism.
   b. Inquire about a recent history of URI.
   c. Hyperemia of one or both eyes, usually one followed by spread to the other in a few days is common. A watery discharge is frequently present.
   d. A palpable preauricular lymph node may be present.
   e. It is usually self-limited, but some patients develop membranous conjunctivitis that requires topical steroids and stripping of the membranes.
2. Bacterial conjunctivitis.
   a. Most commonly caused by *S. aureus* in adults, though other common organisms include *S. pneumoniae, H. influenzae, M. catarrhalis.*
   b. Rapid onset of irritation, hyperemia, and tearing.
   c. Characterized by a mucopurulent exudate with crusting.
3. Chlamydial conjunctivitis—two important forms.
   a. Trachoma (caused by *Chlamydia trachomatis* serotypes A, B, and C)
      - Most common cause of blindness worldwide due to chronic scarring.
   b. Inclusion conjunctivitis (*C. trachomatis* serotypes D to K).
      - Mainly transmitted by genital-hand-eye contact in patients with sexually transmitted infection (STI).
4. Allergic conjunctivitis.
   a. Very common in patients with atopic disease; usually seasonal.
   b. It is typically characterized by redness, itching, tearing, and nasal conjunctivitis. Eyelid edema may also be present. It is typically bilateral.
5. Conjunctivitis secondary to irritants (e.g., contact lenses, chemicals, foreign bodies, dryness).

C. Treatment

1. Viral conjunctivitis: cold compress, strict hand washing; topical antibiotics if bacterial superinfection is suspected
2. Bacterial conjunctivitis
   a. Acute—use broad-spectrum topical antibiotics (e.g., erythromycin, ciprofloxacin, sulfacetamide). Therapy can be altered based on culture results
   b. Hyperacute—Treat gonococcal conjunctivitis with a one-time dose of ceftriaxone, 1g IM, as well as topical therapy.
3. Chlamydial conjunctivitis
   a. Adults and adolescents—oral tetracycline, doxycycline, or erythromycin for 2 weeks
   b. Treat sexual partner(s) for STI
4. Allergic conjunctivitis
   a. Remove the allergen, if possible. Advise the use of cold compresses
   b. Treat with topical antihistamines or mast cell stabilizers
   c. Systemic antihistamines can be effective as well
   d. Topical NSAIDs may be a useful adjunct to treatment

Amaurosis Fugax

- Some variability with how this is defined, but generally refers to sudden, transient loss of vision in one or both eyes
- Causes of transient monocular vision loss include carotid artery disease (cholesterol plaque embolization), cardioembolic phenomenon, giant cell (temporal) arteritis, and others
- Order carotid ultrasonography and cardiac workup (e.g., lipid profile, ECG)

Sleep Disorders

Obstructive Sleep Apnea

A. General characteristics

1. Intermittent obstruction of the air flow (typically at the level of the oropharynx) produces periods of apnea during sleep.
2. Each apneic period is usually 20 to 30 seconds long (but may be longer) and results in hypoxia, which arouses the patient from sleep. This occurs multiple (sometimes hundreds of) times overnight.

B. Risk factors

1. Obesity (especially around the neck)—nonobese patients can also have OSA, however
2. Structural abnormalities—enlarged tonsils, uvula, soft palate; nasal polyps; hypertrophy of muscles in the pharynx; deviated septum; deep overbite with small chin
3. Family history
4. Alcohol and sedatives worsen the condition
5. Hypothyroidism (multifactorial)

C. Clinical features

1. Snoring
2. Daytime sleepiness due to disrupted nocturnal sleep
3. Personality changes, decreased intellectual function, decreased libido
4. Repeated oxygen desaturation and hypoxemia can lead to systemic and pulmonary HTN as well as cardiac arrhythmias
5. Other features: morning headaches, polycythemia

D. Diagnosis: Polysomnography (overnight sleep study in a sleep laboratory) confirms the diagnosis.

E. Treatment

1. All patients should undergo behavior modification, which includes weight loss and exercise, avoiding alcohol and sedatives, and sleeping in a nonsupine position
2. Mild to moderate OSA
   a. Should be offered positive airway pressure therapy
   b. If patient refuses or there are issues with compliance, an oral appliance can be offered
3. Severe OSA
   a. **Continuous positive airway pressure** provides positive pressure, thus preventing occlusion of the upper pharynx. This is the preferred therapy for the majority of patients because it is noninvasive and has proven efficacy. It is poorly tolerated by some due to noise and discomfort
   b. Uvulopalatopharyngoplasty—removal of redundant tissue in oropharynx to allow more air flow
   c. Tracheostomy is a last resort for those in whom all other therapies have failed or who have life-threatening OSA (severe hypoxemia or arrhythmias)

Quick HIT

Complications of OSA
- Increased pulmonary vascular resistance (due to hypoxemia); over time, can lead to pulmonary HTN and eventually cor pulmonale (more likely if the patient is obese)
- Systemic HTN (due to increase in sympathetic tone)

Narcolepsy

A. Inherited disorder (of variable penetrance) of REM sleep regulation (i.e., REM sleep involuntarily occurs at random and inappropriate times)

B. Results in **excessive sleepiness** during the day

C. Characterized by the following features:
1. Involuntary "sleep attacks" at any time of day (during any activity, including driving) that last several minutes
2. Cataplexy, which is loss of muscle tone that generally occurs with an intense emotional stimulus (e.g., laughter, anger)
3. Sleep paralysis, in which patient cannot move when waking up
4. Hypnagogic hallucinations that are vivid hallucinations (visual or auditory)—"dreams" while awake

D. The disorder can range from mild to severe

E. Automobile accidents are a major problem

F. Treatment: modafinil (use is supported by RCTs), methylphenidate (Ritalin), or amphetamines; planned naps during the day may prevent sleep attacks

Insomnia

A. Causes
1. Acute or transient insomnia is usually due to psychological stress or travel over time zones ("jet lag")
2. Chronic causes
   a. Secondary insomnia accounts for over 90% of all cases
      - Psychiatric conditions—depression, anxiety disorders, posttraumatic stress disorder, manic phase of bipolar disorder, schizophrenia, obsessive-compulsive disorder
      - Medications and substance abuse—alcohol, sedatives (with prolonged use, patients develop tolerance and withdrawal rebound insomnia), caffeine, β-blockers, stimulant drugs (amphetamines), decongestants, some SSRIs, nicotine
      - Medical problems—advanced COPD, renal failure, CHF, chronic pain
      - Other—fibromyalgia, chronic fatigue syndrome (CFS)

   b. Primary insomnia is a diagnosis of exclusion. The DSM-5 defines it as dissatisfaction with sleep and one of the following: difficulty initiating sleep, difficulty maintaining sleep, or early-morning awakenings and an inability to fall back asleep
      - Nonrestorative sleep that occurs three nights per week for at least 3 months in the absence of other medical, psychiatric, or other sleep disorders, and that causes clinically significant distress and social or occupational impairment
      - Patients worry excessively about not falling to sleep and become preoccupied with it. The cause is unknown

B. Treatment
1. Treat the underlying cause, if found.
2. Consider a psychiatric evaluation if psychiatric causes or primary insomnia is suspected.
3. Use sedative-hypnotic medications sparingly and with caution for symptomatic relief. Use the smallest dose possible, and avoid use for longer than 2 to 3 weeks.

Quick HIT

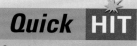

Questions to ask the patient with insomnia—sleep history, timing of insomnia, sleep habits

Miscellaneous Topics

Obesity

A. General
1. Considered to be a global epidemic, particularly in developed nations

2. Health hazards associated with obesity: HTN, heart disease, hyperlipidemia, type 2 diabetes, stroke, heart disease, osteoarthritis, liver disease, cancer, OSA, obesity hypoventilation syndrome, and depression
3. Obesity is associated with a significant increase in mortality
4. Body Mass Index (BMI) = weight divided by height squared (kg/m^2)
   a. Normal: BMI of 18.5 to 24.9
   b. Overweight: 25 to 29.9
   c. Obese: 30 and over
      - Obesity class I: 30 to 34.9
      - Obesity class II: 35 to 39.9
      - Obesity class III: 40 and over

B. Treatment

1. Diet, exercise, lifestyle modification are mainstays of treatment.
2. Drug therapy—for patients who have not succeeded in losing weight with diet and exercise. Orlistat is a first-line agent and can be continued for up to 4 years.
3. Bariatric surgery.
   a. Bariatric surgery is effective in reducing comorbidities associated with obesity, including HTN, diabetes, OSA, and hyperlipidemia. This translates into a 29% reduction in mortality. Only indicated in patients who have earnestly tried other means of losing weight and have been unsuccessful.
   b. Best evidence is for patients with BMI over 40.
   c. Bariatric surgery is based on two mechanisms: restriction of intake (via a small stomach reservoir) and malabsorption (via decreasing small bowel length). Restrictive techniques are technically easier, have lower complication rates, but result in less weight loss than malabsorptive techniques.
   d. Most common procedure is the laparoscopic Roux-en-Y gastric bypass. The laparoscopic adjustable gastric banding (LapBand) has fewer complications, is reversible, but is not as effective in achieving weight loss as compared with the gastric bypass.

Hearing Loss/Impaired Hearing

A. General characteristics—two types of hearing loss

1. Conductive hearing loss
   a. **Caused by lesions in the external or middle ear**
   b. Interference with mechanical reception or amplification of sound, as occurs with disease of the auditory canal, tympanic membrane, or ossicles, creates conductive hearing loss
2. Sensorineural hearing loss—due to lesions in the cochlea or CN VIII (auditory branch)

> **Quick HIT**
>
> **Tympanic Membrane Perforation**
> - History: pain, conductive hearing loss, tinnitus
> - Examination: bleeding from the ear, clot in the meatus, visible tear in the tympanic membrane
> - Ninety percent heal spontaneously within 6 weeks. Surgery is appropriate for larger perforations.

B. Causes

1. Conductive hearing loss
   a. External canal
      - Cerumen impaction—buildup obstructs the auditory canal (most common cause)
      - Otitis externa
      - Exostoses—bony outgrowths of external auditory canal related to repetitive exposure to cold water (e.g., scuba divers, swimmers)
   b. Tympanic membrane perforation
      - Usually due to trauma (direct or indirect)
      - May be secondary to middle ear infection
   c. Middle ear
      - Any cause of middle ear effusion (fluid in middle ear interferes with sound conduction)—otitis media, allergic rhinitis
      - Otosclerosis—bony fusion (immobilization) of the stapes to the oval window; an autosomal dominant condition (variable penetrance); corrected with surgery; rarely progresses to deafness
      - Other—neoplasms, congenital malformation of the middle ear

2. Sensorineural hearing loss
   a. Presbycusis (most common cause)
      - Gradual, symmetric hearing loss associated with aging—most common cause of diminished hearing in elderly patients
      - Pathology—degeneration of sensory cells and nerve fibers at the base of the cochlea
      - Hearing loss is most marked at high frequencies with slow progression to lower frequencies
   b. Noise-induced hearing loss
      - Chronic, prolonged exposure to sound levels >85 dB
      - Hair cells in the organ of Corti are damaged
   c. Infection—viral or bacterial infection of cochlear structures or labyrinth
   d. Drug-induced hearing loss
      - Aminoglycoside antibiotics, furosemide, ethacrynic acid; cisplatin, quinidine
      - Aspirin can cause tinnitus and reversible hearing impairment
   e. Injury to inner ear or cochlear nerve (e.g., skull fracture)
   f. Congenital (TORCH infections)
   g. Ménière disease
      - Fluctuating, unilateral hearing loss
      - Sensorineural hearing loss (usually unilateral), sense of pressure/fullness in ear, tinnitus, vertigo
      - Vertigo usually responds to dietary salt restriction and meclizine, but hearing loss is progressive
   h. CNS causes—acoustic neuromas, meningitis, auditory nerve neuritis (multiple sclerosis, syphilis), meningioma

C. Clinical features

1. Conductive hearing loss
   a. Decreased perception of sound (especially for low-frequency sounds)
   b. Can hear loud noises well
2. Sensorineural hearing loss
   a. Difficulty hearing loud noises; shouting may exacerbate the problem (annoyed by loud speech)
   b. Can hear sounds, but has trouble deciphering words (poor speech discrimination)
   c. More difficulty with high-frequency sounds (doorbells, phones, child's voice, female voice)
   d. Tinnitus is often present

D. Diagnosis

1. Whisper test—Ask the patient to repeat words whispered into the tested ear (mask the other ear) (see Clinical Pearl 12-11)
2. An audiogram is an essential component of the evaluation
3. MRI—in selected cases (e.g., if CNS tumor or multiple sclerosis is suspected)

Quick HIT

Hearing Impairment
- History: medications; history of head trauma, infection (otitis media, otitis externa); noise exposure (occupational or recreational)
- Physical examination: inspect auditory canal (impacted cerumen, exostoses); examine tympanic membrane (inflammation, perforation, scarring); assess middle ear (fluid)

CLINICAL PEARL 12-11

Rinne and Weber Tests

- Conductive loss
  - Abnormal Rinne test—bone conduction is better than air conduction
  - Weber—**sound lateralizes to the affected side** (tuning fork is perceived more loudly in the ear with a conductive hearing loss)
- Sensorineural loss
  - Normal Rinne test—air conduction is better than bone conduction
  - Weber—**sound lateralizes to the unaffected side**

E. Treatment

1. Cerumen impaction is best treated by irrigation after several days of softening with carbamide peroxide (Debrox) or triethanolamine (Cerumenex)
2. Conductive hearing loss
   a. Treat underlying cause
   b. Surgical techniques such as tympanoplasty (reconstructs middle ear) for patients with chronic otitis media; stapedectomy for otosclerosis
   c. Hearing aids
3. Sensorineural hearing loss
   a. Treat underlying cause
   b. Hearing aids
   c. Cochlear implants—transduce sounds to electrical energy, stimulates CN VIII

Urinary Incontinence

Quick HIT

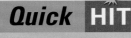

The most common cause of incontinence in elderly patients is urge incontinence. In women <70 years of age, the most common cause is stress incontinence.

A. General characteristics

1. There are five major types of incontinence (urge, stress, overflow, functional, and mixed). Many patients have more than one type.
2. Male incontinence is usually due to BPH or neurologic disease. A urology evaluation is indicated in incontinent male patients.
3. Female incontinence is usually due to hormonal changes, pelvic floor dysfunction or laxity, or uninhibited bladder contractions (detrusor contractions) due to aging.

Quick HIT

Evaluating a Patient with Urinary Incontinence
Inquire about the history of diabetes, multiple sclerosis, Parkinson disease, stroke, spinal cord injury or disease, and pelvic surgery.

B. Risk factors

1. Age—diminished size of bladder, earlier detrusor contractions, postmenopausal genitourinary atrophy
2. Recurrent urinary tract infections
3. Immobility, decreased mental status, dementia, stroke, Parkinson disease, depression
4. DM, CHF
5. Multiparity, history of prolonged labor
6. Pelvic floor dysfunction in women, BPH, and prostate cancer in men
7. Medications
   a. Diuretics increase bladder filling, increasing the episodes of incontinence
   b. Anticholinergics and adrenergics cause urinary retention
   c. β-Blockers diminish sphincter tone
   d. Calcium channel blockers and narcotics can decrease detrusor contraction
   e. Alcohol, sedatives, hypnotics (depress mentation)

Quick HIT

- If urgency of urination is the prominent finding, suspect urge incontinence.
- If increased intra-abdominal pressure (cough, laugh) causes urine loss, suspect stress incontinence.

Quick HIT

Elderly women commonly have both urge and stress incontinence.

Ambulatory Medicine

C. Types of urinary incontinence

1. Urge incontinence (also called detrusor instability)
   a. Most common type in elderly and nursing-home patients
   b. Multiple causes (often idiopathic), including dementia, strokes, severe illness, Parkinson disease
   c. Mechanism: involuntary and uninhibited detrusor contractions result in involuntary loss of urine
   d. Clinical features: This is characterized by a sudden urge to urinate (e.g., patients are unable to make it to the bathroom), a loss of large volumes of urine with small postvoid residual, and nocturnal wetting
   e. Diagnostic study of choice is urodynamic study
   f. Management is initially with bladder-training exercises (the goal being to increase the amount of time between voiding). If this is unsuccessful, medications include anticholinergic medications (oxybutynin) and TCAs (imipramine).
2. Stress incontinence
   a. Occurs mostly in women (after multiple deliveries of children)
   b. Mechanism: Weakness of the pelvic diaphragm (pelvic floor) leads to loss of bladder support (with resultant hypermobility of the bladder neck). This causes the proximal urethra to descend below the pelvic floor so that an increase in

intra-abdominal pressure is transmitted mostly to the bladder (instead of an equal transmission to the bladder and urethra)

c. Clinical features: involuntary urine loss (only in spurts) during activities that increase intra-abdominal pressure (cough, laugh, sneeze, exercise); small post-void volume
d. Rule out infection with a urinalysis
e. Management: Kegel exercises (multiple contractions of pelvic floor muscles as if patient were interrupting flow of urine) to strengthen pelvic floor musculature; estrogen replacement therapy; use of a pessary; surgery (there are various options, and a popular option is the midurethral sling)

3. Overflow incontinence
   a. Common in diabetic patients and patients with neurologic disorders
   b. Mechanism: Inadequate bladder contraction (due to impaired detrusor contractility) or a bladder outlet obstruction leads to urinary retention and subsequent overdistention of the bladder. Bladder pressure increases until it exceeds urethral resistance, and urine leakage occurs
   c. Causes: neurogenic bladder (diabetic patients, lower motor neuron lesions), medications (anticholinergics, α-agonists, and epidural/spinal anesthetics), **obstruction to urine flow** (BPH, prostate cancer, urethral strictures, severe constipation with fecal impaction)
   d. Clinical features: nocturnal wetting, frequent loss of small amount of urine; large postvoid residual (usually exceeds 100 mL)
   e. Management (primarily medical): intermittent self-catheterization is the best management; cholinergic agents (e.g., bethanechol) to increase bladder contractions; α-blockers (e.g., terazosin, doxazosin) to decrease sphincter resistance
4. Functional incontinence—secondary to disabling and debilitating diseases

D. Diagnosis

1. Urinalysis (all patients)—to exclude infection and hematuria
2. Postvoid urine catheterization—record the residual volume. Normal residual volume is less than 50 mL. A urine volume greater than 50 mL may indicate urinary obstruction or a hypotonic bladder
3. Urine cultures—if dysuria and positive urinalysis (WBCs in urine)
4. Renal function studies (BUN/Cr), glucose levels
5. Voiding record is useful—time, volume of episodes, record of oral intake, medications, associated activities
6. Perform further testing in carefully selected patients in whom the cause is not identified. Tests include cystometry, uroflow measurement/urethral pressure profile, imaging studies such as intravenous pyelogram, and voiding cystourethrogram, as needed

Quick HIT

Laboratory studies in workup of fatigue:
- CBC (anemia)
- TSH (hypothyroidism)
- Fasting glucose (diabetes mellitus)
- BMP (electrolyte abnormalities)
- Urinalysis, BUN/creatinine (renal disease)
- LFT (liver disease)

Fatigue

A. General characteristics

1. Fatigue refers to a lack of energy or a sense of being tired—differentiate this from muscular weakness. It is not directly related to exertion
2. Differential diagnosis
   a. Psychiatric causes—depression (most common cause); anxiety and somatization
   b. Endocrine causes—hypothyroidism, poorly controlled DM, apathetic hyperthyroidism of elderly patients, Addison disease, hypopituitarism, hyperparathyroidism, and other causes of hypercalcemia
   c. Hematologic/oncologic causes—severe anemia, occult malignancy (e.g., pancreatic carcinoma)
   d. Metabolic causes—chronic renal failure, hepatocellular failure
   e. Infectious diseases—mononucleosis, viral hepatitis, HIV, syphilis, hepatitis B and C, CMV, parasitic disease, tuberculosis and subacute bacterial endocarditis, Lyme disease
   f. Cardiopulmonary disease—OSA, CHF

Quick HIT

Etiology of Chronic Fatigue
- Only 5% of cases are diagnosed as CFS.
- Most cases of chronic fatigue are due to depression, anxiety, or both (up to two-thirds of cases).
- Between 20% and 25% of cases are idiopathic, yet do not fit the criteria for CFS.
- Less than 5% are due to an unidentified medical illness.

g. Medications—antihypertensive medications (clonidine, methyldopa), antidepressants (amitriptyline, doxepin, trazodone are more sedating), hypnotics, β-blockers, antihistamines, drug abuse/withdrawal
h. Other causes: CFS, fibromyalgia, sleep disturbances (sleep apnea, narcolepsy, insomnia)

3. CFS
   a. CFS is profound fatigue for longer than 6 months that is not due to a medical or psychiatric disorder. More common in women
   b. Cause is unknown. A flu-like illness may act as the triggering event, but infection has not been established as the proven cause. Other theories point to immunologic disturbance or endocrine dysfunction as possible causes
   c. CFS is a diagnosis of exclusion—rule out other causes before making a diagnosis of CFS
   d. Most patients experience partial recovery within 2 years, but relapses can occur at any time
   e. There are specific criteria for diagnosis. The key features include:
      - New or definite onset of unexplained fatigue, not alleviated by rest, not due to exertion, and significantly affecting quality of life
      - Four or more of the following symptoms (for at least 6 months): diminished short-term memory or concentration, muscle pain, sore throat, tender lymph nodes, unrefreshing sleep, joint pain (without redness/swelling), headaches, postexertional malaise for longer than 24 hours
   f. Depression is common in patients with CFS

B. Diagnosis

1. Basic laboratory tests to exclude other causes—consider CBC, LFTs, serum electrolytes, calcium, TSH, erythrocyte sedimentation rate, and HIV testing (if indicated).
2. Extensive testing other than the above is not indicated.

C. Treatment

1. Treat the underlying disorder, if known
2. Treat CFS and patients with idiopathic fatigue as follows:
   a. Cognitive behavioral therapy, including exercise, social, and psychological behavior modifications
   b. Antidepressants, as appropriate
   c. NSAIDs for relief of headache, arthralgias

••• Erectile Dysfunction

A. General characteristics

1. Erectile dysfunction is the recurring inability to achieve and maintain an erection sufficient for satisfactory sexual performance.
2. It is thought that up to half of all men in the United States between the ages of 40 and 70 have some form of erectile dysfunction. Prevalence increases with age.
3. Pathophysiology—once thought to be psychogenic in origin, it is now known that most cases (80%) are organic. A normal erection is largely dependent on the healthy penile and systemic vasculature.
4. Some cases of erectile dysfunction are psychogenic.

B. Risk factors

1. The most important risk factors are those that contribute to atherosclerosis (e.g., HTN, smoking, hyperlipidemia, diabetes)
2. Medications—antihypertensives (may indirectly lower intracavernosal pressure by virtue of lowering systemic BP)
3. Hematologic—sickle cell disease
4. History of pelvic surgery or perineal trauma
5. Alcohol abuse
6. Any cause of hypogonadism/low testosterone state, including hypothyroidism
7. Congenital penile curvature

C. Diagnosis

1. Detailed history and examination, including a digital rectal examination and neurologic examination. Assess for signs of PAD.
2. Laboratory tests—Obtain a CBC, chemistry panel, fasting glucose, and lipid profile. If there is hypogonadism or loss of libido, order serum testosterone, prolactin levels, and thyroid profile.
3. Nocturnal penile tumescence—If normal erections occur during sleep, a psychogenic cause is likely. If not, the cause is probably organic.
4. Consider vascular testing—Evaluate arterial inflow and venous trapping of blood. Tests include intracavernosal injection of vasoactive substances, duplex ultrasound, and arteriography.
5. Psychologic testing may be appropriate in some cases.

D. Treatment

1. Treat the underlying cause. Address atherosclerotic risk factors.
2. First-line treatment is with phosphodiesterase inhibitors such as sildenafil citrate (Viagra), which acts by increasing cGMP levels causing increased nitric oxide release and penile smooth muscle relaxation. It can be taken 30 to 60 minutes before anticipated intercourse. It is contraindicated with use of nitrates because together they can cause profound hypotension.
3. Intracavernosal injections of vasoactive agents (patient learns to self-administer).
4. Vacuum constriction devices are rings placed around the base of the penis that enhance venous trapping of blood; they may interfere with ejaculation.
5. Psychologic therapy may be indicated to reduce performance anxiety and address underlying factors that may be causing or contributing to erectile dysfunction.
6. Hormonal replacement (e.g., testosterone) in patients with documented hypogonadism.
7. Penile implants for patients who have not responded to the above.

Alcoholism

A. General characteristics

1. Ten to fifteen percent of people have alcoholism (alcohol abuse or dependence). There is a **genetic component** to alcoholism—close relatives of alcoholics (especially sons) are at increased risk for alcoholism
2. Screening for alcoholism—ask all patients about alcohol use. If alcoholism is suspected, use one of the following screening methods
   a. CAGE (Any more than one positive answer may suggest alcohol abuse)
      - Cut down? (Have you ever felt the need to cut down on your drinking?)
      - Annoyed? (Have you ever felt annoyed by criticisms of your drinking?)
      - Guilty? (Have you ever felt guilty about drinking?)
      - Eye-opener? (Have you ever taken a morning eye-opener?)

   b. MAST (Michigan Alcoholism Screening Test) questionnaire—a 25-item questionnaire that also helps identify alcoholism

B. Complications

1. GI—gastritis, esophagitis, PUD, alcoholic liver disease (alcoholic hepatitis, cirrhosis, portal HTN), pancreatitis (acute and chronic), Mallory–Weiss tears
2. Cardiac—alcoholic cardiomyopathy, essential HTN (more than three drinks per day significantly increases BP)
3. CNS
   a. **Wernicke encephalopathy**—often reversible
      - Caused by thiamine deficiency
      - Manifests as nystagmus, ataxia, ophthalmoplegia, confusion
      - Can be precipitated by administering glucose in alcoholics without first giving thiamine replacement

   b. **Korsakoff psychosis**—irreversible
      - Caused by thiamine deficiency

Quick HIT

Alcohol and Lipid Levels
Modest alcohol intake (maximum of 1 to 2 drinks per day) is associated with an increase in HDL. On the other hand, alcohol use increases TG levels.

Quick HIT

Laboratory Findings in Alcoholics
- Anemia
- Macrocytic (most common)—due to folate deficiency
- Microcytic—due to GI bleeding
- LFTs—increased GGT; AST–ALT ratio is 2:1
- Hypertriglyceridemia
- Hyperuricemia, hypocalcemia
- Thiamine deficiency
- Decreased testosterone level

CLINICAL PEARL 12-12

Alcohol Withdrawal

- Features include tachycardia, sweating, anxiety, hallucinations.
- Goal is to prevent progression to delirium tremens (DT), which is a medical emergency (mortality rate, 20%). DT occurs in 5% of alcoholic withdrawals.
- DT is delirium developing within a week of the last alcohol intake, usually 2 to 4 days after the last drink. DT is characterized by tactile hallucinations, visual hallucinations, confusion, sweating, increased tachycardia, and elevated BP.
- Risk factors are pancreatitis, hepatitis, or other illness. DT is rare in healthy people.
- Give benzodiazepines if withdrawal symptoms are present. Prevention of DT is the best treatment.
- Diet is important in treatment (high in calorie, high in carbohydrates, multivitamins).

  - Alcohol-induced amnestic disorder
  - Mostly affects short-term memory; confabulation is common

4. Pulmonary—pneumonia, aspiration
5. Nutritional deficiencies (vitamins, minerals)—especially thiamine deficiency, hypomagnesemia, and folate deficiency
6. Peripheral neuropathy—due to thiamine deficiency
7. Sexual dysfunction—impotence, loss of libido
8. Psychiatric—depression, anxiety, insomnia
9. Increased risk of malignancy—esophagus, oral, liver, lung
10. Frequent falls, minor injuries, **motor vehicle accidents**

C. Treatment

1. Alcoholics Anonymous (AA) (see also Clinical Pearl 12-12)
2. Naltrexone is a good first-line drug that improves abstinence rates by reducing the craving for alcohol
3. Acamprosate is another first-line drug that is a good option in patients with liver disease (naltrexone contraindicated)
4. Other options: baclofen, disulfiram, topiramate, gabapentin, SSRIs, and ondansetron
   a. Disulfiram (Antabuse) inhibits aldehyde dehydrogenase and leads to the accumulation of acetaldehyde. A few minutes after drinking alcohol, patient experiences shortness of breath, flushing, palpitations, and tachycardia. If more alcohol is taken, headache and nausea/vomiting ensue. Symptoms last about 90 minutes. It is appropriate for short-term use and should not be taken chronically. It is contraindicated in patients with heart disease
5. Drugs for withdrawal—benzodiazepines—best to use long-acting agents (diazepam)
6. Correction of fluid imbalance, vitamin supplementation (thiamine, folate, multivitamins)

Smoking

A. Health risks associated with cigarette smoking

1. Cardiovascular disease—CAD, acute MI, and stroke; there is a dose-dependent relationship between smoking and cardiovascular disease
2. COPD risk increases with smoking in a dose-dependent manner
3. Malignancy—smoking increases the risk of lung cancer, head and neck cancer, GI cancers (laryngeal/pharyngeal, esophageal, gastric, pancreatic, hepatic, colorectal), GU cancers (renal, ureter, bladder, penile, cervical), and myeloid leukemia
4. PUD
5. Osteoporosis—decreases peak bone mass and increases the rate of bone loss
6. Premature skin aging
7. PAD, Buerger disease

8. Adverse effects during pregnancy—smoking increases the risk of spontaneous abortion, fetal death, neonatal death, sudden infant death syndrome, and low birth weight
9. Infections, especially respiratory

B. Smoking cessation

1. Varenicline—partial agonist at the α-4–β-2 subunit of the nicotinic acetylcholine receptor. Its efficacy has been demonstrated in several randomized controlled trials. Considered first-line therapy (nicotine replacement is the alternative).
2. Nicotine replacement therapy.
   a. Both a long-acting agent (nicotine patch) and a short-acting agent (nicotine gum or lozenge) should be used together for higher quit rates.
   b. Nicotine patch.
      - Quit rates are 2.5 times higher at 6 months than with placebo.
      - Continuous nicotine delivery weans the patient from nicotine, and the dose is gradually decreased. There are no peaks or troughs as associated with smoking, so it eliminates nicotine withdrawal symptoms.
      - The patch should be worn for 16 hours per day (should not be worn during sleep at night because it can cause headaches). The strongest dose (21-mg patch) is used for 1 month or so, then is gradually tapered to a lower dose (14-mg patch) for a few weeks, and finally to the lowest dose (7-mg patch) for a few weeks. Once the habit is broken, the patch use is stopped.
      - **The patient should not continue to smoke while using the patch** (there have been case reports of MIs in these patients).
   c. Nicotine chewing gum or lozenge.
      - Gum is used whenever there is an urge to smoke. Use is continued for 2 to 4 months.
3. Bupropion (Zyban).
   a. Quit rates are similar to that of nicotine replacement therapy (twice that of placebo).
   b. The patient continues treatment for up to 2 months.
   c. The patient can take bupropion in combination with nicotine replacement therapy—combined use may result in higher quit rates than either method alone.
   d. Adverse effects may include dry mouth, insomnia, and headaches.

Quick HIT

Most important causes of smoking-related mortality are lung cancer, COPD, and ASCVD.

Quick HIT

Behavioral modification is crucial for long-term smoking cessation. The patch or gum should be used in conjunction with a smoking withdrawal clinic (behavioral program). Quit rates are higher with this combination.

Health Maintenance

A. Screening for hypertension

1. The United States Preventive Services Task Force (USPSTF) recommends screening all adults 18 years of age and older for HTN. However, other authorities do not recommend screening for HTN until middle age.
2. The recommended interval is 2 years for adults with a normal BP, and 1 year for adults with prehypertension.

B. Screening for hyperlipidemia

1. USPSTF 2008 guidelines recommend screening all men ≥35 and women at risk for CAD ≥45 (grade A); the guidelines also recommend screening men aged 20 to 35 at increased risk for CAD and women aged 20 to 45 at increased risk for CAD (grade B).
2. ACC/AHA 2013 guidelines state that it is reasonable to assess cardiovascular disease risk in healthy patients aged 20 to 79 every 4 to 6 years.
3. **Measure a nonfasting total cholesterol and HDL cholesterol every 5 years.**
   a. If total cholesterol is <200 mg/dL and HDL is >35 mg/dL, repeat screening in 5 years.
   b. If total cholesterol is >240 mg/dL **or** between 200 and 240 with multiple risk factors, get a complete lipoprotein profile (TG levels and calculation of LDL).
   c. Calculating LDL level is not necessary for screening.

Quick HIT

For CRC screening, a colonoscopy is equivalent to flexible sigmoidoscopy plus barium enema but is more expensive.

Quick HIT

Colonoscopy is the best of all colon cancer screening methods. Sigmoidoscopy will miss 40% of cancers. Fecal occult blood testing will detect cancer but if positive, a colonoscopy is needed.

   d. Screen more frequently if the patient has increased risk of CAD (e.g., smokers, diabetic patients, family history of CAD, HTN).
4. Adults with CAD—obtain a complete lipoprotein profile.

C. Colorectal cancer screening/surveillance

1. Average-risk patients 50 to 75 years of age—**any** of the following (USPSTF 2008 guidelines):
   a. Colonoscopy every 10 years
   b. Flexible sigmoidoscopy every 5 years and fecal occult blood test every 3 years
   c. **Fecal occult blood test every year**
2. Moderate-risk patients
   a. Patients with single or multiple polyps, personal history of CRC—initial colonoscopy; repeat at 3 years—if normal, then colonoscopy every 5 years
   b. Family history of CRC or adenomatous polyps in first-degree relatives—colonoscopy at age 40 or 10 years younger than the youngest case in family; if normal, repeat in 3 to 5 years
3. High-risk patients
   a. Families with familial adenomatous polyposis—genetic testing at age 10; consider colectomy if positive genetic testing or polyposis is confirmed; if not, colonoscopy every 1 to 2 years beginning at puberty
   b. Families with hereditary nonpolyposis CRC—genetic testing at age 21; if positive, colonoscopy every 2 years until age 40, and then every year thereafter
   c. Patients with ulcerative colitis—colonoscopy 8 years after disease onset, then every year thereafter

D. Prostate cancer screening

1. **This is controversial**
2. The USPSTF now recommends against prostate cancer screening with prostate-specific antigen (PSA)
3. Other groups state that there is insufficient evidence for or against screening with PSA, and that the physician should engage the patient in the decision to screen

E. Lung cancer screening

1. **USPSTF 2013 guidelines—High-risk adults 55 to 80 years of age should receive an annual low-dose CT scan.**
   a. **High-risk adults are those with a 30 pack-year smoking history and who are currently smoking or quit within the past 15 years; once the patient has stopped smoking for >15 years, annual screening can be discontinued.**

F. Women's health

1. Breast cancer
   a. USPSTF—**Mammogram every 2 years for women 50 to 74 years of age**
      - In agreement with the American College of Physicians and American Academy of Family Physicians
   b. American Cancer Society, National Cancer Institute, National Comprehensive Cancer Network, American College of Obstetricians and Gynecologists, American Medical Association: recommend routine screening every year starting at the age of 40
   c. Recommendations for clinical breast examination (CBE) and breast self-examination (BSE) vary based on expert group recommendations; USPSTF states that there is insufficient evidence to recommend for or against CBE, and some groups (e.g., WHO) recommend against BSE
2. Cervical cancer
   a. **Start at age 21, irrespective of sexual history**
   b. **Age 21 to 29, Pap smear every 3 years**
   c. **Age 30 to 65, Pap smear every 3 years or Pap smear + HPV testing every 5 years**
   d. **Can discontinue screening at age 65 if adequate negative prior screening (3 negative Pap smears or 2 negative Pap smears with negative HPV testing**

TABLE 12-9 Vaccines

Vaccine	Recommended Recipients	Schedule	Contraindications
Influenza	All patients older than 6 mo	Given annually Best time to administer vaccine is October to November, but can also be given any time during flu season	Standard contraindications[a] History of severe anaphylaxis to eggs should receive an egg-free inactivated vaccine. The live attenuated intranasal vaccine should not be given to immunocompromised patients, pregnant patients, or patients above the age of 50.
Pneumococcal polysaccharide (PPSV23) and conjugate (PCV13)	Adults >65 yrs of age (PPSV23) Adults aged 19-64 with an immunocompromising condition, asplenia, advanced kidney disease, CSF leak, or cochlear implants (PCV13 followed by PPSV23 8 wks later) Adults with other chronic medical problems (e.g., COPD, diabetes) should received PPSV23 before the age of 65	Administered as a one-time dose Second dose should be administered 5 yrs after the first dose for patients at highest risk (e.g., those with asplenia, immunodeficiency, kidney disease, etc.)	Standard contraindications
Tetanus/diphtheria (Td) and tetanus/diphtheria/acellular pertussis (Tdap)	Primary series for everyone When indicated in wound management Individuals traveling to countries where risk of diphtheria is high	Primary series: Three doses (1, 1–2, 6–12 mo) After primary series, booster dose q 10 yrs; those aged 19 and older should receive 1 booster dose of Tdap in replacement of Td For the unvaccinated, three doses (0, 1–2 mo, 6–12 mo intervals)	Standard contraindications
Zoster (varicella)	Adults >60 yrs of age	One-time vaccination, regardless of prior herpes zoster episode	Standard contraindications Pregnancy Significant immunocompromise[c]
Hepatitis B	Given as primary series to infants Patients at risk for HBV[b] Healthcare workers	Given as three doses (0, 1, 6 mo)	Standard contraindications
Hepatitis A	Travelers to developing countries Patients with chronic liver disease, HCV MSM	Given in two doses at least 6 mo apart	Standard contraindications
Measles–mumps—rubella (live vaccine)	Given as primary series in children Adults born after 1957 who are ≥18 yrs of age (those born before 1957 are considered immune) if there is no proof of vaccination or immunity All women of childbearing age without proof of rubella immunity or vaccination Healthcare workers	Given as one or two doses Give the second dose at least 4 wks after the first dose	Standard contraindications Pregnancy Significant immunocompromise[c]

(continued)

TABLE 12-9 Vaccines (continued)

Vaccine	Recommended Recipients	Schedule	Contraindications
Varicella (live vaccine)	Given as primary series in children Adults and adolescents who never had chickenpox (chickenpox confers immunity) Susceptible, close contacts of immunocompromised patients Postexposure prophylaxis in susceptible individuals	Given as two doses, with second dose given 4–8 wks after first dose	Standard contraindications Pregnancy Significant immunocompromise[c]
Meningococcus (serotypes A, C, W-135, and Y)	Asplenic individuals Travelers to area where meningococcal disease is epidemic Military personnel All college students Close contacts of patients with sporadic disease	Given as one dose to most Given as two doses to asplenic patients or those with complement deficiencies Repeat vaccination every 5 yrs for those who remain at high risk	Standard contraindications
HPV vaccine (human papilloma virus)	Recommended for men and women aged 9–26 (but should be routinely given at age 11–12) For men, catch up vaccination recommended from ages 13–21, and up to age 26 in MSM	Given as three doses	Standard contraindications
Polio (inactivated)	Given as primary series in children Not routinely given to unvaccinated adults unless they plan to travel to endemic areas	Refer to ACIP guidelines for schedules and dosing information	Standard contraindications
Rabies	See Chapter 10 Postexposure prophylaxis Individuals at high risk for exposure to rabies		

[a]Standard contraindications include a history of anaphylactic reaction to the vaccine as well as moderate to severe illness. Mild illness is not a contraindication. Unless specified, breastfeeding is not a contraindication to vaccine.

[b]Patients at risk for HBV include injection drug users, MSM, heterosexuals who have had more than one sex partner in the past 6 mo, patients recently diagnosed with STIs, sexual partners of HB_sAg-positive patients, and patients with end-stage renal disease.

[c]Note that HIV positivity is not a contraindication to live vaccines unless the patient is severely immunocompromised (CD4 count <200).

Remember that functionally or anatomically asplenic individuals are at risk for infection with encapsulated organisms, so they should receive the *H. influenzae* type B (HIB), meningococcal, and pneumococcal vaccines.

within the previous 10 years, with the most recent test within the previous 5 years)

3. Ovarian cancer
   a. Routine screening is not recommended

G. Sexually transmitted infections

1. All men and women aged 15 to 65 years should be screened for HIV; more frequent screening should be offered for those at risk.
2. All sexually active women <24 years old should be screened for chlamydia and gonorrhea. Insufficient evidence to make these recommendations for men.
3. Asymptomatic men and women with risk factors should be screened for syphilis.

H. Miscellaneous

1. Screening for diabetes mellitus:
   a. The USPSTF in 2008 claimed that there was insufficient evidence to screen nonpregnant, nonhypertensive (<135/80 mm Hg) patients; however, these guidelines are being updated in 2014.
   b. The American Diabetes Association recommends screening all adults with a BMI ≥25 kg/m^2 and at least one risk factor for diabetes every 3 years with hemoglobin A1c, fasting plasma glucose, or a 2-hour oral glucose tolerance test (OGTT). Adults without risk factors should be screened starting at the age of 45.
2. The USPSTF recommends screening for hepatitis B virus in patients at risk—injection drug users, men who have sex with men (MSM), hemodialysis.
3. The USPSTF recommends screening for hepatitis C virus in patients at risk and a one-time screening in patients born between 1945 and 1965.
4. In elderly patients, assess risk factors for PAD, osteoporosis, stroke, and CAD.
5. Osteoporosis—DEXA scan starting at age 65 in women (see osteoporosis section for details).
6. AAA screening with a one-time ultrasound in men aged 65 to 75 who have ever smoked.
7. The USPSTF recommends screening all adults for depression and alcohol misuse (and providing appropriate treatment and follow-up). The USPSTF does not recommend for or against screening for dementia.
8. Routine screening for thyroid disease is not recommended by the USPSTF, though some expert groups recommend it.

Quick HIT

Remember that functionally or anatomically asplenic individuals are at risk for infection with encapsulated organisms, so they should receive the *H. influenzae* type B (HIB) vaccine, and meningococcal and pneumococcal vaccines.

I. Vaccinations

1. Vaccination is most commonly associated with children but is very important in adults as well, especially elderly patients and those with chronic medical problems.
2. The most important vaccinations to know are influenza, pneumococcal polysaccharide, hepatitis B, and tetanus; for who should receive them and when, see Table 12-9.
3. Meningococcal vaccine is indicated for adults with asplenia, military recruits, residents of college dormitories, terminal complement deficiency, travelers to Mecca or Medina in Saudi Arabia for the Hajj.
4. Hepatitis A and B vaccines are indicated in adults with chronic liver disease, homosexual men, injection drug users, and household contacts with hepatitis A or B.
5. There are many misconceptions about contraindications to vaccination. The following are **not** contraindications to vaccination.
   a. Mild illness (e.g., common cold, low-grade fever, mild diarrhea).
   b. Convalescent phase of an illness.
   c. Recent exposure to a communicable disease.
   d. Breastfeeding.
   e. Current antibiotic therapy.
   f. History of a nonspecific reaction to penicillin.

Quick HIT

Most important vaccines in adults are influenza and pneumococcus.

APPENDIX

Radiographic Interpretation

Chest Radiograph

A. Views: Obtain PA and lateral views for all patients who are well enough to be transported to the radiology department and maintain an upright position. Obtain an AP film (i.e., portable chest radiograph [CXR]) for all patients who are too ill to be transported and positioned for a PA film.

B. Always try to compare a patient's CXR with a previous film to note any changes in condition and to assess whether changes are new or chronic.

C. Density: The lower the density, the more radiolucent (or transparent) the object will appear on plain radiographs. Following are structures in the body (main composition) listed from most radiolucent to most radiopaque: Air (lungs, trachea, gastric bubble), fat (breasts), fluid (most of the structures have high fluid content [e.g., vessels, heart, soft tissues]), bone, metallic foreign bodies (e.g., bullets, orthopedic hardware).

D. Assessment of the film's quality.

1. Assess penetration.
   a. The intervertebral spaces should be visible on a good-quality film.
   b. The outline of the vertebral bodies should be visible within (or through) the cardiac silhouette.
2. Assess inspiratory effort.
   a. A CXR is usually taken at the end of a full, deep inspiration. You should be able to see at least nine posterior ribs on the right side above the diaphragm. In general, if the diaphragm is crossing the tenth rib posteriorly (or the eighth rib anteriorly), inspiratory effort is optimal.
   b. Patients who are ill may not be able to hold a full, deep breath for the CXR, leading to a poor inspiratory effort.
   c. The heart appears larger than it actually is when there is poor inspiratory effort, which can be misleading.
3. Assess for rotation.
   a. There should be symmetrical spacing of the clavicles on either side of the sternum, otherwise the patient is probably rotated.
   b. Imagine a horizontal line connecting the clavicular heads and a vertical line down the midline connecting the spinous processes of the vertebrae—these lines should be perpendicular to one another.

E. Examination of the PA/AP CXR (Figure A-1): No one approach is standard. Be sure to observe the following points:

1. Examine bones: shoulders, clavicles, cervical and thoracic spine, and ribs—on PA films, the horizontal ribs are posterior (anterior ribs are angled downward).
2. Evaluate cardiac size: the transverse diameter of the cardiac silhouette should not be more than half the transverse diameter of the thorax; this is the cardiothoracic ratio. (A larger cardiothoracic ratio is acceptable for an AP film because the cardiac silhouette is larger on an AP film.)

Quick HIT

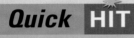

Proper position of lines, tubes, and catheters
- Endotracheal tube—the tip should be approximately 4 to 6 cm above the tracheal carina (this is about the level of the clavicular heads).
- Central line—the tip should be above the right atrium in the superior vena cava.
- Swan–Ganz catheter—the tip should be within the right or left main pulmonary arteries.
- Nasogastric tube—this should be proximal to the gastric pylorus and distal to the esophagogastric junction.

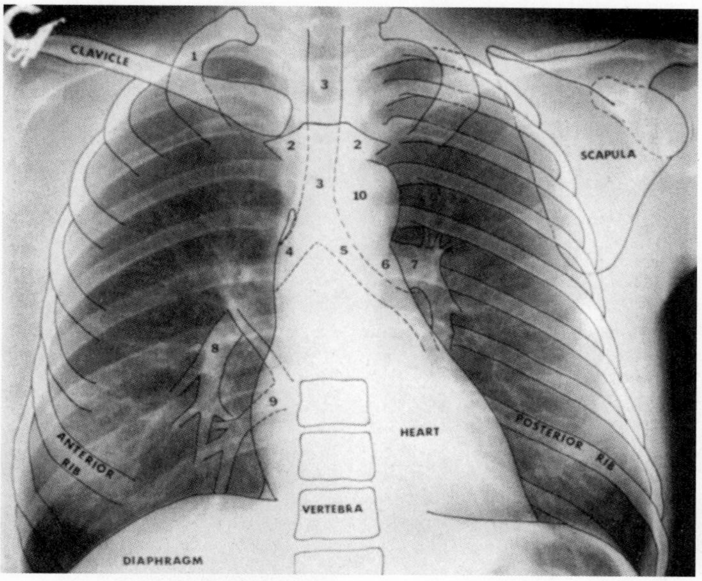

A

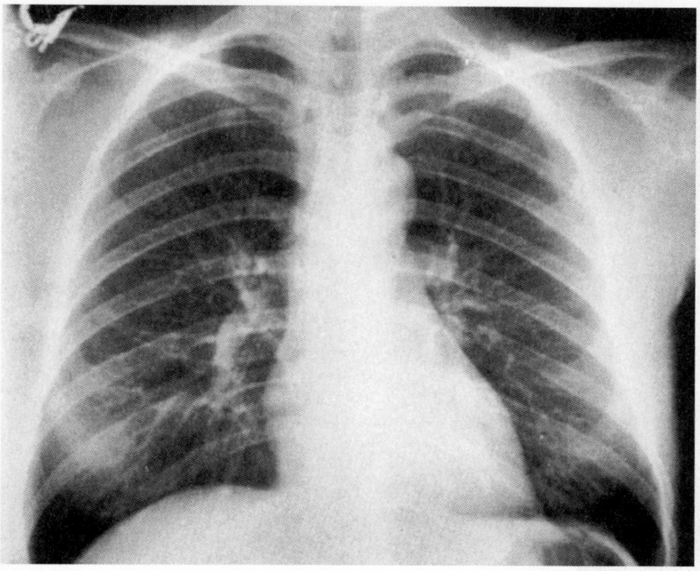

B

FIGURE A-1 **A: PA CXR with diagrammatic overlay: *1,* first rib; *2,* upper portion of manubrium; *3,* trachea; *4,* right main bronchus; *5,* left main bronchus; *6,* main pulmonary artery; *7,* left pulmonary artery; *8,* right interlobar pulmonary artery; *9,* right pulmonary vein; *10,* aortic arch. B: CXR of the same subject without diagrammatic overlay.**

(**A** and **B** from George RB, Light RW, Matthay MA, et al. *Chest medicine—Essentials of Pulmonary and Critical Care Medicine*. 4th ed. Philadelphia, PA: Lippincott Williams & Wilkins, 2000:69, Figure 5.1A and B.)

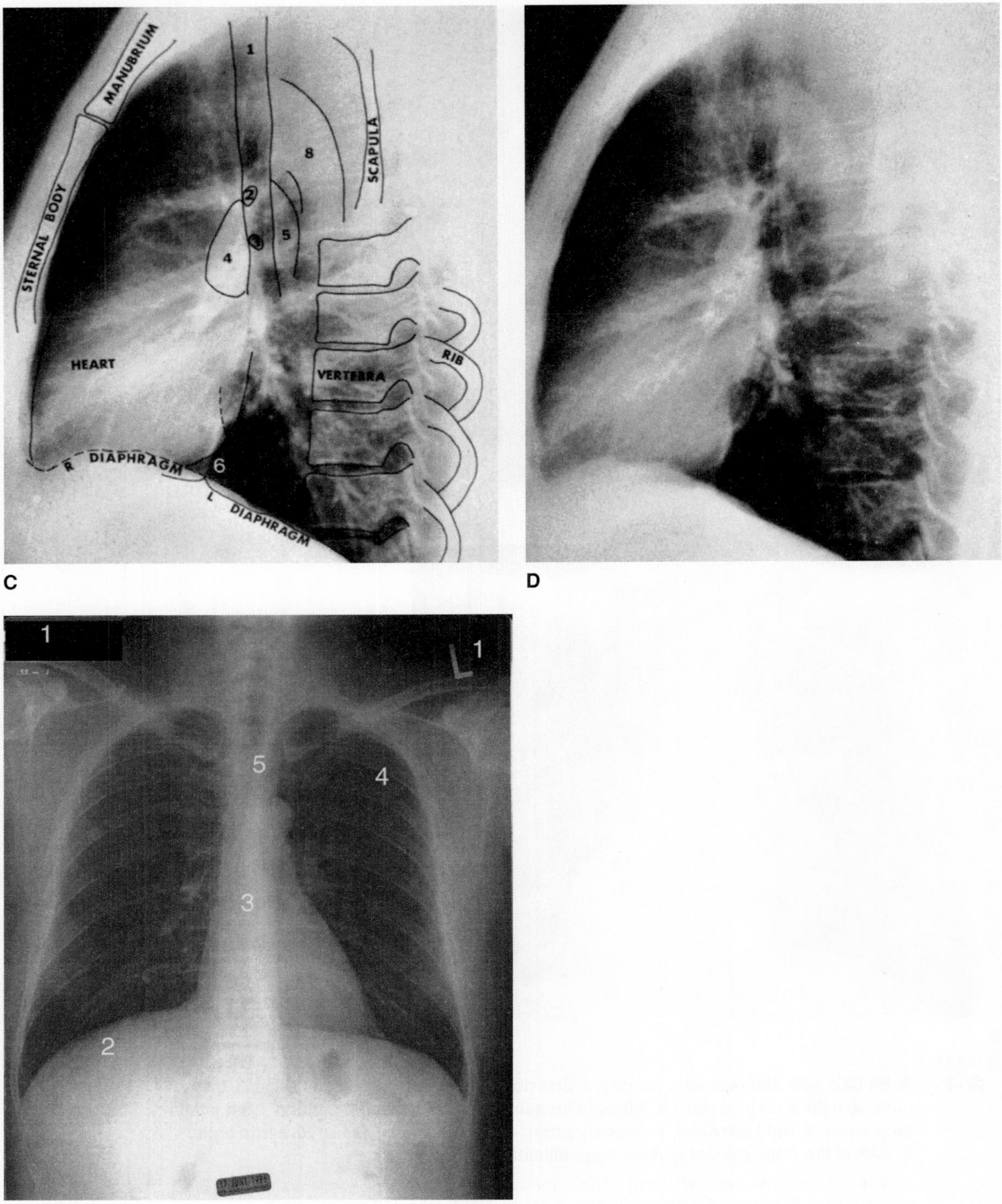

E

FIGURE A-1 **(*Continued*) C: Lateral CXR of the same patient as in A: *1,* trachea; *2,* right upper lobe bronchus; *3,* left upper lobe bronchus; *4,* right pulmonary artery; *5,* left pulmonary artery; *6,* inferior vena cava; *7,* ascending aorta; *8,* descending aorta. D: Same lateral CXR without diagrammatic overlay. E: Technical adequacy of a CXR: *1,* a technically adequate CXR should be labeled with the patient's name, date, and a side marker; *2,* the midportion of the right hemidiaphragm should be below the 10th rib; *3,* vertebral bodies should be visualized throughout the spine; *4,* pulmonary vessels should be visible to the outer third of the lung; *5,* the thoracic spinous processes should be midway between the heads of the clavicle.**

(**C** and **D** from George RB, Light RW, Matthay MA, et al. *Chest Medicine—Essentials of Pulmonary and Critical Care Medicine.* 4th ed. Philadelphia, PA: Lippincott Williams & Wilkins, 2000:70, Figure 5.2A and B.) (**E** from Humes DH, DuPont HL, Gardner LB, et al. *Kelley's Textbook of Internal Medicine.* 4th ed. Philadelphia, PA: Lippincott Williams & Wilkins, 2000:2570, Figure 386.3.)

3. Check for mediastinal widening, which may be present in aortic dissection, trauma, and lymphoma.
4. Evaluate the position of the trachea; it should be in the midline.
5. Compare right and left lung fields. It is best to divide the lung fields into thirds (horizontally) and compare the two sides.
   a. Look for any infiltrates or consolidation.
   b. Congestion—look for signs of CHF; large heart without "shape"; pulmonary vessels are more visible and extend further into the lung field than normal.
   c. Pneumothorax—look for a line demarcating free air (hyperlucent with no pulmonary vascular markings) in the pleural space.
   d. Pleural effusion—examine the costophrenic angles; they should be sharp and clear without any blunting.
   e. Look at the diaphragms—the right diaphragm is normally slightly higher than the left.

F. Examination of the lateral film (see Figure A-1).
1. Look at the cardiac silhouette.
   a. Anterior border—formed by the right ventricle.
   b. Posteroinferior border—formed by the left ventricle.
   c. Posterosuperior border—formed by the left atrium.
   d. The right atrium cannot be seen.
2. Look at the trachea.
3. Examine the retrosternal and retrocardiac spaces for any abnormalities.
4. Examine the diaphragms—note that the anterior portion of the left hemidiaphragm is not visible because of the cardiac silhouette. The entire right hemidiaphragm should be visible, however.

Abdominal Radiographs

A. The standard abdominal film—KUB—is a supine view, which is ideal for seeing the gas pattern.

B. Order an obstruction series (includes PA CXR, as well as supine and upright abdominal films) to evaluate the gas pattern and to look for the following:
1. Free intraperitoneal air (see later)—free air is seen under the diaphragm on the CXR. If the patient is too ill to be upright, order a left lateral decubitus film instead (air rises to the nondependent area).
2. Air–fluid levels—seen on the upright film (see later).

C. Most important things to look for on abdominal films.
1. Air–fluid levels—sign of obstruction; if prominent and multiple, mechanical obstruction is more likely than ileus.
2. Free air under the diaphragm (perforation of a viscous)—this is a surgical emergency.
3. Dilated loops of bowel (obstruction, ileus)—it may be difficult to distinguish mechanical obstruction from ileus. The following may help:
   a. If air is in the small intestine, colon, and rectum, ileus is more likely because ileus distention involves the entire GI tract.
   b. In small bowel obstruction, there are distended loops of small bowel proximal to the site of obstruction and multiple air–fluid levels on upright or decubitus films. Colonic gas is usually minimal.
   c. In large bowel obstruction, look for haustral markings—they span one-half to two-thirds of the diameter of large bowel—as well as the colonic shadow on the periphery or in the pelvis.
   d. In an ileus, the dilated loops are scattered and lack organization (e.g., like a "bag of popcorn"); in mechanical obstruction, dilated loops are stacked on top of one another (e.g., like a "bag of sausages").
   e. Too little gas in the abdomen can be due to high obstruction.

Appendix

Appendix

Electrocardiogram Interpretation

Electrocardiogram Pearls

A. Always look for an old ECG with which to compare the current electrocardiogram (ECG). This is critical in assessing whether any significant changes have occurred.

B. Determine rate

1. Count the number of large blocks (with five little squares) between each R wave. Divide this number by 300 (the distance between large blocks represents 1/300 minute). Therefore, if there are four blocks between each R wave, there is 4/300 or 1/75 minute between each R wave, which means that the rate is 75. (Note that this is the same as the 300-150-75-60-50 rule.)
2. If the rate is irregular, count the number of beats in 6 seconds and multiply by 10.
3. Each block is 1 mm (0.04 seconds), so five boxes equal 0.20 seconds.
4. Tachycardia is defined as a rate >100 beats/min.
5. Bradycardia is defined as a rate of <60 beats/min.

C. Determine rhythm (look at lead II)—is the rhythm regular or irregular? Note that rhythms may be regularly irregular or irregularly irregular as well. (See Chapter 1, Arrhythmias section.)

D. Determine axis

1. Look at the QRS complex in leads I and aVF.
2. If both are mainly positive, then the axis is normal.
3. If mainly positive in lead I and mainly negative in aVF, the axis is deviated to the left.
4. If mainly negative in lead I and mainly positive in aVF, the axis is deviated to the right.
5. If mainly negative in both I and aVF, then there is extreme right axis deviation.

E. Intervals

1. P-R interval—this should be <0.2 seconds.
   a. In **first-degree heart block**, the P-R interval is >0.2 seconds (one large box).
   b. In **second-degree AV block** (Wenckebach or **Mobitz type I**), there is a progressive lengthening of the P-R interval followed by a dropped QRS complex.
   c. In the **Mobitz type II** form of second-degree heart block, the P-R interval is constant, but not every P wave is followed by a QRS complex. There may be two, three, or even more P waves before a QRS, but the ratio of P waves to QRS complexes (e.g., 2:1, 3:1) is constant.
   d. **In third-degree heart** block, there is no relationship between atrial (P waves) and ventricular (QRS) activity.
2. QRS complex—this should be <0.12 seconds.
   a. Prolongation of the QRS complex is seen in bundle branch block, ventricular rhythms, and paced rhythms.
   b. In **right bundle branch block (RBBB)**, look for a widened QRS complex, an rSR wave in the chest leads, and a wide S wave in lead I.
   c. In **left bundle branch block (LBBB)**, look for a widened QRS complex and loss of Q waves with broad, notched R waves in leads I, V_5, or V_6.
3. QT interval—the normal QT interval should be less than half of the R-R interval (<0.42 seconds). Prolongation of the QT interval may be seen in the following.
   a. Medications: tricyclic antidepressants, phenothiazines, nonsedating antihistamines; class IA, IC, and III antiarrhythmics.
   b. Electrolyte disturbances: hypocalcemia, hypokalemia.
   c. Congenital long QT syndromes.
   d. Other: ischemia, significant bradyarrhythmias, and certain CNS lesions.

F. Examine waves

1. P waves—there should be one P wave for each QRS complex in a normal sinus rhythm.
   a. **Left atrial enlargement**—wide P wave (>0.12 seconds) in lead II or a diphasic P wave with a deep terminal component in V_1.
   b. **Right atrial enlargement**—tall P wave (>2.5 mm) in lead II or a diphasic P wave with a large initial component in V_1.
   c. **Multifocal atrial tachycardia**—at least three different P wave morphologies are present.
2. Q waves—indicate myocardial necrosis (acute or old MI).
   a. To be considered significant, they must be >0.04 seconds wide and >25% of the QRS amplitude.
   b. Isolated Q waves in certain leads may be normal, especially in aVR.
3. QRS complex.
   a. Should be narrow (<0.12 seconds) with a regular morphology.
   b. The following are indicators of **left ventricular hypertrophy** (LVH).
      - S wave in V_1 or V_2 ≥30 mm high.
      - R wave in V_5 or V_6 >26 mm high.
      - S wave in V_1 + R wave in V_5 or V_6 >35 mm high in adults (>age 30)
      - Left axis deviation is often present.
   c. The following are indicators of **right ventricular hypertrophy** (RVH).
      - R wave ≥7 mm in V_1.
      - R/S ratio in V_1 ≥1.
      - Progressive decrease in R wave height across the precordial leads.
      - Right axis deviation is often present.
4. ST segments
   a. ST segment depression can occur in the following conditions:
      - Myocardial ischemia
      - Subendocardial MI
      - Digitalis
      - Hypokalemia
      - LBBB
   b. ST segment elevation is a key indicator of myocardial necrosis—it is a hallmark of acute transmural MI, but may persist in an old MI.
      - ST segment elevations in I, aVL, V_5, and V_6 are consistent with a lateral wall MI (circumflex coronary artery).
      - ST segment elevations in V_1 to V_4 are consistent with an anterior wall MI (left anterior descending coronary artery).
      - ST segment elevations in II, III, and aVF are consistent with an inferior wall MI (terminal branches of right or left coronary artery).
      - Diffuse ST segment elevations may be present in pericarditis.
      - Small, concave ST segment elevations may be a normal finding in young people (early repolarization).
      - If LBBB is present, ST segment elevations may be present and are an unreliable indicator of ischemia/infarction.
5. T waves
   a. Peaked T waves may be present in the following situations:
      - Very early stages of MI (before true infarction occurs).
      - Hyperkalemia
      - Hypermagnesemia
   b. T-wave inversions may be present in the following situations:
      - Myocardial ischemia/infarction
      - Pericarditis
      - Cardiomyopathy
      - Intracranial bleeding
      - Electrolyte disturbances, acidosis
      - LBBB, LVH
      - Small T-wave inversions may be normal in the limb leads

Quick HIT

Large R waves and ST segment depressions in V1 or V2 suggest a posterior wall MI.

Appendix

Intravenous Therapy

A. Forms of IV therapy

1. "Intravenous (IV) push"—this is administration of a medication directly into the IV access. It is typically used in emergency situations when a rapid response is needed or when a loading dose of a medication is to be given, followed by a continuous infusion.
2. Continuous administration—electronic devices deliver fluid or medication at a preset volume per hour.
3. Intermittent administration can be accomplished via a number of methods.
   a. Heparin lock or saline lock—this is used when the patient no longer needs IV fluids and IV medications can be given intermittently. The IV line is kept open with saline or heparin when no medication is being given.
   b. Piggyback—a medication or solution is given through another established primary infusion. The first bag that is hung is the primary infusion. Tubes from both the primary bag and the piggyback bag connect to a common tube that feeds into the patient's vein.
   c. Nontunneled central catheter—the exit site of the catheter is at the skin. Locations include internal jugular (IJ), femoral, and subclavian veins.
   d. Tunneled central catheters (e.g., Hickman)—the catheter is inserted into the subclavian vein, but the end of the catheter is then "tunneled" in the subcutaneous tissue so that it exits the skin away from the site of vein insertion. With both nontunneled and tunneled central catheters, there is easy access but also the risk of infection at the exit site.
   e. Ports—the catheter is inserted into a central vein and is tunneled subcutaneously. There is not an exit site because the catheter attaches to the port (chamber) that is placed subcutaneously as well. To administer medication, an anesthetic agent is used to numb the skin, and the needle is inserted into the chamber. Often used for chemotherapy administration. Port-a-Cath is an example. There is less risk of infection (no exit site), but access is more difficult and must be performed by a medical professional.
   f. Peripherally inserted central catheter (PICC) line—these are often used to administer IV antibiotics at home (or blood products, other medications, or chemotherapy). Locations include cephalic, basilic, or brachial veins. A PICC is inserted through the veins of the antecubital fossa, and the tip is advanced into the super vena cava. It can be left in place for weeks to months.

B. Complications of IV therapy

1. Thrombophlebitis—manifested by redness, swelling, and pain at IV site; can be prevented by changing the IV every 2 to 3 days
2. Infiltration—medication/fluid leaks into the surrounding tissue. If it is significant and involves a large area, it may lead to compartment syndrome
3. Blockage
4. Air embolus

Central Venous Line

A. Indications

1. Hemodynamic monitoring (e.g., placement of a pulmonary artery catheter)
2. Transvenous pacing
3. Emergent or short-term hemodialysis
4. Emergent delivery of IV medications (particularly in cardiac arrest)—if feasible, it is generally preferable to have a central venous catheter over a peripheral catheter for the administration of drugs in cardiac arrest because the medication is delivered to the heart and the arterial vasculature more rapidly
5. To administer TPN—the high concentration makes it difficult to administer this through peripheral veins

6. Administration of medications that can be harmful if given peripherally
   a. Irritating medications, which can cause thrombophlebitis in peripheral veins (e.g., high-concentration potassium chloride, chemotherapy)
   b. Vasopressors—they cause arterial vasoconstriction and should not be given through peripheral lines, because if infiltration occurs in a peripheral line, it may cause compartment syndrome or skin necrosis
7. Volume replacement (fluid or blood)—if large volumes of fluid must be given rapidly, large-diameter central catheters are sometimes needed, particularly if the patient does not have adequate peripheral access. (But remember that the flow rate of saline or blood is generally higher in a large-bore peripheral catheter than a central venous catheter because the peripheral catheter is shorter in length.)
8. Although routine or frequent blood draws are not an indication for central venous line placement, an already-existing central line can be used for this purpose

B. Sites

1. IJ vein
2. Subclavian vein
3. Femoral vein

C. Complications

1. Pneumothorax
   a. Can occur with subclavian lines and IJ lines (but more common with subclavian lines); obviously does not occur with femoral lines
   b. Note that patients on PEEP have hyperinflated lungs, and the apex of the lungs is more superior than normal, increasing the chances of an iatrogenic pneumothorax
2. Venous air embolism—if air is sucked into the vena cava, it can be pumped through the right ventricle into the lungs, leading to pulmonary embolism (PE) of air (instead of clot). This is a potentially life-threatening complication. If the patient has a patent foramen ovale, it can result in a paradoxical air embolism to the brain
3. Puncture of adjacent artery (carotid, subclavian, or femoral)—depending on the site, this can lead to complications including hemothorax (subclavian) and hematoma (IJ and femoral). Apply compression if this occurs
4. Infection—central lines very commonly cause infections at the site of entry and often lead to sepsis, which can be life-threatening.
5. Thrombosis and thrombophlebitis

Arterial Lines

- Definition—IV catheters (same ones used for peripheral lines) that are inserted into the radial artery (rarely in ulnar or brachial artery).
- Uses—arterial lines have two major uses.
  - BP monitoring is the most important—arterial lines give more accurate readings than noninvasive blood pressure cuffs. A patient on a pressor or in the ICU generally should have an A-line for proper BP monitoring.
  - Used for frequent blood gas draws.

Nutritional Support

A. Enteral nutrition (administered into the GI tract)

1. Enteral nutrition is preferred over parenteral nutrition because the intestine is used in a physiologic manner.
2. There are two methods of administering enteral nutrition.
   a. Nasoenteric tubes (e.g., nasojejunal tubes)—best for short-term nutrition.
   b. Enterostomy tubes (e.g., PEG/G-tubes, J-tubes)—for long-term support.
3. There are many different formulas available for tube feeds—special formulas can be provided for patients with renal disease, liver disease, CHF, and so on.

Quick HIT

- Immediately after placing a central line (IJ or subclavian), obtain a CXR to check for pneumothorax and to ensure proper position of the catheter tip. The catheter tip should be in the superior vena cava.
- When removing a line, the patient should be supine and should exhale during removal to prevent an air embolism.

Quick HIT

Pulmonary Artery Line

- A central catheter that is inserted through one of the large veins, threaded through the right ventricle, and into the pulmonary artery
- Sometimes called "Swan–Ganz lines" (after the inventors, Dr. Swan and Dr. Ganz)
- Used to measure various hemodynamic parameters, including central venous pressure, PCWP, cardiac index and output, stroke volume, and systemic vascular resistance

Quick HIT

There are two means of providing nutrition for a patient who cannot eat: enteral nutrition and parenteral nutrition.

Quick HIT

- PEG tube—the tube is inserted with the help of an endoscope through the mouth. Alternatively, it can also be done through an open abdominal incision, which is called open gastrostomy.
- The J-tube (jejunostomy) is placed in the intestine and can only be done through an open abdominal procedure.

4. Tube feeds can be delivered intermittently (in boluses) or continuously.
   a. Intermittent feeding (into the stomach) requires close monitoring (by nurses)—gastric residuals should be checked every 4 hours and tube feeds should be held if the residual is >150 mL. Intermittent feeding has a higher risk of aspiration than continuous feeding.
   b. Continuous feeding (into duodenum or jejunum) has a lower risk of aspiration than intermittent feeding and requires less monitoring by nurses.
5. Complications of enteral nutrition.
   a. Intolerance to tube feeds—check for diarrhea, constipation, nausea, vomiting, abdominal pain, or distention.
   b. Malpositioning of tube (in trachea/bronchus).
   c. Aspiration pneumonia.
   d. Overload of solutes—due to high rate of hyperosmolar feedings (can cause diarrhea, electrolyte imbalance, hyperglycemia).

B. Parenteral nutrition (administered into the vasculature)

1. The term TPN is used for a high-concentration solution that can be given alone to meet the body's caloric demands. Parenteral nutrition can also play a supplementary role when enteral feeding alone is inadequate.
2. It is used if the patient cannot eat for prolonged periods or cannot tolerate enteral feedings, and in severely malnourished patients.
3. There are two ways of administration.
   a. Central—via central venous catheter (e.g., subclavian vein)—preferred in patients who require long-term support.
   b. Peripheral—via peripheral line—one cannot administer as much protein or calories with this as with a central line. It should only be used for a short-term period. TPN cannot be administered in a peripheral line.
4. Complications of parenteral nutrition.
   a. Electrolyte imbalances, volume disturbances.
   b. Hyperglycemia
   c. Complications associated with placing a central line (e.g., pneumothorax).
   d. Infection of central (or peripheral) line.

Guide to Antibacterial Antibiotic Therapy

A. Cell wall inhibitors

1. Penicillins (see Table A-1)
   a. Mechanism of action
      - A β-lactam antibiotic
      - Inhibit cross-linkage (transpeptidation step) of bacterial cell walls as they are synthesized
      - Bacterial cell walls lose structural and osmotic integrity
      - Cell lysis ultimately occurs
      - To achieve the desired effect, penicillins must first bind to proteins located inside the bacterial cell wall. These proteins are called penicillin-binding proteins
   b. Antimicrobial coverage (not exhaustive)
      - More effective against **gram-positive** than gram-negative organisms. Effective against viridans group streptococci, *Streptococcus pyogenes,* oral anaerobes, syphilis, Leptospira
      - Acts synergistically with aminoglycosides
      - Penicillin G is a long-acting intramuscular form of penicillin which is the drug of choice to treat syphilis. Because of microbial resistance, it is used less commonly to treat respiratory tract infections caused by streptococcal species, such as pharyngitis secondary to *S. pyogenes* or pneumococcal pneumonia
      - Penicillin V is the oral form of penicillin G which has some anaerobic activity, so it is more useful for dental infections

Quick HIT

Best antibiotics for gram-positive cocci (Staph and Strep):
1. PRPs (oxacillin, nafcillin, etc.)
2. First-generation cephalosporins
3. Fluoroquinolones

Appendix

TABLE A-1 Important Antibiotics

Antibiotic/Antibiotic Category	Mechanism of Action	Most Common Uses	Adverse Reactions Commonly Seen[a]
Penicillins	Cell wall inhibitors (interfere with transpeptidation)	Depends on extension of antimicrobial spectrum Oral and respiratory infections Streptococcal infections Syphilis	Hypersensitivity reactions
Vancomycin	Cell wall inhibitor (see text)	MRSA Enterococcal infections Endocarditis (used with aminoglycoside) Alternative if penicillin allergy present	"Red man" syndrome
Tetracyclines	Inhibit 30 S bacterial ribosomal subunit	Chlamydia Rickettsiae Lyme disease Topical use for acne vulgaris	Deposition in bones and teeth of children >8 yrs old, fetuses
Macrolides	Inhibit 50 S bacterial ribosomal subunit	Atypical pneumonia Alternative to penicillin (i.e., allergy)	GI upset Legionella
Clindamycin	Inhibits 50 S bacterial ribosomal subunit	Anaerobes, staphylococci, streptococci	*C. difficile* colitis, Pseudomembranous colitis
Cephalosporins	Cell wall inhibitors (similar to penicillins)	Depends on generation: First: Similar to penicillins, surgical prophylaxis, streptococci and staphylococci infections Second: Pneumonia in elderly patients, recurrent pneumonia Third: Gonorrhea, meningitis Fourth: Broad-spectrum, including streptococci, staphylococci, and pseudomonads	Possible cross-sensitivity with penicillin A few promote bleeding diathesis, correctable with vitamin K.
Fluoroquinolones	Inhibit bacterial DNA-gyrase	UTIs Diarrhea secondary to gram-negative rods Penicillin-resistant pneumonia Some with anti-Pseudomonas activity	Well tolerated Damage to cartilage in children
Aminoglycosides	Inhibit 30 S bacterial ribosomal subunit	Gram-negative sepsis Endocarditis (with vancomycin) Complicated UTIs	Nephrotoxicity Ototoxicity
TMP/SMX	Blocks bacterial DNA synthesis through action on folate pathway (two steps)	*P. carinii* pneumonia UTIs	Rash Stevens–Johnson syndrome
Metronidazole	Products of reduction reaction kill susceptible bacteria and protozoans	Anaerobes *Trichomonas histolytica* and *Giardia*	Metallic taste Disulfiram-like effect

[a]Note that these are not necessarily the most common side effects.

Appendix

- Penicillins are not good choices for empiric coverage for most infections due to widespread resistance
- Ampicillin and amoxicillin have extended gram-negative activity. Ampicillin is typically given IV, while amoxicillin is an oral drug often used to treat outpatient upper respiratory tract infections caused by streptococcus. They cover same organisms as penicillin, in addition to *Escherichia coli*, Lyme disease and few other gram-negative rods (*Haemophilus influenzae, Listeria, E. coli, Proteus, Salmonella*)
- Penicillinase-resistant penicillins (PRPs) include oxacillin, cloxacillin, dicloxacillin and nafcillin
- Penicillins are generally ineffective against intracellular bacteria

c. Adverse reactions
- **Hypersensitivity reactions**—type I hypersensitivity reaction may present as rash, angioedema, or even anaphylaxis
- Diarrhea
- Interstitial nephritis

d. Other features
- Penicillins are used to treat otitis media, UTI in pregnant women, dental infections, enterococcal infections, Listeria monocytogenes, Lyme disease
- Penicillin is used as prophylaxis against infection in patients with sickle cell disease
- Bacteria gain resistance to penicillins through alterations in penicillin-binding proteins—for example, MRSA
- Resistance is also conferred by β-lactamases, enzymes that hydrolyze the penicillin's β-lactam ring

e. Examples (list of examples is not exhaustive)
- Penicillin G
- Penicillin V
- Ampicillin
- Amoxicillin
- Methicillin
- Nafcillin
- Piperacillin

2. **Cephalosporins**

a. Mechanism of action
- Similar mechanism of action to penicillin
- As with penicillin, the β-lactam ring confers **bactericidal** activity

b. Antimicrobial coverage (not necessarily exhaustive—this applies to the rest of antimicrobial section)
- Cephalosporins are classified according to antimicrobial activity and β-lactamase resistance into "generations"
- First-generation cephalosporins generally serve as substitutes for penicillin, and also have coverage against *Proteus, Klebsiella,* and *E. coli.* Cefazolin is the only parenteral first-generation cephalosporin available in the United States
- Second-generation cephalosporins have more gram-negative activity and less gram-positive activity than first-generation cephalosporins. They are used to treat *H. influenzae, Neisseria gonorrhoeae,* and *Enterobacter* spp.
- Third-generation cephalosporins have even more **gram-negative activity, less gram-positive activity,** and are **able to cross the blood–brain barrier. (First- and Second-generation cephalosporins do not penetrate the CSF and should not be used to treat infections of the central nervous system)**
- Fourth-generation cephalosporins are the most broad-spectrum, including activity against *Pseudomonas, Neisseria,* and methicillin-sensitive *Staphylococcus aureus,* as well as most of the above-mentioned organisms. It has better staphylococcal coverage than third-generation drugs
- Fifth-generation cephalosporins are a new class of drugs which show high activity against MRSA

Quick HIT

Hypersensitivity reactions to penicillin
- Type I hypersensitivity reaction.
- This may present with rash, angioedema, or even anaphylaxis.
- Cross-reactions with other *β-lactam* antibiotics can occur.
- Nausea, vomiting, and diarrhea are not hypersensitivity reactions.
- It may develop at any time, even if past treatments with penicillin were uneventful.

Quick HIT

Best antibiotics for anaerobes:
1. Penicillin (G, VK, amoxicillin, ampicillin)
2. Clindamycin
3. Metronidazole (for abdominal/GI)

Quick HIT

All cephalosporins (every generation) will cover viridans group streptococci, group A, B, and C streptococci, *E. coli, Klebsiella, Proteus mirabilis.*

Quick HIT

Third- and fourth-generation cephalosporins are not useful for treating infections due to gram-positive cocci or Acinetobacter.

c. Adverse reactions
- **Hypersensitivity reactions**—allergic cross-reaction with penicillin can occur in 10% of cephalosporins
- Certain cephalosporins (especially the second generation) promote a bleeding diathesis, which is reversible with vitamin K
- Some second-generation cephalosporins may cause a disulfiram-like reaction to alcohol

d. Other features
- First-generation cephalosporins are used for surgical prophylaxis or minor forms of cellulitis
- Most forms of cephalosporins must be administered intravenously
- Cefuroxime is sometimes used to treat community-acquired pneumonia
- Cefoxitin can be used for abdominal infections, such as peritonitis
- Ceftriaxone can be given as an IM injection to treat gonorrhea. Intravenously it plays an important role in empiric treatment for meningitis
- Third-generation antibiotics are one of the classes of drugs which have been shown to have the highest association with antibiotic-induced *Clostridium difficile* infection
- Because of its broad coverage, cefepime is a good choice for empiric therapy in nosocomial infections as well as febrile neutropenia
- Fifth-generation cephalosporins are currently approved to treat uncomplicated skin and soft tissue infections, though their MRSA activity offers great promise

e. Examples (list of examples is not exhaustive)
- First generation: cefazolin, cephalexin, cefadroxil
- Second generation: cefaclor, cefoxitin, cefuroxime, cefotetan, cefprozil
- Third generation: ceftriaxone, cefixime, cefotaxime, ceftazidime, cefdinir
- Fourth generation: cefepime is the only fourth-generation cephalosporin
- Fifth generation: ceftaroline, ceftobiprole

3. **Miscellaneous cell wall inhibitors**

a. Vancomycin
- Inhibits cell wall synthesis by interfering with cross-linkage of peptidoglycan chains (different site of action from penicillin), also damages cell membranes
- Main use is to treat staphylococcal infections resistant to other β-lactams, such as MRSA, or if penicillin allergy is present; not used for gram-negative organisms
- Oral vancomycin is effective to treat *C. difficile* infections of the bowel
- Acts synergistically with aminoglycosides to treat enterococcal infections
- Adverse reactions include fever, nephrotoxicity, ototoxicity, and "**red man syndrome**" (flushing due to infusion-induced histamine release). Treat red man syndrome by slowing the infusion and giving antihistamines (i.e., diphenhydramine)
- Serum levels must be followed up in prolonged therapy, and doses must be adjusted for renal insufficiency
- Vancomycin resistance is an emerging, ominous phenomenon. Many enterococci have developed resistance to vancomycin creating vancomycin-resistant enterococci (VRE)

Quick HIT

Best antibiotic for MRSA is vancomycin.

b. Carbapenems
- Synthetic β-lactams designed to be more resistant to β-lactamases and penicillinases
- Examples include imipenem, ertapenem, doripenem, and meropenem
- Imipenem is always combed with cilastatin to prevent renal toxicity associated with the metabolism of imipenem
- Carbapenems have broad-spectrum antimicrobial coverage, including penicillin-resistant pneumococci, *Pseudomonas,* anaerobes, and *Enterobacter* infections
- They are used empirically for patients in whom gram-negative sepsis is suspected
- They may cause nausea, vomiting, and sometimes neutropenia
- They reduce the seizure threshold (especially imipenem)

c. Monobactams
- Aztreonam is currently the only available preparation in the United States
- Contains only one of the two structural rings found in other β-lactams, hence the name. It retains resistance to β-lactamases
- Narrow spectrum of activity: Primarily aerobic gram-negative rods, including ***Pseudomonas, Klebsiella,*** and *Serratia*
- Less cross-reactivity with penicillin than other β-lactam antibiotics makes it useful for patients with penicillin allergies

Quick HIT

Piperacillin and ticarcillin are always used in combination with a β-lactamase inhibitor (e.g., tazobactam, clavulanic acid).

d. β-lactamase inhibitors
- Examples include sulbactam, tazobactam, and clavulanic acid
- Not used by themselves, but rather combined with penicillins to enhance antimicrobial activity (e.g., amoxicillin + clavulanic acid = Augmentin)

e. Bacitracin
- Inhibits bacterial cell wall synthesis by inhibiting transport of peptidoglycans
- Effective against gram-positive organisms
- Used **topically** only (because it is so nephrotoxic)

B. Protein synthesis inhibitors

1. **Tetracycline**

a. Mechanism of action
- Inhibits protein synthesis by binding to 30 S subunit of bacterial ribosome
- **Bacteriostatic**

b. Antimicrobial coverage
- Effective against certain intracellular bacteria: Chlamydia, rickettsial diseases (e.g., Rocky Mountain spotted fever), mycoplasma, spirochetes
- Treats gram-negative *Vibrio cholerae*
- Also treats spirochete causing Lyme disease (*Borrelia burgdorferi*)
- Often used to treat uncomplicated respiratory tract infections such as sinusitis and bronchitis
- Tigecycline is broad-spectrum and is able to evade the resistance mechanisms which render the other tetracyclines less active

c. Adverse reactions
- GI—epigastric pain, nausea, vomiting
- **Deposits occur in calcified tissues** (e.g., teeth and bones of the fetus if given during pregnancy and potentially in any child <8 years old). This can result in permanent discoloration of teeth, stunting of growth, and skeletal deformities
- Phototoxicity
- Hepatotoxicity—may occur in pregnant women

d. Cautions
- Do not give to pregnant women or children <8 years old
- Do not give to patients with renal insufficiency (except doxycycline)
- Decreased absorption occurs if taken with milk and antacids
- Resistance is common

e. Examples
- Tetracycline
- Doxycycline
- Minocycline
- Tigecycline is a new antibiotic in a related class of drugs called glycylcyclines.

2. **Macrolides**

a. Mechanism of action
- Inhibit protein synthesis by binding to 50 S subunit of bacterial ribosome
- **Bacteriostatic** (may be bactericidal at high doses)

b. Antimicrobial coverage
- Good at treating intracellular pathogens, such as *Mycoplasma, Chlamydia,* and *Legionella*
- Erythromycin and clarithromycin have activity against staphylococci and streptococci

- Clarithromycin is the treatment of choice for *Mycoplasma* pneumonia ("walking pneumonia") and *Legionella* spp.
- Erythromycin is also appropriate as an alternative to penicillin G if there is a penicillin allergy (e.g., treatment of chlamydia in pregnancy, to avoid tetracycline)
- Due to adverse events and frequent dosing, erythromycin is being used less often as an antibiotic. It is still regularly used as a GI stimulant however
- Clarithromycin is one of the drugs used in therapy for eradication of *Helicobacter pylori*
- Azithromycin and clarithromycin have activity against *H. influenzae*
- Azithromycin also treats *Moraxella catarrhalis*

c. Adverse reactions
- GI side effects are the most common and include epigastric pain, nausea, and vomiting (particularly with erythromycin)
- Cholestasis
- Prolongation of QT interval, especially with erythromycin

d. Cautions
- Erythromycin should not be prescribed to patients with liver failure because it is metabolized in the liver
- Erythromycin and clarithromycin interact with many drugs due to their inhibitory effect on the P-450 system

e. Examples
- Azithromycin
- Clarithromycin
- Erythromycin

3. **Aminoglycosides**

a. Mechanism of action
- Inhibit protein synthesis by binding to 30 S subunit of bacterial ribosome
- **Bactericidal**

b. Antimicrobial coverage
- Treat gram-negative aerobes, such as *E. coli, Pseudomonas, Acinetobacter,* or *Klebsiella*
- Sometimes used in combination with ampicillin or other β-lactams for complicated UTIs, meningitis, or other serious infections
- Used in conjunction with antipseudomonal penicillin to treat penicillin
- No activity against anaerobes

c. Adverse reactions
- **Ototoxicity—may cause irreversible hearing loss,** especially if infused too quickly. Baseline and follow-up hearing tests are required for patients on aminoglycosides long term
- **Nephrotoxicity**—may cause renal insufficiency or acute tubular necrosis Aminoglycoside toxicity is dose-related, so be sure to adjust dose for renal dysfunction

d. Other points
- Most are given parenterally.
- Check peak and trough levels to avoid drug toxicities

e. Examples
- Gentamicin
- Streptomycin
- Tobramycin
- Amikacin
- Neomycin

4. **Miscellaneous protein synthesis inhibitors**

a. Clindamycin
- Binds to 50 S subunit of ribosome, inhibiting bacterial protein synthesis
- Key feature is activity against anaerobic bacteria. In addition to anaerobes, can be used for streptococcal and staphylococcal infections

Quick HIT

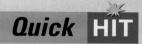

Most common application of aminoglycosides for treating serious infections caused by aerobic gram-negative rods:
- Sepsis
- Complicated UTI
- Pneumonia
- Osteomyelitis
- Complicated intra-abdominal infections

- It can also be used to treat many types of gram-positive cocci. If the patient is allergic to cephalexin (Keflex), clindamycin can be given instead
- The most notable adverse effect is its potential to cause antibiotic-associated diarrhea, including *C. difficile* colitis.

b. Chloramphenicol
- It binds to 50 S bacterial ribosomal subunit, but may also interfere with human ribosomal activity, and so it has the potential to be highly toxic
- Broad-spectrum antimicrobial coverage, including anaerobes and rickettsiae; readily penetrates the CSF
- Adverse effects may be severe and even fatal: **aplastic anemia** and **gray baby syndrome** (cyanosis due to respiratory depression and cardiovascular collapse)
- Inhibits the P-450 system, potentiating the effect of many important drugs

c. Linezolid
- Has great coverage of gram-positive bacteria, including streptococci, enterococci, and MRSA
- Most serious reported adverse effect is thrombocytopenia (monitor blood counts with prolonged therapy). Peripheral neuropathy has also been reported with extended treatment regimens
- Linezolid inhibits monoamine oxidase. This may lead to serotonin syndrome when given with pro-serotonin agents such as SSRIs
- Great oral bioavailability

Appendix

Quick HIT

Fluoroquinolones are only antimicrobial agents in clinical use that are direct inhibitors of bacterial DNA synthesis.

Quick HIT

Best antibiotics for gram-negative rods (*E. coli, Klebsiella, Proteus, Enterobacter, Pseudomonas*):
1. Fluoroquinolones
2. Aminoglycosides
3. Carbapenems
4. Piperacillin
5. Aztreonam
6. Cephalosporins

C. Fluoroquinolones

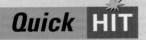

1. Mechanism of action—direct inhibitors of bacterial DNA synthesis
   a. Inhibit bacterial DNA gyrase and topoisomerase IV, blocking replication of bacterial DNA
   b. **Bactericidal**
2. Antimicrobial coverage
   a. Have excellent activity against ***gram-negative organisms***, including *Pseudomonas, E. coli, Proteus, Legionella,* and gonorrhea. Gram-positive coverage is variable. Certain fluoroquinolones (e.g., levofloxacin, moxifloxacin) have good gram-positive coverage and are excellent agents for community-acquired pneumonia. Only moxifloxacin has anaerobic coverage
   b. Commonly used to treat UTIs. Ciprofloxacin also treats acute diarrhea due to enteric bacteria (traveler's diarrhea)
   c. Best therapy for community-acquired pneumonia
3. Adverse reactions
   a. GI—nausea, vomiting, diarrhea
   b. CNS—dizziness, headache, lightheadedness
   c. Nephrotoxicity
   d. Cartilage damage in children has not been shown in humans, although animal studies suggest this
   e. Tendinitis and tendon rupture
   f. Cautions
      - Significantly reduced absorption if consumed with divalent cations, such as antacids that contain magnesium
      - Must be adjusted for renal insufficiency
      - Do not give to nursing mothers and to children (although the latter is evolving, especially in children with cystic fibrosis)
      - Absolutely contraindicated in pregnant patients because animal studies show cartilage damage
   g. Examples
      - Levofloxacin
      - Ciprofloxacin
      - Ofloxacin
      - Moxifloxacin
      - Gemifloxacin

D. Antituberculosis antibiotics

1. Principles of therapy.
   a. **Never treat tuberculosis with only one antibiotic.** Use multidrug therapy because drug resistance is such a problem with *Mycobacterium tuberculosis.*
   b. Treat active tuberculosis with three to four antibiotics (isoniazid [INH], rifampin, pyrazinamide [PZA], and sometimes ethambutol) for 2 months, followed by rifampin and INH for 4 months.
   c. Since *M. tuberculosis* is a slow-growing organism, the required duration of treatment is longer than it is in other bacterial infections.
2. Important first-line antituberculosis agents (many second-line agents also exist).
   a. INH
      - Attacks the enzyme that produces the mycolic acids that comprise the mycobacterial cell walls.
      - Resistance to INH develops rapidly if it is used alone.
      - INH is drug of choice for treatment of latent TB.
      - The most important adverse reaction is **drug-induced hepatitis**, which can be fatal.
      - It may cause a relative pyridoxine (vitamin B_6) deficiency, resulting in peripheral neuropathy. This is reversible with pyridoxine administration.
   b. Rifampin
      - Inhibits bacterial RNA synthesis by blocking RNA polymerase.
      - In addition to its role as an antituberculosis agent, rifampin is used as prophylaxis for close contacts of patients with meningococcal meningitis.
      - Rifampin is also active against *Mycobacterium leprae,* which causes leprosy.
      - May stain tears or urine an orange-red color; induces hepatic microsomal enzymes and decreases the half-life of many medications.
      - Rifampin is a powerful inducer of the cytochrome P-450 enzyme system, so drugs interactions should be monitored carefully.
   c. PZA
      - Inhibits fatty acid synthesis of even slow-growing *M. tuberculosis* at a different step than INH.
      - Active against tubercle bacilli residing in macrophages.
      - May cause hyperuricemia, resulting in a gouty attack.
      - Potentially hepatotoxic
   d. Ethambutol
      - Inhibits an essential component of the mycobacterial cell wall.
      - It may cause **optic neuritis**, resulting in diminished visual ability as well as red-green color blindness. Periodic visual testing may be necessary.
      - It may also precipitate a gouty attack.
      - Also used in the treatment of *Mycobacterium avium intracellulare.*

E. Miscellaneous antibiotics

1. Trimethoprim (TMP)
   a. TMP inhibits dihydrofolic acid reductase, blocking bacterial DNA synthesis.
   b. It works synergistically with sulfonamides.
   c. TMP was formerly used alone to treat UTIs but now is most commonly used in combination with sulfamethoxazole (SMX). SMX inhibits a second, unique step in bacterial folate synthesis, creating a synergistic effect.
   d. TMP/SMX is used both for prophylaxis and treatment of *Pneumocystis jirovecii (formerly carinii).*
   e. It may cause folate deficiency, resulting in megaloblastic anemia.
   f. TMP/SMX is used to treat *S. aureus* (including some MRSA), UTIs, *Pneumocystis carinii* pneumonia, *Shigella,* and *Salmonella,* among other infections.
   g. Side effects of TMP include hematologic (bone marrow suppression), renal (inhibition of creatinine secretion), and hyperkalemia.
2. Sulfonamides
   a. Structural analogues of *p*-aminobenzoic acid that inhibit the enzyme dihydropteroate synthase, which is necessary for folic acid, and thus DNA synthesis.

b. Treat both gram-positive and gram-negative bacteria, although resistance to sulfonamides is increasingly common.
c. Most sulfonamides that were once used alone have been replaced by the combination of TMP/SMX.
d. Some forms of sulfonamides are still given as monotherapy, such as silver sulfadiazine (topical solution) in burn patients to prevent infection, and sodium sulfacetamide (ophthalmic ointment) for bacterial conjunctivitis.
e. The most common adverse reactions are rash, photosensitivity, nausea, vomiting, and diarrhea.
f. A rare but dreaded associated adverse reaction is **Stevens–Johnson syndrome.**
g. **Do not give to patients with G6PD because they can precipitate a hemolytic response.**

3. Metronidazole
   a. Forms a cytotoxic compound through an oxidation–reduction action which damages DNA. Bactericidal.
   b. Effective against anaerobic bacteria as well as certain protozoal organisms such as *Entamoeba histolytica, Giardia,* and *Trichomonas.*
   c. Oral form very useful in the treatment of *C. difficile* diarrheal infections.
   d. Adverse effects—results in a **disulfiram-like reaction** if consumed with alcohol. May also cause headache and a metallic taste. Hepatitis and pancreatitis are extremely rare. Warfarin effects are enhanced with concomitant use of metronidazole due to inhibition of warfarin metabolism—warfarin levels should be closely monitored.
4. Nitrofurantoin
   a. Works by a complex mechanism to inactivate several bacterial enzyme systems including acetyl CoA.
   b. Primary use is for **uncomplicated** lower urinary tract infections caused by *E. coli* or other common community-acquired organisms. Do not use for pyelonephritis or infections outside of the urinary system.
5. Table A-1 lists mechanisms of action, uses, and adverse reactions for important antibiotics.

Appendix

Physical Examination Pearls

Heart Sounds

Quick HIT
- S_1 = mitral valve closure
- S_2 = aortic valve closure (pulmonic valve closure contributes)

A. For murmur of mitral stenosis and to hear S_3 and S_4, use the bell of the stethoscope.

B. For pericardial friction rubs, aortic/mitral regurgitation murmurs, and to hear S_1 and S_2, use the diaphragm of the stethoscope.

Quick HIT
- Aortic area = right second interspace close to sternum
- Pulmonic area = left second interspace close to sternum
- Tricuspid area = left fourth and fifth interspace
- Mitral area = apex

C. Ventricular systole takes place between S_1 and S_2, and ventricular diastole between S_2 and S_1. Remember that diastole lasts longer than systole; this distinction makes it easy to identify the two sounds.

D. How to differentiate S_3 and S_4 (the lines represent duration of pause between sounds): S_3 comes immediately after S_2, and S_4 comes immediately before S_1.
1. S1—S2-S3
2. S4-S1—S2

E. Splitting of S_2 during inspiration and paradoxical splitting of S_2.
1. The second heart sound has two parts: Aortic valve closure, then pulmonic valve closure.
2. With inspiration, there is increased blood return to the right heart. This increased flow delays pulmonary valve closure, which results in the normal splitting of S2 during inspiration.
3. Paradoxical splitting of S2 refers to the narrowing of this split during inspiration (instead of the normal widening that occurs). This can occur as a result of delayed aortic closure (as seen in LBBB, aortic stenosis, and hypertension).

F. It is easier to hear S_3, S_4, and murmur of mitral stenosis if the patient is lying on his or her left side. Use the bell of the stethoscope and apply light pressure at the apical impulse. S_3 disappears if a lot of pressure is applied.

Murmurs

A. Grade 1—very faint; only a cardiologist can hear it

B. Grade 2—quiet

C. Grade 3—moderately loud

D. Grade 4—loud; associated with a thrill

E. Grade 5—very loud; can hear it with stethoscope partially off the chest

F. Grade 6—heard with stethoscope entirely off the chest

Breath Sounds

A. Vesicular breath sounds
1. Soft, low-pitched
2. Audible throughout most lung fields
3. Heard during all of inspiration and first third of expiration

B. Bronchial breath sounds
1. Loud, high-pitched
2. Longer expiratory than inspiratory phase (opposite of vesicular sounds)
3. Hear a gap between inspiration and expiration
4. Heard in central areas (over trachea)
5. Bronchial sounds are abnormal if heard over the peripheral lung areas (where only vesicular sounds should be heard). This suggests an area of consolidation

> **Quick HIT**
> Remember from MCAT that the speed of sound is fastest in solids. Therefore, if air in the lung has been replaced by fluid or solid, sound is transmitted to that area and bronchial breath sounds are heard.

C. Bronchovesicular sounds
1. Intermediate pitch
2. Equal duration of inspiratory and expiratory phases

D. Adventitious breath sounds
1. Rales (also called crackles)
   a. Can be heard during inspiration or expiration; intermittent (discontinuous) sounds
   b. Usually due to excessive fluid in the lungs or atelectasis
   c. Causes include pneumonia, CHF, interstitial lung disease
   d. Sometimes differentiated based on sound—fine crackles are high-pitched, soft, and brief in duration; coarse crackles are lower-pitched, louder, and longer in duration
2. Wheezes have a hissing or musical sound caused by air moving through narrowed airways. Asthma is the most common cause
3. Rhonchi have a snoring quality and lower pitch, and are due to high mucus production in the large airways (e.g., chronic bronchitis)

Abdominal Examination

A. Inspect—look for scars.

B. Auscultate—listen to bowel sounds; this is a nonspecific part of the abdominal examination.

C. Palpate—feel all quadrants, then palpate more deeply in all quadrants.

1. Is the abdomen soft? A rigid abdomen may be a sign of a perforated viscus or peritoneal inflammation (acute abdomen).
2. Check for tenderness in all quadrants.
3. Check for rebound tenderness—does it hurt when you push down or let go? Pain on withdrawal of the hand is **rebound tenderness** and suggests peritoneal inflammation.
4. Is there guarding? **Guarding** refers to an area of rigidity and is significant when it is involuntary (i.e., not due to voluntary muscular contraction).

Neurologic Examination

A. Evaluate the following:

1. **Level of consciousness, speech fluency**
2. **Pupillary size and reactivity, extraocular muscle movement**—give information about function of the brainstem, especially CN III and VI
3. **Complete cranial nerve examination**
4. **Muscle strength testing**
5. **Truncal ataxia, pronator drift of arm** (sensitive test of motor weakness)
6. **Sensation**
7. **Cerebellar testing**—finger to nose and heel to shin; test gait on ambulation, heel-to-toe walking is good for detecting mild ataxia
8. **Deep tendon reflexes**—asymmetry suggests corticospinal tract dysfunction (upper motor neuron lesion)
9. **Babinski sign**—toes should normally flex. If they extend, this is a positive Babinski sign

B. Upper and Lower Motor Neuron Defects (See Table A-2)

1. Deep tendon reflexes
   a. Grading of reflexes
      - 0 = No reflex
      - 1 = Diminished reflexes
      - 2 = Normal
      - 3 = Increased reflexes
      - 4 = Hyperactive reflexes

   b. Locations
      - Biceps (C5)
      - Brachioradialis (C6)
      - Triceps (C7)
      - Patellar (knee jerk) (L4)
      - Ankle (S1)

Quick HIT

If you cannot elicit reflexes, have the patient lock the fingers and pull his or her arms apart as you try again.

TABLE A-2 Upper Versus Lower Motor Neuron Defects

Upper Motor Neuron Signs	Lower Motor Neuron Signs
Spasticity	Flaccid paralysis
Increased deep tendon reflexes (hyperreflexia)	Decreased deep tendon reflexes
Babinski reflex (plantar response extensor)—toes upward (abnormal)	No Babinski reflex (plantar response flexor)—toe downward (normal)
No atrophy	Muscle atrophy
No fasciculations	Fasciculations present

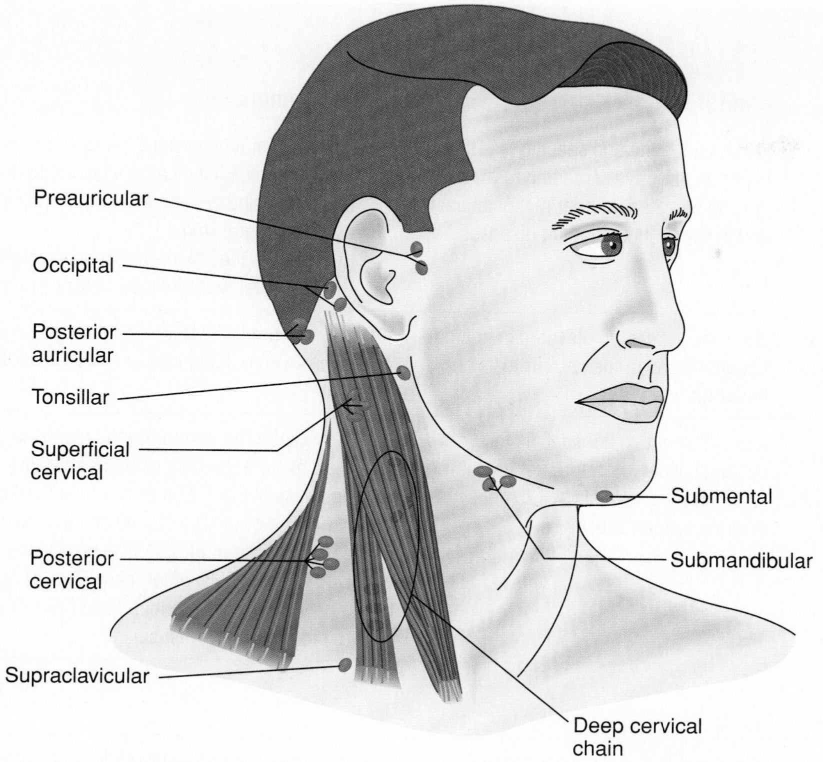

FIGURE A-2 **Palpation of the lymph nodes in a physical examination.**

(From Bickley LS, Szilagyi PG. *Bates' Guide to Physical Examination and History Taking.* 8th ed. Philadelphia, PA: Lippincott Williams & Wilkins, 2003:203.)

c. Muscle strength
- 0 = No contraction
- 1 = Flicker of contraction (muscle is "firing")
- 2 = Moves limb when gravity is eliminated
- 3 = Moves limb against gravity (but not against any resistance)
- 4 = Moves limb against gravity and some resistance
- 5 = Normal muscle strength; moves limb against maximal resistance

C. Palpation of lymph nodes (Figure A-2)

Tumor Markers

Tumor markers and the cancers they differentiate, as well as their usefulness, are covered in Table A-3.

Workup and Management of Common Problems

On The Wards

Refer to respective sections in each chapter for a more thorough discussion.

Hypotension

A. Causes: All causes of shock (sepsis, hypovolemia, cardiogenic, anaphylactic, neurogenic), medication (β-blockers, calcium channel blockers, nitrates, morphine, sedatives, epidural infusion)

TABLE A-3 Tumor Marker

Tumor Marker	Cancer	Limitations	Uses/Comments
CEA	Colorectal cancer	Lacks sensitivity and specificity—this is not an effective screening test; levels may be elevated in other malignancies and in some nonmalignant diseases	• Effective for monitoring disease process—a decrease in CEA indicates a favorable response to surgery, and an increase in CEA indicates disease progression • Prognosis—the risk of recurrence is higher if the CEA level was elevated before surgery
AFP	HCC and nonseminomatous germ-cell tumors of testis (NSGCT)	Not specific; can be elevated in nonmalignant diseases such as cirrhosis and hepatitis	Highly elevated AFP levels are present almost exclusively in primary HCC and NSGCT of the testis
CA-125	Ovarian cancer	Neither sensitive nor specific for ovarian cancer, therefore not useful for screening—a normal CA-125 does not exclude ovarian cancer	• Very useful for monitoring the response to therapy (after surgery or chemotherapy)—a decrease in CA-125 after treatment indicates shrinkage of the tumor, and an increase indicates disease progression or recurrence • From 80% to 90% of women 50 yrs of age with a pelvic mass and an increased CA-125 will be found to have ovarian cancer
Prostate-specific antigen (PSA)	See prostate section		
CA 19-9	Pancreatic cancer	Low specificity—this is elevated in colorectal, pancreatic, and gastric cancer, as well as pancreatitis and ulcerative colitis	73% of patients with pancreatic cancer have CA 19-9 levels greater than 100 U/mL
β-hCG	Gestational trophoblastic disease, gonadal germ cell tumor	Elevated in pregnancy	• This has a high sensitivity for diagnosis of choriocarcinoma and trophoblastic neoplasm after evacuation of a molar pregnancy • Either hCG or AFP is elevated in 90% of patients with NSGCT of the testis • hCG may be elevated in either seminomatous germ cell tumors or NSGCTs, but AFP is only elevated in NSGCTs

Appendix

B. Management

1. Quickly assess mental status—how symptomatic is the patient?
2. Obtain a full set of vitals, including BP in both arms. Expect a compensatory tachycardia. Bradycardia may result in reduced cardiac output.
3. Determine baseline BP (may not be significantly different).
4. Consider ECG, CXR, arterial blood gas (ABG), blood culture (if febrile), and CBC (if bleeding is suspected).
5. Treatment should be directed toward the cause.
6. If patient is symptomatic, the reverse Trendelenburg position may be helpful.
7. Consider NS bolus (500 mL)—repeat this if BP does not improve (but be careful in patients with CHF or cardiogenic shock).
8. Discontinue or hold antihypertensive medications.
9. Vasopressors may be needed if there is no response to IV fluids.
10. If hypotension is profound or persists despite fluid therapy, consider transferring the patient to the ICU.
11. Put the patient on a cardiac monitor.

Hypertension

A. Causes

1. Failure to administer, order, or take antihypertensive medications
2. Pain, agitation
3. Hypertensive emergencies (manifested by MI, aortic dissection, encephalopathy, hemorrhagic CVA, or CHF)
4. Delirium tremens
5. Eclampsia or preeclampsia
6. Cocaine, amphetamine use

B. Management

1. Always recheck the BP with a properly fitting cuff to confirm HTN. Check other vital signs.
2. Check the patient's medication record to ensure appropriate compliance with therapy.
3. Check for signs of end-organ damage due to HTN, which indicate that a hypertensive emergency is occurring: Chest pain/ECG changes, neurologic examination findings/encephalopathy, acute renal insufficiency or failure, papilledema.
4. Consider the following tests as appropriate, given the presentation: ECG, renal function panel, cardiac enzymes, CXR, CT of the head.
5. Treat pain and agitation as needed.
6. If HTN is mild and the patient is asymptomatic, observation with follow-up may be appropriate.
7. Oral antihypertensive medications (e.g., clonidine, ACE inhibitors, or oral β-blockers) can be given for most cases of hypertension. Follow response and repeat medication as needed. Be careful not to over treat hypertension, especially when long standing.
8. **Never ignore symptomatic HTN or hypertensive emergencies.** BP must be reduced quickly but carefully. (Reduce mean arterial pressure by no more than 25% in the first 2 hours.) This should be done in the ICU, with IV labetalol, nitroprusside, or enalapril, or additional doses of the patient's current regimen.
9. Reduce or discontinue IV fluids if volume overload is suspected.

> **Quick HIT**
> With hypotension or hypertension, treat the patient, not the BP reading. Asymptomatic patients with hypotension often do not require treatment.

> **Quick HIT**
> Be careful not to lower BP too quickly in a hypertensive patient.

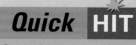

Appendix

Chest Pain

A. Causes

1. **Heart/vascular:** Angina, MI, pericarditis, aortic dissection
2. **GI:** Gastroesophageal reflux disease, diffuse esophageal spasm, peptic ulcer disease, gallbladder disease, acute cholecystitis
3. **Chest wall:** Costochondritis, rib fracture, muscle strain, herpes zoster
4. **Psychiatric:** Anxiety, somatization
5. **Pulmonary:** PE, pneumothorax, pleuritis
6. **Cocaine use:** Can cause angina or MI

B. Management

1. As always, check vital signs. In most cases, obtain a 12-lead ECG. Compare with an old ECG. Get more information about the patient's cardiac history and current history of chest pain.
2. Order cardiac enzymes (creatine kinase; creatine kinase-myocardial bound; troponin) × 3, every 8 hours, if unstable angina or MI is suspected.
3. Consider CXR (pneumothorax, widened mediastinum, pleural effusion). Consider ABG or CT scan/ scan if PE is suspected.
4. If myocardial ischemia is suspected:
   a. Oxygen, 2 L by NC, titrate up as needed.
   b. Nitroglycerin (sublingual) for pain; if pain continues, can give morphine IV.
   c. Keep systolic BP > 90 mm Hg.
   d. Aspirin

e. Heparin—give a loading dose, then start a drip. Check the PTT in 6 hours. Perform a guaiac stool test **before** starting heparin.
f. Put the patient on a cardiac monitor, and consider transfer to a cardiac care unit.

5. Treat other suspected conditions appropriately. See discussions of PE, aortic dissection, pneumothorax, GERD, and PUD.

Tachycardia

A. Types: Determine whether the tachycardia is a narrow or wide complex. Obtain an ECG—is it regular? If wide, treat like ventricular tachycardia (VT). If narrow, determine whether the tachycardia is sinus or nonsinus.

B. Sinus tachycardia

1. HR >100, hardly ever >200 beats/min.
2. Sinus P waves precede each QRS complex.
3. Causes include pain, exercise, anxiety, panic attacks, dehydration, PE, volume loss (bleeding), hyperthyroidism, fever, anemia, albuterol, decongestants, and electrolyte disturbances.
4. Treat the underlying cause. In older patients with cardiac disease, consider a β-blocker to prevent the increase in myocardial O_2 demand that occurs at a high HR.

C. Nonsinus tachycardia

1. Either supraventricular (paroxysmal supraventricular tachycardia, atrial flutter, atrial fibrillation, AV nodal tachycardia) or ventricular (VT, ventricular fibrillation) in origin.
2. Treatments vary according to the arrhythmia.
   a. Paroxysmal supraventricular tachycardia—treat with vagal maneuvers or IV adenosine.
   b. Atrial fibrillation—control the rate with a β-blocker, DC cardioversion, anticoagulation.
   c. Atrial flutter—treat as with atrial fibrillation.
   d. VT—if the patient is stable, give IV amiodarone. If the patient is unstable, perform DC cardioversion.
   e. Ventricular fibrillation—perform immediate defibrillation and CPR.

Oliguria

A. Typically defined as urine output <400 mL/day or <15 mL/hr.

B. Causes

1. Prerenal: hypotension, hypovolemia, CHF, renal arterial occlusion.
2. Renal: glomerulonephritis, acute tubular necrosis, acute interstitial nephritis, vascular insult, and so on.
3. Postrenal: obstruction of lower or upper (bilateral) urinary tract.

C. Management

1. Check other vital signs.
2. Inquire about potential precipitating factors—for example, recent IV contrast administration, new medications (NSAIDs, ACE inhibitors), surgery, recent intake and output, other comorbid conditions (e.g., sepsis, CHF).
3. Palpate the bladder and insert a Foley catheter. If the patient already has a Foley catheter, flush it with 2 to 30 mL of saline to make sure it is not clogged. If urine flows after the Foley placement or flushing, obstruction was most likely the cause.
4. Order serum and urine chemistries and a renal function panel. Calculate the fractional excretion of sodium (<1% is consistent with prerenal causes).
5. Consider a renal ultrasound to exclude hydronephrosis.

6. If prerenal causes are suspected, give an IV fluid challenge (250 to 500 mL of NS). Repeat boluses and maintenance fluids may be required.
7. If CHF is suspected, consider diuresis (e.g., furosemide 20 to 60 mg IV).
8. Stop offending agents (nephrotoxic drugs).
9. Give IV fluids if radiocontrast-induced ATN is suspected.
10. Treat electrolyte disturbances and determine if there is an indication for dialysis.

Fever in the Hospitalized Patient

A. Causes

1. Infection: Likely sources are central lines, peripheral IV lines, pneumonia, Foley catheter, urinary tract, wounds, heart valves, GI tract (diverticulitis), joints (septic arthritis).
2. Noninfectious causes: PE/DVT, medications, neoplasms, connective tissue disorders, postoperative atelectasis.

B. Diagnosis

1. Check vital signs (tachycardia is an expected physiologic response to fever). Hypotension with fever suggests sepsis.
2. Evaluate for signs and symptoms of localizing disease—for example, cough, abdominal pain, meningeal signs, joint pain, diarrhea, cellulitis.
3. Consider CBC, urinalysis, CXR, cultures (blood × 2, urine, sputum, all ports of all lines, any fluid collections), with sensitivity panels.
4. Lumbar puncture if meningitis is a possible cause; CT of the abdomen if intra-abdominal infection is suspected.

C. Therapies

1. Acetaminophen is appropriate in most cases.
2. If the patient is ill-appearing, hemodynamically unstable or neutropenic, start broad-spectrum antimicrobial treatment empirically as soon as cultures are obtained. Transfer to an ICU if patient is in septic shock.
3. If the patient is on an antibiotic and the fever spikes again, consider adding another antibiotic or changing the antibiotic altogether. Antifungal agents may be required.
4. Remove or replace IV lines and indwelling catheters. Culture tips of central lines.
5. If no signs of infection and patient is hemodynamically stable, treat underlying etiology or continue diagnostic workup.

Hypoglycemia

- Usually due to excess insulin or oral hypoglycemic administration (relative to dietary intake) in diabetic patients.
- If the patient can drink and hypoglycemia is mild, give juice. Consider giving 50 mL of D50W intravenously if the patient is symptomatic.
- If the patient is NPO or hypoglycemia persists, start D5W or D10W at 100 mL/hr.
- If there is no IV access and the patient cannot drink/eat, give glucagon (0.5 to 1.0 mg SC or IM).
- Review and modify insulin and oral hypoglycemic regimens.

Change in Mental Status (Confusion)

A. Causes

1. **Medications and intoxications:** sedatives, narcotics, insulin, oral hypoglycemics, H_2 blockers, TCAs, anticholinergics, corticosteroids, hallucinogens, cocaine, alcohol, methanol, ethylene glycol
2. **Hypoxia**—very common
3. **Postoperative delirium**—compounded by pain medications
4. **Hypotension**—with reduced cerebral perfusion
5. **Substance withdrawal**—for example, alcohol, benzodiazepines

Appendix

6. **Hypercapnia**
7. **Infection**— sepsis, meningitis, encephalitis, UTI, intracerebral abscess
8. **Trauma**—head trauma, burns
9. **Metabolic disturbances**—acidosis, hypoglycemia, sodium, calcium, magnesium, hypo/hypernatremia, ammonia (liver failure)
10. **Hyperthyroidism or hypothyroidism, thyroid storm**
11. **Neurologic causes**—CVA, subarachnoid hemorrhage, increased ICP
12. **Dehydration and malnutrition**—deficiencies of thiamine, vitamin B_{12}
13. **ICU psychosis**, sundowning

B. Management

1. Determine if there is a baseline history of dementia—any recent fall?
2. Check vitals; perform a focused examination (including neurologic examination and mental status).
3. Consider pulse oxygen ("pulse ox"), ABG, electrolytes, finger stick, CXR, blood cultures, LFTs, urine toxicology screen.
4. Consider a CT of the head to rule out CVA or intracranial mass or bleed.
5. Correct reversible causes and stop offending medications (if possible).
6. Consider naloxone (2 mg IV), dextrose (D50), and oxygen.
7. If patient is combative or is pulling out IVs, consider haloperidol (Haldol) or possibly restraints if necessary.

Shortness of Breath/Acute Hypoxia

A. Causes

1. Cardiac: PE, CHF exacerbation, MI, arrhythmia
2. Pulmonary: pneumonia, bronchospasm, pleural effusion, pulmonary edema, pneumothorax, upper airway obstruction, hyperventilation
3. Oversedation: narcotics, benzodiazepines (determine exactly how much sedating medication the patient has received)
4. Systemic causes: severe chronic anemia, sepsis, diabetic ketoacidosis
5. Other causes: rib fracture, anxiety, panic attacks

B. Management

1. Perform pulse oximetry immediately. If low, or if the patient appears ill, obtain an ABG and give supplemental oxygen (titrate according to response). Consider biphasic positive airway pressure in cases of COPD.
2. Remember ABCs—intubate if necessary.
3. Consider nebulizer treatments, furosemide, and naloxone as appropriate.
4. Perform portable CXR immediately unless hypoxia is readily resolved (e.g., with naloxone).
5. Consider ECG, CBC (anemia, infection); scan (or spiral CT) if PE suspected.
6. Consider anxiolytics if anxiety-related hyperventilation is suspected and the patient is stable.

Basic Statistics and Evidence-based Medicine

A. Evidence-based medicine has been defined as "the conscientious, explicit, and judicious use of current best evidence in making decisions about the care of individual patients" (Sacket D. *BMJ*. 1996;312:71).

B. Types of research studies

1. Case series—these may describe the results of a specific treatment, determine long-term outcome of a treatment or procedure, or describe the complication rates of a procedure or the natural history of a disease (see also Clinical Pearls A-1 and A-2).
   a. Size of a case series can range from two or three patients to thousands of patients. A case report is the description of a rare or interesting case.

Quick HIT

- Descriptive study designs (case reports, case series, cross-sectional studies) suggest or generate hypotheses.
- Analytic study designs (observational studies, randomized controlled trials) test hypotheses.

Quick HIT

Case-control studies and cohort studies are often referred to as "observational studies."

Quick HIT

Randomization is important because it leaves patient assignment to either experimental or control group completely to **chance.** When any element of human intrusion or judgment enters the process of patient assignment, bias is introduced.

Quick HIT

Hierarchy of evidence (from highest to lowest)
1. Meta-analysis of randomized controlled trials
2. Randomized controlled trials
3. Cohort studies
4. Case-control studies
5. Case series
6. Expert opinion

CLINICAL PEARL A-1

Consolidation of Standards for Reporting Trials (CONSORT) Statement

- Published in 1996, revised in 2001 (*JAMA.* 2001; 285:1987).
- Twenty-one–point checklist of essential items that randomized controlled trial reports should include to facilitate their appraisal and interpretation.
- Many journals have endorsed CONSORT, but the rigor of enforcement varies.

   b. Major disadvantage is the lack of a comparison group so one cannot reach definitive conclusions about treatment efficacy. Case series are prone to many biases.
   c. Very common in surgical research.
2. Cross-sectional studies—subjects are studied at a specific point in time ("snapshot" of a population).
3. Case-control studies.
   a. Patients are selected because they have a certain outcome, and their history is retrospectively reviewed to identify exposures or risk factors that may be associated with that outcome.
   b. By definition, case-control studies can be only retrospective.
   c. Good for rare diseases and for diseases with long latent periods.
   d. Very susceptible to bias because both exposure and disease development occurred prior to initiation of the study.
4. Cohort studies.
   a. Subjects are selected according to exposure (e.g., a new medication, a procedure) and are followed over time to observe the development or progression of disease.
   b. Cohort studies can be prospective or retrospective.
   c. Prospective cohort studies follow patients over time to observe a certain outcome, but patient assignment into the two treatment groups is not randomized, so confounding variables may be unequally distributed (see later).
5. Randomized controlled trial.
   a. A type of cohort study involving a control group and an intervention group.
   b. Patient assignment into either group is left completely to chance (if properly done). Therefore, known and unknown confounders are likely to be equally distributed.
   c. Methodologically superior to other study designs because it is least susceptible to bias.
6. Meta-analyses
   a. Meta-analyses combine data from several individual studies to estimate an overall effect.
   b. The strength of a meta-analysis is only as good as the quality of the primary studies it analyzes (e.g., a meta-analysis of 14 flawed, biased studies will produce a biased estimate of effect).
   c. A meta-analysis of well-conducted randomized controlled trials is the highest level of evidence.

Quick HIT

The basic difference between a randomized controlled trial and a prospective cohort study is the manner in which patients are assigned to either group.
- In a randomized controlled trial, patients are assigned to either the experimental or control group randomly, without input from physician or patient.
- In a cohort study, the treatment decision is not random and is determined by the recommendations of the physician, as well as the wishes of the patient, among other factors.

CLINICAL PEARL A-2

Cochrane Library (www.cochrane.org)

- Regularly updated evidence-based medicine database
- Includes randomized controlled trials and systematic reviews in all specialties of medicine to determine how strong the evidence is for various medical treatments
- Consists of an international network of researchers and physicians who gather and evaluate the evidence in medical research

Quick HIT

The null hypothesis postulates that there is no difference between two groups. This hypothesis is either rejected or not rejected by a study.

Quick HIT

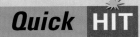

Clinical significance is unrelated to statistical significance. A study may obtain statistical significance for differences that have no clinical significance (e.g., 41% vs. 42% infection rate for two groups). With a large enough sample size, any study will obtain statistical significance.

Quick HIT

If a study has a power of 80%, this means that if a difference of a particular stated magnitude exists between groups, there is an 80% chance of correctly detecting it.

Quick HIT

The lack of statistical power (i.e., sample size too small) invalidates a study because it can lead to statistical insignificance when there actually is a clinically meaningful difference.

Quick HIT

Think of the CI as a weather forecast: a vague forecast of "warm with possibility of rain" (this is a "wide" CI) is more likely to hold true but is not very precise. However, a forecast of "70 degrees with 30% chance of rain" (narrow CI) is much more precise but has a lower likelihood of holding true.

TABLE A-4 Sensitivity and Specificity

	Result of Test Under Investigation	
Result of Gold Standard	**Disease Positive**	**Disease Negative**
Test positive (a 1 b)	True positive (a)	False positive (b)
Test negative (c 1 d)	False negative (c)	True negative (d)

C. Sensitivity and specificity

1. Sensitivity = a/a + c (see Table A-4). Tests with high sensitivity are used for screening. They may yield false-positive results but do not miss people with the disease (low false-negative rate).
2. Specificity = d/b + d. Tests with high specificity are used for disease confirmation.
3. Positive predictive value (PPV) = a/a + b.
   a. If the test is positive, what is the probability that the patient has the disease?
   b. PPV depends on the prevalence (the higher the prevalence, the greater the PPV) and the sensitivity/specificity of the test (e.g., an overly sensitive test yields more false-positive results and has a lower PPV).
4. Negative predictive value (NPV) = d/c + d.
   a. If test is negative, what is the probability that patient does not have the disease? **A high NPV is very important for a screening test.**
   b. NPV also depends on prevalence of disease (higher prevalence = lower NPV) and the sensitivity/specificity of the test (the more sensitive the test, the fewer the number of false-negative results, and the higher the NPV).

D. Type 1 and 2 errors

1. Type 1 (alpha) error: Null hypothesis is rejected even though it is true (false-positive finding).
   a. *P* value is the chance of a type 1 error occurring.
   b. If the *P* value is ≤0.05, it is unlikely that a type 1 error has been made (i.e., a type 1 error is made five or fewer times out of 100 attempts).
2. Type 2 (beta) error: Null hypothesis is not rejected even though it is false (a false-negative finding).
   a. A type 2 error results when the *P* value fails to reach statistical significance **even though the groups being compared are truly different.** A type 2 error usually occurs when sample size is too small.
   b. The likelihood of avoiding a type 2 error is termed the **statistical power** of a study.

E. Statistical power

1. A study with "negative" result (no difference between groups) must have adequate power to detect clinically meaningful differences.
2. Conventionally, a beta error rate of 20% is chosen, which corresponds with a study power of 80%. A study power of less than 80% is believed to have an unacceptably high risk of false-negative results (i.e., a study found no difference between two groups, when there actually was a difference).
3. Factors that affect the power of a study.
   a. Sample size—when sample size is small, a study is susceptible to type 2 error, which is why sample size calculation is done prior to the study being initiated.
   b. Level of statistical significance—conventionally, a *P* value of 0.05 is chosen, although this is somewhat arbitrary.
   c. Variability of the sample data—the lower the variability, the fewer subjects are needed to demonstrate significant differences if they do indeed exist.
   d. Effect size chosen by researcher—this is based on pre-existing data and clinical judgment and is beyond the scope of this discussion.

F. Confidence interval

1. The confidence interval (CI) allows the reader to apply the results of a study to the "true" population from which the sample in the study was taken.
2. The most common CI is 95%, which means that the CI (i.e., the range) reported in the study holds true for 95 of 100 samples similar to the one in the study.
3. A "wider" CI increases the certainty of the estimate (i.e., it is more likely that the population from which the sample was selected would fall within the reported interval), but lowers its precision (see Quick Hit). A very wide CI should be interpreted with caution (a larger sample size may be needed to maintain power).
4. The larger the CI, the less power a study has to detect differences between two groups. The width of the CI depends on sample size; the larger the sample size (more likely to have power), the narrower the CI.

G. Association versus correlation

1. Association is used for describing relationships between categorical variables; correlation describes relationships between continuous variables.
2. Neither association nor correlation implies causation. These terms describe only the relationship and strength of this relationship.
3. Correlation is a matter of "degree." It can range from −1.00 (inverse proportionality) to +1.00 (proportional relationship). Zero signifies no correlation.

H. Causality It is very difficult to prove causality. The following factors help assess causality, but none can give indisputable evidence of a cause-and-effect relationship:

1. Strength of association
2. Biologic plausibility—does the association make biologic sense?
3. Consistency of the association across different studies
4. Dose–response relationship
5. Experimental evidence to support causality—for example, if you eliminate an exposure, does this reduce the incidence of a particular disease?
6. Temporal sequence (very important)—the causative factor must precede the effect.
7. Experimental evidence—has a randomized controlled trial (highest level of evidence) been performed?

I. Bias

1. A study that is biased lacks internal validity. Bias can be introduced in the design of a study or during the statistical analysis because of the lack of statistical power (inadequate sample size). In addition, conflict of interest can introduce bias and affect the validity of a study. Critical appraisal of medical literature essentially requires the ability to identify bias.
2. There are four main types of bias: Selection bias, performance bias, detection bias, and attrition bias (see Clinical Pearl A-3).
3. A **confounding variable** is a factor other than the intervention under investigation that obscures the primary comparison.
   a. Common confounding variables include age, gender, comorbidities, smoking, and socioeconomic status.
   b. A true confounding variable must meet two criteria: It must be associated with the explanatory (independent) variable, **and** it should be a risk factor for the outcome of interest.
   c. Randomized controlled trials control for both known and **unknown** confounders.
4. Minimizing bias in randomized clinical trials hinges on the following:
   a. **Proper randomization**—each patient should have an **equal** chance of receiving either treatment.
   b. **Concealment of allocation**—the person enrolling patients into study should be unaware of next "assignment" into either the experimental or control group. This can be done with sealed opaque envelopes, remote allocation (call made to a separate department to determine patient allocation), or computerized allocation.

Quick HIT

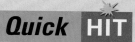

Selection bias refers to differences in characteristics of subjects included/excluded or differences between selected comparison groups.

Quick HIT

Selection Bias
Ideally, comparison groups should be identical in all respects other than factor under investigation. In reality, this comparison group does not exist due to confounding variables. Therefore, randomized controlled trials are preferred to minimize confounding.

Quick HIT

The only inherent advantage of randomized controlled trials over observational studies is the reduction in confounding.

Quick HIT

When evaluating a randomized clinical trial, go through this checklist to assess whether a study is biased:

- Proper randomization
- Concealment of allocation
- Blinding
- Completeness of follow-up and intent-to-treat analysis

Quick HIT

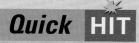

Intent-to-Treat Analysis
Patients are analyzed with the group to which they were randomly assigned, regardless of whether they actually received that treatment or completed the study.

CLINICAL PEARL A-3

Types of Bias

- **Selection bias**—occurs when there are differences in the characteristics of subjects between comparison groups of a study. Unequal distribution of confounding variables among the two groups leads to selection bias.
- **Performance bias**—occurs when subjects in comparison groups are given different care (other than the intervention that is being studied). For example, only one group may receive counseling in addition to the intervention that is being studied (the counseling may affect the outcome in some way). Blinding is important in preventing performance bias (patient and investigators are not aware of the treatment rendered).
- **Detection bias**—refers to inconsistency in outcome assessment. Use of validated outcome measures and blinding of outcome assessors helps prevent detection bias.
- **Attrition bias**—refers to patient drop-outs or exclusion from a study. There is no recognized drop-out rate that is deemed "acceptable." Drop-outs should be kept to a minimum, but if they do occur, *intent-to-treat analysis* is critical to maintain the integrity of randomization (see text).

c. **Blinding**—the higher the level of blinding, the lower the risk of bias. The following participants can potentially be blinded depending on the nature of the study: Patients, physicians, data collectors, assessors of outcome, data analysts. A study should describe precisely which participants were blinded. Terms such as "double" and "triple" blinding, if not defined, are confusing and should be avoided because textbooks and physicians often have varying interpretations of these terms.

d. **Intent-to-treat analysis**—drop-outs are analyzed in groups to which they were initially assigned. Excluding drop-outs from analysis threatens the balance that randomization achieves. Drop-outs often do worse than patients who remain, and excluding them creates bias.

Appendix

J. Glossary of common statistical terms

1. Mean—the average
2. Median—value corresponding to the middle case or middle observation (i.e., 50% of values are less than and 50% of the values are more than the median).
3. Mode—value that occurs most often
4. Standard deviation (SD)—used for normal distributions. An SD of ± 1 includes about 68% of the observations, an SD of ± 2 includes about 95% of the observations, and an SD of ± 3 includes about 99.7% of the observations.
5. Incidence—number of new cases of a disease per year.
6. Prevalence—overall proportion of the population who have the disease.
7. Relative risk—incidence in exposed group/incidence in unexposed group. Relative risk can be calculated only after a prospective or experimental study.
8. Odds ratio—a method of estimating the relative risk in retrospective studies. It is the probability of an event happening divided by the probability of the event not happening.
9. Reliability—ability of a test or measure to reproduce the same results under the same conditions.
10. Validity—extent to which a study correctly represents the relationships being assessed.
    a. Internal validity—a study that suffers from bias lacks internal validity.
    b. External validity—a study may have internal validity but its results may not be generalized to a larger population (lacks external validity).

End of Life Issues and Informed Consent

1. Advance directives are instructions given by patients that specify what actions to take for their health if they are not able to make decisions due to illness.
    a. A living will leaves instructions for treatment, outlining the patient's wishes. A living will may specify that patient does not want to be on a ventilator, or does

not want a blood transfusion. These instructions should be respected even if a family member disagrees with them.

   b. A power of attorney (healthcare proxy)—person appointed by patient to make decisions on their behalf.
   c. Ethics committee is used when patient has lost decision making capacity and there is no advance directive.
   d. Court order—when patient has no capacity to understand and the family is in disagreement and there is no healthcare proxy specified.
2. An adult of sound mind who has capacity to understand has ultimate decision making authority about his or her own medical care. If such an adult refuses a treatment, respect his or her wishes, even if that treatment is clearly indicated or the standard of care. For example, never force a Jehovah's Witness to accept blood products. Patients can refuse medical care even if this refusal results in their death.
   a. All medical interventions (including artificial nutrition and hydration) may be terminated at the patient's request.
   b. If a patient who is mentally incapacitated is in a persistent vegetative state or comatose, family members (even if not formally appointed as proxy decision makers) can withdraw life-sustaining treatments based on prior conversations with the patient or their understanding of the patient's values.
3. Definition of death: An individual who has sustained either (1) irreversible cessation of circulatory and respiratory functions, or (2) irreversible cessation of all the functions of the entire brain, including the brain stem. So to declare an individual dead, either the heart and lungs OR the brain and brain stem stop functioning permanently.
4. Informed consent.
   a. Every procedure needs informed consent. Only the person performing the procedure should obtain consent.
   b. Informed consent should include the following:
      - The diagnosis or medical problem for which the physician is recommending treatment.
      - A description of the proposed treatment or procedure, including its purpose, duration, methods, and implements used, as well as the probability of success.
      - All material risks of the procedure or treatment.
      - Any reasonable alternatives to the proposed procedure
      - The risks of not being treated.
   c. Patient who does not have capacity to consent (comatose, incompetent)—healthcare power of attorney can consent or refuse. If there is uncertainty about a patient's competence, psychiatric evaluation is necessary. If a patient is determined to be incompetent, and if there is no POA, the wishes of family (or next of kin) should be respected. If there is disagreement amongst family members, go to hospital ethics committee.
   d. If an adult regains capacity, then the duty of informed consent returns to the patient and the healthcare POA cannot make decisions.
   e. Emergencies: Consent is not needed in an emergency, it is implied. If a pediatric patient needs emergent treatment and parent is not available for consent, physician may proceed to treat patient without consent.
   f. Remember that minors (under 18) cannot make decisions or consent to or refuse medical treatments. Only parents or legal guardians can consent. Patients under 18 do not require parental consent in the following situations:
      - They are emancipated (married, living on their own and financially independent, raising children, serving in armed forces).
      - Have an STD.
      - Want contraception.
      - Are pregnant and need prenatal care.
      - Want drug tx or counseling (substance abuse treatment).
      - Have psychiatric illness.

Quick HIT

DNR (do not resuscitate)—refers only to withholding cardiopulmonary resuscitation.

QUESTIONS

1. A 61-year-old male presents to your office with the chief complaint of "coughing up blood and weakness" for the past 3 weeks. He reports at least five to six episodes every 2 to 3 days of coughing of bright red blood, approximately one to two tablespoons each time. The patient denies any chest pain, fevers, chills, or recent travel. He has mild dyspnea at baseline. He has recently developed lower extremity muscle cramps and he has difficulty rising from a chair. Past medical history is significant for COPD diagnosed 5 years ago and HTN. He has a 40-pack-year smoking history and currently smokes 1 pack per day. Examination is notable for end-expiratory wheezing and a prolonged expiratory phase on lung auscultation. He has 3/5 hip flexion and decreased deep tendon reflexes bilaterally in lower extremities. Laboratory tests are normal including electrolytes. CXR reveals typical changes seen in COPD (flattened diaphragms, hyperinflation) and a perihilar mass. What is the most likely diagnosis?
   - A. Bronchial carcinoid
   - B. Adenocarcinoma
   - C. Large cell carcinoma
   - D. Squamous cell carcinoma
   - E. Small cell carcinoma

2. A 67-year-old male presents to the ED with LLQ pain that began a few hours ago. His PMH is significant for hypertension, CHF, and renal calculi. He reports one episode of blood in his stools a few months ago. Vital signs are as follows: Temperature = 101.1°F, BP = 130/76 mm Hg, pulse = 70. On physical examination, he has guarding and tenderness to palpation in the LLQ but no epigastric tenderness or flank tenderness. His examination is otherwise unremarkable. His stool is negative for occult blood. Urinalysis reveals no leukocytes or RBCs and Gram stain is negative. Laboratory tests reveal a leukocyte count of 16,000 cells/μL and normal electrolytes and renal function. What is the next step in managing this patient?
   - A. Check a serum lactate
   - B. Obtain a retroperitoneal ultrasound
   - C. Prepare the patient for colonoscopy
   - D. Obtain contrast enhanced CT of the abdomen
   - E. Proceed to the operating room

3. A 64-year-old female with a history of HTN, CAD, and CHF presents to the ED with a chief complaint of left-sided chest pain that began 4 to 5 hours ago. She has a history of periodic episodes of chest pain for which she takes sublingual nitroglycerin, but today's episode has been more severe, has lasted longer, and is not relieved by nitroglycerin. She denies nausea/vomiting, any radiation of the pain, or diaphoresis. Temperature = 97.8°F, BP = 136/76 mm Hg, HR = 105, RR = 20. Physical examination includes clear lungs on auscultation, no JVP elevation, and no LE swelling. EKG shows Q waves in lateral leads and no ST elevation. Troponin is 0.50 ng/mL. Aspirin is given. What is the most important intervention indicated at this time?
   - A. Alteplase
   - B. Heparin
   - C. Hydralazine
   - D. Furosemide
   - E. Digoxin

4. A 64-year-old male presents to the ED with symptoms of RUE weakness and slurred speech. His symptoms started 5 hours ago and have not improved. He has a medical history significant for hypertension and diabetes. Neurologic examination confirms RUE paresis and dysarthria. Rest of examination is normal. Vitals: BP 190/100 mm Hg, HR 75. Labs are notable for glucose of 135 mg/dL, A1c 7.3%. CT head shows an area of ischemia without associated hemorrhage. Home medications include metformin and lisinopril. What is the most important intervention at this point?

A. Insulin
B. Heparin
C. Aspirin
D. Alteplase
E. Labetalol

5. A 58-year-old male presents to your office with weakness in his legs and a history of frequent falls over the past few months. He also complains of fatigue at the end of the day. He denies any back pain. He does not drink alcohol or smoke. His medical history is significant for gastric carcinoma for which he underwent total gastrectomy 2 years ago and there are no signs of recurrence. On physical examination, he is found to have conjunctival pallor, increased deep tendon reflexes, and mild weakness of his lower extremities, along with diminished vibratory sense in his toes. Cerebellar testing is normal. His examination is otherwise unremarkable. What would be the best test in confirming the cause of his symptoms?

A. Folate
B. CBC with mean corpuscular volume
C. Intrinsic factor Ab
D. MRI lumbar spine
E. Methylmalonic acid

6. A 37-year-old nulliparous female presents to your office complaining of weakness, especially with activities that require muscular force, such as climbing stairs. Her symptoms have developed gradually over the past year and she has largely ignored them. She reports a recent weight gain of 25 lb over the past year and has been feeling melancholy for the past few months. She has also had back pain for the past several months. Her medical history is significant for mild HTN, for which she takes metoprolol, and DM that requires insulin therapy. She takes no other medications. Physical examination reveals mild obesity, with fat deposition mainly around the trunk and the posterior neck. You note some facial hair and scattered purple striae on the abdomen. Radiographs reveal a compressed fracture at the level of T11. Vital signs are as follows: BP = 140/85 mm Hg, pulse = 70. What would be the most appropriate next test in this patient?

A. Serum ACTH
B. MRI brain
C. CT abdomen
D. 24-hour urine-free cortisol
E. CRH stimulation test

7. A 56-year-old male with a history of cigarette smoking and hypercholesterolemia is brought to the ED with severe, crushing chest pain that has lasted for 90 minutes. He states that he felt ill all day and then started experiencing pain in his jaw, which progressed to chest pain with radiation to the left arm associated with nausea. Vital signs are as follows: Temperature = 97.4°F, HR = 50, BP = 85/45 mm Hg, RR = 22, pulse oximetry = 98% on room air. Examination reveals JVP without elevation, normal lung examination, and no peripheral edema. An ECG reveals significant ST elevations in leads II, III, and aVF. What is the next step in managing this patient?

A. Nitroglycerin
B. Normal saline
C. Furosemide
D. Metoprolol
E. Morphine

8. A 45-year-old female with history of DM, alcohol abuse, and COPD is evaluated for confusion in the ED. She lives with a roommate who states the patient was acting differently from baseline. The patient is agitated, not oriented, and not responding to questions appropriately. Vitals T 37.5°C, P 110, RR 30. Physical examination reveals lungs with minimal end-expiratory wheezing. Physical examination is otherwise normal. UA is within normal limits. Labs: Na 140 mEq/L, Cl 105 mEq/L, K 5 mEq/L, HCO_3 15 mEq/L, BUN 20 mg/dL, Cr 1 mg/dL. ABG: pH 7.30, PCO_2 25 mm Hg, PO_2 85 mm Hg. What is the next appropriate medical intervention?

A. Fomepizole
B. Acetylcysteine
C. Albuterol
D. Sodium bicarbonate
E. Insulin

9. A 64-year-old male presents to your office for a physical examination. His PMH is significant for HTN, for which he takes metoprolol. He has never had screening for colorectal cancer previously. On examination, there are no palpable masses in the abdomen, no tenderness, and bowel sounds are normal. He denies any change in bowel habits. The remainder of his physical examination is unremarkable. He is given fecal occult blood testing and two of three samples are positive. What is the appropriate next step in managing this patient?

A. Flexible sigmoidoscopy
B. Digital rectal examination
C. Video capsule endoscopy
D. CT colonography
E. Colonoscopy

10. A 55-year-old male presents to the ED with epigastric abdominal pain. He denies nausea/vomiting/diarrhea. His PMH is significant for stroke HTN and osteoarthritis of his knees. Medications include enalapril and a daily aspirin tablet. Vital signs are as follows: RR = 20, BP = 155/90 mm Hg, pulse = 70. His physical examination reveals epigastric tenderness, no abdominal distention, and rectal examination is positive for dark stool that is guaiac positive. Laboratory tests reveal hemoglobin of 10.2 g/dL, hematocrit of 30.0%, platelets $190 \times 10^3/\mu L$. LFT results are normal. Na 135 mEq/L, K 4.5 mEq/L, Cl 105 mEq/L, HCO_3 22 mEq/L, BUN 30 mg/dL, Cr 1.2 mg/dL. What is the next recommended step in managing this patient?

A. IV omeprazole
B. IV octreotide
C. Platelet transfusion
D. RBC transfusion
E. Normal saline

11. A 45-year-old female is admitted to the hospital with abdominal swelling. She has not previously sought medical care and had been well until 3 months ago when swelling began. Swelling gradually began and has worsened to the point that she is now short of breath and has difficulty mobilizing. She was born in Mexico but has been living in the United States for the past 20 years. She denies any use of medications. She admits to social drinking but denies daily use. Lung examination reveals decreased breath sounds at the bases. Cardiac examination reveals no murmurs, JVP 2 cm above sternal angle. Abdomen is moderately distended with a positive fluid wave; liver is unable to be palpated. Skin examination does not reveal telangiectasias. A diagnostic/therapeutic paracentesis is performed which reveals the following: serum albumin 2.5 g/dL, serum total protein 5.0 g/dL, ascites total protein 2.3 g/dL, ascites albumin 1.6 g/dL. What test is the most likely to reveal the cause of her ascites?

A. Echocardiogram
B. Pelvic ultrasound
C. Liver biopsy
D. PPD
E. 24-hour urine protein

12. A 65-year-old man presents to the ED with lower extremity weakness. His symptoms started 1 week prior when he noticed difficulty walking and he tripped once. He now has difficulty raising his legs off the floor and is now using a wheelchair. He denies any pain in his lower extremities but does have paresthesias in both legs. He denies weakness elsewhere. He denies dyspnea or any other associated symptoms. Prior to this he had an episode of nonbloody diarrhea a few weeks prior but that is now resolved. His only past medical history is hypertension for which he takes hydrochlorothiazide. Cardiac examination is normal. Pulmonary examination reveals nonlabored breathing, clear lung fields, and O_2 saturation 98% on room air. Neurologic examination reveals normal speech without dysarthria and cranial nerves without deficits. Strength is 5/5 in bilateral upper extremities in shoulder/elbow/wrist flexion and extension, 1/5 dorsiflexion/plantar flexion bilateral ankles, 1/5 flexion/extension knees, 2/5 hip flexion. Achilles and patellar reflexes are absent bilaterally. Sensory examination is normal. Labs including electrolytes, renal function, and blood counts are normal. CT head is negative for stroke and shows no acute findings. Lumbar puncture is performed and analysis reveals 3 WBC/mm^3, protein 100 mg/dL (normal range <50 mg/dL), Gram stain negative. What is the most appropriate therapy?

A. Prednisone
B. IVIG
C. Ciprofloxacin
D. Pyridostigmine
E. Botulism antitoxin

Questions

13. A 24-year-old female presents to your office for a routine examination. She reports a history of heavy menstrual bleeding since menarche. Her mother had similar symptoms. On further questioning, she states that she has episodes of epistaxis about once every 2 weeks or so and has a tendency to bruise easily. Her physical examination is unremarkable. CBC results are as follows: Hgb = 7.9 g/dL, Hct = 23.9%, MCV = 69 fL. Platelet count is 230,000/μL. PT—12 seconds (normal). PTT—30 seconds (normal). LFTs including bilirubin are normal. What is the most appropriate test to order?

A. Fibrinogen
B. Coombs antibody
C. Factor IX level
D. Mixing study
E. Ristocetin cofactor activity

14. A 43-year-old male presents to the ED with a complaint of headache. Headache developed acutely over the past few hours and is severe in nature. Pain is located bilateral top of his head without radiation elsewhere. He denies any associated weakness. He denies double vision, dizziness, nausea, and vomiting. He denies phonophobia/photophobia. He has no prior history of headaches. Vitals: BP 144/90 mm Hg, T 37.2°C. Examination reveals a middle-aged man in distress related to pain. Neurologic examination is negative for focal weakness or sensory deficit. No nuchal rigidity. CN are intact. CT brain without contrast is obtained and negative for ischemia or hemorrhage. What is the next most appropriate intervention?

A. Sumatriptan
B. MRI brain
C. Cerebral angiogram
D. CT brain with contrast
E. Lumbar puncture

15. A 59-year-old female presents to the office because she is "sick and tired" of this cough she has had for 5 years, and it is getting worse. The cough is often productive of watery mucus. She is also becoming more and more short of breath and cannot climb a flight of stairs without taking a rest. She denies chest pain, paroxysmal nocturnal dyspnea, fevers, chills, and weight loss. PMH is significant for HTN and a 35-pack-year history of cigarette smoking. Vital signs are as follows: Temperature = 99.0°F, HR = 75, RR = 21, BP = 158/82 mm Hg. O_2 saturation is 94% at rest and reaches a nadir of 90% with activity. Physical examination reveals an obese woman in no acute distress. On lung auscultation, there are coarse breath sounds bilaterally but no wheezes or crackles. Chest radiograph is significant for prominent lung markings at the bases. PFTs show FEV_1/FVC ratio 0.60 and FEV_1 65%. What is the most effective long-term intervention for this woman?

A. Smoking cessation
B. Tiotropium inhaler
C. Fluticasone inhaler
D. Oxygen therapy
E. Azithromycin

16. A 56-year-old male comes to your clinic requesting advice after recent cardiac surgery. The patient had a long-standing murmur and was diagnosed with mitral stenosis. He eventually underwent repair with a prosthetic valve and his symptoms of dyspnea have resolved. He has resumed physical activity and seeks to maintain his current health. He wants advice on future procedures and possible risk of infection. Which procedure will you advise warrants such treatment solely for endocarditis prophylaxis?

A. Colonoscopy
B. Wisdom tooth extraction
C. EGD
D. Bronchoscopy without biopsy
E. Dilatation ureteral stricture

17. A 67-year-old African-American male presents to your office with complaint of right hip pain for the last week. He denies any history of falls or injury. The pain came on suddenly as he was getting up from a chair. Prior to this episode, he denies any history of hip pain. PMH is significant for HTN, diabetes, and hypothyroidism. He started using a cane a few days ago but due to increasing pain is now in a wheelchair. On physical examination, he has severe pain with any attempted motion of the right hip joint. Pulses are palpable bilaterally, and neurologic examination is normal. Radiographs of the right hip are obtained and show normal bone density with a displaced fracture of the right femoral neck. Labs: Na+ 135 mEq/L, Cl 105 mEq/L, HCO_3 25 mEq/L, Ca2+ 11.0 mg/dL, Cr 1.9 mg/dL, Hgb 9.5 g/dL, MCV 90 fL. Labs a year ago were completely normal. He is up to date on routine health screening. In addition to obtaining an orthopedic surgery referral for repair of the fracture what other testing would be indicated that would best explain the patient's findings?

A. SPEP
B. ^{99m}Tc bone scan
C. PTHrP
D. PTH
E. DEXA

Questions

18. A 38-year-old female presents to your office with chief complaint of fatigue and weight gain for the past 5 to 6 months. Her fatigue has also affected her performance at work, where she has difficulty concentrating on tasks. She recently began losing hair. She feels more tired than usual after work and has difficulty playing with her children in the evening. She did not have any of these symptoms until 6 months ago. She denies hot/cold intolerance. Weight has been relatively stable but she has gained ~10 pounds in the past 6 months despite attempting to eat healthy and exercise a few times weekly. She is generally happy and denies any recent mood changes. PMH is insignificant. The patient smokes five to six cigarettes a day and drinks alcohol socially. She takes birth control pills. HR 55, BP 120/80 mm Hg, RR 16, BMI 31. Physical examination reveals a pleasant female, oriented and appropriate. ENT examination reveals normal pharynx, no neck fullness, and no palpable thyroid nodules. Abdomen is soft, nontender. Skin examination reveals no lesions/rashes and there is no lower extremity edema. She donated blood last week and was told that her Hgb was normal. What is the appropriate next step in managing this patient?

A. US thyroid
B. TPO
C. Thyroid uptake scan
D. FNA
E. TSH

19. A 38-year-old female presents to the ED with a 2-day history of shortness of breath and chest pain. She states that she has felt tired for the past couple of weeks but is otherwise vague in reporting her history. She denies any history of smoking. PMH is unremarkable. On physical examination, she has diffuse wheezing but no calf tenderness or lower extremity edema. BP = 126/74 mm Hg, pulse = 80, RR = 20, temperature = 98.6°F. D-dimer is elevated. CXR reveals no infiltrate. She subsequently undergoes a CT scan which reveals an 8-mm round nodule without associated lymphadenopathy or effusions and no evidence of pulmonary embolism. There are no calcifications in the nodule. She is treated with albuterol and discharged home in stable condition. What is the appropriate recommendation to this patient upon outpatient follow-up with her primary care physician?

A. Follow-up CT chest
B. Bronchoscopy
C. Needle biopsy
D. Follow-up CXR
E. PET-CT scan

20. A 75-year-old female with a history of two MIs presents to the ED after fainting. She reports fatigue and dyspnea for 2 months. She has mild chest pain and dyspnea. A 12-lead ECG reveals a bradycardia with a ventricular rate of 35 bpm. BP 80/55 mm Hg. Examination reveals: General—mild distress, Heart—regular, bradycardia, no murmurs, Lungs—clear without crackles/effusions, Skin—cold, clammy. Home medications include ASA, metoprolol, atorvastatin, and lisinopril. EKG is as below. Prior echocardiogram from 6 months prior showed EF of 29% with diastolic dysfunction; valves were normal without stenosis or regurgitation. Laboratory testing reveals normal electrolytes including Mg and K. Troponin is elevated. What is the most appropriate management?

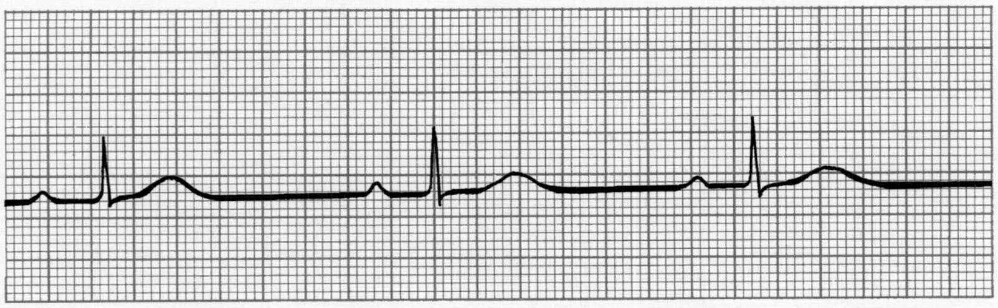

A. Echocardiogram
B. Nitroglycerin
C. Metoprolol
D. Atropine
E. ICD

21. A 40-year-old male presents to your office with a complaint of "chest burning" and cough for the past 5 to 6 months. The pain is not related to meals and is intermittent. Triggers for his symptoms include drinking alcohol and lying flat in bed. He denies food getting stuck upon swallowing. He has tried over-the-counter calcium carbonate and used ranitidine as needed with minimal relief of symptoms. He denies any recent weight loss. He denies any dark or bloody stools. He is a nonsmoker. He denies any history of seasonal allergies, itchy/watery eyes, sneezing, dyspnea, or prior diagnosis of asthma. His PMH is significant for HTN, which is controlled with metoprolol. He does not take any other medications. Physical examination is unremarkable. How would you treat this patient?

A. *Helicobacter pylori* antigen
B. EGD
C. pH monitoring
D. Gastrin level
E. Omeprazole

22. A 32-year-old female presents to your office with a history of diarrhea and intermittent abdominal cramping/bloating with flatus. She reports having loose, watery diarrhea very frequently on and off for several years, but her symptoms have been worse recently. Prior to initial onset she had normal, formed daily bowel movements. Her weight is 75 kg and on review of her records it is 7 kg less than when her symptoms first started. She denies any blood in the stool. There is no family history of IBD or colon cancer. The patient's only past medical history is depression for which she is undergoing counseling. Laboratory evaluation reveals AST 65 U/L, ALT 55 U/L, TSH 3.0 mU/L, and Cr 1.0 mg/dL. Blood counts show Hgb 9.8 g/dL with MCV 70 fL. Vitals: T 37°C, BP 120/85 mm Hg, RR 16. Physical examination reveals a rash on extensor surfaces of both elbows with erythematous vesicles present. A stool test for occult blood is negative. She is a college student and is studying for her midterm examination. What test should be the next intervention?

A. EGD with small bowel biopsy
B. Colonoscopy
C. Loperamide
D. Sertraline
E. Skin biopsy

Questions

23. A 65-year-old Caucasian female with a history of DM, HTN, and a large anterior wall MI 5 years ago presents to the clinic complaining of shortness of breath. At baseline the patient finds it difficult to do any household chores. She has shortness of breath at rest and is homebound because of her symptoms. Vital signs are: Temperature = 98.7°F, HR = 62, RR = 19, BP = 160/85 mm Hg, oxygen saturation = 90% on room air. There are bibasilar crackles with scattered expiratory wheezes. There is also 2+ pitting edema of the lower extremities. JVP is measured just above the clavicle. An ECG reveals left ventricular hypertrophy (LVH), with Q waves and T-wave inversions in V_1 to V_4 and diffuse nonspecific ST segment abnormalities. A CXR shows cardiomegaly and considerable congestion of the pulmonary vasculature. Prior echocardiogram obtained 1 year prior shows EF 30% with wall motion abnormalities. Labs are normal including CBC, Cr, K. The patient's medications include losartan, carvedilol, and aspirin. What is the most important long-term intervention for this patient?

A. Isosorbide dinitrate
B. Spironolactone
C. Hydralazine
D. Digoxin
E. Furosemide

24. A 23-year-old female is in your clinic to be evaluated for wheezing and shortness of breath. She has no history of respiratory problems prior to the past few months. She recently joined a gym and began increasing her physical activity. Every time she runs she has similar symptoms of wheezing and shortness of breath. Symptoms seem to last the duration of the activity but will resolve afterward. She has no dyspnea between episodes. She denies runny nose, sneezing, congestion. She has no fevers/chills or sputum production. She has no known allergies. She does not smoke. Physical examination reveals a young female with no respiratory distress. Cardiac examination reveals normal rate, no murmurs are appreciated, and JVP is not elevated. Lung examination reveals normal expansion, good air movement in all lung fields without rhonchi or wheezing. Peak flow in clinic is normal. PFTs are obtained and show FEV_1/FVC 0.8. FEV_1 is 93% of predicted. TLC is normal. What is the most appropriate management?

A. CXR

B. Inhaled fluticasone

C. Reassurance

D. Inhaled albuterol prn

E. Inhaled salmeterol

25. A 35-year-old female undergoes routine laboratory workup for an insurance physical. Labs reveal WBC 5.0 $10^3/mm^3$, Hgb 12.7 g/dL, Cr 1.0 mg/dL. Urinalysis shows 2+ bacteria and urine culture grows 10^5 CFU *Escherichia coli*. PMH is otherwise negative. She has had occasional UTIs in the past but none for the past year. Her only medication is oral contraceptives. Urine hCG is negative. Vital signs are: Temperature = 98.6°F, BP = 115/60 mm Hg, pulse = 80, RR = 20. Lungs are clear to auscultation bilaterally. Both heart rate and rhythm are regular, without murmurs. The patient appears well and is alert and oriented. She has no tenderness at the right costovertebral angle and no suprapubic tenderness. What is the appropriate next step in managing this patient?

A. Nitrofurantoin

B. Ciprofloxacin

C. Trimethoprim-sulfamethoxazole

D. No treatment

E. Repeat urinalysis and culture

26. A 45-year-old female is brought to the ED complaining of fatigue. The patient has been feeling extremely weak over the past few days. Today she stood up and almost fainted, prompting her visit. She has had cough, rhinorrhea, and nasal congestion for the past week. Today she also began having nausea, vomiting, and severe abdominal pain. Past medical history is significant for hypertension, CKD, and SLE. Home medications are lisinopril, hydroxychloroquine, and prednisone 15 mg daily. Vitals: Temperature = 38.5°C, BP = 85/55 mm Hg, HR = 126. General—appears weak, lethargic. Cardiac—tachycardic, regular, without murmurs. Lungs—occasional rhonchi, no wheezing. Abdomen—diffuse tenderness with normal bowel sounds. Labs: Na 124, K 5.3, Cr 3.0 (baseline 1.8). Hgb is 11.1 g/dL. The patient is diagnosed with influenza and started on IV fluids. After 2 L of normal saline her blood pressure is 90/60 mm Hg. What is the most appropriate next step?

A. Cortisol level

B. IV hydrocortisone

C. CT adrenal glands

D. MRI pituitary

E. Cosyntropin stimulation test

27. A 71-year-old female presents to the ED with a 2-day history of severe abdominal pain. Pain developed suddenly with no clear correlation to meals. Her symptoms were mild at first, becoming severe in the next 6 to 10 hours. She has nausea, but denies vomiting or dysphagia. Her past medical history is significant for GERD, CHF, poorly controlled DM, and atrial fibrillation. She is afebrile. HR 70, BP 135/85 mm Hg. Cardiac examination reveals a 3/6 systolic murmur in L axilla and irregularly irregular heart rate. Her abdominal examination reveals very mild tenderness in the midabdomen. Her stool is positive for blood. Laboratory studies show Hgb 10.0 g/dL, WBC 17.5 $10^3/mm^3$, Na 144 mEq/L, Cl 105 mEq/L, K 4.0 mEq/L, HCO_3 20 mEq/L, Cr 1.1 mg/dL, A1c 12.6%, and INR 1.6. Medications are metoprolol, warfarin, insulin, and enalapril. What is the appropriate next step in evaluation?

A. CT angiography
B. Gastric emptying study
C. Colonoscopy
D. EGD
E. Vitamin K

28. A 43-year-old male presents to your office with a 3-day history of chest pain, which is mostly centrally located and radiates to the right side of his neck. The pain worsens with deep breathing and improves when he sits up. He denies nausea, vomiting, sweating, and SOB. He had an upper respiratory infection about 2 weeks ago which resolved without treatment. PMH is significant for hyperlipidemia. He takes lovastatin. He smokes half a pack of cigarettes a day. Vital signs are: Temperature = 99.4°F, BP = 125/80 mm Hg, pulse = 84. Physical examination is significant for a friction rub over the left sternal border heard best when he leans forward. A 12-lead ECG shows ST elevation in leads I, II, III, aVL, V_2, V_3, V_4, V_5, and V_6. Echocardiogram shows EF 50% with no regional wall motion abnormalities and normal valvular function. There is a small pericardial effusion. What is the most appropriate next step?

A. Coronary angiogram
B. Drainage of pericardial effusion
C. Prednisone
D. Azathioprine
E. Ibuprofen

29. A 55-year-old male with past history of COPD presents to the emergency department with complaint of chest pain and SOB that started last evening. His chest pain is on the right side of the chest and is stabbing in quality, and the pain increases with inspiration. He is short of breath even at rest. He denies any traumatic event or overexertion. He also denies fevers, chills, and sputum. He has a 35-pack-year smoking history. He takes tiotropium and albuterol prn. Temperature = 98.2°F, BP = 130/80 mm Hg, HR = 115, RR = 24. Pulse oximetry shows 84% oxygen saturation on room air. He is 6 ft 2 in and 175 lb, and he otherwise appears healthy. Physical examination reveals absent breath sounds in R upper lung field. There is minimal end-expiratory wheezing in both lungs without crackles. No stridor is appreciated. Heart examination reveals regular tachycardia without murmurs. JVP is flat. There is no lower extremity edema. What is the appropriate next step in managing this patient?

A. Albuterol–ipratropium nebulizer
B. Prednisone
C. Chest tube insertion
D. Azithromycin
E. Pleurodesis

30. A 78-year-old male with a past history of hypertension and diabetes presents to office for evaluation. He is doing well, except for some palpitations over the past few months. He denies associated shortness of breath or syncope. He has never fallen. On physical examination, you note an irregularly irregular heart rhythm and a middiastolic murmur in the L axilla. Examination is otherwise normal. You obtain an ECG, which confirms the irregularly irregular arrhythmia. The patient has no history of bleeding and Hgb is normal. What is the recommended medication to start the patient on?

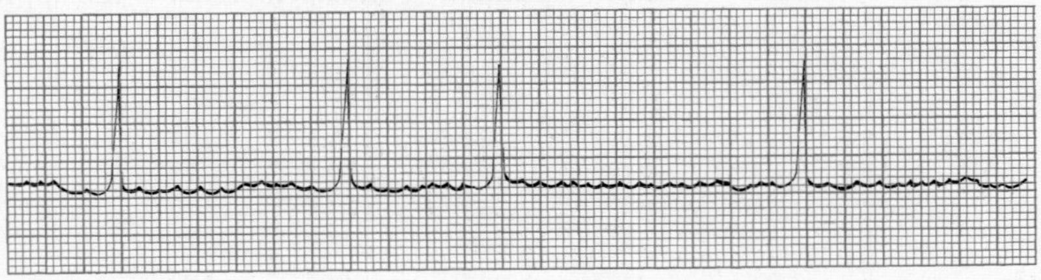

A. Aspirin
B. Dabigatran
C. Clopidogrel
D. Warfarin
E. Fondaparinux

31. A 73-year-old male with HTN presents to the office with a 3-month history of chest pain and dyspnea induced by lifting weights, shoveling snow, and running on a treadmill. Vital signs are as follows: Temperature = 98.3°F, HR = 85, RR = 17, BP = 165/85 mm Hg. Physical examination reveals a 4/6 crescendo–decrescendo murmur heard at the right upper sternal border with radiation to the carotid arteries, weak and delayed carotid pulses, and an S4 gallop. ECG reveals sinus rhythm without arrhythmia. Echocardiogram reveals EF 45% and aortic valve area 0.8 cm^2. Prior coronary angiography 1 year prior showed 20% lesion in the mid-LAD, 30% RCA lesion, and no significant stenosis in the L circumflex artery. What is the most effective intervention strategy for this patient?
A. Nitroglycerin
B. Aortic valve replacement
C. Aspirin
D. Carotid Doppler
E. Coronary artery bypass grafting

32. A 38-year-old female presents to your office complaining of left knee pain for the past 2 to 3 months. She denies any history of injury. PMH is significant for SLE. She was recently increasing her running in an attempt to lose weight but her pain is now limiting her activity. She describes her pain as primarily "around and under my knee cap." She points to her patella and the anterior aspect of her knee as the site of her pain. She especially has difficulty climbing and descending stairs. She has full range of motion without pain. She has no tenderness along medial or lateral joint lines. Examination reveals negative anterior and posterior drawer tests, full ROM in flexion and extension without crepitus, no effusion or erythema present. X-rays of the knee reveal normal alignment with preservation of joint space. Labs: Na 135 mEq/L, K 4.0 mEq/L, Cr 2.3 mg/dL. ANA is positive. ESR 10 mm/hr. What is appropriate next step in the management of this patient?
A. Corticosteroid injection
B. Physical therapy
C. Knee arthroscopy
D. MRI knee
E. Ibuprofen

33. A 57-year-old male had a fasting plasma glucose level of 160 mg/dL 1 month ago. Today, his fasting glucose level is 140 mg/dL. His medical history is significant for CHF and hyperlipidemia. His current medications include aspirin, lisinopril, and metoprolol. He is 5 ft 11 in and weighs 215 lb. BP 142/79. This patient is asymptomatic, and his physical examination is unremarkable. Labs: Na 142 mEq/L, K 4.0 mEq/L, Cr 1.7 mg/dL. Urine microalbumin:Cr ratio >30 mg/g. A1c 7.1 %. In addition to lifestyle changes including increase in physical activity, diet changes, and weight loss, how would you manage this patient?

A. Hydrochlorothiazide
B. Insulin
C. Pioglitazone
D. Metformin
E. Lisinopril

34. A 36-year-old African-American female presents to your office with a 4-month history of dry cough, SOB, and fatigue. She has a 10-pack-per-year smoking history. Vital signs are: Temperature = 98.2°F, BP = 132/79 mm Hg, HR = 74, RR = 16. Pulse oximetry shows 96% O_2 saturation on room air. Examination reveals crackles bilaterally in the lower lung fields. There is no wheezing. She has two tender erythematous nodules on her left leg measuring approximately 3 × 3 cm. CXR shows bilateral hilar adenopathy. What is the next best test in order to confirm the suspected underlying diagnosis that explains the patient's constellation of symptoms?

A. Serum calcium
B. CT chest
C. ACE level
D. Biopsy leg lesion
E. Biopsy hilar adenopathy

35. A 68-year-old male with a history of lung cancer undergoes follow-up labs after recent cycle of chemotherapy. He has mild difficulty with concentration over the past week but is otherwise able to complete all of his daily tasks. He denies any nausea, vomiting, or positional lightheadedness. He has no other significant past medical history. He takes no medications chronically. Vital signs are as follows: Temperature = 99.8°F, RR = 18, BP = 135/88 mm Hg, pulse = 76. On examination, he is alert and oriented. Cardiac examination reveals RRR, no murmurs, JVP not elevated. Lung and abdominal examination is normal. There is no lower extremity edema. Skin turgor is normal. Neurologic examination reveals 5/5 strength in all extremities, no focal deficits and normal gait. Laboratory tests reveal the following: WBC = $8.3 \times 10^3/mm^3$, Hgb = 10.2 g/dL, glucose = 106 mg/dL, serum Na^+ = 121 mEq/L, K^+ = 4.3 mEq/L, BUN 7.0 mg/dL, Cr 0.4 mg/dL. TSH 2.0 mU/L. Serum osmolality 250 mOsm/kg, urine Na 45 mEq/L, urine osmolality 450 mOsm/kg. What would be the most appropriate management of this patient?

A. Administer IV normal (0.9%) saline
B. Initiate fluid restriction
C. Initiate hemodialysis
D. Administer hypertonic (3%) saline
E. Administer hydrochlorothiazide

36. A 20-year-old male presents for evaluation after an episode of dark urine. He felt well up until 2 weeks ago when he had a sore throat and mild fever for which he did not seek medical care. Urinary symptoms started the day prior to evaluation. He denies cough, dyspnea, hemoptysis, joint pains, dysuria, and flank pain. He does have two recent sexual partners but uses condoms. He has no prior medical history and denies any family history of renal diseases. BP 145/90 mm Hg, HR 65, T 37°C. Physical examination reveals a well-appearing male with normal heart sounds, clear lungs, and mild lower extremity edema. There are no skin lesions. Urinalysis that is obtained is dark red in color. Microscopic examination is positive for deformed RBCs and RBC casts. Cr is 1.6 mg/dL. What is the most likely test to help aid in the diagnosis of this patient?

A. ANCA
B. Anti-GBM
C. HIV
D. Antistreptolysin titer
E. IgA levels

Questions

37. A 31-year-old female with hypertension presents to your office complaining of painful joints for the past 4 to 5 months, affecting her wrists, ankles, and knees. She also reports several outbreaks of a rash over her face over the past few months. Her only medications are hydrochlorothiazide and acetaminophen as needed. Vital signs are as follows: Temperature = 99.2°F, RR = 20, BP = 145/83 mm Hg, pulse = 78. Physical examination reveals three ulcers in her mouth and mild swelling of the left wrist and ankle. She has 1+ pitting edema in her lower extremities bilaterally. Examination is otherwise unremarkable. CBC reveals a WBC count of 2,300/mm^3, Hgb 12.2 g/dL, and platelets 82,000/mm^3. What is the most likely diagnosis?

A. Osteoarthritis
B. Reactive arthritis
C. Behçet disease
D. Gout
E. SLE

38. A 62-year-old male presents to your office accompanied by his wife. He complains of a tremor in his hands that disappears when he uses his hands for writing or handling utensils. His wife thinks he stares often and does not show as much emotion as before. He still participates in his usual activities and enjoys gardening with his wife. His appetite and sleep habits have remained unchanged. Weight is similar to his last clinic visit. She notices that he is slower in moving than before and walks steadily. On examination you note a mild resting tremor and a fixed expression on his face. There is resistance on passive range of motion with upper extremities. Gait is slow, without imbalance or falling, and his arm does not swing when walking. He scored 26/30 on Mini-Mental Status Examination. What is the best intervention to improve the patient's symptoms?

A. Fluoxetine
B. Carbidopa–levodopa
C. Propranolol
D. Memantine
E. Deep brain stimulation

39. A 24-year-old male presents to your office having with worsening RLQ cramping abdominal pain for the past 2 months. He reports having diarrhea on and off for the past 1 to 2 years. He previously had colonoscopy with a terminal ileum biopsy showing ulceration, acute inflammation, and noncaseating granulomas. Two months ago he was placed on mesalamine. He has lost 20 lb since then despite attempting to increase his dietary intake. He denies any other medical problems and takes no other medications. His physical examination reveals mild tenderness in the RLQ with normal bowel sounds. There are no anal fissures or fistulae. His stool is negative for occult blood. Vital signs are as follows: Temperature = 98.7°F, RR = 15, BP = 122/78 mm Hg, pulse = 65. BMI 21. Laboratory test results show normal liver/renal function. CBC shows Hgb 9.9 g/dL, MCV 82 fL, WBC 10.1 × 10^3/mm^3. X-ray abdomen reveals nonspecific gas pattern without free air or distended bowel loops. CT enterography reveals thickened mucosa in distal ileum with adjacent mesenteric stranding; there is no fistula, abscess, or free air present. What would be the single most effective intervention recommended to this patient?

A. Loperamide
B. Azathioprine
C. Infliximab
D. Surgical resection
E. Ciprofloxacin and metronidazole

40. A 58-year-old male presents to your office with complaint of left wrist pain for the past 3 months. He cannot recall any history of injury or trauma. He works as a car mechanic. He also has a new granddaughter who is 6 months old that he babysits every weekend. He is an amateur golfer when time allows. He denies neck pain. He has no associated paresthesias or weakness. PMH is significant for mild HTN and chronic kidney disease with a baseline Cr of 2.5 mg/dL. Examination reveals normal sensation throughout bilateral upper extremities. Neck flexion/extension/rotation does not reproduce his symptoms. Strength testing is normal in bilateral upper extremities. There is no evidence of muscle wasting on examination of the hands. With the patient making a fist surrounding the thumb, ulnar deviation of the wrist produces pain over the distal radial styloid. Prolonged wrist flexion does not elicit pain. Palpation over the flexor surface of the wrist base does not reproduce the patient's symptoms. Pain is not elicited with resisted wrist extension or flexion. What is the most appropriate next step in management?

A. Thumb spica splint
B. Wrist splint
C. Counterforce forearm brace
D. Carpal tunnel corticosteroid injection
E. Ibuprofen

41. You are a hospitalist called to evaluate a 74-year-old female for SOB and increasing oxygen requirements. She denies any cough or sputum. The patient was admitted yesterday with multiple leg fractures after a motor vehicle accident. She has been on strict bed rest since admission while a plan is made for surgical repair. She has mild chest pain and feels short of breath. Past medical history is significant for CHF and COPD. She is compliant with her medications which include tiotropium, furosemide, metoprolol, and inhaled fluticasone. Temperature = 100.0°F, BP = 116/74 mm Hg, pulse = 120, RR = 24, oxygen saturation = 91% on 5 L of oxygen via nasal cannula. General examination reveals a patient who is alert to name and year but she does not know where she is. Mental status on admission was normal and she has no history of dementia. She is moderately tachypneic. Lung examination reveals good air movement throughout with no wheezing, crackles, or consolidation. JVP is not elevated. There are scattered petechiae on the upper chest. Bilateral lower extremities have symmetric 1+ edema without calf tenderness. CT chest shows scattered ground glass opacities without consolidation, no segmental or subsegmental emboli, and no effusions. What is the appropriate next step in management?

A. Albuterol
B. Reduction of fracture
C. Furosemide
D. Levofloxacin
E. IV heparin

42. A 38-year-old man is evaluated for palpitations in the ED. He has had these symptoms several times over the past year but this episode is worse. He denies any associated chest pain, lightheadedness, or syncope. He denies any history of medical problems and takes no medications. Examination reveals an adult male in no significant distress. Cardiac examination is significant for regular tachycardia with no JVP elevation. Lungs are clear without crackles or wheezing. There is no lower extremity edema. EKG shows: ____________________. What is the best intervention at this point?

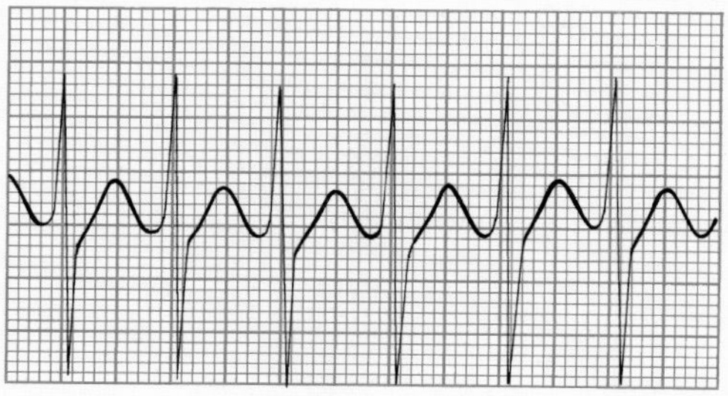

A. Valsalva maneuver
B. Adenosine
C. Metoprolol
D. Digoxin
E. Cardioversion

43. A 38-year-old female presents to your office with pain in her wrists, ankles, and knees bilaterally. She reports noticing numbness and morning stiffness in her hands about 1 year ago, mostly in cold weather. This stiffness gradually spread to her wrists, knees, and ankles, with lesser involvement of her shoulders. The stiffness and pain are worse in the morning but improve as the day wears on. Symptoms have gradually worsened. Some days she cannot go outside her house because of the pain. She denies a history of rash or photosensitivity. She often feels tired and "worn out." Medical history is significant for HTN, for which she takes hydrochlorothiazide. On examination, her metacarpal joints and wrists are swollen and tender, as are her knees and ankles bilaterally. Her examination is otherwise unremarkable. Labs reveal normal liver and renal function. CBC is unremarkable. ESR 65 mm/hr. CCP is positive. ANA is negative. X-rays of hands show erosive changes in MCP joints. What is the most important intervention for this patient to control her disease?

A. Prednisone
B. Corticosteroid injection
C. Indomethacin
D. Hydroxychloroquine
E. Physical therapy

44. A 60-year-old female presents to the ED with a complaint of RUQ abdominal pain that began several hours ago. She has had occasional RUQ pain over the past 3 months but never this severe. Her PMH is only significant for HTN and osteoarthritis. On physical examination, she appears ill. Scleral icterus is present. She has RUQ abdominal tenderness without peritoneal signs and bowel sounds are normal. There are no surgical scars on the abdomen. Initial vital signs are as follows: Temperature = 102.1°F, RR = 16, BP = 95/70 mm Hg, pulse = 120. Laboratory tests reveal ALT 136 U/L and AST 119 U/L, ALP 105 U/L, direct bilirubin 4.5 mg/dL and WBC count $16.8 \times 10^3/mm^3$. Ultrasound of the abdomen shows common bile duct dilatation with gallstones obstructing. Piperacillin-tazobactam is started and the patient is resuscitated with IV fluids. Repeat BP 12 hours after antibiotics and 4 L of IV fluids is BP = 110/82 mm Hg and HR = 85 Temperature = 98.8°F. What is the next step in managing this patient?

A. Cholecystectomy
B. Liver biopsy
C. ERCP
D. MRCP
E. Percutaneous transhepatic cholangiography

45. A 42-year-old female presents to the clinic for pre-employment screening. She is starting a new job as a bus driver and needs to have a physical and TB test before being hired. She denies any fever, chills, sputum, and weight loss. She was born in America and has not traveled outside of the country. She has never received a tuberculosis vaccine. She denies any contact with anyone infected with tuberculosis. She does not use IV drugs. Recent STD testing, including HIV, was negative. Physical examination is normal including lungs. PPD testing is performed and on reevaluation in 48 hours there is 10 mm of induration. What is the best recommendation to the patient?

A. AFB sputum culture
B. Rifampin, isoniazid, pyrazinamide, ethambutol
C. Isoniazid
D. Chest x-ray
E. No further intervention

46. A 64-year-old male presents to your office with left knee pain swelling. He has occasional pain in both knees that is usually dull and resolves with acetaminophen. Over the past few days he has had swelling which has made it difficult to move the joint. He had a similar episode of swelling a year ago that resolved on its own but this episode is much more severe. He denies any preceding trauma. He denies any morning stiffness. He has pain in his right knee as well, but it is mild and does not bother him that much. On physical examination, he has a moderate effusion in his left knee with erythema overlying (no effusion in the right knee). He has crepitus in both knees. Strength is normal, and examination does not indicate any ligamentous instability. X-ray shows mild narrowing of the joint space and calcification of the cartilage. Aspiration of the effusion reveals straw-colored fluid, 25,000 WBCs, 85% PMNs, Gram stain and culture are negative. Evaluation for crystals reveals no intracellular negatively birefringent crystals, but does reveal multiple intracellular positively birefringent rhomboid-shaped crystals. What is the most appropriate laboratory test to obtain?

A. Uric acid
B. TSH
C. ANA
D. ESR
E. HLA-B27

47. A 62-year-old female presents to your clinic with questions regarding her new diagnosis of osteoporosis. She had a hip fracture 6 months ago after a fall. Subsequently, she had a prolonged hospital course complicated by a DVT for which she completed therapy with warfarin. She has had no further falls and is back to her baseline level of activity after a 1 month rehabilitation stay. She had a DEXA scan which showed a T-score of −2.6 in the hip and −2.3 in vertebrae. Her past medical history includes achalasia for which she gets dilatations as needed. Currently she only takes omeprazole on a daily basis. Labs including renal function, calcium, and vitamin D are all normal. She is inquiring about further options to prevent her from having fractures. What is the appropriate management of this patient besides recommending continued supplementation with vitamin D and calcium?

A. Zolendronic acid
B. Alendronate
C. Raloxifene
D. Calcitonin
E. Estrogen

48. A 53-year-old female presents to the hospital with abdominal pain. She is diagnosed with cholecystitis and has a cholecystectomy performed. The following day she complains of palpitations. On questioning she has had an irregular heart beat off/on for the past few months but acutely worsened during this episode. She also notes a 15 lb weight loss over the past month. She denies dizziness, syncope, dyspnea, or chest pain. She has a known history of hyperlipidemia but has otherwise been healthy. Medications include ASA and atorvastatin. Vitals: Temperature = 102.4°F, BP = 155/88 mm Hg, pulse = 134. Oxygen saturation at room air = 96%. Physical examination: patient is agitated and appears confused, sometimes answering questions inappropriately. Skin is diaphoretic. Neck is supple without tenderness and no palpable nodules or enlargement. Cardiac examination reveals an irregular rhythm, tachycardia, and no murmurs. EKG confirms atrial fibrillation with rapid ventricular response. TSH is <0.01 mU/L. What is the most appropriate next step in the management of this patient?

A. Radioactive iodine uptake scan
B. Iodine
C. US thyroid
D. Propranolol
E. Thyroidectomy

49. A 61-year-old male who has been your patient for several years presents to your office with a complaint of two episodes of bloody urine over the past 24 hours. He denies any flank pain, dysuria, fevers, or chills. His urine stream is strong, he is able to void completely and he denies the need to start/stop or strain during urination. PMH is significant for hyperlipidemia, HTN, diabetes, glaucoma, and osteoarthritis. He has smoked one pack of cigarettes per day for the past 35 to 40 years. Physical examination reveals no CVA or suprapubic tenderness. Prostate examination reveals nontender, nonenlarged prostate. Urinalysis shows gross hematuria without proteinuria, pyuria, or RBC casts. Cr 1.1 mg/dL. Urine culture is negative. What is the appropriate next step in managing this patient?

A. CT urography
B. Ultrasound kidneys
C. Renal biopsy
D. PSA
E. Prostate biopsy

50. A 57-year-old male presents to your office with a 2-week history of cough. The cough is associated with clear sputum, occurs daily and has persisted over the past 2 weeks. He has occasional dyspnea and wheezing at times. He denies myalgias, fevers, or chills. He has experienced chest discomfort due to excessive coughing. PMH is negative and he takes no medications and specifically denies any history of pulmonary disease. Temperature is 99.1°F. RR 18. O_2 saturation is 96% on room air. On examination the patient is in no respiratory distress and is breathing comfortably. Auscultation of lungs reveals scattered rhonchi and wheezing but no consolidation, egophany, or crackles. CXR shows normal expansion of the lungs without infiltrates or effusions. Peak flow is 530 L/min (expected 556 L/min). What is the most appropriate management?

A. Prednisone
B. Oseltamivir
C. Azithromycin
D. Albuterol
E. Sputum culture

51. A 32-year-old African-American male, who recently moved to the area, presents to your office for the first time for a routine checkup. PMH is significant for type II DM. He is 5 ft 9 in and weighs 215 lb. The only medication he takes is metformin. He smokes half a pack of cigarettes a day; does not drink alcohol; and exercises sporadically, approximately once every 2 weeks. His mother died at the age of 62 due to an MI. His father is 73 years of age and is healthy. Physical examination is normal. Vital signs are: BP = 146/95, pulse = 73, RR = 19, temperature = 98.2.

Which of the following lifestyle modifications has been shown to result in the greatest reduction in blood pressure?

A. Dietary Approaches to Stop Hypertension (DASH) diet
B. Weight loss
C. Decreasing alcohol consumption
D. Increasing exercise
E. Smoking cessation

52. The patient in the previous question returns to your office in 6 weeks for a repeat evaluation. He has no complaints. He states that he has been walking briskly for 30 minutes four times a week, has lost 10 lb, and has been eating a healthier diet. His laboratory results are within normal limits. Hemoglobin A_{1c} is 7.2. CXR, ECG, and urinalysis are normal. His BP today is between 140/90 and 145/95. Physical examination is unchanged from 2 months ago. What is your recommended treatment?

A. Lisinopril
B. Amlodipine
C. Hydrochlorothiazide
D. Atenolol
E. Propranolol

53. A 17-year-old female is referred to the ED by her primary physician; she presents with a 3-day history of fevers, dysuria, and vomiting. She denies vaginal discharge, abdominal pain, or diarrhea. She is sexually active with her boyfriend. Vital signs are as follows: Temperature = 103 F, RR = 20, BP = 98/65, pulse = 100. She appears ill and is unable to tolerate liquids, but she is alert and oriented. Her examination is positive for suprapubic as well as costovertebral angle tenderness bilaterally. Urinalysis reveals numerous WBCs and bacteria, and it is positive for WBC casts and leukocyte esterase. Other laboratory study results are within normal limits, including a negative urine pregnancy test. What is the likely diagnosis?

A. Pyelonephritis
B. Nephrolithiasis
C. Appendicitis
D. Ectopic pregnancy
E. Acute interstitial nephritis

54. A 32-year-old male presents to the ED with a complaint of severe low back pain for the last 5 weeks. He reports that the pain is most severe when he first wakes up in the morning and gradually improves with exercise throughout the day. He cannot recall any trauma or insult to his back when the pain started. He denies any pain or numbness in the lower extremities. Bowel and bladder function is normal. Physical examination reveals a moderately overweight male in some distress. He has very minimal tenderness on palpation of his low back. Neurologic examination is normal. What is the appropriate next step in managing this patient?

A. Local heat
B. Physical therapy
C. Nonsteroidal anti-inflammatory drugs (NSAIDS)
D. Epidural steroid injection
E. Surgical laminectomy

55. A 29-year-old male with a history of asthma presents to the ED with severe SOB for the past 2 days. He also complains of sore throat, generalized malaise, and a nonproductive cough. He denies chest pain, fever, and chills. Temperature = 98.9, HR = 95, RR = 33, BP = 140/82, and O_2 saturation = 90% on room air. Breathing is labored, and he is speaking in short gasps. Lung auscultation reveals bilateral diffuse expiratory wheezing. There is no urticaria or angioedema on skin examination. ABG is drawn: 7.42/43/70/22. What is the appropriate next step in managing this patient?

A. Cautious oxygen administration, targeting an SaO_2 <94% to prevent hypercapnia
B. IV ceftriaxone and azithromycin
C. Subcutaneous epinephrine for bronchodilation
D. Nebulized ipratropium for bronchodilation
E. Nebulized albuterol for bronchodilation

56. A 22-year-old female presents to the ED with abrupt onset of a rash, high fever, and vomiting. Vital signs are as follows: Temperature = 104, HR = 118, RR = 22, BP = 76/40, and pulse oximetry = 98% on room air. On examination she appears confused and disoriented. Her skin is warm, and there is a diffuse macular rash over her body. She is admitted to the ICU and subsequently develops multisystem organ dysfunction. Which of the following organisms is most likely implicated in this patient's diagnosis?

A. *Streptococcus pyogenes*
B. *Neisseria meningitidis*
C. *Staphylococcus aureus*
D. *Streptococcus pneumoniae*
E. *Rickettsia rickettsii*

57. A 33-year-old Caucasian male comes to the clinic with a 4-day history of chest pain. The pain radiates to the right side of the neck and is worsened by deep inspiration and improved by leaning forward. Several weeks ago he had a fever and cough, which have both since improved. He is afebrile, BP is 130/85, and pulse is 88. On examination, there is a scratching sound heard over the left sternal border on expiration. ECG shows ST elevation in leads I, II, III, avL, and V_2 to V_6. The patient is offered treatment but refuses all medications. Which of the following is the most common complication if this disease remains untreated?

A. Cardiac tamponade
B. Recurrent pericarditis
C. Constrictive pericarditis
D. Ventricular free wall rupture
E. Valvular insufficiency

58. A 52-year-old woman with a history of diabetes mellitus and hypertension presents to the emergency department with fevers, chills, and abdominal pain. The symptoms began about 1 week ago and have been getting worse. The abdominal pain is associated with nausea and vomiting, and she has not been able to eat. On examination, her temperature is 102.1, blood pressure is 104/68 mm Hg, heart rate is 94/min, and respiratory rate is 16/min. Her abdominal examination shows right-sided pain to deep palpation, and she has severe right-sided costovertebral angle tenderness. Laboratories demonstrate a leukocytosis (15,400/mm^3) and urinalysis shows WBCs, WBC casts, protein, and bacteria. Despite IV ceftriaxone for 5 days, the patient remains febrile. The patient's urine culture is positive for *Escherichia coli* and is sensitive to ceftriaxone and ciprofloxacin. What is the appropriate next step in management?

A. Renal biopsy
B. CT scan with contrast
C. Continue the current antibiotic
D. Stop ceftriaxone and start ciprofloxacin
E. Stop ceftriaxone and reculture urine

59. You are paged to come and evaluate a 33-year-old female with SOB and tachycardia. She normally takes inhaled fluticasone and albuterol for asthma, however she is not currently responding to the albuterol. On examination, she appears anxious and is moderately short of breath. There are loud bilateral wheezes on examination, with a prolonged inspiratory and expiratory phase and use of accessory muscles of respiration. Temperature = 99.4, pulse = 116, BP = 116/56, RR = 36. Oxygen saturation is 91% on room air. Examination shows use of accessory muscles on inspiration. An arterial blood gas is obtained and shows a pH of 7.4, PO_2 of 60 mm Hg, and PCO_2 of 40 mm Hg. What is the appropriate next step to be taken in the management of this patient?

A. Increase supplemental oxygen flow rate
B. IV corticosteroids
C. Azithromycin
D. Intubation
E. Nebulized albuterol

60. A 61-year-old man with a history of chronic alcoholism and parathyroid adenoma presents with pain in his left knee for the last 2 days. He denies fevers, chills, night sweats, or any history of trauma to the knee, but does endorse abdominal pain and constipation. Physical examination is significant for tenderness and erythematous skin overlying the left knee. There is also marked swelling of the left knee. Laboratory findings reveal an elevated calcium level (12.1 mg/dL). If joint aspiration is performed, which of the following will be seen on synovial fluid analysis?

A. Negatively birefringent needle-shaped crystals
B. Positively birefringent rhomboid-shaped crystals
C. Neutrophil predominance with gram-positive cocci
D. Negatively birefringent needle-shaped crystals AND gram-positive cocci
E. Normal synovial fluid findings

61. A 26-year-old man presents to his primary care physician complaining of fatigue, headache, and a sore throat for the past week. There is also nausea and diarrhea, but no weight loss, productive cough, or difficulty breathing. He denies any past medical history, does not take any medications, and has no recent sick contacts. He is sexually active and uses condoms inconsistently; he drinks alcohol heavily on the weekends and admits to previous IV drug use. On examination, his temperature is 39°C and the rest of his vital signs are normal. He has nontender cervical and axillary lymphadenopathy, tonsillar exudates, and mild splenomegaly. There are also several painful, well-demarcated ulcers within his mouth and a mild maculopapular rash over his chest and arms. A rapid strep test and a monospot (heterophile antibody) test are negative; further screening for chlamydia, gonorrhea, syphilis, and HIV is negative. What is the likely diagnosis?

A. Hodgkin lymphoma
B. Acute retroviral syndrome
C. Infectious mononucleosis
D. Secondary syphilis
E. Upper respiratory infection

62. A 30-year-old medical student is undergoing medical screening in order to start a rotation at a new hospital. She denies any current symptoms and reports no previous medical problems. She is originally from South Africa and her vaccinations are up to date, including a BCG vaccine she received as a child. A purified protein derivative (PPD) is placed and read 48 hours later, which shows an area of induration that is 11 mm wide. What is the most appropriate next step in management?

A. Start rifampin, isoniazid, pyrazinamide, and ethambutol
B. Obtain a chest x-ray; if normal, reassure the patient
C. Obtain a chest x-ray; if normal, start isoniazid and pyridoxine for 9 months
D. Start isoniazid and pyridoxine for 9 months
E. Reassurance

63. A 35-year-old male presents with complaint of a 6-month history of fatigue and lethargy. His medical history is unremarkable. He denies melena and recent trauma or surgery. He reports that he does not drink alcohol, smoke, or take any medications. His family history is noncontributory. He appears well nourished. Vital signs are as follows: RR = 16, BP = 130/80, pulse = 70. Laboratory test results are as follows: Hb = 7.6, Hct = 22.8%, and MCV = 68. The remainder of his laboratory test results are normal. Which of the following is the best next step in management of this patient?

A. Serum iron studies
B. Hemoglobin electrophoresis
C. Serum lead levels
D. Peripheral blood smear
E. Stool guaiac test

64. A 56-year-old female presents to the ED with a complaint of severe abdominal pain, primarily in the epigastric region. She has had two episodes of vomiting in the past 5 hours. She describes the pain as sharp, with occasional radiation to her back. PMH is significant for DM, HTN, alcoholism, asthma, and chronic low back pain. Her current medications include insulin, atenolol, albuterol inhaler, and oxycodone. She has had abdominal pain several times in the past year, but never this severe and never associated with vomiting. On examination, she has tenderness in the epigastric region. There is mild guarding but no rebound. Physical examination is otherwise unremarkable. Temperature = 101.3, BP = 136/88, pulse = 116. She is alert and oriented and is in obvious distress. Which of the following is the most specific finding in this condition?

A. Elevated amylase
B. Elevated ALT
C. Elevated lipase
D. Positive fecal fat test
E. Calcifications on x-ray

65. A 37-year-old female presents to your office with a history of fatigue for the past few months. She does not have any other complaints. After a thorough medical history, she admits to mild constipation that is not troublesome for her. She reports a 5-lb weight gain over the past 6 months, which she attributes to living a more sedentary life of late due to her fatigue and lethargy. Her physical examination is unremarkable; her thyroid does not seem enlarged, although her face is slightly puffy. Which of the following is the best next step in management?

A. Free T4 levels
B. Thyroid-stimulating hormone (TSH) levels
C. Thyroglobulin levels
D. Radioactive iodine uptake (RAIU) scan
E. Biopsy

66. A 21-year-old male college student is brought to the ED by his friends after developing fever, neck stiffness, confusion, and severe sensitivity to light. Vital signs on admission are as follows: Temperature = 105, RR = 20, BP = 120/75, pulse = 92, and pulse oximetry 99% on room air. Examination reveals a confused male patient with nuchal rigidity. A fundoscopic examination shows bilateral blurring of the optic disk margins and retinal venous engorgement. Which of the following is the next best step in management?

A. CT scan
B. MRI
C. Lumbar puncture
D. Administer empiric antibiotics
E. Administer empiric antiviral therapy

67. A 64-year-old male presents with back pain, constipation, and slight confusion for the past 5 to 6 months. Two days ago he fell while shoveling snow, and he has pain in his right arm as well. Plain films of the spine show several small lytic lesions in the vertebral bodies at the L3 to L4 level. Right humerus films reveal lytic areas in the metaphysis and diaphysis of the right humerus. There is a fracture line through the abnormal area on the humerus film. Physical examination reveals tenderness on palpation of the low back and right humerus, but is otherwise unremarkable. There is no splenomegaly or lymphadenopathy. CBC results are as follows: Hb = 9.1 g/dL, Hct = 27.6%, MCV = 90, platelet count = 150,000/μL. Serum chemistries are as follows: Sodium = 137 mmol/L, potassium = 4.1 mmol/L, chloride = 107 mmol/L, CO_2 = 24 mmol/L, glucose = 89 mg/dL, BUN = 46 mg/dL, Cr = 3.5 mg/dL. Which of the following additional findings do you expect with this patient's condition?

A. Mechanical obstruction
B. Electrolyte abnormality
C. Hormone level abnormality
D. Arterial blood gas abnormality
E. Venous blood gas abnormality

68. A 47-year-old male presents to your office with severe low back pain for the past 2 days. This morning he had an episode of loss of control of his urine, followed by progressive weakness in bilateral lower extremities. His low back pain is severe and sharp, and it radiates into the right lower extremity. PMH is significant for mild asthma. He has had intermittent low back pain for the past 2 years but never this severe and never associated with weakness or urinary symptoms. On physical examination, he has very limited motion of his lumbar spine secondary to pain. He has 3/5 strength in gastrocnemius muscles bilaterally and 2/5 strength with great toe dorsiflexion bilaterally. He has diminished sensation throughout his lower extremities, and reflexes are diminished. Rectal tone is absent as is sensation in the perineal area. What is the next best step in management of this patient's condition?

A. Steroids
B. Surgery
C. MRI lumbar spine
D. Bed rest
E. NSAIDs

69. A 67-year-old female presents to the ED after a transient episode of visual loss in her right eye. She reports that she has had right-sided headache for several months, for which she takes ibuprofen, with some relief. On physical examination, she has tenderness over her scalp in the left temporal region and complains that her jaw "gets tired with chewing." Neurologic examination is normal with no focal deficits. Vital signs are as follows: Temperature = 101.1, HR = 72, RR = 16, BP = 140/82. Which of the following is associated with this condition?

A. Aortic aneurysm
B. Inflammatory bowel disease
C. Hepatitis B
D. Smoking history
E. Alcohol history

70. A 63-year-old female is brought to the ED by the rescue squad after an episode of syncope at home. Her husband witnessed the event. He describes the patient as falling suddenly to the floor from a standing position. She lost consciousness for about 5 seconds, after which she rapidly regained consciousness and was oriented and appropriate. The patient remembers feeling lightheaded, nauseous, and developing "tunnel vision" prior to the event. No bowel or bladder incontinence was noted. PMH is significant for DM, HTN, and depression. She denies any chest pain or SOB. Vital signs are: Temperature = 100.2, BP = 118/68, pulse = 84, RR = 18. Oxygen saturation on room air is 96%. Physical examination is significant only for bruising of her left wrist and thigh. Heart and lung examination is normal. Which of the following is the most likely diagnosis?

A. Arrhythmia
B. Orthostatic hypotension
C. Seizure
D. Vasovagal syncope
E. Aortic stenosis

71. A 63-year-old female presents to your office with complaint of mid to low back pain for the last year, which has become worse over the past 3 months. She denies any weakness or radiating pain in her lower extremities. She currently takes oxycodone for her back pain with inadequate relief. She has difficulty sleeping at night because of the back pain. PMH is significant for HTN, for which she takes a β-blocker. Thoracic and lumbar spine radiographs show multiple compression fractures at T8, T11, L3, and L4, as well as diffuse osteopenia. Laboratory studies are as follows: WBC 8, hemoglobin 9.7, hematocrit 29%, platelets 189, Na^+ 142, K^- 4.1, BUN 43, creatinine 2.3, calcium 14.3. Physical examination reveals tenderness on palpation of thoracic and lumbar spine. She has limited lumbar flexion due to pain. Neurologic examination is normal. Which of the following would be abnormal in this patient's condition?

A. CA-15-3
B. Carcinoembryonic antigen (CEA)
C. Alkaline phosphatase
D. Serum immunoelectrophoresis
E. Bone scan

72. A 62-year-old female is brought to the ED by EMS for confusion, headache, and vomiting over the past 12 hours. Vital signs are as follows: Temperature = 96.9, HR = 100, RR = 22, BP = 220/150. She is disoriented and uncooperative. Examination is otherwise unremarkable. What is the most likely diagnosis, and what is the most appropriate management?

A. Hypertensive urgency; gradual lowering of blood pressure with oral agents
B. Hypertensive urgency; rapid lowering of blood pressure with IV agents
C. Hypertensive emergency; gradual lowering of blood pressure with oral agents
D. Hypertensive emergency; rapid lowering of blood pressure with IV agents
E. Hypertension; gradual lowering of blood pressure with oral agents

73. A 74-year-old male is brought to your office by his daughter, who is having increasing problems caring for him at home. She reports that he has recently had urinary incontinence and has been "clumsier" than usual. She states that he behaves inappropriately at times, and on two occasions he has wandered outside the home and has gotten lost. He misplaces items frequently, and his personality has changed to being more belligerent and demanding. He seems to lack judgment in social situations, and he never had this problem in the past. She states that these problems have become worse gradually over the past 4 months. Physical examination is unremarkable. What is the likely diagnosis?

A. Pseudotumor cerebri
B. Alzheimer disease
C. Normal pressure hydrocephalus
D. Multi-infarct dementia
E. Lewy body dementia

74. A 73-year-old female is brought to the ED by EMS with a complaint of SOB and progressive dyspnea. Her medical history is significant for a previous MI 5 years ago and mild CHF. The patient has also had several episodes of ventricular tachycardia that ultimately required cardioversion. She is currently taking a prophylactic medication and has not had any recurrent arrhythmias. On physical examination, she is in moderate respiratory distress and she has dry rales throughout her lung fields. Temperature = 99.1, BP = 138/75, pulse = 96, RR = 28. CXR is normal, but CT scan of the chest shows diffuse ground-glass opacities. Which of the following is contributing to this patient's symptoms and clinical findings?

A. Digoxin
B. Lisinopril
C. Amiodarone
D. Bleomycin
E. Losartan

75. A 39-year-old female presents to your office with a 3-year history of headaches. They occur once or twice per week, lasting several hours. The headaches are throbbing and are usually on her left side. During these episodes, the patient is incapacitated and must lie down in a dark room for several hours. She is sensitive to light during the episodes and cannot move because of the pain. She is often nauseated and has vomited on several occasions. Medical history is significant for hypothyroidism, for which she takes levothyroxine (Synthroid). Her physical examination is unremarkable, however the patient endorses another similar headache and begins vomiting near the end of the examination. What is the appropriate next step in managing this patient?

A. Propranolol
B. Amitriptyline
C. Chlorpromazine
D. Verapamil
E. Sumatriptan

76. A 55-year-old female presents to your office for a routine follow-up examination. Medical history is significant for poorly controlled DM (20-year history), HTN, and osteoarthritis of bilateral knees. She also has had chronic renal insufficiency for the past 5 years. Her current medications include hydrochlorothiazide, lisinopril, insulin, and metoprolol. She has been taking increasing amounts of NSAIDs for the past several weeks for her painful knees. She is obese with 2+ peripheral pitting edema. She appears weak with dry mucous membranes and is tachycardic. Laboratory tests reveal the following: Na^+ = 138, K^+ = 4.6, Cl^- = 104, HCO_3^- = 27, Cr = 3.6, WBC = 7.9, Hgb = 8.2, Hct = 24.6, MCV = 75. On her last visit 3 months ago, her Cr was 2.3. Which of the following would be most helpful in determining the etiology of this patient's renal failure?

A. Urine dipstick
B. Urine sodium
C. Fractional excretion of sodium (FENa)
D. Renal ultrasound
E. No further workup is necessary

77. A 64-year-old female presents to the ED with sudden onset of severe chest pain that occasionally radiates to her back. She has a history of angina and takes nitroglycerin, but this time the pain is much worse and is not relieved with nitroglycerin. PMH is significant for HTN. She is afebrile, and HR = 105, BP = 160/105, RR = 17. Cardiac enzymes are negative. CXR shows a widened mediastinum. What is the likely diagnosis?

A. Myocardial infarction
B. Aortic dissection
C. Stroke
D. Acute aortic regurgitation
E. Hypertensive emergency

78. A 17-year-old male presents to the ED with severe pain in his right leg and back that began suddenly a few days ago. The pain is sharp and throbbing. He has a history of sickle cell disease with frequent painful crises requiring hospitalization once or twice per year. He has no other medical problems. Vital signs are as follows: Temperature = 101.6, HR = 94, RR = 20, BP = 132/84. Oxygen saturation is 97% on room air. His right shin is very tender, as is his low back in the midline. His examination is otherwise unremarkable. CBC results are as follows: Hb = 7, Hct = 21%, MCV = 94. Osteomyelitis of the right tibia is ultimately diagnosed.

What is the most likely cause of this patient's osteomyelitis?

A. *Listeria*
B. *Salmonella*
C. *Shigella*
D. *Cryptosporidium*
E. *Campylobacter*

79. A 42-year-old male presents to your office because he noticed a "lump" in his neck 1 month ago. He endorses weight loss and palpitations, but denies pain or dysphagia. On physical examination, you note a nontender, firm nodule about 2 cm in size to the left of the midline in the region of the thyroid gland. Vital signs are as follows: BP = 125/82, pulse = 75. He does not take any medications and has no significant medical history. He denies any family history of thyroid disease or cancer. His routine serum laboratory values (CBC, electrolytes, BUN, creatinine) are normal. The physician decides to do a radioactive iodine uptake (RAIU) scan.

Which of the following features is not associated with an increased risk of malignancy?

A. Hard and immobile mass
B. Cold nodule on RAIU
C. Cervical lymphadenopathy
D. Hot nodule on RAIU
E. Microcalcifications

80. A 65-year-old female presents to your office with a 1-month history of intermittent neck and shoulder pain with SOB that normally occurs when she does chores around the house or climbs stairs. She is previously healthy and denies any medical conditions. She does not smoke or drink alcohol. The patient is up to date on vaccinations and had a mammogram done at her previous appointment 1 year ago that was normal. BP = 148/86 and pulse = 88. She had a colonoscopy performed 6 years ago that was normal. You order an ECG, CXR, CBC, and electrolytes. What should be recommended to the patient at her visit today?

A. Mammogram
B. Colonoscopy
C. Calcium and phosphorus levels
D. Dual-energy x-ray absorptiometry (DEXA)
E. CT scan of the chest

Questions

81. A 54-year-old male with a history of parathyroid adenoma presents to the ED with severe pain in his right knee. He says that the pain is extreme and intolerable, and he is in obvious distress. On examination, there is exquisite tenderness, erythema, and swelling of the right knee joint and it feels very warm to the touch. The pain began suddenly a few hours ago. He denies any previous episodes or pain in any other joints. He denies any trauma. Medical history is significant for osteoarthritis of his left knee, for which he takes ibuprofen. He drinks 6 to 7 glasses of wine per day. He does not take any other medications. Vital signs are as follows: Temperature = 100.5, RR = 16, BP = 140/85, pulse = 78. Which of the following is the best next step in management for this patient?

A. Indomethacin
B. Joint aspiration with synovial fluid analysis
C. Uric acid levels
D. Knee x-ray

82. A 41-year-old male presents to your office with a complaint of epigastric pain for the past several months. He takes over-the-counter antacids, but symptoms have been worse over the past month. He denies any weight loss, vomiting, hematemesis, or melena. The discomfort is worse after eating. Medical history is noncontributory. He takes no other medications. He smokes half a pack a day of cigarettes and drinks alcohol socially about once per week. Physical examination is unremarkable except for mild epigastric tenderness. What is the appropriate next step in managing this patient?

A. Continue antacids
B. Barium swallow evaluation
C. Empiric 1-month trial with proton pump inhibitor (PPI)
D. Upper GI endoscopy
E. Observation

83. An 81-year-old female was in a motor vehicle accident 3 days ago and suffered a left femur fracture, for which she had surgery on the same day. She has been hospitalized since the day of surgery and has been taking part in daily physical therapy without difficulty. Her family (husband and daughter) report that she has not been "acting like herself" at times when they come to visit her. She becomes agitated and is belligerent toward them, and she sometimes wonders why she is in the hospital. She reports seeing "creatures." At other times, the patient is doing very well, and they do not notice these inconsistencies. The patient has a history of borderline HTN. Current medications include a stool softener and morphine for pain control. On examination, the patient is alert and oriented to time/place/person and is appropriately responding to questions. She denies any hallucinations. Neurologic examination is normal. Which of the following is true of this patient's condition?

A. Anticholinergic medications are first-line treatment
B. Pathologic findings include neurofibrillary tangles and β-amyloid plaques
C. Long-term memory is intact, but short-term memory is affected
D. This is an irreversible condition
E. Etiologies include infection and polypharmacy

84. A 49-year-old female presents to the ED with complaint of severe epigastric and RUQ abdominal pain. Her symptoms started 3 days ago but have progressively worsened over the past 12 hours. Her symptoms are worse with meals. She has had two episodes of vomiting in the past 12 hours and is nauseous currently. PMH is significant for diabetes, osteoarthritis, and HTN. Temperature = 102.3, BP = 146/80, pulse = 110, RR = 16. On physical examination, there is severe right upper quadrant pain on deep palpation, most pronounced on palpation after deep inspiration. Bowel sounds are diminished. The patient is lying on her side holding an emesis basin. Which of the following is causing this patient's disorder?

A. Alcoholic liver disease
B. Gallstone obstruction in the cystic duct
C. Obstruction from carcinoma of the head of the pancreas
D. Gallstone obstruction in the common bile duct
E. Pancreatic inflammation

85. A 31-year-old female presents to your office with multiple musculoskeletal aches and pains including, but not limited to, her shoulders, elbows, knees, neck, and buttocks. She has had these symptoms for at least the past year. She does not sleep very well when the pain is severe and has no relief with NSAIDs. She has tried exercising more, but the pain is persistent. On palpation, she has marked tenderness over both lateral epicondyles, the anterior aspect of her left shoulder, the medial aspect of her right knee, her posterior neck, and her left greater trochanter. There are no effusions at any of the above sites. Routine laboratory test results are normal. What is the appropriate next step in managing this patient?

A. Prednisone
B. Naproxen
C. Amitriptyline
D. Colchicine
E. Steroid injections

86. A 52-year-old male with a long-standing history of alcohol abuse is brought to the ED by his wife for vomiting blood. He vomited bright red blood at least twice this morning. PMH is significant for cirrhosis, HTN, and arthritis. He has never vomited blood before. On examination, the patient is awake but appears nervous and is in moderate distress. Delayed capillary refill is present. You are able to determine that he has vomited approximately 2 L of blood over the past 6 hours. Vital signs are: Temperature = 99.2, BP = 90/58, HR = 134, RR = 20. Pulse oximetry shows 98% oxygenation on room air. What is the appropriate next step in managing this patient?

A. Immediate upper GI endoscopy
B. Administration of fluids
C. *Helicobacter pylori* serologic testing
D. Intravenous (IV) proton pump inhibitor
E. Reassurance

87. A 57-year-old female presents to the ED with a complaint of abdominal pain and vomiting. The pain is diffuse and poorly localized. She has had these symptoms for the past month and has been constipated during this time. She has not had a bowel movement or passed gas in 3 days. She has no significant PMH. Vital signs are: Temperature = 99.2, BP = 128/78, HR = 78, RR = 16. On physical examination, there is abdominal distention and no guarding or rebound tenderness. The remainder of the examination is normal. What is the next appropriate step in the management of this patient?

A. Abdominal ultrasound
B. Colonoscopy
C. Abdominal x-ray
D. Sigmoidoscopy
E. CT scan of abdomen

88. A 43-year-old female with a history of Crohn disease presents to the ED with a 4-hour history of left flank pain radiating to her left groin. The pain was sudden in onset but was mild at first. However, it has been increasing in severity over the past 2 to 3 hours. The pain is now constant and excruciating. It was associated with nausea and vomiting, but the patient denies fevers/chills. She denies seeing any gross blood in his urine. Medical history is insignificant. Vital signs are as follows: Temperature = 98.1, RR = 24, BP = 148/88, pulse = 93. On physical examination, the patient is in obvious distress, writhing in pain. She has marked tenderness along the left flank, but the examination is otherwise unremarkable. Urinalysis reveals 2+ heme. Urine sediment reveals no casts but many RBCs and few WBCs per HPF. Laboratory tests reveal the following: WBC 8.2, Hgb 11.9, Hct 36.1, BUN 14, Cr 0.9. A urine pregnancy test is negative. What is the most likely diagnosis?

A. Pyelonephritis
B. Nephrolithiasis
C. Appendicitis
D. Ectopic pregnancy
E. Pancreatitis

89. A 39-year-old female is brought to the ED by her husband with the chief complaint of acute SOB and anxiety that started suddenly 2 to 3 hours ago while she was working around the house. Last night she drank seven glasses of wine with her husband. She denies chest pain. Her PMH is unremarkable, however she uses diuretics to help "prevent bloating." She also takes oral contraceptives. Vital signs are: Temperature = 99.1, RR = 34, BP = 148/90, pulse = 100. Oxygen saturation is 94% on room air. On examination, the patient appears healthy although in moderate respiratory distress. Her examination is otherwise unremarkable. Laboratory tests reveal: WBC = 7.1, Hgb = 12.2, Hct = 37.3, Na^+ = 138, K^+ = 4.7, Cl^- = 109, HCO_3^- = 25, BUN = 14, Cr = 0.9, glucose = 106. ABGs are obtained and reveal: pH = 7.52, HCO_3^- = 20, $PaCO_2$ = 26, PaO_2 = 70. CXR and ECG are normal. Which of the following is the etiology of her acid–base disturbance?

A. Accumulation of unmeasured anions due to hepatic metabolism of alcohol
B. Vomiting due to alcohol toxicity
C. Hyperventilation secondary to anxiety
D. Electrolyte imbalance due to diuretic use
E. Hypoventilation from respiratory depression due to alcohol intoxication

90. A 63-year-old male is brought to the ED by his wife for altered mental status. The patient regularly drinks alcohol and has a long-standing history of alcohol use. Over the past 24 hours, he has become more confused and is not "acting like himself" according to his wife. She states that he has never acted like this before. On further questioning, the patient had an episode of massive hematemesis last year that required admission to the hospital, necessitating blood transfusion and other treatment that the wife does not recall. On physical examination, the patient is arousable and is alert to person but not to place or time. He is cachectic, with prominent veins over his abdomen. He has a significant ascites. There are several dilated superficial arterioles scattered throughout his body. When the patient extends his arms out in front of him, a jerking movement of the limbs is observed. Which of the following is the most appropriate next step in management?

A. Furosemide
B. Thiamine
C. Lactulose
D. Morphine
E. Hydromorphone

Questions

91. A 65-year-old obese female presents to your office with a chief complaint of low back pain and bilateral knee pain that is worse with activity and relieved by rest. She has had this pain for 6 or 7 months. She denies any recent trauma or any event that she recalls precipitating the pain. One year ago she suffered a distal radius fracture when she tripped in her bedroom and landed on her outstretched left arm. Medical history is significant for HTN, for which she takes hydrochlorothiazide. She smokes approximately 12 cigarettes per day and has a 25-pack-per-year history of smoking. She denies any alcohol use. She does not exercise. On physical examination, she has no radicular symptoms, and the straight-leg test is negative. What is the appropriate next step in managing this patient?

A. Intra-articular corticosteroid injection
B. Acetaminophen
C. Naproxen
D. Allopurinol
E. Observation

92. A 46-year-old male presents to your office with the complaint of fatigue for the past 2 months. He does not abuse alcohol. His medical history is significant for HTN, for which he takes metoprolol. He denies melena, hematochezia, or any other blood loss. His family history is noncontributory. He has no symptoms other than fatigue. He admits he does not have a good diet. Vital signs are: BP = 135/85, pulse = 70. Physical examination is unremarkable except for mild pallor. Stool is negative for occult blood. Laboratory test results are: Hb = 9.2, Hct = 27.6, MCV = 117. ECG is normal. The patient is started on folic acid and 4 weeks later presents with a hemoglobin level of 10.1 mg/dL. However, he reports a new "pins and needles" sensation in his distal toes and fingers. Which of the following is the underlying cause of the patient's current symptoms?

A. Inadequate treatment with folic acid
B. Iron deficiency
C. Glucose intolerance
D. Vitamin B_{12} deficiency
E. Peripheral neuropathy from diabetes mellitus

93. A 41-year-old female with history of hypertension presents to your office for a routine checkup. She is new to your office as she recently moved and presents to establish care. She takes blood pressure medications but cannot recall the names. On today's visit, her BP is 142/96. She is asymptomatic except for leg swelling. Physical examination reveals bilateral edema of the lower extremities. She smokes one pack of cigarettes per day and has a 20-pack-per-year history. Family history is negative. Her total serum cholesterol concentration is 175 mg/dL and HDL is 40 mg/dL. Routine laboratory test results are within normal limits. Which medication is most likely responsible for the patient's complaint?

A. Amlodipine
B. Metoprolol
C. Hydrochlorothiazide
D. Metformin
E. Glipizide

94. A 73-year-old male is brought to the ED in a coma. He was delivered to the ED from a nursing home and was reported by the nursing home staff to have had a seizure that lasted less than 1 minute. He was subsequently confused and soon thereafter entered a comatose state. His medical history is significant for type II DM requiring insulin, HTN, and mild CHF. In the ED, the patient is very lethargic and responds only to pain stimuli. His vital signs are stable, and CBC and electrolyte levels are normal. Serum glucose is 16 mg/dL and serum insulin is elevated. C-peptide is 0.2 ng/mL (normal range, 0.5 to 3 ng/mL). Urine sulfonylurea level is undetectable. What is the likely cause of this patient's condition?

A. Factitious hypoglycemia from surreptitious injection of insulin
B. Insulinoma
C. Somatization disorder
D. Glucagonoma
E. Dehydration

95. A 78-year-old female presents to your office for a routine checkup. Her only complaint is burning when she urinates that she has had for several weeks. Her medical history is significant for HTN and DM. She has four children, all delivered vaginally. Medications include hydrochlorothiazide for her HTN, insulin, and a daily aspirin. She wears adult pads because she loses large volumes of urine throughout the day and usually cannot reach the bathroom in time. Physical examination is unremarkable. Vital signs are unremarkable. Routine laboratory test results are within normal limits except for a random blood glucose level of 210. Urinalysis shows positive nitrites and bacteria. She receives oral antibiotics for a urinary tract infection. After completing the course of antibiotics, she goes on a run, and feels a "pop" above her heel that is associated with severe pain. She has pain and difficulty with plantar flexion of the affected foot.

Which of the following antibiotics is most likely responsible?

A. Trimethoprim-sulfamethoxazole
B. Metronidazole
C. Tobramycin
D. Ciprofloxacin
E. Azithromycin

96. A 33-year-old female presents to your office with the complaint of insomnia and difficulty concentrating at work for several weeks. She reports a 20-lb weight loss over the past 2 to 3 months, despite eating more. When questioned, she reports that she frequently feels "hot and sweaty" at work and at home. She denies chest pain or palpitations but does have diarrhea frequently. Vital signs are: Temperature = 98.9, RR = 15, BP = 130/80, pulse = 98. She appears worried. On physical examination, she has warm and moist skin. She has a slight hand tremor. On palpation of her thyroid, you note a diffusely enlarged thyroid gland that is nontender. Which of the following is the best next step in management?

A. Free T4 levels
B. Thyroid-stimulating hormone (TSH) levels
C. Thyroglobulin levels
D. Radioactive iodine uptake (RAIU) scan
E. A fine-needle aspiration (FNA) biopsy

97. A 26-year-old medical student is injured via needle stick while drawing blood from a patient with chronic hepatitis B. The patient received his final hepatitis B vaccination of the series 7 years ago. The patient had his titers checked before clinical rotations 6 months ago and was found to be positive for anti-hepatitis B surface antibodies (HBsAbs). Which of the following is the best next step in the management of this patient?

A. Hepatitis B immunoglobulin (HBIG) now
B. Serologic testing for HBsAg
C. Hepatitis B vaccination
D. Reassurance

98. A 71-year-old female is brought to the ED by her husband for increased confusion over the past 3 days. The husband reports that the patient fell 4 days ago and immediately after the fall she was asymptomatic but over the ensuing days has become lethargic and more confused. PMH is significant for hyperlipidema. She underwent a right total hip replacement 5 weeks ago and was diagnosed with a DVT 2 weeks after the operation. Medications include warfarin and atorvastatin. Two weeks ago, her INR was 2.7. On examination, patient has slurred speech and appears confused. She is oriented to person but not to place or time. Neurologic examination is normal. The remainder of physical examination is normal. A head CT is ordered which confirms the diagnosis. Which of the following is the etiology of this patient's condition?

A. Tearing of the middle meningeal artery
B. Tearing of the bridging veins
C. Ruptured aneurysm
D. Hypertensive hemorrhage
E. Alzheimer disease

Questions

99. A 66-year-old male is brought to your office by his wife with complaint of productive cough, fever, and chills for the past 2 days. The patient lives with his wife and is retired. PMH is significant for DM, for which he takes insulin; CHF, with an ejection fraction of 40%; and a history of renal insufficiency. He is alert and oriented. There is no history of smoking or alcohol use. On physical examination, the patient is lethargic. He has crackles over the left lower lung. Cardiovascular examination is normal. Vital signs are: Temperature = 103.3, BP = 82/54, HR = 128, RR = 24. Oxygen saturation on room air is 97%. CXR shows infiltrates and consolidation in the left lower lobe of the lung. Laboratory test results show WBC 15, hematocrit 36, Na 142, glucose 167, BUN 36, creatinine 1.5. Lactate is elevated. What is the likely diagnosis in this patient?

A. Cardiogenic shock
B. Pulmonary embolism
C. Sepsis
D. Severe sepsis
E. Septic shock

100. You are called to see a 69-year-old male with acute SOB. Vital signs are: Temperature = 100.1, BP = 166/88, pulse = 130, RR = 33. You rush to see the patient and on your arrival, oxygen saturation is 79% on a 100% oxygen nonrebreather face mask. The nurse informs you that his oxygen saturation was 68% on room air. He currently has heavily labored breathing and appears cyanotic. The nurse informs you that the patient was admitted 2 days ago for a severe COPD exacerbation. You decide to emergently intubate the patient. Which of the following will reduce the risk of developing pneumonia in this patient?

A. Place the patient in a supine position
B. Avoid daily attempts to wean the patient from the ventilator
C. Administer oral chlorhexidine solution twice daily
D. Administer daily omeprazole
E. Avoid any instrumentation of the airway, including endotracheal suctioning

ANSWERS

1. **Answer: E. Small cell carcinoma.** The patient most likely has small cell carcinoma given the main risk factor of a strong smoking history, a mass located in the central/proximal airways and the weakness suggestive of paraneoplastic Lambert–Eaton syndrome. Other associated paraneoplastic syndromes with small cell include Cushing and SIADH.

   Bronchial carcinoid is not clearly associated with smoking or Lambert–Eaton, although usually presents as a central/proximal lesion. Large cell carcinoma is not associated with Lambert–Eaton. Squamous cell carcinoma is not associated with Lambert–Eaton but is typically a central lesion; this lung malignancy is also the most likely lung cancer associated with paraneoplastic hypercalcemia.

2. **Answer: D. Obtain contrast enhanced CT of the abdomen.** The patient is presenting with typical signs/symptoms of acute diverticulitis—fever, leukocytosis, LLQ location of pain. Further suggestion is made by the fact that the patient had a prior episode of rectal bleeding, likely from underlying diverticulosis. CT scan will help not only confirm the diagnosis but also to rule out other processes and assess for any complications of diverticulitis.

   Checking the serum lactate will help assess for ischemia but will not help you confirm the diagnosis of diverticulitis. Retroperitoneal ultrasound will assess for hydronephrosis and pyelonephritis but urinalysis/chemistry are normal and there is no suggestion of obstruction/infection regardless of his history of renal stones. Colonoscopy would be contraindicated in a patient with acute diverticulitis because of the risk of perforation. Proceeding to the operating room would be premature unless the patient had surgical indications such as fistula, stricture, large abscess, or perforation related to the diverticulitis.

3. **Answer: B. Heparin.** IV UFH (unfractionated heparin) and subq LMWH are shown to decrease mortality in UA/NSTEMI. In addition, statins, ASA, β-blockers are shown to do so as well. ACE inhibitors have evidence of benefit and are recommended in the acute setting after an MI as well.

   Alteplase is NOT indicated for UA/NSTEMI but ONLY for STEMI when PCI is *not* available. Hydralazine, furosemide, and digoxin offer no mortality benefit in this setting either.

4. **Answer: C. Aspirin.** Aspirin is shown to reduce recurrent stroke and to decrease mortality and should be administered within 48 hours.

   Insulin is not necessary as the level of glucose elevation is not contributing to the current presentation; in fact, aggressive glycemic control is associated with worse outcomes. Heparin has not been shown to improve outcomes and is not recommended as an acute treatment for ischemic stroke. Alteplase can be considered but only for significant deficits when the patient presents within 3 hours of symptom onset and has no contraindications; this patient presented too late for this to be a treatment option. Labetalol would not be used despite the elevated BP as permissive hypertension is allowed in the setting of an acute ischemic stroke; BP up to 220/120 mm Hg is generally tolerated initially.

5. **Answer: E. Methylmalonic acid.** The other answers will help narrow down your differential but will not definitely give your diagnosis. The patient has a gastrectomy and thus loss of intrinsic factor leading to impaired absorption of B12. The neurologic symptoms are a result of this deficiency and the fatigue/pallor are related to macrocytic anemia. Laboratory assessment of B12, methylmalonic acid, or homocysteine would all be useful to confirm deficiency; however, homocysteine is also elevated in folate deficiency and thus not as specific.

   Folate level could help confirm a deficiency in this vitamin which does cause a macrocytic anemia but this deficiency is not associated with neurologic deficits; in addition, folic acid is absorbed in the small intestine not the stomach. CBC with mean corpuscular volume may help confirm macrocytic anemia but this is not always present with B12 deficiency; in addition, there are multiple causes of macrocytosis and anemia and this will not confirm his diagnosis. Intrinsic factor Ab is present in pernicious anemia; it is not a sensitive test but regardless, a positive test would not confirm the cause of his symptoms. MRI lumbar spine has nonspecific findings in B12 deficiency; it may help assess for central/foraminal stenosis but without back pain this is unlikely and would this test would not assess his pallor/anemia.

6. **Answer:** D. **24-hour urine-free cortisol.** The patient likely has Cushing syndrome given the constellation of weight gain, striae (without prior history of pregnancy), new onset diabetes, hypertension, and vertebral compression fracture indicative of osteoporosis. 24-hour urine-free cortisol, dexamethasone suppression test, and late night salivary cortisol are the screening tests that are indicated at this point.
   Serum ACTH is not used for screening and is only helpful in determining the etiology once the diagnosis of Cushing syndrome has been made. MRI brain and CT abdomen may help identify pituitary adenoma and adrenal adenoma respectively but this test is premature at this point as the diagnosis of Cushing has not yet been confirmed. CRH stimulation test is only used once hypercortisolism has been established and ACTH is elevated as it helps distinguish Cushing disease versus ectopic ACTH production.

7. **Answer:** B. **Normal saline.** The patient is presenting with an inferior MI as evidenced by the location of the ST elevations on ECG. Because the patient also has bradycardia and hypotension he also has evidence of an associated right ventricular MI, which is strongly associated with inferior wall MIs and importantly is treated much differently than L-sided MI. It is important to remember that hemodynamic instability can result from increased vagal tone and sinus node dysfunction. The patient is preload dependent and IV fluids are indicated and will increase the patient's systemic blood pressure. Treatment with ASA, fibrinolysis versus PCI, heparin are all indicated as well.
   Nitroglycerin will decrease preload and worsen the patient's hemodynamics. Furosemide is not indicated as the patient has no signs of fluid overload and diuresis will decrease preload. Patient is already showing signs of hemodynamic instability and metoprolol will cause further bradycardia and hypotension. Morphine may cause vasodilation and further hypotension.

8. **Answer:** D. **Sodium bicarbonate.** The patient has evidence of an anion gap metabolic acidosis (HCO_3 is decreased and AG is 15) as well as a respiratory alkalosis (CO_2 is decreased) consistent with salicylate toxicity. This involves using Winter's formula and the expected PCO_2 in this example is 31 ± 2; however, the actual PCO_2 is 25 confirming there is a respiratory alkalosis as well. Treatment options include alkalinization of urine and hemodialysis.
   Fomepizole is indicated for methanol or ethylene glycol toxicity; however neither of these would also cause respiratory alkalosis. Albuterol will treat a COPD exacerbation although this usually leads to retention of CO_2 from inability to expire sufficiently and respiratory acidosis would be the dominant finding in that scenario. Insulin will help treat DKA if that was the underlying diagnosis but ketones are not mentioned thus assumed to be negative and not treating salicylate toxicity in a timely fashion will be detrimental.

9. **Answer:** E. **Colonoscopy.** The patient has not had colorectal cancer screening and this would certainly be indicated at this time given his age (>50). Initial choices for screening include FOBT, flexible sigmoidoscopy, or colonoscopy. In this example, the patient had a positive screening test and requires a colonoscopy as it will allow full visualization of the entire colon for diagnostic and therapeutic (biopsy if needed) purposes.
   Flexible sigmoidoscopy will miss more than half of the colon and therefore is not the best answer. Digital rectal examination has no role as it will not be sensitive enough to check anything but the rectum. Video capsule endoscopy is not the best next step; it will allow visualization of the entire GI tract but will not allow for biopsy if needed. CT colonography will not be sensitive enough to detect small lesions and again will not allow for intervention of necessary.

10. **Answer:** A. **IV omeprazole.** The patient likely has an upper GI bleed as evidenced by epigastric abdominal pain, melena, and labs showing an elevated BUN:Cr ratio of 25 in the setting of ASA use. Acid suppression and upper endoscopy (EGD) are the indicated interventions.
    IV octreotide is not indicated as the patient has no signs of liver disease to suggest esophageal varices as the cause of bleeding. Platelet transfusion will not reverse the effect aspirin has had on platelets and the platelet level presented is not low enough to lead to bleeding. RBC transfusion is not necessary as the patient is hemodynamically stable and the Hgb is not low enough that the patient is symptomatic. Normal saline is not necessary as the patient is already hypertensive and does not have hypovolemia.

11. **Answer:** E. **24-hour urine protein.** The patient has ascites in the setting of a low SAAG (<1.1 g/dL) indicating a lack of portal hypertension, and low ascitic protein (<2.5 g/dL) indicating low protein overall. The expected diagnoses would be severe malnutrition or protein-losing disorder such as nephrotic syndrome; thus, 24-hour urine protein is the most appropriate test.
    Echocardiogram would be helpful if the patient had hepatic congestion in the setting of elevated SAAG and elevated ascitic protein. Pelvic ultrasound to assess for potential ovarian malignancy would be indicated if

patient had low SAAG and elevated ascitic protein. Liver biopsy would be helpful to assess for causes of cirrhosis if patient had elevated SAAG and low ascitic protein. PPD would be indicated if patient had low SAAG and elevated ascitic protein.

12. Answer: B. IVIG. The patient is presenting with an ascending paralysis, absent reflexes, and albuminocytologic dissociation consistent with a diagnosis of Guillain–Barré syndrome in the setting of a preceding diarrheal illness. IVIG and plasmapheresis are the recommended treatments.

Prednisone is not recommended as steroids have not shown benefit. Ciprofloxacin is not indicated as there are no signs of infection; there are many precipitating illnesses that can trigger this disorder. Pyridostigmine would be indicated in myasthenia gravis. Botulism antitoxin would be beneficial if the patient has symptoms suggestive of botulism, a DESCENDING paralysis.

13. Answer: E. **Ristocetin cofactor activity.** The patient is presenting with mucocutaneous bleeding suggestive of von Willebrand disease. vWD is an autosomal dominant disorder and can be associated with factor VIII deficiency, sometimes manifested by an increased PTT level. Ristocetin testing is the only test mentioned that assess platelet aggregation.

Fibrinogen levels can be low in DIC but these patients are usually acutely ill and PT/PTT would also be elevated. Coombs testing will assess for causes of anemia but not for bleeding; in addition, bilirubin is normal suggesting against hemolysis. Factor IX level would be testing for hemophilia B but this is X linked recessive so unlikely to see in successive generations of females; in addition, hemarthrosis or hematomas would be more prominent. Mixing study is not indicated as the PT/PTT times are normal so unlikely to have a factor deficiency.

14. Answer: E. **Lumbar puncture.** The patient has acute headache in "thunderclap" fashion and subarachnoid hemorrhage is the worrisome consideration. CT brain showed no hemorrhage but LP would be the next step to evaluate for RBCs/xanthochromia and for increased opening pressure.

Sumatriptan would be used for migraines but symptoms are not suggestive and ruling out SAH is necessary. MRI brain may have comparable sensitivity to CT scan but regardless a negative scan demands a lumbar puncture for definitive evaluation. Cerebral angiogram will be useful once SAH is confirmed, but is invasive and will not be the next step. CT brain with contrast is unlikely to visualize a small aneurysm and is not the next step.

15. Answer: A. **Smoking cessation.** She has evidence of obstructive pulmonary disease as indicated by her FEV_1/FVC ratio <0.70. Not only will smoking cessation decrease the rate of decline in lung function it has also been shown to decrease mortality.

Tiotropium inhaler and fluticasone inhaler are likely to decrease her symptoms but will have no effect on mortality. Oxygen therapy has been shown to decrease mortality but is only indicated if O_2 saturation is 88% or below, otherwise if 89% and evidence of cor pulmonale, pulmonary hypertension or elevated hematocrit. Azithromycin would be indicated for a COPD exacerbation if a bacterium was thought to be the cause but there is no suggestion of infection in the provided scenario.

16. Answer: B. **Wisdom tooth extraction.** Endocarditis prophylaxis requires a high risk situation PLUS a qualifying procedure which is high risk for bacteremia and resultant endocarditis (see Cardiology chapter text). Wisdom tooth extraction involves cutting of the oral mucosa and would thus require prophylaxis.

Colonoscopy, EGD, as well as GI procedures in general do not require prophylaxis. Bronchoscopy only requires prophylaxis if mucosa will be broken, such as with biopsy. Dilatation ureteral strictures as well as GU procedures in general do not require antibiotics solely for the purpose of endocarditis prophylaxis.

17. Answer: A. SPEP (**serum protein electrophoresis**). The patient is presenting with a pathologic fracture indicating that there is weakening of the underlying bone prior to a low impact injury. Given the laboratory findings (hypercalcemia, normocytic anemia, renal failure, and low anion gap) it is most suggestive of the patient having multiple myeloma; thus, SPEP would be the ideal test to confirm.

Bone scans detect osteoblastic activity and can be falsely negative in myeloma. PTHrP is cancer related of which there is no suggestion of a separate primary malignancy; in addition, this would explain only the hypercalcemia. PTH elevation in hyperparathyroidism would explain only the hypercalcemia. DEXA would be useful if evaluating for osteoporosis but cortical bone was described as normal in density thus this is unlikely, and the injury was most likely related to a lytic lesion at the site of fracture.

18. Answer: E. TSH. The patient has symptoms suggestive of hypothyroidism (bradycardia, fatigue, weight gain, hair loss) and TSH is the best initial screening test.

US thyroid is not necessary when the physical examination is normal. TPO would help confirm Hashimoto's as a potential cause of hypothyroidism but would not help confirm hypothyroidism itself as patients may have elevated antibodies but normal thyroid function. Thyroid uptake scan would be more helpful in evaluating hyperthyroidism, such as thyroiditis or Graves disease. FNA is only indicated if a patient has a nodule with size or features worrisome for malignancy and in need of tissue diagnosis.

19. Answer: A. **Follow-up CT chest.** The patient has an indeterminate nodule discovered incidentally and this requires further follow-up. The patient is low risk (<5%) as evidenced by her lack of smoking history and young age. CT scan would be the most appropriate follow-up (Fleischner guidelines and ACCP guidelines). Of note, if the patient clearly has benign properties such as popcorn calcification suggesting hamartoma no further follow-up is required.

Bronchoscopy and needle biopsy would be indicated if the patient had an intermediate/high malignancy risk, it was enlarging or the patient desired a tissue diagnosis. CXR would not be sensitive enough to follow changes in size. PET-CT scan would also be indicated if there is intermediate/high risk of malignancy.

20. Answer: D. **Atropine.** The patient has symptomatic bradycardia with hypoperfusion leading to her symptoms; she requires increase in heart rate to maintain cardiac output and atropine is the only choice that would be able to provide this. If this medication was ineffective then epinephrine, dopamine or transcutaneous pacing would all be alternative treatments.

Echocardiogram will not help treat the patient in the acute setting as the patient demands urgent intervention; obtaining this test will only delay treatment. Nitroglycerin can be used for chest pain in the setting of angina to cause vasodilation, but will cause worsened hypotension and is contraindicated in this patient. ICD is a consideration for this patient for long-term primary prevention of VF/VT given her sustained decreased EF; however, it is not an acute treatment for the patient's life-threatening condition.

21. Answer: E. **Omeprazole.** His symptoms are suggestive of gastroesophageal reflux with a component of laryngeal reflux as well. Treatment failure is not considered until there have been at least several months of scheduled PPI use; he is currently only using as needed. PPIs are more effective than H2 blockers and if a patient fails empiric treatment then one can consider workup for other causes of his symptoms.

H. pylori antigen would be useful if evaluating for abdominal pain if gastritis/ulcers were the suspected diagnoses. EGD would be indicated if patient was following lifestyle changes and taking scheduled PPI but having no relief in symptoms, or if he had alarm symptoms (melena, anemia, weight loss, or dysphagia). pH monitoring can also be used for refractory symptoms after appropriate empiric therapy. Gastrin level would only be indicated if evaluating for suspected gastrinoma or with multiple gastroduodenal ulcers.

22. Answer: A. **EGD with small bowel biopsy.** The patient has chronic symptoms suggestive of celiac sprue (iron deficiency, transaminitis, anemia, and dermatitis herpetiformis). There is also an association with psychiatric issues with celiac sprue. TTG serology would be reasonable and duodenal biopsy is necessary for confirmation.

Colonoscopy would not be able to evaluate for a diagnosis of celiac sprue. Loperamide may help diarrhea but will not address the underlying cause of her symptoms and is therefore not the best answer. Sertraline would not help in diagnosing or treating her condition; there is a link of IBS with mood disorders but IBS is a diagnosis of exclusion and only considered when labs/examination is normal. Skin biopsy may confirm dermatitis herpetiformis but small bowel biopsy would still be needed for the diagnosis of celiac sprue, as one may have this skin condition without having sprue.

23. Answer: B. **Spironolactone.** The patient has stage IV systolic heart failure and spironolactone is shown to decrease mortality in these patients as it is cardioprotective. β-Blockers, ACE inhibitors, and ICDs are also shown to decrease mortality in patients with systolic heart failure.

Isosorbide dinitrate and hydralazine are shown to decrease mortality in class III/IV heart failure in African Americans but this patient is Caucasian and not expected to receive that same benefit. Digoxin and furosemide do not decrease mortality in any heart failure patients.

24. Answer: D. **Inhaled albuterol prn.** The patient has classic symptoms of exercise induced bronchoconstriction and would benefit from pre-exercise inhaler usage to prevent symptoms. It is important to remember that PFTs may be normal between episodes when the patient is asymptomatic; a challenge may be needed to objectively evaluate the bronchoconstriction.

CXR is not necessary as the lung examination is clear and she has no symptoms at baseline. Inhaled fluticasone is not the best answer as the patient only has intermittent symptoms related to activity, not any symptoms between episodes to suggest chronic asthma. Reassurance is not appropriate as the patient clearly has symptoms that limit her lifestyle and are causing airway constriction. Inhaled salmeterol is not appropriate as the patient has no baseline symptoms between episodes; in addition, treatment of asthma with LABA alone, without cotreatment with corticosteroids, is associated with increased mortality.

25. Answer: D. No treatment. It is not recommended to screen for asymptomatic bacteriuria as treatment does not offer benefit but does include potential harm from side effects, etc. The only population in which to screen and treat asymptomatic bacteriuria is pregnancy.

Nitrofurantoin would be the drug of choice for a patient with uncomplicated cystitis. Ciprofloxacin and TMP-SMX would be considerations for cystitis or for pyelonephritis. Repeat urinalysis and culture would not be indicated as screening and treating asymptomatic patients does not offer clinical benefit.

26. Answer: B. IV hydrocortisone. The patient is presenting with acute adrenal insufficiency and this is a medical emergency. The patient must be adequately resuscitated with aggressive IV normal saline in addition to replacement of corticosteroids. The most likely cause for the patient's adrenal insufficiency is her long-term use of corticosteroids and inadequate response in the setting of her acute illness.

Cortisol level can be checked but medical treatment is the most important intervention and is mandatory. CT adrenal glands and MRI pituitary are unlikely to yield further information regarding the diagnosis in the patient; in addition, they would be inappropriate as they would delay the treatment of the patient and lead to higher morbidity/mortality. Cosyntropin stimulation test can be used to confirm the diagnosis of adrenal insufficiency but should NOT delay treatment; dexamethasone could be used if the diagnosis is in question as it will not interfere with interpretation of this test.

Answers

27. Answer: A. CT angiography. The patient has pain out of proportion to examination in the setting of atherosclerotic risk factors for thrombosis as well as atrial fibrillation with a subtherapeutic INR which would be risk factors for embolism; the most likely diagnosis is acute mesenteric ischemia and CT angiography would be helpful in confirming this diagnosis.

Gastric emptying study would be helpful in evaluating for gastroparesis which the patient is at risk for with uncontrolled DM; however, this patient is presenting with acute abdominal pain and not consistent with that diagnosis. EGD and colonoscopy would help evaluate for many causes of abdominal pain but will delay the time to diagnosis of mesenteric ischemia which is needed urgently to prevent infarction/necrosis. Vitamin K will reverse warfarin in the setting of the patient's bleeding but given the scenario suggestive of mesenteric ischemia and stable hemodynamics (INR is also therapeutic) this is not indicated and anticoagulation will be used if thrombosis/embolism is confirmed.

28. Answer: E. Ibuprofen. NSAIDs are the mainstay of treatment for acute pericarditis. Colchicine can be added to this regimen for added benefit.

Coronary angiogram is not indicated as there are no focal ST elevations or wall motion abnormalities suggestive of an acute MI. Drainage of pericardial effusion is only indicated in large effusions causing hemodynamic compromise or for diagnostic purposes. Prednisone is not indicated unless the patient fails NSAIDs or has contraindications to receiving them. Azathioprine would only be used if the patient had recurrent pericarditis and was unable to wean off of steroids.

29. Answer: C. Chest tube insertion. It is important to recognize that the above patient is presenting with a symptomatic pneumothorax, in this setting related to his underlying COPD and likely bleb rupture. CXR can confirm the diagnosis but this can also be made clinically. Supplemental oxygen would be appropriate followed by needle aspiration or chest tube insertion to remove air from the pleural space.

Albuterol–ipratropium nebulizer and prednisone would help treat COPD exacerbation but this is not the diagnosis presented. Azithromycin would not be the best answer as there is no suggestion of infection in this patient. Pleurodesis is only indicated if there are recurrent pneumothoraces.

30. Answer: D. Warfarin. The patient has valvular atrial fibrillation and a CHADS2 score of 3, thus warranting systemic anticoagulation. Warfarin is indicated and the most appropriate choice.

Aspirin is not adequate as warfarin has superior efficacy in stroke prevention in comparison to aspirin. Dabigatran is one of the newer oral anticoagulants that could be considered as an alternative to warfarin but it is only used in the setting of nonvalvular afib; this patient has evidence of mitral stenosis on examination and this is the presumed cause of his atrial fibrillation. Clopidogrel is inferior to warfarin for stroke prevention in the setting of atrial fibrillation. Fondaparinux is used in treatment/prophylaxis for DVT, not for afib stroke prevention.

31. Answer: B. Aortic valve replacement. The patient has symptomatic aortic stenosis which is an indication for surgery.

Nitroglycerin would be indicated if his symptoms were related solely to atherosclerotic disease; however, vasodilation may worsen his systemic blood pressure. Aspirin will prevent further atherosclerotic disease but will not fix his valvular disease. Carotid Doppler will assess for carotid stenosis; however, the murmur heard in the neck is referred from the aortic valve. Coronary artery bypass grafting is sometimes done at the same time as a valve replacement if significant atherosclerotic disease is present; however, he has very mild disease on prior angiogram and this is not indicated.

32. Answer: B. Physical therapy. The diagnosis here is patellofemoral pain syndrome and PT is the most appropriate intervention.

Corticosteroid injection would be unlikely to be helpful as the cause of pain is not intra-articular; she does have an underlying autoimmune disease but there is no effusion and markers do not show significant inflammation to heighten suspicion of SLE as the cause. Knee arthroscopy and MRI knee are also unwarranted at this time given the normal examination and lack of trauma to suggest meniscal or ligamentous injury. Ibuprofen is contraindicated given CKD.

33. Answer: E. Lisinopril. The patient has a new diagnosis of type 2 diabetes and requires not only control of his glucose but also treatment for complications related to his disease. An ACE inhibitor or ARB would be indicated for hypertension, CKD, or microalbuminuria and thus lisinopril is the best answer.

Hydrochlorothiazide is not the best answer as it does not have renoprotective features that ACE inhibitors do; in addition, efficacy decreases as GFR decreases. Insulin is not necessary given relatively controlled A1c and lack of a lifestyle intervention trial yet. Pioglitazone is contraindicated in setting of CHF. Metformin is contraindicated with CKD.

34. Answer: E. Biopsy hilar adenopathy. The patient's clinical picture is consistent with possible sarcoidosis. Tissue biopsy showing noncaseating granulomas along with ruling out other diseases is essential for the diagnosis. One of the major risk factors of sarcoidosis is being African American.

Serum calcium will be elevated in a subset of sarcoid patients but this is not sensitive enough to make the diagnosis. CT chest will yield more information in regard to lung imaging but will not confirm a diagnosis. ACE level is not sensitive enough to confirm a diagnosis. Biopsy of a leg lesion which is easily accessible will reveal inflammation as the patient has findings consistent with erythema nodosum; however, this will NOT show noncaseating granulomas so this will not confirm a diagnosis of sarcoid.

35. Answer: B. Initiate fluid restriction. The patient is euvolemic and has lung cancer, low serum osmolality, and high urine osmolality all suggestive of SIADH as the cause. He has very mild symptoms and can be managed with fluid restriction and increased salt intake.

Administering IV normal (0.9%) saline is not the appropriate answer as sodium will be excreted but water will be retained; thus, worsening hyponatremia. Initiating hemodialysis is not appropriate as the patient has minimal symptoms, has not failed other therapies, and because it is invasive. Administering hypertonic (3%) saline is not necessary as the patient has minimal symptoms; if the patient had more severe symptoms such as confusion, lethargy, nausea, or vomiting this would be appropriate. Administering hydrochlorothiazide is not correct as this medication itself is a cause of hyponatremia; loop diuretics such as furosemide can be used to correct sodium levels in SIADH.

36. Answer: D. Antistreptolysin titer. The patient is presenting with hematuria in the setting of a recent infection and the most likely diagnosis is poststreptococcal glomerulonephritis. Antistreptolysin titer can help confirm recent strep infection.

ANCA is unlikely to be helpful as the patient does not have other symptoms suggestive of a systemic vasculitis. Anti-GBM is also unlikely to assist in the diagnosis as the patient has no other symptoms to suggest Goodpasture's and the time course fits best with PSGN. HIV is associated with renal disease, most specifically collapsing variant of FSGS but this is nephrotic in presentation. IgA levels are unnecessary as serum IgA levels are not useful in the diagnosis of IgA nephropathy; in addition, the glomerulonephritis associated with IgA deposits happens much quicker after the infection, usually within several days.

37. Answer: E. SLE. This patient has multiple symptoms and examination findings consistent with a likely diagnosis of SLE—oral ulcers, malar rash, arthritis, edema suggestive of renal impairment, as well as hematologic abnormalities.

Osteoarthritis is unlikely given the patient's young age and would not explain the patient's multiple other symptoms. Reactive arthritis usually follows a GI/GU infection and includes arthritis, urethritis, and uveitis. Behçet disease can include many symptoms, most notably oral/genital ulcerations but would be unlikely to include the classic malar rash and is very rare in the United States. Gout is possible given her use of HCTZ and potential for hyperuricemia but this would not explain the other findings.

38. **Answer: B. Carbidopa–levodopa.** The patient is presenting with symptoms consistent with Parkinson's and medical treatment would be recommended with dopamine agonist.

Fluoxetine is not appropriate as the patient does not have a clinical diagnosis of depression; his psychomotor slowing alone should not be misinterpreted as depressive symptoms unless there are other symptoms such as sadness, appetite changes, sleep disturbance, or disinterest in activities. Propranolol would be beneficial in patients with essential tremor. Memantine would be indicated only if patient had moderate to severe dementia. Deep brain stimulation is invasive and would not be considered unless there were severe symptoms in which the patient had failed other medical therapy.

39. **Answer: C. Infliximab.** The patient has moderate to severe Crohn disease (anemia, abdominal tenderness, and weight loss) and demands appropriate therapy to prevent complications. Infliximab is an anti-TNF antibody that is indicated for moderate to severe Crohn disease.

Loperamide should not be used in active inflammatory bowel disease. Azathioprine is less likely to offer control of the patient's symptoms than infliximab; in addition, this medication takes up to 6 weeks to reach a therapeutic effect and needs to be given alongside steroids. Surgical resection is not indicated as the patient has no evidence of abscess, perforation, or fistula. Ciprofloxacin and metronidazole is more useful in mild disease and will not treat the underlying inflammatory process responsible for the patient's symptoms.

40. **Answer: A. Thumb spica splint.** The patient has risk factors for several causes of pain related to overuse in the upper extremity but examination reveals a positive Finkelstein test which confirms a diagnosis of de Quervain tenosynovitis. This is related to a combination of repetitive motions a mechanic but also associated with caring for and lifting his grandchild. Immobilization of the thumb is the most appropriate intervention.

Wrist splint would be helpful if the patient had carpal tunnel syndrome. Counterforce forearm brace would be helpful if patient had lateral/medial epicondylitis. Carpal tunnel corticosteroid injection is not helpful as this is not the source of his pain. Ibuprofen is contraindicated given his known chronic kidney disease.

41. **Answer: B. Reduction of fracture.** The patient has the classic triad diagnostic for fat embolism: hypoxia, petechial rash, and neurologic abnormalities. Treatment is supportive and given the source is the multiple long bone fractures; these should be repaired when the patient is stabilized.

Albuterol is not indicated as the patient has no evidence of obstruction (e.g., wheezing) as a cause for her acute decline. Furosemide is not indicated as the patient has no evidence of volume overload in the pulmonary vasculature. Levofloxacin is not indicated as there is no evidence of pulmonary infection. IV heparin will be ineffective in improving the patient's symptoms as it cannot dissolve fat, only thrombi.

42. **Answer: A. Valsalva maneuver.** The patient has SVT likely related to AVNRT and he has no concerning symptoms. Initial attempt at termination should use vagal maneuvers such as Valsalva maneuver or carotid sinus massage.

Adenosine is very short acting and can be used if vagal maneuvers fail to terminate the arrhythmia. Metoprolol would also be considered if the above measures failed. Digoxin would also inhibit the AV node but has more potential side effects than the other medications and is rarely used for this purpose. Cardioversion would be reserved for hemodynamic instability including hypotension, heart failure, or angina.

43. **Answer: D. Hydroxychloroquine.** The patient is presenting with signs/symptoms fulfilling criteria for a diagnosis of rheumatoid arthritis. The most important intervention is DMARD therapy (disease-modifying antirheumatoid drugs), especially given the patient already has evidence of joint damage.

Prednisone, corticosteroid injections, and indomethacin will all help control symptoms but not control joint damage. Physical therapy will help improve function for the patient but without DMARD therapy her joint damage will continue to worsen.

44. **Answer: C. ERCP.** The patient has cholangitis secondary to obstructing common bile duct stone and is presenting with severe sepsis. The patient needs hemodynamic support, antibiotics, and control of the source of infection. ERCP is the next step in order to relieve the obstruction and allow drainage of the biliary system.

Cholecystectomy is recommended eventually to prevent recurrence but not in the acute setting given the high morbidity and mortality. Liver biopsy will not aid in diagnosis or treatment; the cause of transaminitis is evident. MRCP will not aid in management as the diagnosis is already confirmed. Percutaneous transhepatic cholangiography is second line to ERCP as it carries higher morbidity in regard to bleeding or peritonitis.

45. Answer: E. No further intervention. There is no further workup or treatment that is required at this point. The patient is in a low-risk category with no identifiable risk factors and a PPD would only be considered positive if 15 mm or greater.

AFB sputum culture is not necessary to rule out active pulmonary TB because the patient is asymptomatic and has a negative PPD test. Rifampin, isoniazid, pyrazinamide, ethambutol would be indicated only if the patient had active pulmonary TB. Isoniazid would be indicated for prophylaxis if the patient had a positive TB test without any pulmonary symptoms and a negative CXR. Chest x-ray would be indicated to screen for evidence of pulmonary TB if the PPD was positive.

46. Answer: B. TSH. The patient has calcium pyrophosphate dehydrate deposition disease (CPPD, pseudogout). This is confirmed by the inflammatory arthrocentesis with CPPD crystals and imaging findings showing deposition. Associated disorders include hemochromatosis, hypothyroidism, and hyperparathyroidism so labs including ferritin/transferrin/TSH/Ca are all reasonable to screen for as treatment of underlying disorder can improve symptoms.

Uric acid would be helpful in determining initial treatment for gout but this is not the underlying diagnosis. ANA and ESR are nonspecific and would not be helpful in guiding therapy. HLA-B27 is not indicated as the diagnosis of CPPD is confirmed and this will not screen for any associated disease.

47. Answer: A. Zolendronic acid. The patient has osteoporosis and a history of a fracture; thus, every attempt would be made to start the patient on a medication to reduce her risk of fractures. Zolendronic acid is a bisphosphonate which will reduce both vertebral/nonvertebral fractures; in addition, it is given intravenously and is most appropriate in this patient with achalasia.

Alendronate is a PO bisphosphonate and would be contraindicated given achalasia and the risk of pill esophagitis. Raloxifene is a SERM and has evidence only for reduction of vertebral fractures and would thus not be an ideal choice; in addition, it is contraindicated given the prior history of thromboembolic disease. Calcitonin is inferior to bisphosphonates and is not the correct choice. Estrogen is no longer used for management of osteoporosis given many risks, one of them DVT/PE, and this medication would be contraindicated in this patient.

48. Answer: D. Propranolol. The patient is presenting with thyroid storm, an endocrine emergency, and requires treatment without delay. This was likely triggered by her recent surgery. Adrenergic effects of thyroid hormone (e.g., tachycardia) as well as T4→T3 conversion are blocked with this treatment.

RAIU at this point will delay treatment which is not appropriate given the morbidity/mortality associated with thyroid storm. Iodine is a treatment option used in thyroid storm; however, it should be given AFTER methimazole or PTU to avoid its use as a substrate for more thyroid hormone synthesis. US thyroid is also unnecessary and will delay treatment. Thyroidectomy should only be performed once the hyperthyroidism is treated given the mortality rate associated with surgery in thyroid storm.

49. Answer: A. CT urography. The patient has hematuria and whether it be gross or microscopic demands further workup. Infection has been ruled out and by the fact that casts are not seen, a glomerular cause has been ruled out. To evaluate the rest of the GU tract one must perform urine cytology, cystoscopy, and CT urography.

Ultrasound of kidneys will evaluate the kidneys relatively well but miss small tumors and will be less sensitive in evaluating the ureters. Renal biopsy is not indicated in this scenario as a glomerular source of bleeding is unlikely; RBC casts or dysmorphic RBCs on microscopy would be suggestive of glomerular cause. PSA and prostate biopsy are unlikely to yield a cause of the patient's bleeding and would not evaluate the rest of the GU tract.

50. Answer: D. Albuterol. The patient has a diagnosis of acute bronchitis and this is most likely viral in nature. Symptoms are related to hyperreactive airways and should self-resolve in a few weeks; treatment is symptomatic. Because of the wheezing associated with his symptoms albuterol would be the appropriate choice.

Prednisone is not indicated as the patient has no underlying reactive lung disease, is not in distress, and his peak flow is normal. Oseltamivir is not indicated because the patient does not have symptoms suggestive of influenza; in addition, he is well outside the appropriate window of treatment given his risk factors. Azithromycin or any antibiotics is NOT indicated as most bronchitis is caused by viruses; antibiotics would be indicated if pertussis was suspected or pneumonia was confirmed. Sputum culture is not necessary as a viral cause is much more likely.

51. Answer: B. Weight loss. The seventh report of the Joint National Committee (JNC 7) on Prevention, Detection, Evaluation, and Treatment of High Blood Pressure recommends *all* patients with hypertension (blood pressure of 140/90 mm Hg or higher) or prehypertension (blood pressure of 120/80 to 139/89 mm Hg) execute five lifestyle modifications: *Reducing dietary sodium* to less than 2.4 g per day; *increasing exercise* to at least 30 minutes per day (4 days per week); *limiting alcohol consumption* to 2 drinks or less per day for men and 1 drink or less per day for women; following the *Dietary Approaches to Stop Hypertension (DASH) diet* (high in fruits, vegetables, potassium, calcium, and magnesium; low in fat and salt); and achieving a *weight loss* goal of 10 lb (4.5 kg) or more. Of these, weight loss has shown to have the highest reduction in systolic blood pressure (reduction from 5 to 20 mm Hg) in overweight patients. **(A, C, D)** These three lifestyle modifications are also recommended and do have a substantial effect on reduction of systolic pressure, just not as much as weight loss does. **(E)** Smoking cessation should always be encouraged as part of any comprehensive lifestyle modification plan.

52. Answer: C. Hydrochlorothiazide. For most patients with hypertension, thiazide diuretics are the best proven first-line treatment in reducing morbidity and mortality. Thiazide diuretics are especially effective in preventing secondary cardiovascular events in patients with hypertension. **(D, E)** Current evidence does not support the use of β-blockers, particularly atenolol, as first-line treatment for hypertension. **(A, B)** Although there is increasing evidence that ACE inhibitors (lisinopril) and possibly calcium channel blockers (amlodipine) may be equivalent to thiazide diuretics in reducing morbidity and mortality, the relative expense of these medications makes thiazide diuretics an ideal first-line choice.

Answers

53. Answer: A. Pyelonephritis. Pyelonephritis produces flank pain, but is also suggested by fever, leukocytosis, and a urine dipstick showing infection (e.g., positive nitrites, positive leukocyte esterase). The presence of WBC casts is also seen in pyelonephritis, as is the physical examination finding of costovertebral angle tenderness (CVA) tenderness. **(B)** Nephrolithiasis (kidney stones) produces a colicky pain that shoots down into either groin region. It does not produce fever, leukocytosis, or urine dipstick findings suggestive of infection (however it often is positive for blood). Calcium stones are the most common type of kidney stones, and patients with these stones are encouraged to increase their dietary intake of calcium (in order to decrease oxalate absorption in the GI tract). **(C)** Appendicitis if a very important diagnosis to consider in young patients with abdominal pain, however does not produce positive urinalysis findings. **(D)** Ectopic pregnancy can often mimic the pain produced in nephrolithiasis, however this diagnosis is unlikely given the negative pregnancy test. **(E)** Acute interstitial nephritis (AIN) can indeed produce WBC casts in the urine, but also produces urine eosinophils. AIN is a type of intrinsic renal acute kidney injury (AKI) that produces fever, rash, arthralgias, and/or eosinophilia. The most common cause is an allergic reaction to medications.

54. Answer: C. Nonsteroidal anti-inflammatory drugs (NSAIDS). Back pain is a high-yield topic on the USMLE. Back pain that improves with exercise, but worsens with rest in an otherwise healthy patient lends credence to the diagnosis of ankylosing spondylitis (AS). AS is a seronegative spondyloarthropathy (rheumatoid factor is negative) that is a systemic rheumatic disease. Ninety percent of people express the HLA-B27 genotype. It is also three times more common in males than females. In addition to back pain, patients can also experience anterior uveitis causing eye redness and pain, in addition to cardiovascular and lung involvement. The first-line treatment for all seronegative spondyloarthropathies is NSAIDS but biologics and disease-modifying antirheumatic drugs (DMARDs) are effective in treating the progression of the disease. **(A, B)** Local heat and physical therapy are especially effective in back pain caused by disc herniation. Disc herniation typically causes an electricity-like shooting lower back pain. **(D, E)** Epidural steroid injections and surgical laminectomy are typically reserved for advanced refractory back pain that does not respond to more conservative measures initially.

55. Answer: E. Nebulized albuterol for bronchodilation. This patient is likely suffering from an asthma exacerbation caused in part by his recent exposure to a viral illness. There were wheezes on examination with no urticaria or angioedema, making an anaphylactic reaction unlikely. **(C)**. Management of an acute asthma exacerbation involves oxygen administration as well as intermittent or continuous nebulized albuterol, which is the first-line treatment. If the patient fails to respond to albuterol, then ipratropium and magnesium are additional options to promote bronchodilation. Oral corticosteroids should also be given to reduce airway inflammation during and after the exacerbation. Response to therapy can be monitored by following the SaO_2 as well as either the FEV_1 or the peak expiratory flow (PEF). Arterial blood gases may also be useful; be concerned about the finding of a normal $PaCO_2$, which is often indicative of respiratory fatigue leading to the requirement of intubation (hypoxemia should cause hyperventilation and hypocapnia). **(A)** Oxygen should be administered to asthmatics with a target SaO_2 >90%. In COPD, the target is 90% to 94% due to the concern for the development of hypercapnia, however this is not seen in asthma. **(B)** This patient is unlikely to have pneumonia given that he is afebrile and has no suggestive findings of pneumonia on lung examination. (C) Subcutaneous epinephrine is useful in anaphylaxis, but has no benefit over inhaled β_2-agonists in asthma for bronchodilation. (D) Ipratropium is an anticholinergic and is the first-line treatment for COPD exacerbation (although albuterol is often used too); it may be used as an adjunctive therapy in asthma exacerbation, but albuterol is the first-line therapy.

56. Answer: C. ***Staphylococcus aureus*****.** This patient's clinical presentation and subsequent deterioriation are consistent with a diagnosis of toxic shock syndrome (TSS), which is caused by preformed *S. aureus* exotoxin, TSST-1. TSS is associated with prolonged tampon use. For the purposes of your Step, always suspect prolonged tampon use in young women. The toxin acts as a superantigen, which activates T cells leading to massive cytokine release. TSS typically presents with fever, vomiting, diarrhea, and the development of a diffuse macular erythematous rash. Complications of TSS include acute respiratory distress syndrome (ARDS), hypotension, disseminated intravascular coagulation (DIC), and hemorrhage. (A) *Streptococcus pyogenes* is very rarely associated with TSS (only group A Strep species are associated with TSS), but when it is, it is not associated with tampon use. (B) *Neisseria meningitidis* can certainly present with fever and diffuse rash, however it is not associated with such a high fever or tampon use. (D) *Streptococcus pneumoniae* is a type of group B Strep species, and accordingly, does not cause TSS. (E) Rocky Mountain spotted fever presents with fever and a rash that is first apparent in the extremities and moves centrally.

57. Answer: B. Recurrent pericarditis. The chest pain and ECG are typical of acute pericarditis, which commonly presents with fever, pleuritic chest pain, new onset pericardial effusion, and diffuse concave ST elevations on ECG. Most cases have an infectious etiology, including coxsackie viruses, HIV, influenza, *Staphylococcus aureus, Streptococcus pneumoniae,* tuberculosis, and various fungi. Other important causes include cancer, autoimmune diseases, post-MI or cardiac surgery, radiation therapy, and uremia. All patients should be treated with NSAIDs and colchicine to improve symptoms and prevent complications. Patients who are not treated are much more likely to develop recurrent pericarditis, which is defined as a recurrence of symptoms after the inciting event (e.g., virus) has passed. (A) Pericardial effusions commonly accompany acute pericarditis, however cardiac tamponade is a rare complication. (C) Constrictive pericarditis is a possible outcome of any cause of acute pericarditis, however it is not the most common complication. (D) Free wall rupture is a complication of acute myocardial infarction. (E) Pericarditis affects the pericardium although the myocardium is sometimes affected as well. However, the rate of valve involvement and complications is low.

58. Answer: B. CT scan with contrast. This patient has pyelonephritis that likely progressed to a renal or perinephric abscess, which is indicated by the persistent fever. Patients with this complication will present with symptoms typical of pyelonephritis (fevers, chills, flank pain, abdominal pain, anorexia, nausea/vomiting), but will continue to be febrile despite treatment with appropriate antibiotics. Most cases of renal/perinephric abscesses are caused by urologic pathogens (e.g., *E. coli* and other enteric gram-negative bacilli), however *Staphylococcus aureus* is also common and arrives at the kidneys by hematogenous spread. The best diagnostic test is a CT scan of the abdomen with contrast, although a renal ultrasound can also identify many renal/perinephric abscesses. If the abscess is small (<5 cm), it can be observed with antibiotics alone; if the patient does not respond to antibiotics, or if the abscess is large (≥5 cm), both antibiotics and drainage are necessary. Antibiotic therapy should always be based on culture and sensitivity data when available, however empiric therapy for renal/perinephric abscesses is the same as for pyelonephritis. Options include a fluoroquinolone, ceftriaxone, ampicillin–sulbactam, an aminoglycoside, or antistaphylococcal antibiotics if *S. aureus* is suspected. (A) WBC casts do not necessarily indicate acute interstitial nephritis or glomerulonephritis; they may also indicate an upper urinary tract infection such as pyelonephritis. Therefore, a renal biopsy is not the next step. (C) Failure to defervesce after treatment with antibiotics raises the concern for a complication of pyelonephritis, such as a renal or perinephric abscess, and therefore further diagnostic workup should be pursued. (D, E) The organism is sensitive to both antibiotics, so there is no benefit of changing antibiotics or stopping antibiotics.

59. Answer: D. Intubation. The patient in this vignette is experiencing an acute asthma exacerbation with worrisome symptoms/signs: loud wheezes, use of respiratory accessory muscles, tachycardia, tachypnea, and poor oxygen saturation. In addition, the arterial blood gas shows a normal $PaCO_2$ which is not a good sign; hypoxic patients should hyperventilate to maintain oxygenation, which causes hypocapnia and a respiratory alkalosis. When a patient has a normal $PaCO_2$, this is a sign that the patient is tiring and decompensating. Even though intubation should be avoided if possible, there is a low threshold for intubating patients that are showing signs of respiratory fatigue. (A) Increasing the oxygen flow rate might improve oxygenation, but the patient is likely starting to develop hypercapnic respiratory failure, which is due to inadequate ventilation. Once the patient is on a ventilator, ventilation is controlled primarily by adjusting the respiratory rate or tidal volume. Oxygenation can be maintained by adjusting the FiO_2 and positive end-expiratory pressure (PEEP). (B) IV corticosteroids are used in acute exacerbations but will not act immediately to prevent this patient from further decompensation. (C) Azithromycin and other antibiotics are used in acute COPD exacerbations, not acute asthma exacerbations. (E) This arterial blood gas shows a normal $PaCO_2$ which is not a good sign. Although nebulized albuterol is typically first-line treatment for acute asthma exacerbation, this patient is decompensating as evidenced by the arterial blood gas and intubation must be pursued next.

60. Answer: B. Positively birefringent rhomboid-shaped crystals. This patient has a history of parathyroid adenoma which is likely causing hypercalcemia secondary to hyperparathyroidism. Patients with hypercalcemia are at risk for developing pseudogout, a rheumatologic disease with diverse symptoms and signs arising from the accumulation of calcium pyrophosphate dihydrate crystals in the connective tissues. It commonly presents with acute onset, painful monoarthropathy of the knee. Joint aspiration with synovial fluid analysis confirms the diagnosis, showing rhomboid-shaped crystals that are positively birefringent. (A) Negatively birefringent needle-shaped crystals describe *gout,* which also presents with acute onset monoarthropathy, but usually affects the first metatarsophalangeal joint of the foot. Furthermore, gout is not triggered by hypercalcemia. (C, D) Neutrophil predominant synovial fluid with gram-positive cocci is diagnostic of septic arthritis. This patient has no fever, making septic arthritis highly unlikely from the clinical picture alone. (E) Normal synovial fluid findings are not the norm in the setting of pseudogout.

Answers

61. Answer: B. Acute retroviral syndrome. Acute HIV infection can present in a variety of ways, but typical symptoms of the "acute retroviral syndrome" include a mononucleosis-like syndrome with fever, lymphadenopathy, headache, myalgias/arthralgias, sore throat, and a maculopapular rash. Another less sensitive but more specific finding is painful, well-demarcated mucocutaneous ulcerations. Additional clues to the diagnosis in this case are the patient's high-risk behaviors (unprotected sex, IV drug use) and negative test results for other conditions on the differential diagnosis (mononucleosis due to EBV, syphilis, and other STIs, etc.). During the acute phase of HIV infection, there may be a negative screening test (ELISA may take weeks to become positive) with high viral RNA levels. Typically, the diagnosis of HIV is made with a highly sensitive screening test (e.g., ELISA) followed by a more specific confirmatory test (e.g., Western blot). (A) The finding of diffuse nontender lymphadenopathy is more consistent with a systemic process such as a viral infection rather than Hodgkin lymphoma, which often presents with focal or asymmetric lymphadenopathy. (C) Though heterophile-negative mononucleosis due to CMV is a possibility, the findings of both a maculopapular rash and mucocutaneous ulcerations make HIV more likely (both may occur in CMV infection but are less common manifestations, and GI ulcerations usually occur in the setting of immunosuppression). (D) Secondary syphilis is less likely to have mucocutaneous ulcerations and the screening test was negative. Although false negatives are possible with RPR and VDRL tests, the constellation of findings makes HIV infection much more likely than a false-negative syphilis test. (E) These clinical findings are much more severe than typical upper respiratory infection symptoms.

62. Answer: C. Obtain a chest x-ray; if normal, start isoniazid and pyridoxine for 9 months. There are a couple important teaching points in this vignette. First, screening for TB is often performed with a PPD, and it is important to know what the threshold is for a positive test result. In patients with close contact to a patient with active TB, a concerning chest x-ray, or who are immunosuppressed (via medications, HIV infection, etc.), a positive test is >5 mm. For those patients at high risk (healthcare workers, jail workers, the homeless, IV drug users, uncontrolled diabetes, chronic kidney disease, etc.), a positive test is >10 mm. And for all others without risk factors, a positive test is >15 mm. This patient has an induration of 11 mm and is a healthcare worker, therefore she warrants further workup to differentiate active from latent TB. (Note: prior BCG vaccination rarely produces an induration >10 mm as an adult, and the CDC recommends that BCG vaccination status should not influence the workup and treatment of TB.) If the chest x-ray is negative, then the patient has latent TB and should be treated with 9 months of isoniazid and pyridoxine (vitamin B_6, which helps to prevent isoniazid-induced neuropathy). (A) Treatment of active TB is becoming complicated with MDR TB, however active TB is generally treated with a 4-drug regimen (rifampin, isoniazid, pyrazinamide, ethambutol) for 2 months followed up a 2-drug regimen (rifampin, isoniazid) for 4 months. (B) Because this patient is a healthcare worker, she should be treated for latent TB given the risk of reactivation and exposure to other patients. (D) A chest x-ray should be performed before starting treatment to differentiate latent from active TB. (E) Reassurance would only be appropriate if the PPD result was negative.

63. Answer: A. Serum iron studies. The patient in this question is presenting with a microcytic anemia (MCV <80 fL). The differential diagnosis of microcytic anemia can be remembered by the mnemonic "*TAILS*" (*T*halassemia, *A*nemia of chronic disease, *I*ron-deficiency anemia, *L*ead poisoning, *S*ideroblastic anemia). The most common cause of microcytic anemia is iron deficiency and the best next step is ordering iron studies: serum iron, total iron-binding capacity (TIBC), and serum ferritin. In iron-deficiency anemia, serum iron is typically low, TIBC is increased, and serum ferritin is low. After iron-deficiency anemia is confirmed, the underlying cause should be determined. Iron deficiency is by far the most common cause of microcytic anemia, so a trial of iron supplementation is often performed instead of an extensive workup.

(B) Hemoglobin electrophoresis would be useful for diagnosing thalassemia. β-Thalassemia trait usually has reduced or absent HbA, elevated levels of HbA2, and increased HbF. Clinical manifestations generally arise very early in life. (C) Although lead poisoning is a cause of microcytic anemia, it is uncommon and should only be sought after iron-deficiency anemia has been ruled out. (D) Peripheral blood smear is often used to exclude sideroblastic anemia, but this is an uncommon cause of microcytic anemia. (E) Stool guaiac test should most likely have been performed on initial presentation, but this patient's young age makes malignancy an unlikely diagnosis. Considering this patient's already known microcytic anemia present on CBC, serum iron studies should be performed in order to evaluate the cause.

64. Answer: C. Elevated lipase. The patient in this question is presenting with signs and symptoms of acute pancreatitis (epigastric abdominal pain radiating to the back, nausea, and vomiting). The vast majority of cases (80%) result from gallstones and alcohol. However, other causes of acute pancreatitis can be remembered with the mnemonic *GET SMASHED* (Gallstones, Ethanol, Trauma, Steroids, Mumps, Autoimmune, Scorpion bite, Hyperlipidemia, ERCP, Drugs [specifically diuretics, gliptins, azathioprine, salicylates, steroids]). Acute pancreatitis can be diagnosed through several modalities: physical examination demonstrating epigastric pain radiating to the back, elevated amylase and lipase levels (typically 3× higher than the normal limit), and abdominal imaging (CT) showing pancreatic enlargement with heterogeneous enhancement with IV contrast. Ultrasound is also helpful in diagnosing gallstone pancreatitis by visualizing gallstones in the gallbladder. Lipase has the greatest *specificity* of all possible tests and is usually more elevated than amylase in acute pancreatitis. (A) Amylase can sometimes be normal in acute pancreatitis (particularly if the etiology is hyperlipidemia). Furthermore, amylase is not specific to the pancreas as there is not only pancreatic amylase, but also salivary amylase. (B) Although elevated ALT is very useful in suggesting *gallstone* pancreatitis, it does not encompass all the causes of acute pancreatitis and therefore is not a specific test. (D) Positive fecal fat test is typically positive (>7 g/day) in *chronic* pancreatitis, however chronic pancreatitis presents with symptoms of malabsorption (as opposed to pain) and is typically due to alcohol use (neither of which this patient endorses). (E) Pancreatic calcifications are seen in chronic pancreatitis, not acute pancreatitis.

65. Answer: B. Thyroid-stimulating hormone (TSH) levels. The patient in this question is demonstrating clinical manifestations of hypothyroidism. In approaching the diagnosis of thyroid disorders, the first step is to order a TSH level. TSH is the *most sensitive* test to detect primary hypothyroidism and hyperthyroidism. Based on the TSH level, additional tests can be performed. (A) Free T4 is important in the diagnostic workup of thyroid disorders and should be the next test ordered if TSH comes back decreased. If free T4 is increased with a decreased TSH level, this is diagnostic of primary hyperthyroidism. If free T4 is decreased with a decreased TSH level, then central hypothyroidism is the diagnosis and the etiology involves the pituitary gland or the hypothalamus. Finally, if free T4 is normal with a decreased TSH, then this is subclinical hypothyroidism. (C) Thyroglobulin is often increased in goiter and hyperthyroidism and is also a tumor marker for thyroid cancer. It is not the best first test in working up thyroid disorders. (D) Radioactive iodine uptake (RAIU) scan is the next best step once primary hyperthyroidism is diagnosed (increased free T4 with decreased TSH) as it can help differentiate causes of hyperthyroidism (Graves vs. multinodular goiter vs. silent thyroiditis). (E) Thyroid biopsy is far too invasive of a test without a baseline TSH level.

66. Answer: A. CT scan. The suspected diagnosis here is meningitis, and a CT scan should be performed first to rule out mass effect before a lumbar puncture is performed. He has a high fever, as well as other symptoms/signs of meningitis (including the most sensitive test for meningitis: the jolt accentuation sign, in which a patient's headache intensifies after a quick head jolt). Kernig and Brudzinski signs are not sensitive, but they are fairly specific. Once a diagnosis of meningitis is suspected and a lumbar puncture needs to be performed, a CT scan should be performed in patients thought to be at high risk for cerebral herniation. Risk factors include papilledema, previous CNS disease, a seizure in that past week, immunosuppression, altered mental status, and focal neurologic signs. (C) This patient has both papilledema and immunosuppression (methotrexate), and therefore a CT scan should be performed before a lumbar puncture to assess the risk for cerebral herniation during lumbar puncture. (B) An MRI provides better visualization of the brain, however it is costly and time-consuming. Because the purpose here is to rule out mass effect, a CT scan can do this adequately and quickly. (D, E) It is most appropriate to administer empiric antibiotics (and antivirals if HSV encephalitis is suspected) shortly after blood and CSF cultures are sent, however the lumbar puncture has not been performed yet.

67. **Answer: B. Electrolyte abnormality.** The patient in this question is presenting with anemia, low back pain, increased erythrocyte sedimentation rate (ESR), and renal dysfunction, suggesting the diagnosis of multiple myeloma. A peripheral smear often shows the rouleaux formation (stacked appearance of RBCs). This patient additionally is presenting with constipation and confusion, both symptoms of hypercalcemia (>10.2 mg/dL), which is seen in about one-third of patients with multiple myeloma. The etiology of hypercalcemia in multiple myeloma is bone lysis from humoral factors released by the plasma cells. (A) Mechanical obstruction secondary to malignancy also can cause constipation, but the patient's signs and symptoms do not lend credence to colon cancer. (C, D, E) Hormone level and blood gas abnormalities are typically not seen in multiple myeloma and are not associated with constipation.

68. **Answer: B. Surgery.** This patient is presenting with signs and symptoms consistent with a diagnosis of cauda equina syndrome, a serious neurologic condition in which damage to the cauda equina (a bundle of spinal nerves originating in the conus medullaris) causes acute loss of function of the lumbar plexus. The management of this condition is urgent surgical decompression. However, there are several physicians who advocate for steroids prior to surgical decompression. (A) Nonetheless, there is no evidence that steroids are useful in treatment of cauda equina syndrome. (C) Imaging will only delay the diagnosis of cauda equina syndrome and increase the likelihood of long-term neurologic damage. (D, E) Given the finding of absent rectal tone and saddle anesthesia, conservative management with NSAIDs and bed rest should be avoided as cauda equina syndrome is a neurologic emergency.

Answers

69. **Answer: A. Aortic aneurysm.** The patient in this question is presenting with signs, symptoms, and laboratory values consistent with a diagnosis of giant-cell arteritis (GCA), also known as temporal arteritis. Symptoms can include headache, visual problems, jaw claudication, fever, and temporal scalp tenderness. GCA is a vasculitis most commonly involving large and medium arteries of the head, predominantly the branches of the external carotid artery. A decreased temporal artery pulse can be noted as well. ESR and C-reactive protein are commonly elevated. High-dose corticosteroids should be started as soon as the diagnosis is suspected (even before confirmation by temporal artery biopsy) to prevent irreversible blindness secondary to ophthalmic artery occlusion. GCA can involve branches of the aorta leading to aortic aneurysm, thus patients should have serial chest x-rays performed. (B) Inflammatory bowel disease includes ulcerative colitis and Crohn disease and is not associated with GCA. (C) Hepatitis B is associated with polyarteritis nodosa (30% of the time), a vasculitis of medium and small-sized arteries. (D) A smoking history is seen in thromboangiitis obliterans (Buerger disease), which presents with progressive inflammation and thrombosis of small and medium arteries of the hands and feet. Ulceration and gangrene are common complications. (E) Alcohol has never been shown to be associated with the development of temporal arteritis.

70. **Answer: D. Vasovagal syncope.** Syncope is defined as loss of consciousness that results from cerebral hypoperfusion. The most common cause of syncope is neurocardiogenic (vasovagal) syncope, which is caused by a sudden surge of sympathetic activity that transiently increases the contractility of the left ventricle. Mechanoreceptors in the left ventricle sense this increased contractility and cause an excessive vagal response, which lowers heart rate and contractility. This transiently drops the blood pressure and causes syncope. These patients typically have symptoms of lightheadedness, nausea, and narrowing vision before losing consciousness and can usually brace their fall somewhat. Diagnosis can be made with the tilt table test. (A, E) Cardiovascular causes of syncope include arrhythmias, mechanical heart disease (e.g., aortic stenosis and hypertrophic cardiomyopathy), pulmonary embolism, aortic dissection, and cardiac tamponade. Patients with sudden onset syncope and trauma to the face (indicating an inability to brace the fall) should increase the reader's suspicion for a cardiac etiology. (B) Orthostatic hypotension usually occurs in the presence of hypovolemia, dysautonomia, and/or certain medications (e.g., diuretics and β-blockers). Diagnosis can be made if systolic blood pressure decreases by ≥20 mm Hg or diastolic blood pressure decreases by ≥10 mm Hg when going from a sitting to a standing position, which was not seen in this patient. (C) Seizures technically do not meet the definition of syncope, since they are not caused by a disruption in cerebral blood flow. History that would indicate a seizure includes a preceding aura, tonic–clonic movements during the episode, and a postictal state (confusion with gradual improvement in neurologic function).

71. **Answer: D. Serum immunoelectrophoresis.** The patient in this question is presenting with signs and symptoms consistent with a diagnosis of multiple myeloma. *CRAB* can be a useful mnemonic in diagnosing multiple myeloma: Hyper*C*alcemia, *R*enal failure, *A*nemia, *B*one lesions (often punched out lesions in the skull). Serum and urine electrophoresis with immunofixation may reveal a monoclonal spike and is useful for confirmation of the diagnosis. (A) CA-15-3 is a tumor marker for breast cancer. (B) CEA is a tumor marker for adenocarcinomas,

particularly colon (but also lung, breast, and stomach). **(C)** Alkaline phosphatase would be elevated in Paget disease, however Paget disease is not characterized by hypercalcemia (as seen with this patient). Furthermore, Paget disease is characterized by a *mixed* osteolytic and osteoblastic phage (where multiple myeloma is purely osteolytic). As a result, rather than showing punched out skull lesions as seen in multiple myeloma, Paget disease will show a "cotton wool" appearance due to irregular areas of sclerosis. **(E)** An abnormal bone scan is certainly not diagnostic of multiple myeloma; rather it is useful in diagnosing cancer of the bone or cancers that have metastasized to the bone.

72. Answer: D. Hypertensive emergency; rapid lowering of blood pressure with IV agents. Hypertensive urgency is defined as a systolic blood pressure >180 mm Hg and/or a diastolic blood pressure >120 mm Hg with no end-organ damage. Hypertensive emergency is the same definition with the addition of end-organ damage. Many organs are acutely affected by high blood pressure, including the brain (stroke), eyes (papilledema), heart (aortic dissection), lungs (pulmonary edema), and kidneys (renal failure). Within the umbrella term of hypertensive emergency, there are additional terms for specific end-organ involvement: malignant hypertension refers to hypertensive emergency in the presence of papilledema (other ophthalmologic findings include retinal exudates and hemorrhage), and malignant nephrosclerosis refers to renal damage. This patient has a hypertensive emergency with end-organ involvement including the brain (headache) and the eyes (papilledema). **(A, B, C, E)** The management of hypertensive urgencies and emergencies is slightly different. In hypertensive urgency, the goal is to gradually lower the blood pressure to achieve a normal value within a couple of days. Oral antihypertensive agents are given while monitoring the reduction in blood pressure over hours. Some options for oral medications include labetalol, captopril, clonidine, furosemide, and hydralazine. In hypertensive emergency, there is ongoing end-organ damage and therefore blood pressure needs to be lowered quickly. The goal in this setting is to immediately lower blood pressure using IV agents, targeting a decrease in mean arterial pressure by 25% within minutes to hours. Some options for IV medications include nitroprusside, nitroglycerin, calcium channel blockers (e.g., nicardipine), labetalol, hydralazine, fenoldopam, and phentolamine. Because adaptive mechanisms occur with chronically elevated blood pressure, rapid lowering of blood pressure is not always tolerated and can cause cerebral hypoperfusion. If this happens, the blood pressure must be lowered more gradually.

73. Answer: C. Normal pressure hydrocephalus. The patient in this question is presenting with dementia, urinary incontinence, and gait disturbance. This triad, often remembered by "wet, wacky, wobbly," is characteristic of normal pressure hydrocephalus (NPH). NPH is diagnosed by MRI, which will show dilated ventricles. As one would expect from the name, the opening pressure measured during lumbar puncture is normal. Treatment generally consists of repeated spinal taps to improve the symptoms (by decreasing the pressure exerted on the adjacent cortical tissue by the enlarged ventricles). **(B)** Alzheimer disease is not associated with gait problems or urinary incontinence. **(A)** Pseudotumor cerebri is associated with headaches, not memory impairment or dementia. Furthermore, it is typically seen in young, obese females. **(D)** Although this patient has a history of hypertension, it is well-controlled and thus her symptoms are unlikely to be a result of multi-infarct dementia. This type of dementia tends to be very abrupt in onset and show multiple areas of increased T2-weighted density on MRI in the periventricular regions. **(E)** Lewy body dementia is the second most common form of dementia (after Alzheimer) closely associated with Parkinson disease.

74. Answer: C. Amiodarone. Amiodarone is an antiarrhythmic medication that may be used for prophylaxis or treatment of serious arrhythmias, especially ventricular arrhythmias. This patient has a history of ventricular tachycardia, and therefore has an indication to be taking amiodarone. This drug has many toxicities, and therefore when started the patient must have baseline pulmonary function tests, thyroid function tests, and liver function tests due to the toxicity involving each of these organs. Other notable side effects include blue-gray discoloration of the skin, corneal deposits, and peripheral neuropathy. This patient developed pulmonary fibrosis as a result of chronic amiodarone use. **(A, B, E)** Digoxin, lisinopril, and losartan are not associated with pulmonary fibrosis. **(D)** Bleomycin can cause pulmonary fibrosis, but it is an antineoplastic drug and the patient has no reason to be taking this medication.

75. Answer: C. Chlorpromazine. The patient in this question is likely having an acute episode of a migraine headache. Migraines are characterized by unilateral, pulsating pain that is often associated with photophobia and an aura of neurologic symptoms prior to the onset of the headache. Acute attacks can range in duration from 4 to 72 hours. Acute treatment and primary preventive treatment vary in migraine headaches. Acute attacks are best treated with intravenous antiemetic medications (chlorpromazine and prochlorperazine) and/or triptans (sumatriptan). **(E)** Given that this patient presents with vomiting, chlorpromazine is the best choice since it can be given in IV form, unlike sumatriptan. **(A, B)** Propranolol and amitriptyline are both excellent medications used for migraine *prophylaxis,* not for acute episodes. These would be appropriate to give to the patient after her acute migraine episode resolves to prevent further attacks. **(D)** Verapamil is a calcium channel blocker that is the first-line medication for cluster headache prophylaxis. However, this patient is having a migraine, not a cluster headache. Cluster headaches typically involve pain around the eye with eye watering, nasal congestion, and swelling.

76. Answer: C. Fractional excretion of sodium (FENa). Acute kidney injury (AKI) is defined as an abrupt rise (within 48 hours) in serum creatinine by ≥0.3 mg/dL from baseline, a ≥50% increase in serum creatinine from baseline, or oliguria of <0.5 cc/kg/hr for >6 hours. Once AKI is recognized, the next step in diagnosis is determining whether the etiology is prerenal, intrinsic renal, or postrenal. These terms reflect the perceived sight of pathology; prerenal AKI is caused by decreased blood flow to the kidneys, intrinsic renal AKI is caused by direct damage to the kidney parenchyma (i.e., to the renal vasculature, tubules/interstitium, or glomeruli), and postrenal AKI is caused by an obstruction in the urinary tract leading away from the kidneys. The patient in this question is hypovolemic (tachycardia and dry mucus membranes). In response to hypovolemia, the renal arterioles vasoconstrict, decreasing blood flow to the kidneys and decreasing the glomerular filtration rate (GFR). Prerenal AKI is a result of ischemia from poor perfusion, however it can progress to acute tubular necrosis (ATN), which is a form of intrinsic renal AKI. Besides hypovolemia, her daily NSAID may also be contributing to the AKI since NSAIDs cause renal vasoconstriction. One of the best tests for differentiating between prerenal AKI and ATN is the FENa. In prerenal AKI, sodium is reabsorbed in an attempt to maintain circulating blood volume, and therefore there will be little sodium in the urine. **(B)** Although this is often reflected by the urine sodium, this value is affected by renal water handling and urine output. FENa is a better test, since it only measures the fraction of sodium excretion and is not affected by urine output. In general, low FENa values indicate prerenal AKI and high values indicate intrinsic renal AKI (tubular damage leads to salt wasting). The FENa will be <1% in prerenal AKI and >2% in ATN. (Note: FENa should not be used in the setting of diuretics, but the fractional excretion of urea may be used instead.) **(A)** A urine dipstick is a helpful screening tool for things like proteinuria or infection, but it will not help to differentiate between prerenal and intrinsic renal AKI. **(D)** A renal ultrasound would be helpful in excluding postrenal AKI, which is not suspected in this case. **(E)** The diagnosis of prerenal AKI versus ATN cannot be made by history alone.

77. Answer: B. Aortic dissection. The most important risk factor for aortic dissection in the general population is hypertension, however there is a high incidence in patients with connective tissue disease (e.g., Marfan and Ehlers–Danlos syndromes). Sharp chest pain radiating to the back is the first clue to this diagnosis. Other symptoms may occur based on which arteries are occluded by the dissected flap. Finally, a widened mediastinum is seen on chest x-ray. Other potential manifestations not seen in this patient are cardiac tamponade and Horner syndrome (from compression of the superior cervical ganglion). Dissections involving the proximal aorta require immediate surgical intervention. **(A, C, D)** All of these diagnoses are a result of the patient's aortic dissection, but are not the underlying (primary) diagnosis. Acute coronary syndromes (ACS) may occur during an aortic dissection as a result of involvement of one or more coronary arteries, and stroke can occur with involvement of the carotid arteries. Aortic regurgitation is common in patients with Marfan syndrome, and this can also occur as a result of a dissection in the ascending aorta. In either situation, it is not the primary diagnosis. **(E)** Hypertensive emergency requires a systolic blood pressure >180 mm Hg and/or a diastolic blood pressure >120 mm Hg.

78. Answer: B. ***Salmonella.*** Patients with sickle cell disease have functional asplenism from infarction. This often results in impaired immunologic response to encapsulated organisms, such as *Streptococcus pneumoniae, Haemophilus influenzae,* and *Neisseria meningitidis.* Furthermore, they are more prone to invasive *Salmonella* infections which, when localized, can result in osteomyelitis. In addition to treatment with antibiotics here, this patient should immediately be treated with oxygen, aggressive hydration, and analgesics (morphine). **(A, C, D, E)** These organisms do not cause osteomyelitis in sickle cell patients.

79. Answer: D. Hot nodule on RAIU. Thyroid nodules are fairly common with a 5% to 10% prevalence. Approximately 5% of thyroid nodules are malignant. **(A, B, C, E)** Factors associated with malignancy include history of radiation to the neck, male sex, hard and immobile mass, age greater than 70 years, worrisome ultrasound findings such as irregular borders and microcalcifications, cervical lymphadenopathy, and cold nodule on RAIU. Cold nodules are nonfunctional and do not absorb the radioiodine. Hot nodules, on the other hand, are autonomous (toxic) and readily absorb the radioiodine. However, hot nodules are benign and not associated with malignancy.

80. Answer: D. Dual-energy x-ray absorptiometry (DEXA). Risk factors for osteoporosis include smoking, family history, low body weight, excessive alcohol use, and secondary organic causes such as premature menopause, among others. Regardless of symptoms, the USPSTF recommends a one-time screening for osteoporosis in *all* women aged 65 years or older with DEXA scan of the spine and hips. A bone density with T-score <2.5 standard deviations below the mean is associated with osteoporosis and a T-score between 1 and 2.5 standard deviations below the mean is associated with osteopenia. (A) The patient had a normal mammogram the year before. Mammograms should be performed every 2 years in her age group. (B) The patient had a colonoscopy 6 years ago that was normal. She is due for another colonoscopy in 4 years (reaching the 10-year mark after her previous one). (C) Calcium and phosphorus levels are normal in patients with osteoporosis and have no value in screening for the condition. (E) There is no history or clinical suspicion here for lung cancer, so a CT scan of the chest is not warranted.

81. Answer: B. Joint aspiration with synovial fluid analysis. This patient is presenting with signs and symptoms consistent with an acute gout attack. The patient's alcohol use lends credence to the history of gouty arthritis. Furthermore, the patient is presenting with acute right knee pain, swelling, and low-grade fever, all confirming the likely diagnosis of gout. Given that septic arthritis and pseudogout can show clinical similarities to gout, it is imperative to first perform joint aspiration and synovial fluid analysis. Synovial fluid analysis of gout will demonstrate a leukocyte count of 2,000 to 50,000/mm^3 and negatively birefringent needle-shaped crystals with a negative Gram stain and negative culture. (A) Indomethacin (an NSAID) is very helpful in treating acute gout. Nonetheless, the diagnosis of gout must first be confirmed before administering indomethacin especially with its side effect profile. (C) Uric acid levels will certainly be elevated in gout (elevated uric acid is the underlying cause of the clinical manifestations), however uric acid levels do not have a high degree of sensitivity or specificity for diagnosing gout. (D) An x-ray of the knee is not as specific as synovial fluid analysis for diagnosing gout.

82. Answer: C. Empiric 1-month trial with proton pump inhibitor (PPI). The patient in this question is presenting with dyspepsia (characterized by epigastric pain and early satiety). Dyspepsia is a common presentation, and only a minority of patients are diagnosed with an underlying etiology contributing to the dyspepsia. The most common etiologies of dyspepsia are GERD, NSAIDs, peptic ulcer disease (PUD), and malignancy. (D) Importantly, if a patient presents with any "alarm symptoms" such as unexplained weight loss, persistent vomiting, blood loss, dysphagia, or family history of gastrointestinal cancer, then he/she should undergo an upper GI endoscopy to evaluate for malignancy. In patients without the "alarm symptoms," current recommendations are to test for *Helicobacter pylori* in regions where there is a high prevalence of the bacteria and begin treatment with a proton pump inhibitor (PPI). In regions where there is a low prevalence of *H. pylori,* some physicians will treat empirically with a PPI. The most important thing to note here is that patients who fail either of these treatment options after 4 to 8 weeks should undergo endoscopy. (A) Antacids have not alleviated this patient's symptoms and therefore are not the correct answer here. (B) Barium swallow evaluation is not helpful in diagnosing the etiology of dyspepsia. (E) This patient is symptomatic and clearly not responding to over-the-counter antacids. Observation is inappropriate.

83. Answer: E. Etiologies include infection and polypharmacy. This patient is presenting with signs and symptoms consistent with a diagnosis of delirium, which has several etiologies including infection, surgery, trauma, or polypharmacy side effects. Acute onset of symptoms, fluctuating level of consciousness, and presence of visual hallucinations favor a diagnosis of delirium over dementia. Additionally, sleep-wake cycle disturbance is a prominent feature of delirium. (D) Delirium is reversible, while dementia, by contrast, is often irreversible. Clinically, patients with dementia show gradual decline in cognition with preserved level of consciousness. Given the reversibility of the disease, the confused patient should be assumed to have delirium until proven otherwise. Reversible causes of delirium should be considered, including metabolic disorders, infections, medications, normal pressure hydrocephalus, vitamin deficiencies, or thyroid dysfunction, which may be potentially reversible causes of dementia-like symptoms. Delirium occurs in up to 20% of acute hospital inpatients and up to 60% of surgical patients in the perioperative period. Identifying and treating the cause of delirium is critical. (A) Anticholinergic medications will *worsen* delirium. (B) Neurofibrillary tangles and β-amyloid plaques seen on pathology are consistent with Alzheimer dementia, not delirium. (C) If long-term memory is intact, but short-term memory is affected, then this is more consistent with dementia.

84. Answer: B. Gallstone obstruction in the cystic duct. The patient in this question is presenting with acute cholecystitis. He is presenting with fever, right upper quadrant pain after a fatty meal that radiates to the right scapula, and positive Murphy sign (pain on palpation in the right upper quadrant with cessation of inspiration). Additional nonspecific findings include vomiting, leukocytosis, and mild elevation in transaminases. Acute cholecystitis usually arises from gallstone formation that obstructs the cystic duct. The symptoms occur after eating a fatty meal because the fat stimulates gallbladder contraction, and in the presence of cystic duct obstruction, this leads to colicky pain. Infection results from stasis that contributes to bacterial growth in the gallbladder. (D) Importantly, alkaline phosphatase is *not* elevated in this patient with acute cholecystitis. Assume if laboratories are not shown, they are normal. If it were elevated (in addition to total bilirubin and direct bilirubin), this might indicate common bile duct obstruction in the setting of jaundice (choledocolithiasis). (A) Alcoholic liver disease does not present with this constellation of symptoms. (C) Similar to common bile duct obstruction, obstruction from a carcinoma of the head of the pancreas would cause severely elevated alkaline phosphatase levels and would normally present with weight loss and painless jaundice. (E) Pancreatitis should definitely be ruled out with a lipase check, but pain typically is only epigastric in nature and radiates to the back.

85. Answer: C. Amitriptyline. The patient in this question is presenting with signs and symptoms consistent with a diagnosis of fibromyalgia (FM). FM is more common in middle-aged women and is characterized by chronic widespread pain and allodynia (a heightened and painful response to pressure). Physical examination is typically normal except for point muscle tenderness in several areas including the mid trapezius, lateral epicondyle, and greater trochanter, among others. Of note, FM has no laboratory findings that are diagnostic of the condition. The first-line treatment for FM is patient education, aerobic exercise, and good sleep hygiene. This patient has clearly attempted those recommendations based on the history she provides, so the first-line *medication* is a tricyclic antidepressant (TCA) such as amitriptyline. Several other drugs (pregabalin and duloxetine) can be attempted if TCAs fail to alleviate the patient's symptoms. (A, B, E) Corticosteroids and NSAIDs are useful in treating *inflammatory* conditions, but FM is not an inflammatory condition (not associated with elevated inflammatory markers such as ESR). (D) Colchicine is useful in treating gout, not FM.

86. Answer: B. Administration of fluids. This is a common question on the USMLE that emphasizes the importance of airway, breathing, and circulation (ABCs) in the management of patients (regardless of the underlying disorder). This patient presents with hypotension and delayed capillary refill, indicating that there is compromise of his circulation. The best next step in management of circulatory compromise (in this case from an upper GI bleed) is fluid resuscitation. After the patient is hemodynamically stable, treatment for the actual underlying condition can be initiated. (A, C, D) All these answer choices address the underlying cause of the upper GI bleeding (likely peptic ulcer bleeding); however, the patient must be stabilized before these modalities are pursued. (E) This is a life-threatening condition and reassurance is inappropriate.

87. Answer: C. Abdominal x-ray. The patient in this question is presenting with signs and symptoms concerning for a small-bowel obstruction (SBO). The typical constellation of symptoms includes abdominal pain, vomiting, obstipation, abdominal distention, and diffuse tenderness. A mild leukocytosis and elevated amylase is often found in an SBO. The best initial test is an abdominal x-ray because it often reveals dilated bowel loops and several air–fluid levels. Treatment involves supportive care, bowel rest, and decompression with a nasogastric tube. Surgery is reserved for those patients who fail to improve with the aforementioned treatments and/or develop findings consistent with strangulation. (A, B, D, E) These options are not the best *initial* test in diagnosing an SBO.

88. Answer: B. Nephrolithiasis. This patient is presenting with the typical symptoms of a kidney stone. Patients with Crohn disease are at risk of developing calcium oxalate stones due to increased absorption of oxalate in the GI tract (and therefore increased oxaluria), which has two causes. First, malabsorption of bile salts and GI tract inflammation increase mucosal permeability. Second, fatty acids (also a result of malabsorption) bind intestinal calcium, and so less calcium is available to bind and trap intestinal oxalate. This causes an increase in free oxalate that can be absorbed, eventually making it back to the kidneys to be excreted. Calcium stones are the most common type of kidney stones, and patients with these stones are encouraged to increase their dietary intake of calcium (in order to decrease oxalate absorption in the GI tract). Ammonium magnesium phosphate (struvite) stones are caused by urinary tract infections with urease-positive organisms (e.g., *Proteus, Klebsiella*) and can form staghorn calculi. Uric acid stones are associated with hyperuricemia (e.g., leukemia, gout). Cystine stones are seen in the genetic disease cystinuria and are treated by alkalinizing the urine with acetazolamide. (A) Pyelonephritis would also produce flank pain, but unlike nephrolithiasis it would also produce fever, leukocytosis, and a urine dipstick showing infection (e.g., positive nitrites, positive leukocyte esterase). (C) Appendicitis is important to consider in any young patient with abdominal pain, however it would be unusual for appendicitis to cause hematuria. (D) Ectopic pregnancies can mimic the pain of a kidney stone, however this diagnosis is unlikely given the negative pregnancy test. (E) This would be an unusual presentation of abdominal pain seen in pancreatitis, which is usually epigastric and radiating to the back.

89. Answer: C. Hyperventilation secondary to anxiety. According to the ABG, this patient has an acute respiratory alkalosis (caused by loss of CO_2 which is balanced by increased excretion of HCO_3). Respiratory alkalosis can only be caused by an increase in ventilation (commonly caused by high altitudes or sympathetic stimulation like anxiety or pain). **(A)** Accumulation of unmeasured anions due to hepatic metabolism of alcohol would cause an anion gap metabolic acidosis (*low* pH with *low* HCO_3 and *low* CO_2 and an increased gap, calculated by subtracting ($Cl^- + HCO_3^-$) from Na^+). **(B)** Vomiting causes a *metabolic* alkalosis from loss of acid and chloride. Metabolic alkalosis is characterized by *high* pH, *high* HCO_3, and *high* CO_2 (respiratory compensation by hypoventilating). **(D)** Diuretics are associated with a *metabolic* alkalosis from volume contraction. **(E)** Hypoventilation causes a *low* pH from CO_2 retention. This will cause a *respiratory* acidosis, not alkalosis as seen with this patient.

90. Answer: C. Lactulose. This patient is presenting with signs and symptoms of cirrhosis (ascites, spider angiomata) and hepatic encephalopathy (altered mental status and asterixis). In hepatic encephalopathy, the liver is unable to convert ammonia into urea and it therefore accumulates, in addition to other toxins the liver is unable to clear. It is often precipitated by illness or gastrointestinal bleed (as in this patient with hematemesis). Increased ammonia levels can assist in making the diagnosis, but the diagnosis is ultimately clinical and can cause confusion in the correct setting of end stage liver disease (ESLD). Treatment involves treating the precipitant and decreasing serum ammonia levels (however, even if one uses ammonia to help with diagnosis, it is not necessary to follow ammonia levels; rather, one should follow clinical improvement). Lactulose, a nonabsorbable disaccharide, is used because bacteria in the gut metabolize it into acidic compounds (lactic acid, acetic acid) that permit the *absorbable* ammonia to be converted into the *nonabsorbable* ammonium, thereby enabling excretion from the body. **(A)** Furosemide would improve the ascites and volume status in a cirrhotic patient, but is not helpful in the management of hepatic encephalopathy. **(B)** Thiamine is useful in the treatment of *Wernicke encephalopathy*, another form of encephalopathy characterized by altered mental status, ataxia, and nystagmus and is associated with thiamine deficiency. Of note, asterixis is *not* present in Wernicke encephalopathy. **(D, E)** Morphine and hydromorphone are narcotics that would be challenging for a cirrhotic patient to metabolize.

91. Answer: B. Acetaminophen. This patient is obese, greater than 40 years of age, and is presenting with bilateral knee and back pain. The fact that the pain is worsened with activity and relieved by rest suggests that it is most likely secondary to osteoarthritis (OA). If she reported morning stiffness lasting greater than 30 minutes and had systemic symptoms, rheumatoid arthritis would have been the likely diagnosis. OA is a *noninflammatory* arthritis that results in eroding cartilage in the intra-articular joints. This causes joint crepitus (a "grating" or popping sound) that occurs when the surfaces of the joint grind against each other. Although the diagnosis is usually made clinically, the typical changes seen on x-ray include joint space narrowing, subchondral sclerosis (increased bone formation around the joint), subchondral cyst formation, and osteophytes. Acetaminophen is the first-line treatment for mild to moderate OA. It is just as efficacious as NSAIDs in alleviating the pain in OA with considerably fewer side effects. **(A)** Intra-articular corticosteroid injections lead to short-term pain relief that lasts up to a few months. This should not be the initial treatment in OA. **(C)** Naproxen is an NSAID and although NSAIDs have been shown to be efficacious in the treatment of OA, their side effect profile consists of gastrointestinal and renal consequences that make them second-line treatments. **(D)** Allopurinol is used in the prophylactic treatment of gout. It acts via inhibition of xanthine oxidase which decreases production of uric acid. It is not used in the treatment of OA. **(E)** This patient is clearly in pain and would benefit from medication, so observation is inappropriate.

92. Answer: D. Vitamin B_{12} deficiency. The patient in this question likely has cobalamin (vitamin B_{12}) deficiency. This results in a megaloblastic anemia. Long-term consequences of vitamin B_{12} deficiency include peripheral neuropathy and posterior column defects from abnormal myelin synthesis. Importantly, folic acid deficiency is another cause of macrocytic anemia and treatment with folic acid can improve the actual *anemia* of vitamin B_{12} deficiency since both folate and vitamin B_{12} are involved in the conversion of homocysteine to methionine. However, neurologic symptoms can be worsened in vitamin B_{12} deficiency with the treatment of folic acid since vitamin B_{12} is used in other biologic processes as well. As a result, it is critical to rule out vitamin B_{12} deficiency before initiating folic acid. Vitamin B_{12} deficiency results from inadequate vitamin B_{12} intake (diet lacking in animal products) and autoimmune gastritis. The loss of gastric parietal cells secondary to autoimmune gastritis causes intrinsic factor deficiency (which is necessary for vitamin B_{12} absorption in the terminal ileum). **(A)** The patient's underlying disorder is vitamin B_{12} deficiency and no amount of folic acid supplementation will improve his neurologic symptoms. **(B)** Iron deficiency is a microcytic anemia (MCV <80 fL) and is not associated with peripheral neuropathy. **(C, E)** Although glucose intolerance commonly causes peripheral neuropathy, this patient does not have a history that suggests diabetes.

93. Answer: A. Amlodipine. Amlodipine is a calcium channel blocker that is often used as an antihypertensive agent. It has a high incidence of peripheral edema as a side effect. **(B)** Metoprolol is a selective β_1-blocker used

Answers

in hypertension, heart failure, and rate control for atrial fibrillation. It can cause bradycardia and hypotension, but avoids some of the adverse effects of nonselective β-blockers (e.g., bronchospasm). It rarely causes peripheral edema. (C) Hydrochlorothiazide blocks the Na-Cl channel in the distal convoluted tubule, leading to sodium and water excretion. It is used as an antihypertensive agent, and can cause orthostatic hypotension, hypercalcemia, hypokalemia, hyperlipidemia, and hyperglycemia. (D) Metformin is a biguanide drug used in diabetes and acts by decreasing hepatic glucose secretion and increasing insulin sensitivity. It causes GI symptoms, vitamin B_{12} deficiency, and lactic acidosis in patients with renal failure. (E) Glipizide is a sulfonylurea antidiabetic drug. It blocks potassium channels in islet cells of the pancreas, leading to increased insulin release that can result in hypoglycemia.

94. Answer: A. Factitious hypoglycemia from surreptitious injection of insulin. The patient in this question is presenting with clinical symptoms and laboratory findings consistent with surreptitious injection of insulin (elevated insulin, decreased glucose, and decreased C-peptide). **(B)** Since this patient presents with a decreased C-peptide level, this is not consistent with an ENDOGENOUS source of insulin since pancreatic β-cells produce proinsulin (which breaks down into insulin and C-peptide). Therefore, insulinoma is not the diagnosis since there are decreased levels of C-peptide in this patient. Note that surreptitious sulfonylurea use will also produce elevated insulin and C-peptide levels (similar to insulinoma) since this drug essentially stimulates proinsulin secretion. That is why it is critical to order a urine sulfonylurea level, which is undetectable in this patient. **(C, D)** Somatization disorder and glucagonoma do not produce hypoglycemia. **(E)** Dehydration cannot explain the severe hypoglycemia seen in this patient.

95. Answer: D. Ciprofloxacin. One reported adverse reaction of fluoroquinolone antibiotics is tendinopathy, and the Achilles tendon is most often affected. Fluoroquinolones can also cause GI upset, dizziness, rash, and a prolonged QT interval. **(A)** Trimethoprim-sulfamethoxazole may cause Stevens–Johnson syndrome, leukopenia, hyperkalemia, hypoglycemia, and hepatitis. The incidence of adverse reactions is much higher in HIV patients. **(B)** Metronidazole can cause a disulfiram-like reaction with alcohol. **(C)** Tobramycin and other aminoglycosides may cause renal failure and ototoxicity. **(E)** Azithromycin and other macrolides can cause a prolonged QT interval and hepatitis.

Answers

96. Answer: B. Thyroid-stimulating hormone (TSH) levels. The patient in this question is demonstrating clinical manifestations of hyperthyroidism. In approaching the diagnosis of thyroid disorders, the first step is to order a TSH level. TSH is the *most sensitive* test to detect primary hypothyroidism and hyperthyroidism. Based on the TSH level, additional tests can be performed. **(A)** Free T4 is important in the diagnostic workup of thyroid disorders and should be the next test ordered if TSH comes back decreased. If free T4 is increased with a decreased TSH level, this is diagnostic of primary hyperthyroidism. If free T4 is decreased with a decreased TSH level, then central hypothyroidism is the diagnosis and the etiology involves the pituitary gland or the hypothalamus. Finally, if free T4 is normal with a decreased TSH, then this is subclinical hypothyroidism. **(C)** Thyroglobulin is often increased in goiter and hyperthyroidism and is also a tumor marker for thyroid cancer. It is not the best first test in working up thyroid disorders. **(D)** Radioactive iodine uptake (RAIU) scan is the next best step once primary hyperthyroidism is diagnosed (increased free T4 with decreased TSH) as it can help differentiate causes of hyperthyroidism (Graves vs. multinodular goiter vs. silent thyroiditis). **(E)** A fine-needle aspiration (FNA) biopsy is far too invasive of a test without having basic laboratory values.

97. Answer: D. Reassurance. This patient demonstrates immunity to hepatitis B (positive for HBsAb) and therefore reassurance should be offered. Immunity to hepatitis B occurs when anti-hepatitis B surface antibodies (HBsAbs) develop against the recombinant hepatitis B surface antigen. Given the patient's documented hepatitis B vaccination and positive titers for HBsAb, reassurance is appropriate. **(A, C)** If the patient had unknown vaccination history, he should receive *both* HBIG (passive immunity) and hepatitis B vaccine (active immunity). **(B)** The patient has documentation already revealing positivity for HBsAb. Therefore, a hepatitis B panel is unnecessary.

98. Answer: B. Tearing of the bridging veins. This patient is suffering from a subdural hematoma, which is caused by blunt trauma that tears the bridging veins, which connect the cortical superficial veins to the sagittal sinus in the dura. This blood will *slowly* extravasate into the subdural space, which is why this patient's fall was recorded 4 days prior to admission. Epidural hematomas, on the other hand, become immediately symptomatic (although the classic description of epidural hematomas is that of a "lucid" phase followed by rapid decline). Subdural hematomas manifest symptomatically with headache and gradual confusion and loss of consciousness. Of note, subdural hematomas are much more common in elderly patients and alcoholic patients (brain atrophy and fragility of vasculature). Radiologic findings of a subdural hematoma include a white crescent on noncontrast CT of the head. Also, a midline shift is commonly appreciated. Treatment is neurosurgical hematoma evacuation. (A) Tearing of the middle meningeal artery is the underlying cause of most epidural hematomas. (C) Ruptured aneurysm is the underlying cause of a subarachnoid hemorrhage. (D) In addition to the radiologic evidence, this particular patient has an insignificant past medical history and therefore hypertensive hemorrhage is not the right answer. (E) Alzheimer disease would not present with this acute presentation. This patient clearly endorses trauma making a hematoma much more likely than underlying dementia.

99. Answer: D. **Severe sepsis.** This patient has severe sepsis secondary to pneumonia. It is important to know the definitions related to the topic of sepsis. Systemic inflammatory response syndrome (SIRS) is defined by 2 or more of the following: (1) temperature >38°C or <36°C; (2) a heart rate >90/min; (3) a respiratory rate >20/min or a $PaCO_2$ <32 mm Hg; and (4) a serum leukocyte count >12,000/mm^3 or <4,000/mm^3 or >10% bands. (C) When there is a suspected source of infection, the definition becomes sepsis. Severe sepsis is the definition for sepsis with end-organ dysfunction, signified by hypotension or hypoperfusion (e.g., oliguria, elevated serum lactate, etc.). Septic shock is severe sepsis that does not respond to adequate fluid resuscitation. This patient meets SIRS criteria with a suspected source of infection (pneumonia) and hypotension; (E) IV fluids have not been administered yet, so the definition of septic shock is not met. Septic shock is one type of distributive shock, which is characterized by hypotension with flat neck veins and warm extremities (low systemic vascular resistance). (A, B) Both cardiogenic shock and pulmonary embolism (a type of obstructive shock) are ruled out by the flat neck veins. Lastly, hypovolemic shock would present with flat neck veins and *cool* extremities, since systemic vascular resistance increases in an attempt to maintain blood pressure.

100. Answer: C. **Administer oral chlorhexidine solution twice daily.** Mechanical ventilation is the biggest risk factor for developing HAP, and the risk can be decreased with certain measures. (A) Patient should be placed in a semirecumbent position (head of the bed elevated 30 degrees to 45 degrees) to prevent aspiration events. (B) Daily attempts to wean a patient from the ventilator should be performed to minimize the duration of mechanical ventilation. (D) Omeprazole and other agents that increase the pH of gastric contents have been shown to increase the rate of HAP. They should be avoided if possible. (E) Endotracheal suctioning of subglottic secretions reduces the risk of VAP. Other important preventive measures include following proper hand hygiene protocols, avoiding gastric overdistention, and using orotracheal intubation rather than nasotracheal intubation.

INDEX

Page numbers followed by b, f, and t indicates boxed material, figure, and table respectively.

B

C

Index

Index

CCS0915